ADVANCED PRACTICE IN ONCOLOGY NURSING

Case Studies & Review

ONCOLOGY NURSING SOCIETY

ADVANCED PRACTICE IN ONCOLOGY NURSING

Case Studies & Review

Esther Muscari Lin, RN, MSN, CS, ACNP, AOCN

Oncology Clinical Nurse Specialist

Acute Care Nurse Practitioner

Lymphedema Therapies

Charlottesville, Virginia

W.B. SAUNDERS COMPANY

A Harcourt Health Sciences Company

Philadelphia   London   New York   St. Louis   Sydney   Toronto

W.B. Saunders Company
A Harcourt Health Sciences Company

The Curtis Center
Independence Square West
Philadelphia, PA 19106

Library of Congress Cataloging-in-Publication Data
Advanced practice in oncology nursing : case studies and review / [edited by] Esther Muscari Lin.
p. ; cm.
Includes bibliographical references and index.
ISBN 0-7216-7394-5
1. Cancer—Nursing—Case studies. 2. Cancer—Nursing—Examinations, questions, etc. I. Muscari Lin, Esther. II. Oncologic Nursing Society.
[DNLM: 1. Oncologic Nursing—Case Report. 2. Oncologic Nursing—Examination Questions. WY 18.2 A2447 2001]
RC266 .A286 2001
610.73′698—dc21
2001020398

Vice President and Publishing Director, Nursing: Sally Schrefer
Executive Editor: Barbara Nelson Cullen
Managing Editor: Sandra Clark Brown
Project Manager: Catherine Albright Jackson
Designer: Amy Buxton

Printed in the United States of America

01 02 03 04 05 GW/MVY 9 8 7 6 5 4 3 2 1

CONTRIBUTORS

Jennifer L. Aikin, RN, MSN, AOCN
National Surgical Adjuvant Breast Program
   Operations Center
Pittsburgh, Pennsylvania

Deborah Boyle, RN, MSN, AOCN, FAAN
Oncology Clinical Nurse Specialist
Inova Fairfax Cancer Center
Falls Church, Virginia

Nancy Jo Bush, RN, MN, MA, AOCN
Lecturer, UCLA School of Nursing
Nurse Practitioner, Hematology
   Oncology Associates
Los Angeles, California

Mary E. Cooley, PhD, CRNP, AOCN
Research Associate
Adult Nurse Practitioner
Harvard Medical School/Harvard School
   of Dental Medicine
Smoking Cessation Research Program
Boston, Massachusetts

Constance Engelking, RN, MS, OCN
Executive Director
Zalmen A. Arlin Cancer Institute
Westchester Medical Center
Valhalla, New York

Jeanne Erickson, RN, MSN, AOCN
Clinical Instructor
Oncology Clinical Nurse Specialist
University of Virginia School of Nursing
Charlottesville, Virginia

**Annette Wilkening Kuck, RN, MS,
   CNP, AOCN**
Minnesota Oncology Hematology, P.A.
Minneapolis, Minnesota

**Esther Muscari Lin, RN, MSN, CS,
   ACNP, AOCN**
Oncology Clinical Nurse Specialist
Acute Care Nurse Practitioner
Lymphedema Therapies
Charlottesville, Virginia

Leslie Mathews, RN, MS, NP, AOCN
Adult Nurse Practitioner, Oncology/
   Hematology Division
Winthrop-University Hospital

Sarah McCaffery, RN, MS
Nurse Fellow
City of Hope National Medical Center
Duarte, California

Sandra A. Mitchell, CRNP, MScN, AOCN
Lead Nurse Practitioner
Stem Cell Transplant Program
Greenebaum Cancer Center
Faculty Associate, School of Nursing
University of Maryland
Baltimore, Maryland

Dana N. Rutledge, RN, PhD
Nurse Consultant
Irvine, California

Janet Van Cleave, RN, ACNP-CS, AOCN
Acute Care Nurse Practitioner
Oncology Care Center
The Mount Sinai Medical Center
New York, New York

Rita Wickham, PhD, RN, AOCN
Oncology/Palliative Care Clinical
   Nurse Specialist
Rush Presbyterian St. Luke's Medical Center
Associate Professor, Rush College of Nursing
Chicago, Illinois

REVIEWERS

Laura A. Fennimore, RN, MSN
Director of Education
Oncology Nursing Society
Pittsburgh, Pennsylvania

This book is dedicated to:

My two little girls: Samantha and Carly Lin, who think I'm famous.

My mother, Anneliese Baumberger Muscari, who has always believed in me, like no other; who has taken such pride in my work and profession as a nurse; who has read everything I have written, even my nursing school papers; and who has set such a high standard by embracing every day with simplistic joy and happiness. I will always remember.

And finally,
My husband Kant, who holds my hand (sometimes tighter at times than others) with concern and humor, as we traverse this journey of life together.

PREFACE

IMPORTANT in using this book is recognizing the philosophy regarding advanced practice from which it was designed and written. This advanced practice book can serve as a resource and reference for advanced practice nurse (APN) practitioners, educators, and consultants to apply the information in clinical and educational settings.

The oncology APN is unique. The APN requires a wide berth of knowledge to practice nursing at such a high level and in so many different roles, all of which are extremely challenging and often high powered. It is generally agreed that the APN has an oncology knowledge base that encompasses the information necessary to pass the Oncology Certification Generalist (OCN) examination. However, the APN knowledge extends beyond the generalist content and into advanced practice role functions. APN practice extends to how the content is used—the decision making involved; the analytical and critical thinking; and the intentional, thoughtful plan of action and evaluation. It is impossible to cover all of the information or knowledge the APN requires to practice competently. Reflective of a major adult learning principle, the APN's high level of functioning, expertise, and training has taught the APN to continuously identify what areas he or she is deficient in and then to search for the answers or solutions.

This book is not intended as a quick reference. As a study guide for the AOCN examination, this approach departs from the norm of other review books that present material only for review or memorization. The unique approach presented here validates the APN's understanding of the material and provides the reasoning for choosing the advanced practice interventions necessary to achieve the most effective clinical outcomes. It requires active participation on the part of the APN reader. The richness of advanced practice, which includes the comprehensive knowledge base, the integration of multiple concepts, and the synthesis of biopsychosocial perspectives, are woven into the cases, the questions, the answers, and the rationales unique to this book's format. The information and "facts" are integrated throughout. Although there are numerous question formats, such as multiple-choice questions or open-ended questions, they are intended only to reach the highest level of questioning possible and are not reflective of the actual AOCN examination developed and administered by the Oncology Nursing Certification Corporation (ONCC).

This book builds on the *Core Curriculum Oncology Nursing*. It is assumed that the APN planning to take the AOCN examination is familiar with basic oncology nursing practice and the content of the review books for the OCN examination. This book is designed to "pull" the reader into the cases and challenge those higher areas of thinking, which are tapped into every day in every APN role. This book demands use of critical thinking skills in cases reflective of many oncology situations that APNs finds themselves in. It is *how* the APN applies the basic oncology nursing knowledge that this book is intended to exemplify.

Specific topics such as nutrition, symptom management, and physical assessment may be covered in more than one section of the book. Although the table of contents lists the role components of advanced practice, it is the index that will provide the most help in locating the aspects you are interested in. The index lists the specific problems, symptoms, and issues of oncology nursing. The index should help identify the pages containing the sought-after content.

Esther Muscari Lin

ACKNOWLEDGMENTS

As everyone knows, nothing of quality is accomplished in this world without the input of intelligent, giving people. I have had that rare experience with this book. Although my name is on the cover, it should really contain the names of each of the contributors. Each contributor worked with me repeatedly, over time, to articulate my vision of advanced practice nursing. It is the sum of the parts that has resulted in the unique contribution I believe this book brings to oncology nursing. The experiences, insights, and talents each contributor brings to this book are simultaneously humbling and inspiring to me. It is because of their excellence as advanced practice oncology nurses in different roles that this book has resulted. So, to give credit where credit is due, thank you:

Jennifer Aikin
Debi Boyle
Nancy Jo Bush
Mary Cooley
Connie Engelking
Jeanne Erickson
Nette Kuck
Leslie Mathews
Sandy Mitchell
Rita Wickham

I'd like to thank:

Rose Mary Carroll-Johnson, for her honest helpfulness and support as I began this project, and which dramatically turned into compassionate, intelligent strategizing as I worked my way toward completion. Rose Mary's generosity of time, insight, and experiences "jump-started" me on the right track from the very beginning. I am grateful for her global vision, her integrity, and all that I learn every time we interact.

Susan Baird, for her willingness, kindness, and professional generosity; for teaching me how to write and edit 13 years ago; for being happily available for my mentoring needs; and for guiding me through a unique aspect of this book process. Sue has been and always will be the ultimate mentor.

Sandy Mitchell, my dear friend and confidant, who has had to suffer through my incessant discussions of advanced practice, who allowed me to bounce ideas off of her, and who, through it all, still laughed with me.

Laura Fennimore and the Oncology Nursing Society for their support. Laura has "stayed the path," believing in my vision, even during times of doubt, for which I have been very grateful.

Jonathan Truitt, MD, and Kant Lin, MD, for their 24-hour "on-call" medical consultative services.

Peter Cassileth, MD, and Edward Stadtmauer, MD, who always supported me as I operationalized the first oncology advanced practice nursing position at PENN. In many ways, their belief in my abilities allowed me to stretch the boundaries of what nursing had traditionally done. I will always hold my memories of those years in high regard, with respect for the intelligent care we provided as a team and an appreciation for their sense of humor at some of the oddest moments!

Sandra Brown and Barbara Cullen at WB Saunders for their faith in what this book could look like and all the support in making it happen.

Finally, in a nonprofessional vein, my warmhearted and fun-loving brother Butch, who influenced me like no other. I would never have reached my professional goals without the standards he set while we were growing up. While teaching me that the sky is the limit and that working hard will get you whatever you set your sights on, he taught me to laugh at the silliest things. "God love you" Butch for supporting me in my efforts as I tried to define myself, for sharing pride in my accomplishments, and after all these years, for still making me feel like I'm "the next best thing to sliced white bread."

CONTENTS

PART II

Administrator/Coordinator Role, 375

PART III

Consultant, Researcher, and Educator Roles, 411

Direct Caregiver Role

1 Breast Cancer

Jennifer L. Aikin

CASE STUDY

Nancy Smith is a 42-year-old Caucasian woman who presents to the breast care clinic for a mammogram. She states that she has some breast tenderness that seems to be more pronounced before her menstrual period and that when she examines her breasts, they feel "lumpy." She says, "I am concerned because my mother and sister have both been diagnosed with breast cancer. I want to be certain that everything is okay."

Medical History
First menstrual period at age 11
One pack of cigarettes each day
Cervical dysplasia (CIN I) diagnosed 3 years previously
Hypertension for 2 years

Medications
Triamterene and hydrochlorothiazide (Maxzide) 25 mg daily
Norethindrone acetate and ethinyl estradiol (Loestrin) 1.5/30

Social History
Married, with one son (age 2 years). Works as a cashier at the local grocery store.

Vital Signs
T: 37° C
P: 88 beats/min
R: 14 breaths/min
BP: 160/100 mm Hg
Height: 5 feet, 2 inches
Weight: 230 pounds

QUESTIONS

1. Based on her age and screening guidelines from the American Cancer Society and the National Cancer Institute (NCI), what screening activities should Nancy engage in, in addition to monthly breast self-examination?
   a. Yearly mammogram, yearly clinical breast examination
   b. Annual clinical breast examination, mammogram every other year
   c. Clinical breast examination and mammogram every other year
   d. Annual mammogram and clinical breast examination every 6 months

ANSWERS

1. According to the American Cancer Society Recommendations for the Early Detection of Cancer in Average Risk, Asymptomatic People (Smith, Mettlin, Davis, et al., 2000), breast cancer screening for women should be conducted as follows:

Age 20-39:   Monthly breast self-examination
              Clinical breast examination every 3 years
Age 40+:   Monthly breast self-examination
              Yearly clinical breast examination
              Yearly mammography

In the 1990s there was controversy about whether screening mammograms were effective in reducing cancer mortality in the group of women age 40 to 49. The NCI referred to pooled data from eight randomized trials demonstrating that a reduction in breast cancer mortality did not occur until about 15 years after screening was initiated (when women were in their 50s) and that the sensitivity of mammography was lower for younger women. For this reason, the NCI decided to defer decisions about screening mammography in this age group to individual women and their physicians.

Because Nancy is 42 years old, she falls into the 40- to 49-year-old category, where there is debate about the value of screening mammography. However, given her family history of breast cancer, it may be wise to follow the more conservative American Cancer Society recommendations, which involve monthly breast self-examinations, with yearly clinical breast examinations and mammograms. *Answer 1:* **a.**

QUESTIONS

2. What factors in Nancy's medical history suggest that she may be at increased risk for developing breast cancer?

a. Her age and weight
b. Family history and pregnancy history
c. Use of oral contraceptives
d. History of smoking and hypertension

3. What additional information should be gathered to more fully evaluate Nancy's risk for developing breast cancer?

1. Number of previous breast biopsies
2. Alcohol intake
3. Other family members with breast cancer
4. Personal history of atypical hyperplasia or lobular carcinoma in situ
  a. 1 & 2
  b. 1 & 3
  c. 2 & 3
  d. All of these

ANSWERS

2. Known risk factors for breast cancer are outlined in Box 1-1. Primary risk factors include age, family history of breast cancer, and biopsy

---

BOX **1-1**   Risk Factors for Breast Cancer

PRIMARY RISK FACTORS

Age >50
Country of origin: North America
                              Northern Europe
Family history: Personal history of breast cancer
                        Two or more first-degree
                            relatives with breast cancer
                        Bilateral/premenopausal breast
                            cancer in first-degree relative
Biopsy histology: Atypical hyperplasia
                          Lobular carcinoma in situ
                              (LCIS)
                          Ductal carcinoma in situ
                              (DCIS)

SECONDARY RISK FACTORS

Early menarche (<12) coupled with late menopause (>55)
First term pregnancy >30 years of age or nulliparity
Ionizing radiation to chest
Postmenopausal obesity

POSSIBLE RISK FACTORS

Alcohol intake >2 drinks/day
Oral contraceptives (before age 20 and persisting for ≥6 years)
Estrogen replacement therapy
High-fat diet

Adapted from Chapman, D. D., & Goodman. M. (2000). Breast cancer. In Yarbro, C. H., Frogge, M. H., Goodman, M., Groenwald, S. L. (Eds.). *Cancer nursing principles and practice*, 5th ed (p. 918). Boston: Jones and Bartlett.

histology. Secondary risk factors include early menarche, late menopause, nulliparity or term pregnancy after age 30, and ionizing irradiation to the chest. Other possible risk factors include a history of estrogen replacement therapy, use of oral contraceptives before age 20 and persisting for 6 years or more, alcohol intake, and a high-fat diet.

Because Nancy is relatively young (younger than 50), her age in and of itself does not put her at increased risk for breast cancer. There are no data suggesting that overweight premenopausal women are more at risk for developing breast cancer. Data regarding the use of oral contraceptives and risk for breast cancer are inconclusive; therefore this is not a definitive risk factor. Smoking and hypertension are not associated with an increased risk for breast cancer. Nancy's family history of breast cancer, combined with early menarche (age 11) and first pregnancy after the age of 30 (she had her son at age 40) increase her risk of developing breast cancer. *Answer 2:* **b.**

3. Additional information is needed to fully understand Nancy's risk for developing breast cancer. It is important to determine whether Nancy has had any previous breast biopsies and the resulting histologic diagnoses. A diagnosis of atypical hyperplasia, lobular carcinoma in situ (LCIS), ductal carcinoma in situ (DCIS), or a personal history of invasive breast cancer would significantly increase Nancy's breast cancer risk. Some studies have linked increased alcohol consumption with an increase in breast cancer risk. It is also important to ascertain whether other family members have been diagnosed with breast cancer or other related cancers (i.e., breast cancer/ovarian cancer syndrome associated with BRCA1 mutations). All of these issues should be assessed. *Answer 3:* **d.**

Case Study continued

Upon further questioning, you learn more about Nancy's family history:

- Maternal grandmother: ovarian cancer at age 62 (deceased)
- Mother: breast cancer at age 56
- Maternal aunt: colon cancer at age 62
- Paternal grandmother: uterine cancer
- Father: heart disease (deceased at age 52)
- Sister: breast cancer in right breast at age 41 and in left breast at age 45

Using the Gail Model risk assessment tool, you calculate Nancy's risk for developing breast cancer to be 2.2% over the next 5 years and 28.6% over her lifetime.

QUESTIONS

4. The Gail Model may be useful in assessing Nancy's risk because it:

1. Is a linear regression model used to determine breast cancer risk in the general population
2. Considers both first- and second-degree relatives with breast cancer
3. Makes it feasible to calculate breast cancer risk in the clinical setting
4. Considers both the maternal and paternal family history of breast cancer
   a. 1 & 2
   b. 1 & 3
   c. 2 & 3
   d. 2 & 4

5. What three factors in Nancy's history suggest that she may benefit from genetic counseling?

1. _____
2. _____
3. _____

6. Which of the following statements are true with respect to hereditary breast cancer?

1. Only 5% to 10% of breast cancers are caused by an inherited breast cancer gene.
2. Women who inherit the BRCA1 or BRCA2 genes are also at increased risk for ovarian cancer.
3. The breast cancer genes BRCA1 and BRCA2 are expressed in an autosomal-recessive pattern.
4. BRCA1 is most often associated with male breast cancer.
   a. 1 & 2
   b. 1 & 4
   c. 2 & 3
   d. 2 & 4

7. Before Nancy undergoes genetic testing, what factors should you and Nancy consider?

1. Whether genetics counseling services are available
2. Whether Nancy's sister or mother agree to testing
3. What the impact of testing will be on health insurance and employment
4. How the test results will affect Nancy's decisions about screening and steps to reduce risk
   a. 1 & 2
   b. 1, 2, & 3
   c. 2, 3, & 4
   d. All of these

ANSWERS

4. The Gail Model, a statistical linear regression model, was developed to calculate breast cancer risk in the general population of women, whereas other models, such as the Claus Model, are more accurate for risk prediction in high-risk families. Box 1-2 outlines the risk factors assessed in the Gail Model. The Gail Model is available as a computer disk that can be used on a personal computer, as a slide rule, or as a handheld calculator, all of which are easily used in the clinical setting. The Gail Model considers only maternal first-degree relatives (mothers, sisters, and daughters) who have had breast cancer. *Answer 4:* **b.**

5. Box 1-3 lists the indications for genetics counseling in women at high risk for breast cancer. *Answer 5:* **Any three of the following responses are correct: Nancy may benefit from genetics counseling because her family history shows (1) breast cancer in two generations, (2) bilateral breast cancer, (3) breast cancer at a young age, and (4) a number of cancers on her mother's side of the family, including ovarian cancer and colon cancer.**

6. Because breast cancer susceptibility genes account for only 5% to 10% of all breast cancers, many women overestimate their risk for developing breast cancer. Inherited breast cancer has several unique features: younger age of onset; greater likelihood to present as bilateral cancer; and its association with other cancers, such as ovarian, colon, prostate, and uterine cancers, as well as sarcomas.

Two breast cancer susceptibility genes have been identified thus far: BRCA1 and BRCA2. These two genes are transmitted in an autosomal-dominant pattern. During gametogenesis, both parents contribute one chromosome from each

BOX 1-2	Risk Factors Assessed by the Gail Model

Race*
Age
Age at first menses
Age at first live birth, or nulliparity
Number of first-degree female relatives with breast cancer (mother, sisters, daughters)
Number of breast biopsies
Diagnosis of atypical hyperplasia

*In the National Cancer Institute's "Risk Assessment Tool," available for use in the clinical setting, the Gail Model was adapted to include race.

BOX **1-3** | **Indications for Genetics Counseling**

Family history of the following:
Bilateral breast cancer
Multiple primary cancers
Young age of onset
Breast and ovarian cancers
Cancer in two or more generations
Multiple childhood sarcomas

Adapted from Tranin, A. S. (1996). Genetics and breast cancer risk. In Dow, K. H. (Ed.). *Contemporary issues in breast cancer* (pp. 14-15). Boston: Jones and Bartlett.

chromosome pair to the germ cell. If, for example, the mother is affected or carries a breast cancer susceptibility gene, there is a 50% likelihood that she will contribute this gene to her offspring (Figure 1-1). Female carriers of the BRCA1 gene are estimated to have an 87% cumulative risk of developing breast cancer by age 70 and a 62% risk of developing ovarian cancer by the age of 70. The BRCA1 gene is located on chromosome 17, and BRCA2 is located on chromosome 13. Both BRCA1 and BRCA2 are associated with the breast/ovarian cancer syndrome, with BRCA2 more commonly associated with male breast cancer. *Answer 6:* **a.**

7. Predictive (genetic) testing should not be done without the support of a qualified genetics counselor. The first step in breast cancer risk counseling involves the construction of a family pedigree that includes both the maternal and paternal sides of the family, going back at least two generations. Medical records are obtained to verify cancer diagnoses when possible. Predictive testing for the BRCA1 or BRCA2 genes should not be recommended without careful consideration of a number of issues: cost, potential harm to individuals and families in terms of insurance coverage and employment, confidentiality, and what course of action the individual will take as a result of the genetic information. Ideally, predictive testing begins with a family member who has been diagnosed with breast cancer; so in Nancy's case, her mother or sister need to be involved in decisions about genetic testing. In addition, this information will affect other family members. *Answer 7:* **d.**

QUESTIONS

8. What are the *two most effective* interventions that can be recommended to reduce Nancy's risk for developing breast cancer?

1. Yearly screening
2. Bilateral prophylactic mastectomy
3. Discontinuation of oral contraceptives
4. Chemoprevention with tamoxifen
    a. 1 & 2
    b. 1 & 3
    c. 2 & 3
    d. 2 & 4

9. Before recommending that Nancy take tamoxifen for chemoprevention, what additional information should you consider?
1. Whether she has a history of deep vein thrombosis (DVT) or pulmonary embolus (PE)
2. The report from her last electrocardiogram (ECG)
3. A complete gynecologic examination
4. Whether she plans on having more children
    a. 1 & 2
    b. 2 & 3
    c. 3 & 4
    d. 1, 3, & 4

ANSWERS

8. As you consider interventions to reduce Nancy's risk for developing breast cancer, it is important to determine which will be most effective based on her level of risk. In 1999 Hartmann, Schaid, Woods, et al. published the results of a case-control study that looked at women who underwent bilateral prophylactic mastectomies, comparing them with their sisters who did not. After about 14 years follow-up, the women who had bilateral prophylactic mastectomies had a 1.4% incidence of breast cancer, compared with 38.7% of their sisters who did not have the surgery. This translated into a 90% reduction in both the risk of developing breast cancer and the risk of death for the women who had bilateral prophylactic mastectomies. In another landmark study, Fisher, Costantino, Wickerham, et al. (1998) published the results of the Breast Cancer Prevention Trial (BCPT) in which women at high risk for developing breast cancer (women with LCIS, women 60 years of age or older, and women with a breast cancer risk of 1.66% as calculated by the Gail Model) were randomly assigned to receive tamoxifen or a placebo for 5 years. In this study there was a 49% reduction in the incidence of invasive breast cancer among the women who received tamoxifen, compared with those who received placebo.

Although it is not clear whether Nancy has

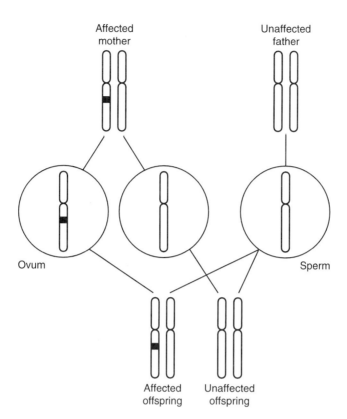

Affected
mother

Unaffected
father

Ovum

Sperm

Affected
offspring

Unaffected
offspring

Figure 1-1 Autosomal-dominant inheritance. (From Weber, B. L., & Garber, J. E. [1996]. Familial breast cancer. In Harris, J. R., Lippman, M. E., Morrow, M., et al. [Eds.]. *Diseases of the breast* [p. 172]. Philadelphia: Lippincott-Raven.)

inherited a breast cancer susceptibility gene, her breast cancer risk is substantial. Without question, based on the preceding results, bilateral prophylactic mastectomy is an effective means of reducing breast cancer risk. However, this is a drastic and disfiguring approach that must be considered carefully. Based on her 5-year risk for developing breast cancer calculated by the Gail Model, Nancy may also benefit from tamoxifen. Yearly screening is an appropriate intervention but not likely to be as effective as either bilateral prophylactic mastectomy or tamoxifen. It is not known whether discontinuing oral contraceptives will have much effect on reducing breast cancer risk. *Answer 8:* **d.**

9. A number of factors must be taken into account when considering tamoxifen for chemoprevention. In the BCPT tamoxifen was associated with a reduction in osteoporotic hip fractures, a reduction in both invasive and noninvasive breast cancer, and an increased incidence of endometrial cancer, DVT, PE, and stroke (Fisher et al., 1998). The most notable side effects of tamoxifen in this study were hot flashes and vaginal discharge. All of these risks and benefits must be considered. A thorough history must be conducted to determine whether Nancy has a history of DVT, PE, or stroke, and Nancy's risk factors for these thromboembolic events (i.e., inactivity, obesity, uncontrolled hypertension, or diabetes) must be assessed. In addition, a thorough gynecologic history should be obtained, and Nancy should be referred to her gynecologist for a bimanual pelvic examination. It is also important to assess whether Nancy and her husband plan to have more children. If so, tamoxifen should not be considered because the drug is teratogenic. Although tamoxifen lowers serum cholesterol, in the BCPT the drug was not associated with a reduction in cardiovascular events. An ECG would not provide any important information as to the risks and benefits of tamoxifen for Nancy. *Answer 9:* **d.**

CASE 2 STUDY

Joan Miller is a 67-year-old African American woman who presents to the comprehensive breast care center with a palpable mass in her right breast. She is accompanied by her daughter. She states that she performs breast self-examinations "almost every month" and that she found this lump the previous week while she was taking a shower. She is very anxious and states, "I've done everything that I can to live a healthy lifestyle so that I wouldn't get cancer. I'm very conscientious about eating a low-fat diet and exercising regularly."

Medical History
First menstrual period at age 12
First of four children at age 22
Hysterectomy at age 47
Hormone replacement therapy (HRT) for 20 years

Medications
Multiple vitamin supplement
Conjugated estrogens/medroxyprogesterone acetate tablets (Prempro) (0.625 mg/2.5 mg) one tablet daily

Breast Examination
There is a palpable, 2-cm mass in the upper outer quadrant of her right breast. There is no tethering or dimpling of the breast, no redness or skin thickening, and no nipple discharge. The left breast is without masses. There are no palpable nodes in either axilla.

Mammogram
A bilateral mammogram shows a spiculated mass in the upper outer quadrant of the right breast. The radiologist recommends that a biopsy be performed on the mass.

1. How can you be most supportive?
    1. Reassure Joan that most breast lumps are benign
    2. Describe the different methods for performing breast biopsies
    3. Explain that these findings represent cancer
    4. Ensure that Joan's insurance will cover the biopsy and that the surgeon participates in her insurance plan
    a. 1 & 2
    b. 1 & 4
    c. 2 & 4
    d. 2, 3, & 4

ANSWERS

1. Although the clinical examination and mammogram are suspicious for cancer, these findings need to be followed up with a biopsy. Therefore it is premature to explain that these findings are either benign or likely to be cancer. You can honestly say that the biopsy will reveal important information about the breast mass, and then prepare Joan for the biopsy. You can describe the different methods for performing breast biopsies and ensure that Joan's insurance will cover both the biopsy and the surgeon visit. *Answer 1:* **c.**

QUESTIONS

2. Describe the difference between a fine-needle aspiration (FNA) biopsy, a core-needle biopsy, an excisional biopsy, and an incisional biopsy. *Answer 2:* **See Table 1-1.**

Case Study continued
A core-needle biopsy of the palpable lump determines that the mass is an invasive ductal carcinoma. Joan returns to the breast center with her husband and daughter to meet with the surgeon and discuss her surgical options. The surgeon explains that the tumor must be removed and that, based on the size of the tumor, a lumpectomy is feasible. He also explains that Joan will need an axillary dissection to determine whether her axillary nodes show signs of cancer or that she can participate in a clinical trial evaluating the sentinel lymph node procedure. Following this discussion with the physician, you meet with Joan and her family.

QUESTIONS

3. Joan is visibly upset. She asks, "How did this happen? I don't have a family history of breast cancer, and I've always taken care of myself. Did I get breast cancer because I was taking hormones?" Which of the following responses is the most appropriate?
    a. "Yes, the hormone replacement therapy probably caused your breast cancer."
    b. "No, its unlikely that hormone replacement therapy caused your breast cancer."
    c. "It is difficult to say whether the hormone replacement therapy contributed to your diagnosis. Most women who develop breast cancer have few or no risk factors for the disease."

TABLE 1-1 **Overview of Biopsy Methods to Diagnose Breast Cancer**

Fine-needle aspiration (FNA): An FNA is generally performed on a palpable mass to determine whether it is cystic or solid. The procedure is easily performed by a surgeon in the office using a 21- to 27-gauge needle, without anesthetic. A drop of the aspirate is placed on a glass microscope slide, and the specimen is sent for cytopathologic evaluation. An FNA cannot always distinguish between an invasive carcinoma and noninvasive ductal carcinoma. Advantages include low morbidity, convenience, low cost, and immediate availability.

Core-cutting needle biopsy: A core-needle biopsy is obtained using a disposable needle, such as the Tru-Cut needle, or a spring-loaded biopsy device. This type of biopsy obtains enough histologic material to process for permanent sections or for frozen section, making it possible to distinguish between invasive and noninvasive carcinoma. A core biopsy may be performed on mammographically detected lesions using a stereotactic device, which is a more costly procedure.

Excisional biopsy: An excisional biopsy involves the complete removal of a tumor with or without a rim of normal tissue surrounding the lesion. It is generally performed with local anesthesia, with or without additional sedation. For benign lesions, an excisional biopsy is all that is required; furthermore, an excisional biopsy may be sufficient for some malignant lesions as long as the margins are not involved. This type of biopsy is more costly because anesthesia is required.

Incisional biopsy: An incisional biopsy may be performed when complete removal of a mass is unnecessary and when removal may jeopardize a future mastectomy. In this procedure, only a portion of the mass is removed for pathologic examination.

Adapted from Foster, R. S. (1996). Biopsy techniques. In Harris, J. R., Lippman, M. E., Morrow, M., et al. (Eds.). *Diseases of the breast* (pp. 133-138). Philadelphia: Lippincott-Raven.

d. "It is more likely attributable to your race. African American women are more likely to develop breast cancer than Caucasian women."

ANSWERS

3. Although estrogen replacement therapy is a possible risk factor for breast cancer, it is impossible to say whether this contributed to Joan's diagnosis. Joan has few other risk factors: She has no family history of breast cancer, she had her first child at an early age, and she had an earlier age of menarche. Furthermore, the incidence of breast cancer is lower in African American women than in Caucasian women, although a greater percentage present at more advanced stages. To alleviate any concerns that Joan may have caused her own breast cancer by taking HRT, the best approach for the advanced practice nurse (APN) to take is to explain that most women who develop breast cancer have few or no risk factors for the disease and that it is difficult to determine whether HRT caused her breast cancer. *Answer 3:* **c.**

QUESTIONS

4. Joan states that she has a friend who had a modified radical mastectomy and that perhaps it would be best if she had the surgeon remove the entire breast so that she did not have to worry about breast cancer returning. What additional information does Joan need to know as she makes a decision about her surgical treatment?

1. Studies have shown that in early-stage breast cancer, a lumpectomy with radiation is as effective as a modified radical mastectomy.
2. An axillary dissection will be performed with either procedure (lumpectomy or modified radical mastectomy).
3. If she has a lumpectomy, she will need to have about 5 weeks of radiation therapy. The most common side effect is skin redness.
4. There is a much greater degree of lymphedema associated with a modified radical mastectomy compared with a lumpectomy and axillary dissection.
   a. 1 & 2
   b. 1, 2, & 3
   c. 1, 3, & 4
   d. 2 & 4

5. Joan asks, "What is the difference between an axillary dissection and sentinel lymph node biopsy?" When answering this question, you should include all of the following information *except:*
   a. A description of the anatomy of the axilla and role of the lymph nodes
   b. A discussion of the sentinel node procedure
   c. An explanation of the morbidity associated with axillary dissection
   d. The rationale for the clinical trial

10 PART I Direct Caregiver Role

4. Joan is deciding whether to have a modified radical mastectomy or a lumpectomy. A modified radical mastectomy involves the removal of the entire breast, the pectoral fascia, and an axillary node dissection. Only one transverse incision is required for this procedure. A total mastectomy involves the removal of the entire breast with the preservation of both pectoral muscles and axillary nodes.

A number of types of breast reconstruction may be performed, either at the time of the mastectomy or later. These include saline implants and flap procedures (e.g., latissimus dorsi musculocutaneous flap, transverse rectus abdominis myocutaneous [TRAM] flap, gluteus maximus flap).

The goal of a lumpectomy and other breast-conserving procedures (e.g., segmental mastectomy, quadrantectomy) is to preserve the breast in a way that is cosmetically acceptable. With a lumpectomy, a curvilinear incision is made directly above the tumor and the tumor is removed with a margin of uninvolved tissue. This is generally performed as an outpatient procedure under local anesthesia (with or without sedation). For patients with invasive breast cancer, a lumpectomy is followed by a course of radiation therapy (usually about 5 weeks for a total of about 5000 cGy).

An axillary dissection is performed to complete the surgical staging, determine postoperative therapy, and obtain local control. The number of involved axillary nodes is probably the most important prognostic factor for breast cancer. When performed in conjunction with a lumpectomy, a separate incision is made for the axillary dissection.

Studies have shown that a lumpectomy, axillary dissection, and radiation therapy are equivalent to a modified radical mastectomy in terms of survival. In 1990 the NCI Consensus Conference on the treatment of early-stage breast cancer advocated breast-conservation treatment because it preserved the breast while providing equivalent survival to a total mastectomy and axillary dissection.

Between 15% and 20% of women experience lymphedema after breast cancer treatment. This condition is the result of the axillary dissection, not the primary breast surgery (lumpectomy or total mastectomy). Lymphedema may be mild and barely noticeable, or it may be severe, causing disfigurement, discomfort, and disability. *Answer 4:* **b.**

5. When describing the difference between a traditional axillary dissection and the sentinel lymph node biopsy procedure, first you need to describe the anatomy of the axilla, determine the purpose of the lymph nodes, and define *sentinel node*. The sentinel node is the first node that drains lymphatic fluid from the breast tumor. (There may be more than one sentinel node.) You can then go on to describe the procedure. Before surgery, the patient receives a number of injections of a radioactive tracer with or without a blue dye; these are injected into the skin surrounding the tumor. Within 10 to 20 minutes, a radiation detection device called a *gamma probe* is used to find the "hot spot," which guides the surgeon to the location of the sentinel node so that it can be removed. It is important to explain that the levels of radiation are extremely low and therefore not dangerous for the patient or health care professionals. If the sentinel node is negative, there is a great likelihood that the remaining lymph nodes are also negative. Generally, if a woman has positive nodes, she will go on for a full axillary dissection.

You need to objectively describe the potential risks and benefits of both procedures. The axillary dissection provides important prognostic information that may not be obtained from a sentinel node biopsy; however, there may be more morbidity (e.g., lymphedema, decreased range of motion) associated with the axillary dissection. Clinical trials are under way to compare the accuracy of predicting the presence or absence of lymph node involvement and to compare survival rates in patients who undergo sentinel lymph node biopsy versus axillary dissection. Until the results of these clinical trials are available, one procedure should not be endorsed over another. *Answer 5:* **c.**

Case Study *continued*

Joan chooses to undergo a modified radical mastectomy. When she returns to the breast center for her first postoperative visit, she states that she has pain at the site of her incision, that her right arm is stiff, and that she still has some drainage, although the amount is less every day.

QUESTIONS

6. To rule out postoperative complications, all of the following should be included in your assessment *except:*
- **a.** Homans' sign to rule out DVT
- **b.** Volume of drainage from drain over the past 24 hours
- **c.** Signs and symptoms of wound infection
- **d.** Right shoulder and arm range of motion and strength

7. What teaching will Joan require during the postoperative period?
1. Drain care
2. Arm exercises to maintain mobility
3. Types of prostheses and how to use them
4. Arm care following an axillary dissection
   a. 1 & 2
   b. 2 & 3
   c. 3 & 4
   d. All of these

ANSWERS

6. Your postoperative assessment should target potential complications. (Complications of surgical procedures for breast cancer are outlined in Box 1-4.) You should assess the location, intensity, and duration of pain; determine the volume of drainage from the drainage tube over the past 24 hours; observe for signs and symptoms of wound infection; and evaluate the range of motion and

| BOX **1-4** | **Complications of Breast Cancer Surgery** |

MASTECTOMY
Wound infection (6%-14%)
  Cellulitis (early postoperative period)
  Abscess (later postoperative period)
  Seroma formation (100%)
Necrosis of skin flap (uncommon)
Phantom breast syndrome
  Pain
  Itching
  Nipple sensation

LUMPECTOMY
Wound infection (uncommon)

AXILLARY DISSECTION
Major Complications (Uncommon)
Injury or thrombosis of the axillary vein
Injury to motor nerves

Minor Complications
Seroma formation
Shoulder dysfunction
Loss of sensation
Edema of the arm and breast
Other subjective symptoms
  Pain
  Numbness
  Weakness

Adapted from Harris, J. R., & Morrow, M. (1996). Treatment of early-stage breast cancer. I In Harris, J. R., Lippman, M. E., Morrow, M., et al. (Eds.). *Diseases of the breast* (pp. 487-547). Philadelphia: Lippincott-Raven.

strength in Joan's right shoulder. Although Joan may be at risk for axillary vein thrombosis as a result of the axillary dissection, there is not a prolonged period of immobilization following breast cancer surgery. Therefore Homans' sign (used to detect a DVT in the lower extremities) would not be a routine part of a postoperative assessment. *Answer 6:* **a.**

7. To prevent seroma formation, the surgeon inserts one or more drains (attached to closed suction) during the mastectomy and/or axillary dissection. When the total volume of drainage in 24 hours decreases to less than 40 ml or at the first postoperative visit, the drain is removed. During the immediate postoperative period, Joan will need to learn how to care for her drain at home: how to strip the drainage tubing daily to prevent blockage and collapse, how to empty it and record the volume of drainage in each 24-hour period, and what complications to report to the surgeon (e.g., air in the tubing, drainage of 200 ml or more in 24 hours.)

After an axillary dissection, arm exercises are important to prevent immobility of the shoulder. You may be responsible for this teaching, or it may be taught by an American Cancer Society Reach to Recovery volunteer or a physical therapist. Joan should begin to perform arm exercises on the second or third postoperative day.

After the axillary dissection, Joan will be more at risk for lymphedema. Without causing undue concern or alarm, the nursing staff should teach Joan about arm and hand precautions that will help prevent lymphedema (Box 1-5).

In the immediate postoperative period after a mastectomy, Joan may wear a bra with a soft prosthesis. She should not use a permanent prosthesis until complete wound healing has occurred. This teaching may be performed by the APN, a staff nurse, or a Reach to Recovery volunteer. *Answer 7:* **d.**

Case Study continued

During the postoperative visit the surgeon discusses the results of the pathology report with Joan. The report reads as follows:

RIGHT BREAST (mastectomy)
- Infiltrating ductal carcinoma, NOS type, histologic grade 2/3, nuclear grade 2/3, measuring 1.5 cm in maximum diameter, with foci of ductal carcinoma in situ, solid and cribriform type within the infiltrating tumor mass, WITH: all margins, including anterior (skin), inferior, superior, lateral, medial, and posterior, free of tumor.

BOX **1-5** | Arm and Hand Precautions after an Axillary Dissection

1. Do not ignore any increased swelling in the arm, hand, fingers, neck, or chest wall.
2. Never allow an injection (intravenous) or blood to be drawn in the affected arm(s). Wear a lymphedema alert bracelet.
3. Check blood pressure on the unaffected arm.
4. Keep the affected arm, or "at-risk" arm, clean. Use lotion after bathing. When drying, be gentle but thorough. Dry any creases and between the fingers.
5. Avoid vigorous, repetitive movements against resistance with the affected arm (e.g., scrubbing, pushing, pulling).
6. Avoid heavy lifting with the affected arm. (Do not lift more than 15 pounds.) Never carry heavy handbags or bags with over-the-shoulder straps.
7. Do not wear tight jewelry or elastic bands around affected fingers or arm(s).
8. Avoid extreme temperature changes when bathing and washing dishes. Do not sit in saunas or hot tubs. Keep the arm protected from the sun.
9. Avoid any type of trauma, such as bruising, cuts, sunburn or other burns, sports injuries, insect bites, and cat scratches.
10. Wear gloves while doing housework, gardening, or any type of work that could result in injury.
11. When manicuring your nails, avoid cutting the cuticles.
12. Exercise is important but do not overtire an arm at risk. Recommended exercises are walking, swimming, light aerobics, and bike riding.
13. When traveling by air, patients with lymphedema should wear a compression sleeve. Additional bandages may be required on a long flight. Increase fluid intake while in the air.
14. Patients with large breasts who have a mastectomy should wear a light breast prosthesis because heavy prostheses put too much pressure on the lymph nodes above the collarbone. Wear a well-fitting bra without an underwire, and soft padded shoulder straps.
15. Use an electric razor to remove hair from the axilla. Maintain the electric razor properly, replacing heads as needed.
16. Patients with lymphedema should wear a well-fitted compression sleeve during waking hours.
17. Symptoms such as rash, itching, redness, pain, and increased temperature of the skin on the arm should be reported to the physician immediately.
18. Maintain an ideal weight with a well-balanced, low sodium, high-fiber diet. Avoid smoking and alcohol consumption.

Adapted from National Lymphedema Network (NLN). (1999). *18 steps to prevention for upper extremities.* Oakland, CA: NLN.

- Fibrocystic changes, mainly fibrosis, in the background breast tissue.

RIGHT AXILLARY LYMPH NODES (dissection)
All 13 lymph nodes identified are free of tumor; they show reactive follicular, parafollicular, and sinusoidal hyperplasia.

ESTROGEN RECEPTOR IMMUNOASSAY (ER-ICA):
Positive nuclear staining in more than 75% of tumor cells

PROGESTERONE RECEPTOR IMMUNOASSAY:
Positive nuclear staining in more than 75% of tumor cells

QUESTIONS

8. Based on the preceding information and your knowledge about breast cancer, you know that:
1. Joan has a stage II, estrogen receptor–positive breast cancer
2. Infiltrating ductal carcinoma is a common type of breast cancer
3. Joan will benefit from tamoxifen therapy
4. Joan should see a medical oncologist to discuss the need for chemotherapy
   a. 1 & 2
   b. 2, 3, & 4
   c. 3 & 4
   d. All of these

ANSWERS

8. Joan's pathology report indicates that her tumor is 1.5 cm and that she does not have positive axillary lymph nodes. Therefore, based on the staging system for breast cancer (Table 1-2), Joan has a $T_1N_0M_x$ breast cancer. Given her positive estrogen receptors, she is considered to have stage I, estrogen receptor (ER)–positive breast cancer.

Invasive (infiltrating) ductal carcinoma is the most common type of breast cancer, accounting for 65% to 80% of breast cancer diagnoses (Rosen, 1996). Ductal carcinomas may show features of tubular, medullary, papillary, or mucinous differentiation. The next most common histology is invasive lobular carcinoma, constituting 10% to 14% of invasive carcinomas. Other rare types of

TABLE **1-2**   **TNM Staging of Breast Cancer**

STAGE	CHARACTERISTICS
PRIMARY TUMOR (T)	
T_X	Primary tumor cannot be assessed
T_0	No evidence of primary tumor
Tis	Carcinoma in situ: intraductal carcinoma, lobular carcinoma in situ, or Paget's disease of the nipple with no tumor
T_1	Tumor ≤2 cm in greatest dimension
T_{1mic}	Microinvasion ≤0.1 cm in greatest dimension
T_{1a}	Tumor >0.1 but not more than 0.5 cm in greatest dimension
T_{1b}	Tumor >0.5 cm but not more than 1 cm in greatest dimension
T_{1c}	Tumor >1 cm but not more than 2 cm in greatest dimension
T_2	Tumor >2 cm but not more than 5 cm in greatest dimension
T_3	Tumor >5 cm in greatest dimension
T_4	Tumor of any size with direct extension to (a) chest wall or (b) skin, only as described below
T_{4a}	Extension to chest wall
T_{4b}	Edema (including peau d'orange) or ulceration of skin of the breast or satellite skin nodules confined to the same breast
T_{4c}	Both (T4a and T4b)
T_{4d}	Inflammatory carcinoma

Note: Paget's disease associated with a tumor is classified according to the size of the tumor.

STAGE	CHARACTERISTICS
REGIONAL LYMPH NODES (N)	
N_X	Regional lymph nodes cannot be assessed (e.g., previously removed)
N_0	No regional lymph node metastasis
N_1	Metastasis to movable ipsilateral axillary lymph node(s)
N_2	Metastasis to ipsilateral axillary lymph node(s) fixed to one another or to other structures
N_3	Metastasis to ipsilateral internal mammary lymph node(s)
DISTANT METASTASIS (M)	
M_X	Distant metastasis cannot be assessed
M_0	No distant metastases
M_1	Distant metastasis (includes metastasis to ipsilateral supraclavicular lymph node[s])

STAGE GROUPING

Stage 0		Tis	N0	M0
Stage I		T1*	N0	M0
Stage IIA	T0	N1	M0	
		T1*	N1†	M0
		T2	N0	M0
Stage IIB	T2	N1	M0	
		T3	N0	M0
Stage IIIA	T0	N2	M0	
		T1*	N2	M0
		T2	N2	M0
		T3	N1	M0
		T3	N2	M0
Stage IIIB	T4	Any N	M0	
		Any T	N3	M0
Stage IV	Any T	Any N	M1	

From the American Joint Committee on Cancer (AJCC®), Chicago, IL. The original source for this material is the *AJCC® Cancer Staging Manual*, 5th ed (1997) published by Lippincott-Raven Publishers, Philadelphia, PA.
*T_1 includes T_{1mic}.
†The prognosis of patients with N_{1a} is similar to that of patients with pN_0.

TABLE 1-3	Indications for Tamoxifen	
Metastatic breast cancer	Effective for both women and men. For premenopausal women with metastatic disease, tamoxifen is an alternative to oophorectomy or ovarian irradiation. Evidence indicates that patients whose tumors are estrogen receptor positive are more likely to benefit from tamoxifen therapy.
Adjuvant treatment of breast cancer	Node-positive breast cancer in postmenopausal women; node-negative breast cancer. Insufficient data to predict whether tamoxifen provides benefit for women with tumors <1 cm. Reduces the occurrence of contralateral breast cancer.
Reduction in breast cancer incidence in high-risk women	*High-risk* is defined as women at least 35 years of age with a 5-year predicted risk of breast cancer ≥1.67% as calculated by the Gail Model.

From Aikin, J. L. (2000). Adjuvant therapy for breast cancer: Choices and challenges. *Innovat Breast Cancer Care, 5*(1), pp. 3-8.

breast cancer include lymphoma, sarcoma, and melanoma.

Tamoxifen citrate is the most widely prescribed agent for the treatment of breast cancer. Indications for tamoxifen are outlined in Table 1-3. Because Joan is postmenopausal and ER positive, she is a candidate for tamoxifen therapy.

Recent data suggest that women with stage I, ER-positive breast cancer may benefit from chemotherapy in addition to tamoxifen; however, the margin of benefit is small (Fisher, Dignam, Wolmark, et al., 1997). Joan should be referred to a medical oncologist to discuss this treatment option. *Answer 8:* **b.**

QUESTIONS

9. Joan's medical oncologist recommends that she consider chemotherapy. She calls to ask for advice about whether she should take chemotherapy. How can you be supportive during this decision-making process?
   1. Identify gaps in Joan's knowledge about the risks and benefits of chemotherapy.
   2. Arrange for Joan to meet with another patient who has received the chemotherapy regimen recommended by Joan's oncologist.
   3. Caution that side effects of chemotherapy are generally more severe in older patients.
   4. Reassure Joan that the side effects of chemotherapy are very manageable.

   a. 1 & 2
   b. 1, 2, & 3
   c. 2 & 3
   d. 3 & 4

ANSWERS

9. You can play a key role in helping women weigh the benefits, risks, and side effects of chemotherapy. First you must identify what information Joan has been given, identify any gaps in information, and provide missing information. Written educational materials and helpful websites are useful resources. Joan may benefit from meeting with another patient of a similar age and diagnosis who has had the recommended chemotherapy regimen so that she can hear first-hand about side effects and effect on lifestyle. However, it is important that you explain that the response to chemotherapy varies from individual to individual.

Studies have shown that age is not a factor in determining how patients tolerate chemotherapy; rather performance status is a more important indicator. Therefore Joan should not be expecting more severe side effects based on her age. Finally, you should not raise expectations that chemotherapy side effects will be easily manageable. Certainly you can mention that there are a number of effective symptom management strategies for side effects such as nausea and vomiting, but there are no guarantees that Joan will have an easy treatment experience. *Answer 9:* **a.**

CASE 3 STUDY

Judy Smith is 36-year-old woman who presents to the outpatient chemotherapy department for chemotherapy. Accompanied by her husband, Judy says that she is very nervous about her treatment and is afraid of being very sick.

Medical History
First menstrual period at age 12
First child at age 29
Appendectomy at age 21
Tubal ligation at age 33
Four weeks postlumpectomy and axillary dissection. She had a 4-cm invasive lobular carcinoma in her left breast with 1 of 22 positive lymph nodes. Her tumor was positive for estrogen receptors.

Medications
Loratadine and pseudoephedrine sulfate (Claritin-D) orally daily for allergies

Social History
Judy and her husband have two sons, ages 7 and 3. She works as an accountant for a small construction company. Her older son is active in soccer and baseball, so her evenings and weekends are spent going to games. She lives in the same small community where she grew up, and her mother and sister live nearby. Her husband is self-employed as a computer consultant.

Physical Examination
Her breast and axillary incisions are healing without signs of infection. Lung sounds are clear. Left breast is tender but without masses; right breast and axilla are without masses. No palpable supraclavicular or cervical lymph nodes present.

The medical oncologist writes the following chemotherapy orders:
- Ondansetron (Zofran) 0.15 mg/kg IV 30 minutes before chemotherapy then 8 mg PO q8h for 2 days
- Dexamethasone (Decadron) 10 mg IV 30 minutes before chemotherapy
- Doxorubicin (Adriamycin) 60 mg/m^2 IV push q3wk for 4 cycles
- Cyclophosphamide (Cytoxan) 600 mg/m^2 in 250 ml normal saline (NS) over 1 hour q3wk for 4 cycles
- Prochlorperazine (Compazine) 10 mg PO q6h prn nausea or vomiting
- Tamoxifen citrate (Nolvadex) 20 mg PO daily

QUESTIONS

1. In addition to the aforementioned chemotherapy regimen, what other regimens are routinely used in the adjuvant therapy of breast cancer?

2. Before beginning treatment, you visit with Judy to determine whether her educational

needs have been met. Which of the following issues should be addressed?
1. The need to take antiemetics as prescribed
2. Preparing for alopecia associated with this regimen
3. Self-administration of growth factors to combat anemia
4. Effect of agents on menopausal status and fertility
   a. 1 & 2
   b. 1, 2, & 3
   c. 1, 2, & 4
   d. All of these

ANSWERS

1. The most common chemotherapy regimens used in the adjuvant treatment of breast cancer are AC (Adriamycin [doxorubicin]/cyclophosphamide), CMF (cyclophosphamide/methotrexate/5-fluorouracil), and CAF (cyclophosphamide/Adriamycin [doxorubicin]/5-fluorouracil). Paclitaxel (Taxol) may also be given based on a study published in 1998 by Henderson, Berry, Demetri, et al. that showed additional benefit for disease-free survival and survival when Taxol was added to AC in women with node-positive breast cancer. *Answer 1:* **See text.**

2. It is important that you assess Judy's understanding of the side effects of the AC chemotherapy regimen and the resulting impact of chemotherapy on her lifestyle. The AC regimen is moderately to highly emetogenic, so it is important that the antiemetic regimen include a 5HT$_3$ serotonin antagonist agent. The effects of the 5HT$_3$ antagonists are enhanced by steroids. Alopecia is a side effect of doxorubicin, so Judy needs to be prepared for its occurrence. Generally, hair loss occurs before the second cycle of chemotherapy. Although the AC regimen is associated with neutropenia, prophylactic granulocyte colony-stimulating factor (G-CSF) or granulocyte-macrophage colony-stimulating factor (GM-CSF) is not routinely used unless severe neutropenia or febrile neutropenia occurs. Anemia is rarely significant enough to require the administration of growth factors.

Alkylating agents such as cyclophosphamide cause ovarian dysfunction in premenopausal women. Irregular menses and amenorrhea may result. Ovarian dysfunction may be temporary or permanent, depending on the woman's age at the time of chemotherapy, resulting in infertility and menopausal symptoms such as hot flashes and vaginal dryness. Because Judy is premenopausal, she needs to be prepared for these changes.

Although tamoxifen does not cause ovarian dysfunction, this drug may cause menopausal symptoms such as hot flashes and vaginal dryness. If Judy had not had a previous tubal ligation, she would need to be counseled to use a form of barrier contraception because there is still a chance that she could become pregnant.

In addition to these side effects, fatigue may result. Judy may need to take time off work. Furthermore, based on her age and her husband's being self-employed, there may be insurance issues to consider. *Answer 2:* **c.**

QUESTIONS

3. Judy asks you when she will have her radiation therapy. What is the best response to this question?

    a. "Because you are receiving chemotherapy, you will not need radiation."

    b. "You will receive radiation therapy at the same time as your chemotherapy."

    c. "Your radiation will be sandwiched between your first and second cycle of chemotherapy."

    d. "You will receive radiation when you have recovered from your chemotherapy."

ANSWERS

3. Because Judy had a lumpectomy, she will require radiation therapy. With the AC and CAF regimens, radiation therapy is often given following recovery from all chemotherapy because there can be increased skin sensitivity when radiation is given concurrent with or before Adriamycin (Harris & Morrow, 1996). With the CMF regimen, radiation therapy may be given concurrently or "sandwiched" between cycles. *Answer 3:* **d.**

Case Study continued

Judy has very few side effects with her first two cycles of chemotherapy. On the day of her third cycle, she states that her menstrual periods have become irregular and that she has been having severe hot flashes. She says that she is frequently awakened at night and then has difficulty going back to sleep. She says, "I can handle the queasiness I feel for the first few days after chemotherapy, but these hot flashes are awful."

QUESTIONS

4. Judy asks what she can do about the hot flashes. Which of the following should you recommend for managing her menopausal symptoms?

    1. Estrogen replacement therapy

    2. Herbal remedies such as black cohosh root, oil of evening primrose, or ginseng

    3. Avoidance of caffeine, spicy foods, and alcohol

    4. Pharmacologic agents such as clonidine (Catapres-TTS), phenobarbital/belladonna/ergotamine (Bellergal-S), and venlafaxine hydrochloride (Effexor)

    a. 1 & 2

    b. 2 & 3

    c. 2 & 4

    d. 3 & 4

ANSWERS

4. Although estrogen replacement therapy is by far the most effective treatment for menopausal symptoms, it is usually contraindicated for women with breast cancer. However, a number of nonhormonal agents may provide relief from hot flashes (Lin, Aikin, & Good, 1999). These agents include vitamin E, clonidine, Bellergal-S (a combination of ergotamine and phenobarbital), and antidepressants such as Effexor and Paxil (paroxetine hydrochloride). Other practical suggestions for coping with hot flashes include physical exercise and avoidance of caffeine, spicy foods, and alcohol. Herbal remedies such as black cohosh root, oil of evening primrose, ginseng, and soy foods contain "phytoestrogens," naturally occurring plant estrogens. These have not been studied sufficiently to determine whether they cause harm in women with estrogen-sensitive tumors such as breast cancer. *Answer 4:* **d.**

QUESTIONS

5. On day 10 following her third cycle of treatment, Judy calls in to the office to report that she "just isn't feeling well." She says that she has a fever of 100.3° F and is very tired. What should you do in response to this information?

    1. Tell Judy to rest and call if her temperature climbs above 101° F

    2. Question Judy about signs and symptoms of infection

    3. Arrange for Judy to have a complete blood count (CBC) with differential and a platelet count drawn

    4. Phone in a prescription for an oral antibiotic

    a. 1 & 2

    b. 2 & 3

    c. 2 & 4

    d. 3 & 4

ANSWERS

5. It is important that you gather more information about Judy's situation. You know to question Judy about any signs and symptoms of infection because she is 10 days posttherapy when her white blood cells (WBCs) are at their nadir. You have anticipated her high risk of infection and are monitoring her counts by having a CBC with differential and platelet count drawn. Once you have conducted a thorough assessment and obtained the results of her blood work, the decision can be made whether to bring the patient in for intravenous (IV) antibiotics or order oral antibiotics. *Answer 5:* **b.**

Case Study *continued*

As the day progresses, Judy's temperature continues to climb and her blood work comes back as follows: WBCs, 400/mm³; segments, 30%; bands, 2; platelets, 102,000/µl. She is admitted to the hospital for antibiotics, with a diagnosis of febrile neutropenia. She is discharged 2 days later.

QUESTIONS

6. When Judy presents for cycle 4, she states that she is still very tired but that she is feeling better. How will Judy's hospitalization for febrile neutropenia affect this final course of chemotherapy?

ANSWERS

6. First, it is important to determine whether Judy has fully recovered from her episode of febrile neutropenia. A CBC with differential and platelets should be drawn before beginning chemotherapy. According to the American Society of Clinical Oncology (ASCO) guidelines for the administration of colony-stimulating factors (CSFs) (1994), Judy should receive G-CSF or GM-CSF prophylactically with cycle 4 to protect her from infection without compromising the dose intensity of the chemotherapeutic agents. It will be important to find out what insurance coverage Judy has for growth factors and to teach her how to perform the injections. In addition, she will need more frequent blood work during this final cycle. *Answer 6:* **See text.**

QUESTIONS

7. At this final chemotherapy visit, Judy says, "I'm relieved that this is my final dose of therapy, but it's kind of scary to think that I'm finished with treatment. I'm afraid that my cancer will come back when the chemotherapy is finished." What is the best response to this statement?
   a. "You received standard therapy, so you have a very good chance of being cured."
   b. "It's time to move on with your life."
   c. "You're taking tamoxifen, so you don't have to worry about the cancer coming back."
   d. "What you're feeling is common. It can be frightening to finish chemotherapy."

ANSWERS

7. Because this is a common concern of women who are completing adjuvant therapy, it is important that the APN listen to Judy's concerns and not minimize them. *Answer 7:* **d.**

CASE 4 STUDY

Mary Thompson is a 59-year-old Caucasian woman who was first diagnosed with adenocarcinoma of the breast at the age of 48. At that time she had a modified radical mastectomy for a 2-cm tumor in her right breast. Of 14 lymph nodes, 4 were positive for cancer. She was treated with six cycles of CMF and tamoxifen. She presents to her oncologist's office with a skin nodule at the site of her mastectomy scar. She says, "At first I thought it was a pimple that wouldn't heal, but now I'm not sure. Has the cancer come back?"

Medical History
Breast cancer history (see previous discussion). She was in an automobile accident at age 43 in which she broke her femur and was in traction. She was diagnosed with emphysema at age 52.

Medications
Theophylline (Theo-Dur) 300 every 12 hours

Social History
Mary is divorced with three adult children, two of whom still live at home. She worked as a housekeeper at a local hospital for 20 years but was recently laid off because of cutbacks. She has 1 to 2 drinks a day and a 37 pack/year smoking history.

1. In addition to performing a physical examination of the chest wall, breast, and axilla, what should you do?
   1. Auscultate lung sounds
   2. Palpate the supraclavicular and cervical lymph nodes
   3. Palpate the liver
   4. Assess the presence or absence of pain (location, quality, and precipitating factors)

TABLE 1-4	Sites of First Breast Cancer Recurrence	
FREQUENCY (%)	SITE(S)
15-40	Local or regional
	Chest wall
	Axillary nodes
	Supraclavicular nodes
30-60	Bones
10-15	Bone in combination with other sites
5-15	Lung or thorax
3-10	Liver
<5	Central nervous system

Adapted from Hayes, D. F., & Kaplan, W. (1996). Evaluation of patients after primary therapy. In Harris, J. R., Lippman, M. E., Morrow, M., et al. (Eds.). *Diseases of the breast* (pp. 634-635). Philadelphia: Lippincott-Raven.

a. 1 & 2
b. 1, 2, & 3
c. 2, 3, & 4
d. All of these

2. On review of systems, Mary describes a non-productive cough and some aching in her left upper leg. In addition to a biopsy, what diagnostic tests should be conducted to complete Mary's workup?
1. Liver function tests
2. Computed tomography (CT) scan of the head
3. Chest x-ray study
4. Bone scan
 a. 1 & 2
 b. 2 & 4
 c. 1, 3, & 4
 d. All of these

ANSWERS

1. Because Mary has signs of a breast cancer recurrence, it is important to conduct a more global physical assessment to determine whether there are other sites of recurrence. Breast cancer can metastasize to almost every organ in the body. At first recurrence, between 50% and 75% of patients relapse at a single site, and the remainder have multiple sites of recurrence (Hayes & Kaplan, 1996). Table 1-4 outlines the most common sites of first recurrence. Your assessment should include the regional lymph nodes and a thorough pain assessment to determine whether the patient has clinical signs of bone metastases. Bone metastases typically present with pain that is described as dull, gradually progressive, and constant. This pain may occur at night, may not be relieved by rest, and may be referred to adjacent joints. The next most

common site of metastasis is the lungs; liver and brain metastases are less common. All of these organ systems should be assessed. *Answer 1:* **d.**

2. A number of diagnostic tests may be performed to rule out metastatic disease. A bone scan should be performed on patients with bone pain. If bone scan results are not definitive, magnetic resonance imaging (MRI) may be more accurate in detecting bone metastases. In addition to hepatic enzyme elevations, a CT scan of the abdomen detects approximately 90% of all liver metastases (Hayes & Kaplan, 1996). A chest radiograph is the choice for screening to rule out pulmonary metastases. Abnormal or suspicious results are followed up with a CT scan of the thorax. Screening for brain metastases is not routinely done because of the low incidence of nervous system metastases. In high-risk patients or patients with symptoms, a CT scan may be ordered. *Answer 2:* **c.**

Case Study continued

A biopsy of the nodule on her mastectomy scar reveals adenocarcinoma. No palpable axillary, supraclavicular, or cervical lymph nodes are present. A chest radiograph shows a new solitary 2-cm lung nodule in the right lower lobe. On a follow-up CT of the thorax, this is confirmed to be consistent with cancer. Mary's bone scan reveals an area of increased uptake in her left femur, consistent with the injury caused by the automobile accident, but otherwise there is normal uptake. The CT scan of the abdomen is negative, and liver function tests are within normal limits.

QUESTIONS

3. Based on this information, what conclusions can be drawn?
1. Mary has a local breast cancer recurrence.
2. Mary has lung metastasis.
3. A biopsy needs to be performed on the lung nodule to characterize the pathology.
4. Mary has bone metastasis.
 a. 1 & 2
 b. 1 & 3
 c. 1, 2, & 4
 d. 3 & 4

ANSWERS

3. Based on the biopsy of the nodule at the mastectomy scar, Mary has a local recurrence of her breast cancer. A single pulmonary nodule visible on a chest radiograph may represent either cancer or benign granulomas (Mentzer & Sugarbaker, 1996). CT is more sensitive but cannot distinguish between primary and metastatic disease. Based on Mary's breast cancer and smoking history, the lung nodule may represent either metastatic breast cancer or a primary lung cancer, so a biopsy is required. The abnormal uptake on Mary's bone scan is consistent with the fracture caused by her previous automobile accident, so there is no evidence of bone metastasis. *Answer 3:* **b.**

Case Study *continued*

A lung biopsy reveals adenocarcinoma consistent with a primary breast cancer. A review of Mary's original tumor block from her mastectomy specimen shows that the Her2-neu assay is positive.

QUESTIONS ─────────────────

4. What can be concluded from this information?
   a. Mary may benefit from immunotherapy with trastuzumab (Herceptin).
   b. Mary has a less aggressive type of breast cancer.
   c. Patients who are Her2-neu negative are likely to benefit from Herceptin.
   d. Because of Mary's history of lung disease, she is not a candidate for Herceptin.

───────────────── **ANSWERS**

4. Approximately 25% of all breast cancer patients overexpress the Her2-neu protein, signifying a more aggressive type of breast cancer (Press, Bernstein, Thomas, et al., 1997). Her2-neu overexpression is detected in tumor tissue by immunohistochemical assay. In 1999 the drug Herceptin (trastuzumab) was approved for the treatment of metastatic breast cancer in patients whose tumors overexpress Her2-neu. Herceptin is given as a single agent to patients who have received one or more chemotherapy regimens for metastatic disease, and Herceptin is given with Taxol to women who have not received chemotherapy for metastatic breast cancer. Because Herceptin can cause cardiac dysfunction, patients with history of heart disease are not candidates for this treatment. Mary has no cardiac history, and her tumor is positive for Her2-neu overexpression; therefore she meets the criteria to receive Herceptin. *Answer 4:* **a.**

QUESTIONS ─────────────────

5. The medical oncologist recommends that Mary receive Taxol and Herceptin. To prepare Mary for this chemotherapy regimen, what issues must be addressed?
   1. The need for a vascular access device must be assessed because Mary will require Herceptin weekly.

2. Mary must be taught about side effects of Herceptin, such as first infusion reactions.
3. Mary must be taught about the need for periodic radionuclide angiography to evaluate ejection fractions and wall motion.
4. Social work should be consulted to assist with insurance and payment issues.
   a. 1 & 2
   b. 1, 2, & 3
   c. 3 & 4
   d. All of these

6. While Mary is receiving therapy, what should you be assessing regularly?
   1. Vibratory sensation and deep tendon reflexes
   2. Cranial nerves
   3. Heart sounds and presence of peripheral edema
   4. Lung sounds
      a. 1, 2, & 3
      b. 1, 3, & 4
      c. 2 & 4
      d. All of these

───────────────── **ANSWERS**

5. Because Herceptin is given weekly until complete response or disease progression, a vascular access device may be desirable. Although Herceptin has few side effects, unique first infusion reactions may occur, which are characterized by fever and chills. Mary also needs to know that the first Herceptin infusion is a loading dose of 4 mg/kg given over 90 minutes, and if that infusion is well tolerated, all subsequent doses will be given at 2 mg/kg over 30 minutes. Teaching should also include the side effects of Taxol (hypersensitivity reactions, arthralgias/myalgias, peripheral neuropathy, and alopecia) and the need for frequent radionuclide angiography to evaluate cardiac status. Finally, because Mary was recently laid off from her job at the hospital, there may be insurance or payment problems, so a referral to social services is indicated. *Answer 5:* **d.**

6. To assess for peripheral neuropathy associated with Taxol, you should assess vibratory sense with a tuning fork and evaluate deep tendon reflexes. Any report of symptoms such as changes in gait, problems with fine motor function, and sensory changes such as numbness and tingling should be noted. Abnormalities in cranial nerve function are not usually associated with peripheral neuropathy. Because of the risk of heart failure associated with Taxol and Herceptin, it is important that you check heart sounds and assess for symptoms of heart failure, such as dyspnea, orthopnea, fatigue, edema, weight gain, chest pain, nocturia, and impaired mental function, and physical signs such as sinus tachycardia, ventricular or S_3 gallop, neck vein distension, hepatojugular reflux, and peripheral pitting edema. Because Mary has a lung nodule, lung sounds, respirations, and presence of cough and shortness of breath should be assessed at each visit. *Answer 6:* **b.**

Case Study *continued*

After a port placement, Mary begins her chemotherapy. When she returns to the outpatient chemotherapy unit for her eighth cycle of Taxol, she states that she has been having problems buttoning her clothes and that she feels "burning and prickling" in her fingers and toes. During the neurologic examination, you note that Mary has lost vibratory sense in her great toe and forefinger but is able to sense vibration in her wrists and ankles. Her Achilles deep tendon reflexes were 3+ before chemotherapy and are now reduced to 1+. She has difficulty picking up a coin from a smooth surface and difficulty writing her name. Her gait is slightly unsteady. Mary states that the burning and prickling in fingers and toes is intermittent, but she rates this discomfort as a "6" on a 0 to 10 scale.

QUESTIONS

7. Which of the following interventions should you consider?

1. Discussing the safety measures to reduce falls and injuries
2. Delaying Taxol until neurologic symptoms improve
3. Treating neuropathic pain with a tricyclic antidepressant
4. Preventing further neurotoxicity with amifostine (Ethyol)

   a. 1 & 2
   b. 1, 2, & 3
   c. 3 & 4
   d. All of these

ANSWERS

7. Mary is at risk for falls and injuries as a result of her peripheral neuropathy. You need to teach Mary about the safety measures outlined in Box 1-6. When patients have severe neuropathy that interferes with activities of daily living, it is best to delay treatment until symptoms improve or to discontinue Taxol entirely. Neuropathic pain may respond to a tricyclic antidepressant. Although

---

BOX **1-6**	**Safety Measures for Patients with Peripheral Neuropathy**

Ensure that rooms are well lit to prevent falls.
Use handrails on stairways.
Eliminate clutter that may cause falls.
Use a nonbreakable water thermometer to check the temperature of bath water and dishwater to be sure that it is no hotter than 101° F (43.3° C).
Use potholders when cooking.
Wear gloves when washing dishes or gardening.
Avoid the use of motorized yard and garage equipment.

Adapted from Almadrones, L. A., & Arcot, R. (1999). Patient guide to peripheral neuropathy. *Oncol Nurs Forum, 26,* pp. 1359-1362.

---

amifostine reduces renal toxicity associated with cisplatin, studies have not shown the drug to protect against neurotoxicity associated with Taxol. *Answer 7:* **b.**

QUESTIONS

8. On her next follow-up visit, Mary complains of a dull, aching pain in her back. She says, "It's probably nothing, I think I did too much around the house last week." What additional history do you need to obtain?

ANSWERS

8. Because back pain is the first sign of epidural spinal cord compression, it is essential that the APN conduct a thorough assessment of the pain and associated neurologic symptoms (Table 1-5). *Answer 8:* **See text.**

Case Study *continued*

Upon further questioning, you learn that Mary's pain is localized in the region of her thoracic spine, is intermittent, and is more severe when lying in the supine position. She has some weakness of her extremities. She denies bowel or bladder problems but has some residual neuropathy from her Taxol treatments.

QUESTIONS

9. What conclusions can you make based on this information?

   a. These symptoms are most likely caused by overexertion and residual effects of the Taxol.
   b. Mary has a spinal cord compression.
   c. Plain radiographs of the spine and/or an MRI are indicated.

| TABLE **1-5** | Assessing Back Pain in Women with Breast Cancer |

PAIN

Pinpoint the location of the pain: localized or radicular?

Determine when the pain started and the quality of pain (intermittent versus continuous)

Evaluate the intensity of the pain (on a 0-10 scale)

Question the patient about precipitating factors:
Lying supine
Coughing, sneezing, or straining at stool
Stretching

MYELOPATHY

Evaluate for the presence of the following:
Motor weakness
Sensory changes (numbness and tingling)
Hyperreflexia
Urinary retention, urgency, or incontinence
Bowel incontinence or constipation
Gait disturbances

Adapted from Freilich, R. J., & Foley, K. M. (1996). Epidural metastasis. In Harris, J. R., Lippman, M. E., Morrow, M., et al. (Eds.). *Diseases of the breast* (pp. 779-789). Philadelphia: Lippincott-Raven; and Belford, K. (2000). Central nervous system cancers. In Yarbro, C. H., Frogge, M. H., Goodman, M., Groenwald, S. L. (Eds.). *Cancer nursing principles and practice*, 5th ed (pp. 1088-1089). Boston: Jones and Bartlett.

d. Mary will need radiation therapy to her spine.

ANSWERS

9. The thoracic spine is the most common location for epidural spinal cord compressions in women with breast cancer (Freilich & Foley, 1996). Pain may be localized, radicular (shooting), or referred. Pain associated with epidural metastasis is made worse by lying in the supine position, by performing the Valsalva maneuver (coughing, sneezing, or straining at stool), or by stretching. Neurologic symptoms such as weakness, numbness, and bowel and bladder control problems (see Table 1-5) are later signs. Mary's history is complicated by residual neurologic symptoms from Taxol; however, her symptoms must be evaluated. Spine radiographs or an MRI is required to determine whether Mary has epidural metastasis that may be causing her spinal cord compression. If spinal cord compression is suspected, Mary may receive steroids; however, it would be premature to say whether Mary would benefit from radiation therapy until a diagnosis is confirmed. *Answer 9:* **c.**

Case Study continued

Mary is diagnosed with thoracic spine metastasis and treated with radiation therapy to relieve her spinal cord compression. Over the next few months, Mary is diagnosed with new lung and liver metastases. Her condition deteriorates, and she is referred to hospice. She expresses a desire to stay in her own home for as long as possible, and her children agree to take turns caring for her.

QUESTIONS

10. Based on Mary's condition, what are the goals for the hospice care providers?
  1. To help Mary come to peace with her terminal condition
  2. To provide pain relief
  3. To support Mary and her family as her condition deteriorates
  4. To ensure that Mary has adequate nutrition and hydration
    a. 1 & 2
    b. 2 & 3
    c. 2, 3, & 4
    d. 3 & 4

ANSWERS

10. According to Martinez and Wagner (1997), the interdisciplinary hospice team has a number of goals, including patient and family understanding of home death protocol, comfort, prevention of injuries, adaptation to partial independence, support for family members, and enhanced spiritual support. Maintaining nutrition and hydration are not always feasible and not necessary for comfort. Although it would be ideal if Mary were to come to be at peace with her terminal condition, that is not a realistic goal for all hospice patients. *Answer 10:* **b.**

REFERENCES

Aikin, J. (2000). Adjuvant therapy for breast cancer: Choices and challenges. *Innovat Breast Cancer Care,* 5(1), pp. 3-8.

Almadrones, L. A., & Arcot R. (1999). Patient guide to peripheral neuropathy. *Oncol Nurs Forum,* 26, pp. 1359-1362.

American Joint Committee on Cancer (AJCC). (1997). *AJCC cancer staging manual,* 5th ed. Philadelphia: Lippincott-Raven.

American Society of Clinical Oncology. (1994). American Society of Clinical Oncology recommendations for the use of hematopoietic colony-stimulating factors: Evidence-based, clinical practice guidelines. *J Clin Oncol,* 12, pp. 2471-2508.

Belford, K. (2000). Central nervous system cancers. In Yarbro, C. H., Frogge, M. H., Goodman, M., Groenwald, S. L. (Eds.). *Cancer nursing principles and practice*, 5th ed (pp. 1088-1089). Boston: Jones and Bartlett.

Chapman, D. D., & Goodman, M. (2000). Breast cancer. In Yarbro, C. H., Frogge, M. H., Goodman, M., & Groenwald, S. L. (Eds.). *Cancer nursing principles and practice*, 5th ed. (pp. 994-1047). Boston: Jones and Bartlett.

Fisher, B., Costantino, J. P., Wickerham, D. L., et al. (1998). Tamoxifen for prevention of breast cancer: Report of the National Surgical Adjuvant Breast and Bowel Project P-1 Study. *J Natl Cancer Inst, 90*, pp. 1371-1388.

Fisher, B., Dignam, J., Wolmark, N., et al. (1997). Tamoxifen and chemotherapy for lymph node-negative, estrogen receptor-positive breast cancer. *J Natl Cancer Inst, 89*, pp. 1673-1682.

Foster, R. S. (1996). Biopsy techniques. In Harris, J. R., Lippman, M. E., Morrow, M., et al. (Eds.). *Diseases of the breast* (pp. 133-138). Philadelphia: Lippincott-Raven.

Freilich, R. J., & Foley, K. M. (1996). Epidural metastases. In Harris, J. R., Lippman, M. E., Morrow, M., et al. (Eds.). *Diseases of the breast* (pp. 779-789). Philadelphia: Lippincott-Raven.

Harris, J. R., & Morrow, M. (1996). Treatment of early-stage breast cancer. In Harris, J. R., Lippman, M. E., Morrow, M., et al. (Eds.). *Diseases of the breast* (pp. 487-547). Philadelphia: Lippincott-Raven.

Hartmann, L. C., Schaid, D. J., Woods, J. E., et al. (1999). Efficacy of bilateral prophylactic mastectomy in women with a family history of breast cancer. *N Engl J Med, 340*, pp. 77-84.

Hayes, D. F., & Kaplan, W. (1996). Evaluation of patients after primary therapy. In Harris, J. R., Lippman, M. E., Morrow, M., et al. (Eds.). *Diseases of the breast* (pp. 629-647). Philadelphia: Lippincott-Raven.

Henderson, I. C., Berry, D., Demetri, C., et al., for CALGB, ECOG, SWOG, and NCCTG. (1998). Improved disease-free (DFS) and overall survival (OS) from the addition of sequential paclitaxel (T) but not from the escalation of doxorubicin (A) in the adjuvant chemotherapy of patients (pts) with node-positive primary breast cancer. *Proc Am Soc Clin Oncol, 17*, p. 10a. Abstract 390A.

Lin, E. M., Aikin, J. L., & Good, B. C. (1999). Premature menopause after cancer treatment. *Cancer Pract, 7*, pp. 114-121.

Martinez, J., & Wagner, S. (1997). Hospice care. In Groenwald, S., Frogge, M. H., Goodman, M., Yarbro, C. H. (Eds.). *Cancer nursing principles and practice* (pp. 1531-1549). Boston: Jones and Bartlett.

Mentzer, S. S., & Sugarbaker, D. J. (1996). Management of discrete pulmonary nodules. In Harris, J. R., Lippman, M. E., Morrow, M., et al. (Eds.). *Diseases of the breast* (pp. 853-858). Philadelphia: Lippincott-Raven.

National Lymphedema Network (NLN). (1999). *18 steps to prevention for upper extremities*. Oakland, CA: NLN.

Press, M. F., Bernstein, L., Thomas, P. A., et al. (1997). HER-2/neu gene amplification characterized by fluorescence in situ hybridization: Poor prognosis in node-negative carcinomas. *J Clin Oncol, 15*, pp. 2894-2904.

Rosen, P. P. (1996). Invasive mammary carcinoma. I In Harris, J. R., Lippman, M. E., Morrow, M., et al. (Eds.). *Diseases of the breast* (p. 393). Philadelphia: Lippincott-Raven.

Smith, R. A., Mettlin, C. J., Davis, K. J., et al. (2000). American Cancer Society guidelines for the early detection of cancer. *CA Cancer J Clin, 50*, pp. 34-49.

Tranin, A. S. (1996). Genetics and breast cancer risk. In Dow, K. H. (Ed.). *Contemporary issues in breast cancer* (pp. 3-18). Boston: Jones and Bartlett.

Weber, B. L., & Garber, J. E. (1996). Familial breast cancer. In Harris, J. R., Lippman, M. E., Morrow, M., et al. (Eds.). *Diseases of the breast* (p. 172). Philadelphia: Lippincott-Raven.

2   Lung Cancer

Janet Van Cleave
Mary E. Cooley

CASE | STUDY

Nancy, an advanced practice oncology nurse, is working as a consultant for the state Department of Public Health. The Department of Public Health would like to initiate a cancer control effort within the state. Lung cancer has been identified as one of the priority cancer sites, and the focus of the plan will be directed toward primary and secondary prevention.

QUESTIONS

1. What are the most effective primary prevention strategies for lung cancer?
   1. Tobacco smoking prevention
   2. Tobacco smoking cessation
   3. Dietary modification
   4. Chemoprevention
      a. 1 only
      b. 1 & 3
      c. 2 & 3
      d. 4 only

2. What screening examinations are recommended for the early detection of lung cancer?
   1. Sputum cytology every 6 months
   2. Chest radiograph every 6 months
   3. Chest computed tomography (CT) scan
   4. Annual physical examination
      a. 1 & 2
      b. 1, 3, & 4
      c. 4 only
      d. None of these

ANSWERS

1. Tobacco smoking is responsible for approximately 85% of lung cancer. Primary prevention, which is the prevention of smoking, is the most effective means of decreasing the incidence of lung cancer. Smoking cessation efforts, also known as *secondary prevention,* are also important and can decrease the rate of developing lung cancer. The risk of developing lung cancer is 10 to 25 times greater in heavy smokers than in those who do not smoke (Ingle, 2000). Benefits associated with smoking cessation have been noted such that the risk of developing cancer begins to decrease 5 years after quitting and continues to decrease over time. Although epidemiologic evidence suggests an inverse relationship between lung cancer and consumption of vitamins A, C, and E and selenium, further study is needed. Chemoprevention, a secondary prevention intervention, is the use of agents that may prevent or reverse the process of carcinogenesis. Clinical trials using oral beta-carotene as a chemoprevention agent did not demonstrate benefit in those at high risk of developing lung cancer (Omenn, Goodman, Thornquist, et al., 1996). Additional chemoprevention trials are under way. *Answer 1:* **a.**

2. There is no proven role for lung cancer screening in the high-risk population. Early clinical trials that investigated screening procedures of chest radiograph and sputum cytology to detect early lung cancer did not find a survival advantage for those undergoing screening (Fontana, Sanderson, Woolner, et al., 1986). Screening for lung cancer, however, is undergoing reexamination. A recent clinical trial, The Early Lung Cancer Action Project, was designed to evaluate the use of low-radiation-dose CT scans as a potential screening method for detecting early-stage lung cancer in those at high risk for the disease. Adults 60 years of age and older with at least a 10-pack/year history of cigarette use and no previous cancer were selected as participants in this study. Preliminary results from the study suggest that yearly screening with low-dose radiation CT scans increased the diagnosis of lung cancer at earlier and potentially more curable stages (Henschke, McCauley, Yankelevitz, et al., 1999). Further study is needed, and screening is not currently recommended. *Answer 2:* **d.**

Case Study continued

Nancy is working with a multidisciplinary team to develop a plan and identify priorities for lung cancer within the state. Smoking prevention, cessation, and tobacco control were identified as priorities. Given the rising prevalence of youth smoking within the state, the team discusses the need to implement educational programs directed toward smoking prevention.

QUESTIONS

3. Which of the following groups would be best to target for a smoking prevention program?
   a. Grade school students
   b. Seniors in high school
   c. College students
   d. Pregnant women

4. Which of the following interventions are most effective to decrease youth smoking?
   1. Increasing the cost of cigarettes
   2. Enforcing age restrictions on access to tobacco
   3. Initiating hospital-based programs
   4. Restricting use of tobacco by adolescents in public places
      a. 1 & 2
      b. 1 & 4
      c. 1, 2, & 3
      d. All of these

ANSWERS

3. It is important to begin smoking prevention education *early* because the incidence of tobacco use among school-age children is becoming widespread. It is best to target children *before* they start smoking. The addictive potential of nicotine is the same in children and adolescents as it is in adults. Programs may start as early as kindergarten and continue through grade 12. Most adults start smoking before age 18. Moreover, the younger one starts to smoke, the more likely he or she is to continue smoking as an adult. Recent data suggest that the rates for smoking tobacco have increased progressively among eighth, tenth, and twelfth graders (18%, 26%, 35%, respectively) (U.S. Department of Health and Human Services, 2000). Although interventions directed toward pregnant women are needed, the focus of interventions would be smoking cessation rather than smoking prevention. Smoking during pregnancy increases the risk of having a low-birth-weight baby. Because it is best to initiate interventions before children and adolescents start smoking, it would be best to target grade school students for smoking prevention education (Cataldo, Cooley, & Giarelli, 2000). *Answer 3:* **a.**

4. Increasing the cost of cigarettes and enforcing age restrictions are the most effective strategies to

decrease rates of smoking among youth (Ingle, 2000). Although physician office–, clinic-, and hospital-based interventions have been advocated as opportunities for smoking prevention counseling among youth, many youths may not be reached through these systems. Similarly, although restriction on the use of tobacco by adolescents in public places has been advocated as a method to decrease use, studies have not demonstrated the efficacy of this approach (Cataldo, Cooley, & Giarelli, 2000). *Answer 4:* **a.**

Case Study continued

The group discusses the need to target special populations who have been disproportionately affected by tobacco use as another priority.

QUESTIONS

5. List special populations that have been disproportionately affected by tobacco use.

ANSWER

5. A comprehensive tobacco control program should be designed to meet the needs of high-risk groups and those who have been disproportionately affected by tobacco. These groups include any of the following: women, racial and ethnic minorities, persons of low socioeconomic status, and children and adolescents. These groups are targeted because their smoking prevalence rates have remained relatively steady or have declined less slowly as compared with white males, whose rates are on the decline (Wingo, Giovino, Miller, et al., 1999). *Answer 5:* **See text.**

QUESTIONS

6. Prevalence of smoking varies among various ethnic minority groups. Which of the following groups has the highest prevalence of smoking?
   a. African American
   b. American Indian/Alaska Native
   c. Hispanic
   d. Asian/Pacific Islander

7. Although fewer African Americans smoke than Caucasians, they have a more difficult time quitting. Which of the following factors may help explain why this disparity exists?
   1. Higher nicotine content in brands preferred by African Americans than brands preferred by whites
   2. Greater concern about weight gain associated with smoking cessation
   3. Greater addiction to tobacco

4. Cultural practices that incorporate tobacco into ceremonies
   a. 1 & 2
   b. 1, 2, & 3
   c. 1 & 3
   d. All of these

ANSWERS

6. A wide range of diversity exists within each cultural group regarding smoking behaviors. Between 1978 and 1995 the prevalence of smoking declined among African American, white, Asian American/Pacific Islander, and Hispanic adults but remained stable for American Indians/Alaska Natives (AI/AN) (Wingo, et al., 1999). Overall, AI/AN have the highest smoking prevalence among the various ethnic and minority groups. In contrast to other ethnic groups, smoking prevalence is highest for both adults and adolescents and there are not significant gender differences (Cataldo, Cooley, & Giarelli, 2000). Tobacco use differs in AI/AN according to geographic area and among various tribes. Unique challenges to change tobacco use exist among American Indians because cultural practices incorporate tobacco into ceremonies and rituals. *Answer 6:* **b.**

7. African American smokers may have more difficulty with smoking cessation and relapse as compared with white smokers because of differences in patterns of tobacco use. In particular, African American smokers choose to smoke brands that are high in nicotine and mentholated. In addition, African Americans who are light to moderate smokers are more likely to smoke shortly after awakening, which is a sign of increased physiologic addiction. This addiction can make it difficult for even light smokers to quit and stay quit. Women are more likely to be concerned about weight gain after smoking cessation (Cataldo, Cooley & Giarelli, 2000; Cooley & Jennings-Dozier, 1998). *Answer 7:* **c.**

Case Study continued

During the planning meetings Nancy voiced the concern that morbidity associated with lung cancer treatment is also an important issue. Various members of the team discounted this issue and stated that this is not a focus for the plan.

QUESTIONS

8. Because Nancy is working as a consultant, she should be aware of which of the following key characteristics of consultation?

1. Because Nancy is the expert, the relationship between the consultant and consultee is hierarchical.
2. The problem is always identified by the consultee.
3. The consultee is free to accept or reject the ideas and recommendations of the consultant.
4. The outcome of the plan is Nancy's responsibility.
   a. 1, 2, & 3
   b. 2 & 3
   c. 2, 3, & 4
   d. 3 & 4

9. What characteristics and skills are necessary for advanced practice nurses (APNs) who are involved in consultation process?

ANSWERS

8. Caplan and Caplan (1993) define *consultation* as the interaction between two professionals. They identify four key characteristics associated with this process: (1) The problem is always identified by the consultee, (2) the relationship between the consultant and consultee is nonhierarchical, (3) professional responsibility for the outcome lies with the consultee, and (4) the consultee is free to accept or reject the recommendations of the consultant. *Answer 8:* **b.**

9. APNs have a long tradition of providing consultation services. Certain characteristics and skills are necessary to implement effective consultation. First and foremost, the APN should possess the clinical expertise needed to solve the problem identified by the consultee. Other important characteristics are self-awareness, excellent interpersonal skills, and a desire to develop the practice of others. It is essential for a good consultant to be aware of his or her personal issues and motives because he or she must be able to suspend judgments and avoid stereotyping (Barron & White, 1996). Consultees often seek consultation when a fresh perspective is needed to solve a problem. Moreover, it is not uncommon that the consultant is called to intercede in highly charged emotional situations, underscoring the need to be able to remain objective and clear about the situation. Additional skills needed for effective consultations are the ability to develop warm, respectful, and accepting relationships and communicate issues clearly and concisely. *Answer 9:* **See text.**

CASE 2 STUDY

Paul Jones is a 51-year-old African American who is recovering from a motor vehicle accident. He has no sustained injuries. A routine chest radiograph in the emergency room has revealed a left apical 2-cm lung mass. Mr. Jones then underwent a CT scan of the chest that again showed the 2-cm apical lesion. A CT-guided needle biopsy was performed and revealed non–small cell lung cancer suggesting adenocarcinoma. You are called to see Mr. Jones regarding his new diagnosis as part of the thoracic oncology team.

QUESTIONS

1. You begin taking Mr. Jones's history. Which of the following are key components to focus on?
   1. Potential risk factors
   2. Infections
   3. Weight loss
   4. Use of laxatives
      a. 1 only
      b. 1 & 3
      c. 1, 3, & 4
      d. 1, 2, & 3

ANSWERS

1. The history and physical examination are important components in the evaluation of a patient and should include potential risk factors such as personal and family smoking history and past exposure to environmental carcinogens (in-

cluding occupational history, radon exposure, and family history of lung cancer). Common risk factors for lung cancer are listed in Table 2-1. The patient should also be asked about new symptoms, including a change in cough, hemoptysis, or history of recurrent respiratory infection suggestive of postobstructive pneumonia. In addition, involuntary weight loss often indicates the presence of systemic disease and is an important prognostic indicator in lung cancer. Patients with chest pain may have tumors involving the parietal pleura or other extension beyond the lung. History of laxative use would be more appropriate for patients who have signs and symptoms indicating colorectal problems. The most common presenting clinical features of lung cancer are presented in Table 2-2 (Hoffman, Mauer, & Vokes, 2000). *Answer 1:* **d.**

Case Study continued

From your interview you find that Mr. Jones has chronic obstructive pulmonary disease. He is a temporary worker who has held multiple jobs, including working in a shipyard with known asbestos exposure. He has no regular primary care provider. He has never been married but has a sister who lives close by. His parents are deceased; his mother passed away at age 55 from lung cancer, and his father died at age 65 from a myocardial infarction. He has a 50-pack/year history and drinks three to six beers per day.

TABLE 2-1	Risk Factors Associated with Lung Cancer
RISK FACTOR	**INCIDENCE AND EFFECT**
Smoking tobacco	~90% incidence. Dose-response relationship noted such that an increased amount and longer duration of smoking increases the risk of lung cancer. In particular, those who have a history of a 10 pack/year* of smoking are at greater risk for developing lung cancer.
Occupation	~3%-4% incidence. Exposure to radon, bis(chloromethyl)ether, polycyclic aromatic hydrocarbons, chromium, nickel, inorganic arsenic compounds, asbestos.
Dietary factors	An inverse relationship exists between the intake of foods high in vitamin A (specifically the retinoids/carotenoids), raw fruits and vegetables, and vitamin E supplements and the incidence of lung cancer.
Family history	Incidence greater in smokers with a family history than in smokers without a family history. Inconclusive evidence.

Adapted from Ihde, D. C. (1992). Chemotherapy of lung cancer. *N Engl J Med, 327*, pp. 1434-1441; Mayne, S. T., Janerich, D. T., Greenwald, P., et al. (1994). Dietary beta carotene and lung cancer risk in U.S. nonsmokers. *J Natl Cancer Inst, 86*, pp. 33-38; and Mayne, S. T., Redlich, C. A., & Cullen, M. R. (1998). Dietary vitamin A and prevalence of bronchial metaplasia in asbestos-exposed workers. *Am J Clin Nutr, 68*, pp. 630-635.
*Pack/year = pack per day × number of years.

Medications
Albuterol 2 puffs every 6 hours as needed
Ipratropium 2 puffs four times daily
Thiamin 100 mg daily
Folate 1 mg daily
Oxazepam 15 mg every 6 hours

Mr. Jones has no known drug allergies. He smokes 1 pack of cigarettes per day. He has tried to quit several times but has been unsuccessful.

Also during the interview, you ask Mr. Jones about symptoms that may indicate metastatic disease. Mr. Jones tells you that he has not lost weight; that does not have any pain, headaches, or visual problems; but that he notices slight shortness of breath when he walks 5 blocks. He also has a chronic nonproductive cough. He denies fevers, chills, or night sweats. A review of medical systems reveals no known heart disease, kidney disease, or liver disease.

Mr. Jones's physical examination is recorded as follows:

Mr. Jones is a healthy looking male in no acute distress.

HEENT
Ecchymosis above right eye, PEARL (pupils equal and reactive), EOMI, (extraocular muscle intact) no cervical or supraclavicular lymph nodes palpated.

THORAX
Lungs with slight midinspiratory crackles, hyperresonant on percussion, decreased pulmonary excursion bilaterally.

HEART
S_1, S_2, no murmurs/rubs/clicks.

ABDOMINAL
(+) bowel sounds, nontender/nondistended, no masses, no hepatosplenomegaly.

EXTREMITIES
No cyanosis/clubbing/edema.

NEUROLOGIC
CN II-XII intact.

DATA:
Chest radiograph: 2-cm left apical lung mass
CT scan: 2-cm spiculated peripheral left upper lobe (LUL) mass not involving the bronchus. No abnormalities seen in the liver, spleen, adrenal glands, or kidneys. No mediastinal, pretracheal, or carinal adenopathy noted.

TABLE 2-2	Presenting Clinical Features in Adults with Lung Cancer
EXTENT OF LUNG CANCER	**PRESENTING CLINICAL FEATURES**
Primary tumor	• Cough • Dyspnea • Hemoptysis • Postobstructive pneumonia • Chest pain from parietal pleural involvement • Shoulder, arm, brachial plexopathy or Horner's syndrome* from superior sulcus tumors
Mediastinal spread of tumor	• Hoarseness from left recurrent laryngeal nerve injury by tumor or nodes • Obstruction of superior vena cava • Elevation of hemidiaphragm from phrenic-nerve paralysis • Dysphagia from esophageal obstruction • Pericardial tamponade
Metastatic spread of tumor	• Mental status changes, headaches, double vision from brain metastases • Bone pain • Weight loss
Associated paraneoplastic syndromes	• Hypertrophic pulmonary osteoarthropathy • Hypercalcemia • Syndrome of inappropriate antidiuretic hormone secretion • Cushing's syndrome *hypersecretion adrenal cortex* • Encephalomyelitis • Subacute sensory neuropathy • Opsoclonus and myoclonus • Cerebellar degeneration • Limbic encephalitis • Eaton-Lambert myasthenic syndrome *muscular weakness*

Adapted from Hoffman, P. C., Mayer, A. M., & Vokes, E. E. (2000). Lung cancer. *Lancet, 355*, pp. 479-485.
*Horner's syndrome is characterized by dry forehead, small pupil, and ptosis of eyelid on affected side.

paralysis of sympathetic nerves
caused by tumors in neck, TB, neuritis cervical plexus, etc

Mr. Jones underwent a percutaneous CT-guided fine-needle aspiration, and it was determined that he had lung pathology favoring adenocarcinoma.

QUESTIONS

2. What are the other histopathologic classifications in non–small cell lung cancer?
   a. Squamous cell, large cell
   b. Neuroendocrine, small cell
   c. Sarcoma, schwannoma
   d. Squamous cell, schwannoma

3. What other tests can be done to obtain tissue for diagnosis?

4. What additional diagnostic examinations are commonly used to determine the location and spread of lung cancer?
   1. Liver function tests
   2. Bone scan
   3. Brain CT
   4. Bronchoscopy
      a. 4 only
      b. 1, 2, & 3
      c. 2, 3, & 4
      d. All of these

5. Mr. Jones states that he is continuing to smoke and that because he has lung cancer, he sees no reason to quit. Which of the following would be the best response to Mr. Jones?
   1. Provide information about the health benefits associated with smoking cessation
   2. Suggest that he pick a quit date
   3. Advise him to quit
   4. Suggest that he switch to low-tar, low-nicotine cigarettes and wean himself
      a. 1 only
      b. 1, 2, & 3
      c. 4 only
      d. 1 & 3

ANSWERS

2. The three histopathologic classifications in non–small cell lung cancer are squamous cell, adenocarcinoma, and large cell. Adenocarcinoma is increasing in occurrence and now is the most common type of tumor, accounting for 40% of all cases of lung cancer. Most adenocarcinoma tumors originate in the periphery of the lung. These tumors form glands and produce mucin, which can be seen on tissue slides. Generally, adenocarcinoma has a worse prognosis stage for stage than squamous cell carcinoma (Ginsberg, Vokes, & Raben, 1997). Bronchoalveolar is a pathologic

subtype of adenocarcinoma. It may be unifocal or multifocal, which can mimic pneumonia (Hoffman, Mauer, & Vokes, 2000). Squamous cell carcinoma previously was the most prevalent lung cancer, but it now accounts for approximately 30% of all lung cancer. The tumor is commonly located in the proximal segmental bronchi. It is generally a slow-growing tumor in which metaplasia may occur for 3 to 4 years before a clinically apparent tumor develops. Large cell carcinoma is the least common type of all non–small cell lung cancer (NSCLC) tumors, accounting for approximately 10% of all lung cancers. They usually develop in the peripheral lung and metastasize early, commonly to the gastrointestinal tract (Ingle, 2000). The prognosis is similar to adenocarcinoma (Ginsberg, Vokes, & Raben, 1997). *Answer 2:* **a.**

3. An accurate tissue diagnosis is essential in treating lung cancer to determine whether it is a non–small cell lung cancer or a small cell lung cancer (Hoffman, Mauer, & Vokes, 2000). Overall, pattern of growth, staging systems, and treatment options differ greatly between these two types of lung cancer. Fine-needle aspiration biopsy of pulmonary nodules can be performed either with ultrasound or CT guidance. Sputum cytology is a simple method for diagnosis; however, the yield is variable depending on the patient's ability to produce an adequate sample, the size of the tumor, the proximity of the tumor to major airways, and to a lesser degree, the histology of the tumor. Bronchoscopy can examine the proximal tracheobronchial tree up the second or third subsegmental division. During this procedure cytologic or histologic specimens can be obtained from abnormal lesions. In the event of no visible lesion, an irrigation and lavage of the bronchus draining the suspicious area is performed to obtain a cytology tissue sample. Peripheral lesions can be reached by cytology brushes, needles, or biopsy forceps. Video-assisted thoracoscopy can be used to obtain tissue for diagnosis as well as for staging. Thoracotomy is used in a small percentage of patients whose tumor is positioned in an area too difficult to be reached by other methods (Ginsberg, Vokes, & Raben, 1997). *Answer 3:* **Bronchoscopy, video-assisted thoracoscopy, sputum cytology and ultrasound-guided fine-needle aspiration, thoracotomy.**

4. In NSCLC, surgical resection of the tumor offers the highest likelihood for cure. Therefore further examinations are needed to identify patients with localized disease who can be resected. Often, the history and physical examination with liver function tests and serum lactate dehydrogenase concentration can point to suggestion of metastatic spread of the cancer. CT of the chest is performed to evaluate for tumors involving adjacent structures as well as hilar and mediastinal lymphadenopathy. The CT scan should also include the upper abdomen to evaluate the liver and adrenal glands for metastatic disease. Radionuclide bone scanning and CT or magnetic resonance imaging (MRI) of the brain are also commonly performed, but their use is controversial in asymptomatic patients. If resection is planned, a bronchoscopy is always performed preoperatively to evaluate for proximal bronchial disease and to rule out additional lesions unseen on other tests. Positron emission tomography (PET) is highly sensitive and can be used for questions in mediastinal staging. Mediastinoscopy is used for lymph node sampling to document initially unresectable disease by proving the involvement of ipsilateral mediastinal or contralateral mediastinal nodes. Video-assisted thoracoscopy can be used for assessment of the pleura and mediastinum, as well as for biopsy of suspicious contralateral and peripheral lesions (Hoffman, Mauer, & Vokes, 2000). It can also be used for resection of nodules for curative surgery. Box 2-1 provides information about common surgical procedures that may be used in non–small cell lung cancer (Ginsberg, Vokes, & Raben, 1997). *Answer 4:* **d. All of these tests are used to evaluate for metastatic disease to determine stage of the cancer.**

5. It is important to provide smokers with a clear message that they should consider quitting. Information about the health benefits associated with quitting should also be provided. Although patients may think that the damage is done and that quitting will not benefit them, evidence suggests that quitting will decrease the chance for cancer recurrence, improve their tolerance for therapy, and lower their risk for pulmonary infections. If patients are not ready to quit, a note should be made to ask them about their smoking status in the future. They may not be ready at this point, but this may change in the future. It is not recommended to suggest that smokers switch to lower-dose tar and nicotine cigarettes. Similarly, a nonjudgmental approach should be used with those who are not ready or cannot quit, and the nurse should not push them to pick a quit date until they are ready to make a commitment. Smoking cessation guidelines for health care providers to use in clinical practice have recently been updated and published (Tobacco Use and Dependence Clinical Practice Guideline Panel, 2000). Table 2-3 provides an overview of strategies used to promote smoking cessation. *Answer 5:* **d.**

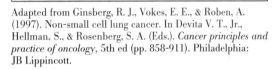

BOX **2-1** **Surgical Procedures for NSCLC**

PNEUMONECTOMY
Performed for tumor involving the proximal bronchus

LOBECTOMY
Most common surgical procedure
Confined to a single lobe of the lung

SLEEVE RESECTION WITH BRONCHOPLASTIC RECONSTRUCTION
When tumor is confined to bronchus or pulmonary artery

SEGMENTAL RESECTION
Partial removal of a lobe of the lung

WEDGE RESECTION
Removes small peripheral nodule
Performed in patients with limited pulmonary reserve

Adapted from Ginsberg, R. J., Vokes, E. E., & Roben, A. (1997). Non-small cell lung cancer. In Devita V. T., Jr., Hellman, S., & Rosenberg, S. A. (Eds.). *Cancer principles and practice of oncology,* 5th ed (pp. 858-911). Philadelphia: JB Lippincott.

Case Study continued

The thoracic oncology team reviewed the results of Mr. Jones's tests and found that his tumor is less than 3 cm in greatest dimension and does not involve the main bronchus; he has no other involvement, so he has stage I lung cancer. The physician has provided information about his stage of cancer and treatment options, but Mr. Jones has additional questions. You are called to provide additional information and implement teaching.

6. Based on the knowledge that Mr. Jones has stage I lung cancer, what would be the best treatment option for Mr. Jones?
    a. Chemotherapy
    b. Surgery
    c. Radiation therapy
    d. Combination therapy

ANSWERS

6. Table 2-3 provides information about the staging system for non–small cell lung cancer. This staging system was revised in 1997 to provide greater specificity for identifying patient groups with similar prognoses and treatment options with the least disruption of the previous classification (Mountain, 1997). The staging system assesses the primary tumor, presence of involved lymph nodes,

| TABLE **2-3** | **Smoking Cessation Strategies** |

THE 5 A's

Ask about tobacco use	• Identify and document tobacco use for every patient at every visit.
Advise to quit	• In a clear, strong, and personalized manner, urge every tobacco user to quit.
Assess willingness to make a quit attempt	• Is the tobacco user willing to make a quit attempt at this time?
Assist in quit attempt	• For the patient willing to make a quit attempt, use counseling and pharmacotherapy (first-line agents are Bupropion SR and/or nicotine replacement therapy) to assist him or her to quit. • Set a quit date—ideally within 2 weeks. • Tell family and friends about the quit date and request understanding and support. • Anticipate challenges to planned quit attempt. • Remove tobacco products from environment.
Arrange follow-up	• Schedule follow-up contact, preferably within the first week after the quit date. A second follow-up is recommended within the first month. • Congratulate success if abstinent. • Review circumstances and elicit recommitment to total abstinence if tobacco use has occurred. A lapse can be used as a learning experience to identify problems that occurred and anticipate challenges for the future.

THE 5 R's FOR THOSE UNWILLING TO QUIT

Relevance	• Provide information about quitting that is relevant to the patient's specific situation (e.g., disease status, having children in the home).
Risks	• Identify potential negative consequences or risks of tobacco use that are most relevant to patient (e.g., shortness of breath, cancer recurrence, impotence, infertility).
Rewards	• Identify potential benefits associated with quitting smoking (improved health, food will taste better, set a good example for children).
Roadblocks	• Identify barriers or impediments to quitting and note elements of treatment (problem solving or pharmacotherapy) that could address barriers. • Common barriers may include withdrawal symptoms, fear of failure, weight gain, depression, lack of support.
Repetition	• The motivational intervention should be repeated when the unmotivated person visits the clinic setting. • Tobacco users who have failed in previous quit attempts should be told that most people make repeated quit attempts before they are successful.

From Frank-Stromborg, M. & Cohen, R. R. (2000). Assessment and interventions for cancer detection. In Yarbro, C. H., Frogge, M. H., Goodman, M., & Groenwald, S. L. (Eds). *Cancer nursing: Principles and practice* (p. 159). Boston: Jones and Bartlett.

and metastases (TNM). According to this system, the primary tumor is subdivided into four T categories depending on size, site, and local involvement (T_1 to T_4). Lymph node spread has been subdivided into no lymph node involvement (N_0); bronchopulmonary (N_1); ipsilateral, mediastinal, and/or subcarinal (N_2); and contralateral or supraclavicular disease (N_3). Metastatic disease is absent or present (M_0 or M_1). See Tables 2-4 and 2-5.

In non–small cell lung cancer when the tumor is limited to a hemithorax and can be totally excised, surgery provides the best chance for cure. By definition, this would include stage I and II disease in which the tumor has not extended beyond the bronchopulmonary lymph nodes and a complete

excision of the tumor is possible without compromising the patient. Patient evaluation for surgery includes clinical staging of the disease to assess its resectability and cardiopulmonary assessment of the patient to determine perioperative risk and to ensure that there is adequate pulmonary reserve after the lung resection. A bronchoscopy may also be performed to rule out occult lesions.

Patients with stage III disease pose a treatment challenge because clinically distant metastases are absent. Patients with stage IIIA disease are considered marginally respectable. Small, randomized clinical trials have suggested a survival advantage with induction chemotherapy added to radiation or surgery. Surgery is usually excluded for stage IIIB disease because of the spread of the

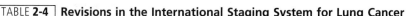

TABLE 2-4 | Revisions in the International Staging System for Lung Cancer

STAGE	1973 TNM	1986 TNM	1997 TNM
Occult	n/a	T_x, N_0, M_0	Delete
Stage 0	n/a	T_{is}, N_0, M_0	T_{is}, N_0, M_0
Stage I(A)*	T_{is}, N_0, M_0	T_1, N_0, M_0	T_1, N_0, M_0
	T_1, N_0, M_0	T_2, N_0, M_0	
	T_2, N_0, M_0		
Stage I(B)*	n/a	n/a	T_2, N_0, M_0
Stage II(A)*	T_2, N_1, M_0	T_1, N_1, M_0	T_1, N_1, M_0
		T_2, N_1, M_0	
Stage II(B)*	n/a	n/a	T_2, N_1, M_0
			T_3, N_0, M_0
Stage III(A)†	T_3, with any N or M	T_3, N_0, M_0	Any T, N_2, M_0
	N_2, with any T or M	T_3, N_1, M_0	
	M_1, with any T or M	T_1-T^3, N_2, M_0	
Stage III(B)†	n/a	Any T, N_3, M_0	T_4, any N, M_0
		T_4, any N, M_0	Any T, N_3, M_0
Stage IV†	n/a	Any T, any N, M_1	Any T, any N, M_1

Data from Mountain, C. F. (1997). Revisions in the international system for staging of lung cancer. *Chest*, *111*, pp. 1710-1717.
n/a, Not applicable, the stage did not exist at the time. For example, stages in 1973 were stage I, II, and III, whereas the stages in 1986 were occult, 0, I, II, IIIA, IIIB, and IV, and the stages in 1997 are 0, IA, IB, IIA, IIB, IIIA, IIIB, and IV. Revisions in the staging system created more specific categories as knowledge about lung cancer progressed.
*1997 revision.
†1986 revision.

TABLE 2-5 | TNM Definitions

PRIMARY TUMOR (T)

T_x: Tumor proven by the presence of malignant cells in bronchopulmonary secretions but not visualized roentgenographically or bronchoscopically, or any tumor that cannot be assessed as in a re-treatment staging.

T_0: No evidence of primary tumor.

T_{is}: Carcinoma in situ.

T_1: A tumor that is ≤3.0 cm in greatest diameter, surrounded by lung or visceral pleura, and without evidence of invasion proximal to a lobar bronchus at bronchoscopy.*

T_2: A tumor ≥3.0 cm in greatest diameter, or a tumor of any size that either invades the visceral pleura or has associated atelectasis or obstructive pneumonitis extending to the hilar region. At bronchoscopy, the proximal extent of demonstrable tumor must be within a lobar bronchus or at least 2.0 cm distal to the carina. Any associated atelectasis or obstructive pneumonitis must involve less than an entire lung.

T_3: A tumor of any size with direct extension into the chest wall (including superior sulcus tumors), diaphragm, or the mediastinal pleura or pericardium without involving the heart, great vessels, trachea, esophagus, or vertebral body; or a tumor in the main bronchus within 2 cm of the carina without involving the carina.

T_4: A tumor of any size with invasion of the mediastinum or involving the heart, great vessels, trachea, esophagus, vertebral body or carina, or presence of malignant pleural effusion.† Multiple tumor lesions in the same lobe of the lung.

NODAL INVOLVEMENT (N)

N_0: No demonstrable metastasis to regional lymph nodes.

N_1: Metastasis to lymph nodes in the peribronchial or the ipsilateral hilar region, or both, including direct extension.

N_2: Metastasis to ipsilateral mediastinal lymph nodes and subcarinal lymph nodes.

N_3: Metastasis to contralateral mediastinal lymph nodes, contralateral hilar lymph nodes, ipsilateral or contralateral scalene, or supraclavicular lymph nodes.

DISTANT METASTASIS (M)

M_0: No (known) distant metastasis.

M_1: Distant metastasis present (specify sites). Multiple tumor lesions in more than one lobe of the lung.

From Mountain, C. F. (1997). Revisions in the international system for staging lung cancer. *Chest*, *111*, p. 1711.
*The uncommon superficial tumor of any size with its invasive component limited to the bronchial wall, which may extend proximal to the main bronchus, is classified as T_1.
†Most pleural effusions associated with lung cancer are caused by tumor. However, there are a few patients in whom cytopathologic examination of pleural fluid (on more than one specimen) is negative for tumor and the fluid is nonbloody and is not an exudate. In such cases when these elements and clinical judgment dictate that the effusion is not related to tumor, the patient should be staged T_1, T_2, or T_3, excluding effusion as a staging element.

cancer to the lymph nodes on the opposite side of the mediastinum from the original tumor. Stage IIIB patients who have received curative treatment with radiation therapy have shown early progression of systemic disease because of the presence of micrometastatic disease at the time of initial diagnosis. Randomized clinical trials and meta-analyses have shown a survival benefit with induction chemotherapy before radiation therapy. In stage IV disease the patient is not a candidate for surgery secondary to distant spread of the disease but may be a candidate for palliative chemotherapy. Clinical trials and meta-analyses of palliative chemotherapy in this population have demonstrated a survival benefit in those who have a good performance status (Hoffman, Mauer, & Vokes, 2000). *Answer 6:* **b.**

QUESTIONS

7. Mr. Jones has been judged to be a good candidate for surgery. You are preparing to talk to Mr. Jones about his surgery. What information about Mr. Jones should you consider before providing him with information about his surgery?
   a. Ethnicity and occupation
   b. Occupation and education
   c. Education and ethnicity
   d. Income and education

8. To best prepare Mr. Jones for surgery, his patient education should include which of the following?
   1. Effective breathing and coughing exercises
   2. Postoperative range-of-motion shoulder exercises
   3. Leg exercises
   4. Need for additional treatment
      a. 1 only
      b. 1 & 3
      c. 1, 2, & 3
      d. 1 & 4

ANSWERS

7. Recent research suggests that a lower surgical treatment rate among African Americans exists in early-stage non–small cell lung cancer as compared with white patients; this results in lower survival rate among African Americans (Bach, Cramer, Warren, & Begg, 1999). The authors could not determine from their study the reasons for the racial disparity of treatment. However, the authors cited alternative explanations in the literature. One explanation was that African American patients may view the risks of surgical therapy differently. Another explanation was that white patients might be offered optimal treatment more often than African American patients. Therefore, when providing information to patients about potential treatment options, one must consider the patients' ethnic background and educational level so that the information provided is culturally relevant and understandable. *Answer 7:* **c.**

8. The most common thoracic surgical postoperative complications are pain and atelectasis. Postthoracotomy incisional pain can be severe and is aggravated by the presence of chest tubes used after a thoracotomy. Inadequate pain control prevents effective coughing and mobilization, and atelectasis may result. Although intravenous or epidural infusion of narcotics is often used for pain control, preoperative education should include coughing and breathing exercises. Because patients will be immobilized after surgery, providing information about leg exercises is also important. Shoulder immobility or a frozen shoulder can result after surgery. Thus teaching patients how to do range-of-motion exercises should be incorporated into the plan (Ingle, 2000). Teaching would not include providing information about additional therapy because Mr. Jones has stage I lung cancer and no further treatment is planned. *Answer 8:* **c.**

QUESTIONS

9. Mr. Jones is getting ready to be discharged after his surgery, and you notice that he seems to have trouble concentrating, reports decreased interest and pleasure in his usual activities, feels sad and hopeless, and is sleeping more than usual. You are concerned that Mr. Jones is suffering from which of the following?
   a. Attention deficit disorder
   b. Anxiety
   c. Depression
   d. Normal grief response after surgery

ANSWERS

9. Although a grief response can occur after the diagnosis of a life-threatening illness, a careful assessment is needed to identify those who may be at risk for depression. Depression occurs in 25% of patients with cancer and often goes undiagnosed, which results in higher heath care costs, decreased compliance, and decreased quality of life (Sivesind & Rohaly-Davis, 1998). Signs of depression include insomnia or hypersomnia, weight loss or gain, psychomotor retardation or agitation, decreased self-esteem, crying spells, feeling hopeless or helpless, suicide ideation, decreased pleasure in usual activities, lack of energy, and inability to concentrate (Sivesind & Rohaly-Davis, 1998). Because somatic symptoms commonly occur in cancer patients, the presence of psychologic symptoms are more reliable indicators of depression. Patient assessment should include current medications, unmet spiritual needs, unrelieved pain or other distressing symptoms, anxiety, psychosis, history of depression or alcoholism, and need for psychotherapy (Wrede-Seaman, 1996). If depression is suspected, assessment of its depth and any risk of suicide should be made (Sivesind & Rohaly-Davis, 1998). Suicidal ideation may represent a medical emergency and must be further evaluated by the health care provider. It is important to understand that anxiety and depression often occur together. Assessment tools are available to assist in identification of those who may be at risk. In particular, the mini-assessment for screening for anxiety and depression may be useful in clinical practice (Gobel & Donovan, 1987). Mr. Jones has several symptoms that are characteristic of depression; decreased interest and pleasure in his usual activities and feeling hopeless are two important symptoms that may indicate depression. *Answer 9:* **c.**

Case Study *continued*

Two years later Mr. Jones returns to the thoracic oncology clinic with a complaint of right hip pain. His pain is rated at 8 on a 0 to 10 scale. He has slight dyspnea on exertion. He also notes a weight loss of about 20 pounds over the past 6 months without dieting.

On physical examination, his temperature is 97.8° F, his pulse is 120 beats/min, his blood pressure is 116/76 mm Hg, and his pulse oximetry is 98%. His heart rate is fast but regular. He has no spine tenderness on palpation. He has full range of motion in his hips and lower extremities, and his motor examination shows that he has normal muscle bulk and tone. His strength is 5/5 throughout. His gait is normal.

The sensory examination of his lower extremities shows that pinprick, light touch, position sense are intact. His knee, ankle, and plantar reflexes are all 2+.

QUESTIONS

10. What further information should you gather about Mr. Jones's pain?

11. What symptom management recommendations should you suggest for Mr. Jones?

  1. Initiate a nonsteroidal antiinflammatory drug (NSAID)

  2. Initiate a short-acting opioid around the clock and begin a bowel regimen

  3. Wait to start pain medication until a diagnosis is established

  4. Initiate guided imagery and relaxation therapy

   a. 1 & 4
   b. 2 only
   c. 3 only
   d. 1, 2, & 4

ANSWERS

10. A comprehensive assessment is the first step in addressing pain and being able to provide adequate relief. Initial assessment of pain should include gathering a detailed history of the pain, performing a physical examination, and ordering further diagnostic tests to understand the cause of the pain. The nurse should gather more information about the onset of the pain, location, duration, characteristics, associated or aggravating factors, relieving factors, and therapeutic interventions used by the person with pain. In addition, a psychosocial assessment is performed. Important factors to consider in the psychosocial assessment include the meaning of the pain, impact of pain on mood, cognition, and ability to perform everyday activities. Many assessment tools and flowsheets are available and should be used to monitor pain in clinical practice. The physical examination focuses on examining the site of pain, examining common referral patterns, and performing a pertinent neurologic evaluation (Paice, 1999). Finally, further diagnostic testing is conducted to identify the underlying cause of the pain. In adults with cancer pain, it is critical to conduct an evaluation for cancer recurrence and/or progression of their disease. *Answer 10:* **See text.**

11. Treatment of cancer-related pain involves using a multimodality approach consisting of anticancer therapy and pharmacologic and nonpharmacologic interventions. Anticancer therapies are often effective in relieving cancer pain by decreasing the size of the tumor. Surgery, chemotherapy, radiation therapy, or a combination may be used depending on the type of cancer.

Pharmacologic interventions often provide the foundation for effectively treating cancer pain. The World Health Organization has developed an approach for titration of cancer pain therapy. The approach is based on a three-step analgesic ladder. The first step in this approach is to use nonopioids such as acetaminophen, aspirin, or another NSAID for mild to moderate pain. Adjuvant medicines, such as corticosteroids, antidepressants, anticonvulsants, biphosphonates, and antiemetics, may be used to enhance analgesic efficacy and/or treat concurrent symptoms that increase pain at any step of the ladder. When pain persists or increases, an opioid such as codeine or hydrocodone should be added to the NSAID as the second step of the ladder. If pain persists or is moderate to severe at the outset, increasing opioid potency (morphine, hydromorphone, methadone, fentanyl, or levor-phanol) or using higher dosages of the opioid should be used to treat the pain as the third step of the ladder. Oral medications for persistent cancer-related pain are preferred, if possible, and should be used around the clock, with additional "as-needed" doses to maintain a constant serum drug level. Long-acting pain medication is best for chronic, persistent pain. The type of long-acting pain medication should be selected based on cost-effectiveness and past experience with ad-verse reactions with opioids (Agency for Health Care Policy and Research, 1994).

Nonpharmacologic interventions can also be added to provide additional relief if the patient so chooses. The use of these methods allows patients to take an active role and participate in their care. It is important to recognize, however, that these methods should be used in combination with drugs and other modalities to manage cancer pain. Relaxation and imagery exercises are simple to use and may be used during brief episodes of pain, such as during procedures, as well as when patients experience severe pain. It is recommended that nonpharmacologic interventions be initiated early in the course of illness so that patients can learn and practice these techniques (Agency for Health Care Policy and Research, 1994).

Constipation is a common side effect with the use of opioids and, unless medically contraindi-cated, can be avoided with an effective bowel regimen. Generally, mild constipation can be managed with the use of a mild laxative (e.g., Milk of Magnesia) and increased fiber consumption. Inhibition of peristalsis by opioids causes severe constipation and can be treated with a stimulating cathartic drug (e.g., standardized senna concen-trate) or hyperosmotic agents (e.g., lactulose). Mr. Jones should be started on a "potent" opioid because his pain is 8 on a 0 to 10 scale and an NSAID. NSAIDs decrease inflammation and enable one to use lower dosages of opioids when treating moderate to severe pain. A bowel regimen should be initiated prophylactically and monitored closely, especially in the elderly be-cause they are at risk for constipation. Relaxation and imagery would also be started if he is inter-ested in using nonpharmacologic techniques. See Figure 2-1. *Answer 11:* **d.**

Case Study continued

Mr. Jones has a bone scan, which shows an abnormal focal area of accumulation in the posterior aspect of the right iliac crest. Follow-up plain films confirm a diagnosis of metastatic disease. He is referred for palliative radiation therapy of his right hip.

QUESTIONS

12. Which of the following side effects should you monitor during Mr. Jones's treatment with an NSAID?
    1. Leukocytosis
    2. Renal toxicity
    3. Gastric ulceration
    4. Sedation
      a. 1 only
      b. 1, 2, & 3
      c. 2 & 3
      d. All of these

13. Which of the following side effects should you expect from Mr. Jones's treatment with radia-tion therapy?
    1. Myelosuppression
    2. Skin erythema
    3. Nausea and vomiting
    4. Cystitis
      a. 1 & 2
      b. 2 only
      c. 2, 3, & 4
      d. None of these

ANSWERS

12. Patients who take NSAIDs, especially the elderly, must be monitored closely for adverse side effects, the most common of which are renal and hepatic toxicity, bleeding, and gastric ulceration. NSAIDs should be avoided in patients with thrombocytopenia and clotting disorders because many NSAIDs interfere with platelet aggregation. Sedation is not an expected side effect of NSAID use. In fact, lower dosages of an opioid may be given when combined with NSAIDs because of its antiinflammatory action. *Answer 12:* **c.**

13. Research shows that palliative radiation ther-apy produces significant benefit that can be sustained over a proportion of the patient's survival (Ginsberg, Vokes, & Raben, 1997). Radia-tion therapy is used to treat pain, prevent pathologic fractures, and prevent spinal cord compression in patients with bone metastasis. Acute side effects occurring during the course of radiotherapy are organ specific and related to the treatment field and dose of radiotherapy. Radia-

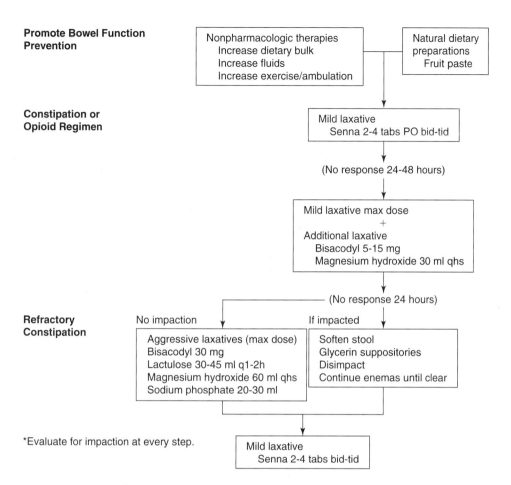

Promote Bowel Function
Prevention

Nonpharmacologic therapies
Increase dietary bulk
Increase fluids
Increase exercise/ambulation

Natural dietary
preparations
Fruit paste

Constipation or
Opioid Regimen

Mild laxative
Senna 2-4 tabs PO bid-tid

(No response 24-48 hours)

Mild laxative max dose
+
Additional laxative
Bisacodyl 5-15 mg
Magnesium hydroxide 30 ml qhs

(No response 24 hours)

Refractory
Constipation

No impaction

Aggressive laxatives (max dose)
Bisacodyl 30 mg
Lactulose 30-45 ml q1-2h
Magnesium hydroxide 60 ml qhs
Sodium phosphate 20-30 ml

If impacted

Soften stool
Glycerin suppositories
Disimpact
Continue enemas until clear

*Evaluate for impaction at every step.

Mild laxative
Senna 2-4 tabs bid-tid

Figure 2-1 Constipation algorithm.* (From Lin [in press].)

tion for bone metastasis of the extremities generally results in few acute toxicities because of the minimal surrounding structures. Radiation of the hip may result in diarrhea depending on the extent of the field (Maher, 2000). In general, however, patients experience few acute side effects. Skin changes are common side effects no matter where the treatment is administered but may vary in intensity depending on the site and dose. Erythema and itching are common side effects and should be expected with Mr. Jones's treatment. Acute myelosuppression is usually not seen unless the radiation field includes a substantial portion of active bone marrow. Patients at high risk for myelosuppression include those who are receiving concurrent chemotherapy and radiation or whole abdominal, splenic, and/or total body irradiation. Nausea and vomiting are not expected to occur in this case because the whole abdomen, extended pelvis fields, epigastric, or paraaortic area are not within the treatment field. Similarly, cystitis is not expected because the

bladder is not within the treatment field (Maher, 2000). Pain relief in bony metastasis can be enhanced by the use of radiopharmaceuticals such as Strontium-89 and Samarium-153-lexidronam (Janjan, 1997). *Answer 13:* **b.**

Case Study continued

Mr. Jones's pain is well controlled after treatment with radiation therapy. One month later he arrives in the oncology clinic in a wheelchair pushed by his sister because he was unable to walk farther than 10 feet without assistance. He is complaining of shortness of breath.

QUESTIONS

14. What additional information do you need to evaluate Mr. Jones's dyspnea?
   1. Onset and duration of dyspnea
   2. Presence of fevers or chills
   3. Sputum color/quality
   4. Chest pain

a. 1 only
b. 2 & 3
c. 1, 3, & 4
d. All of these

14. In obtaining a patient's history, it is important to determine when the dyspnea first occurred and how long it lasts. If this is a sudden onset without fever or chills, the dyspnea may represent an effusion versus a slow onset without fever, which may signal lymphangitic spread of a tumor (Enck, 1994). A patient with a pulmonary embolism may experience sudden dyspnea with chest pain. It is important to also assess for precipitating factors and reversible causes of dyspnea. The presence of fever and/or sputum production that has changed in color and quantity should be assessed because it may be related to a reversible problem such as infection. Common causes of dyspnea are listed in Box 2-2. *Answer 14:* **d.**

Case Study continued

Mr. Jones has difficulty talking because of his dyspnea. Between breaths, however, he states that

---

BOX **2-2**	**Common Causes of Dyspnea in Adults with Advanced Cancer**

CARCINOMA OF THE LUNG
Obstructing lesions with atelectasis and
   pneumonia
Restrictive ventilatory defect
Lymphangitic spread
Metastases
Impaired diaphragmatic function
Pleural effusion
Superior vena caval syndrome
Bleeding
Pneumothorax
Pericardial effusion

ADVANCED CANCER EFFECTS
Massive ascites
Hepatomegaly

PRIOR CANCER THERAPY
Postpneumonectomy
Postradiation fibrosis
Chemotherapy

COMORBIDITIES
Congestive heart failure
Chronic obstructive pulmonary disease
Anxiety
Aspiration pneumonia

Adapted from Enck, R. E. (1994). *The medical care of the terminally ill patients* (p. 42). Baltimore: The Johns Hopkins University Press.

---

his dyspnea started suddenly without fever or chills. He has a chronic productive cough of yellow-white sputum that has not changed. Vital signs show Mr. Jones's temperature to be 99.1° F, his pulse to be 130 beats/min, his blood pressure to be 94/64 mm Hg, his respirations 40 breaths/min, and his oxygen saturation 86%. On physical examination, he has decreased breath sounds in the lower left lung, dullness to percussion, and decreased tactile fremitus; his heart rate is rapid yet regular, and his abdomen is flat and non-tender. His lower extremities show no signs of cyanosis or edema. A chest radiograph is obtained and shows a large left pleural effusion. Mr. Jones states that he wants to be kept comfortable and does not wish to undergo any further treatment. He is admitted to the hospital for management of his dyspnea.

QUESTIONS

15. Which of the following interventions are appropriate to promote comfort for Mr. Jones?
   1. Relaxation exercises
   2. Breathing exercise/desensitization techniques
   3. Oxygen therapy
   4. Morphine
      a. 1 & 3
      b. 1, 3, & 4
      c. 3 only
      d. 3 & 4

15. A multimodal approach to the treatment of severe dyspnea is best (Harwood, 1999). Oxygen therapy often provides relief of hypoxemia and dyspnea in adults with cancer. The use of morphine to treat severe dyspnea in terminally ill patients is an important component of therapy and may be administered either orally, intravenously, or by nebulizer. It may be combined with other medications to improve response or treat unwanted side effects. For example, dexamethasone may be added for patients with lymphangitic spread of tumor, and/or prochlorperazine may be added for those who experience nausea or vomiting from morphine. Relaxation exercises may also be used to decrease anxiety associated with dyspnea and to promote comfort. Breathing exercises and desensitization techniques may be too difficult for patients at this point because of the time and energy required to learn these techniques. Similarly, physical exercise retraining can be useful to improve activity tolerance for those with pulmonary and cardiac comorbidity but is not an appropriate intervention at this time. *Answer 15:* **b.**

CASE 3 STUDY

Mrs. Sarah Hogan is 44 years old. About 2 months ago, she noticed swelling of her entire neck and a sensation that her neck was being cut off. For the last week she noticed a light-headed and dizzy feeling when she leaned forward. For 2 days, her right hand was swollen but has since resolved. She has also noticed difficulty swallowing; she can eat and drink but has the sensation that something is stuck in her throat. She lost 40 pounds over the past 6 months without dieting. She reports no other symptoms and has no other medical problems. She smoked 1 pack of cigarettes a day for 20 years but quit 4 years ago. She is married, works full-time as an accountant, and has two teenage children: Matthew and Ann. You are struck by a bluish hue to her face and neck from numerous dilated cutaneous veins. On physical examination, you find a full neck with engorged veins.

QUESTIONS

1. What are probable differential diagnoses for Mrs. Hogan?
  1. Esophageal cancer
  2. Superior vena cava syndrome (SVCS)
  3. Syndrome of inappropriate antidiuretic hormone secretion (SIADH) with fluid overload
  4. Lymphedema
     a. 1 & 2
     b. 1, 2, & 3
     c. 2 & 3
     d. All of these

2. What would be indications for *not* ordering a barium swallow immediately?
  1. There are accompanying symptoms.
  2. A chest radiograph is quicker and easier.
  3. Cigarette use is a cause behind lung cancer, not esophageal cancer.
  4. The barium could be constipating.
     a. 1 only
     b. 1 & 2
     c. 2 & 4
     d. All of these

3. What symptoms are consistent with SVC obstruction?
  a. Shortness of breath and hypotension
  b. Headaches and dyspnea
  c. Depression and confusion
  d. Anxiety and weight gain

4. What other clinical findings should you expect with SVC obstruction?
  1. Flushed face
  2. Chest wall vein distension
  3. Periorbital edema
  4. Cyanosis
     a. 1 only
     b. 1 & 2
     c. 1, 2, & 4
     d. All of these

ANSWERS

1-4. Mrs. Hogan has fullness in her neck with engorged veins, which are signs of SVCS. The SVC is a thin-walled vessel that produces unique signs and symptoms when blood flow is obstructed, resulting in SVCS. The symptoms of SVCS include dyspnea; nonproductive cough; and head, upper trunk, or extremity fullness. Clinical findings include venous distension of neck and chest wall; edema of the face, periorbital area, and/or extremities; facial flushing; cyanosis; and tachypnea. The signs and symptoms are classic for SVCS and not many other problems. The physical examination can help in the determination of hypervolemia and cardiac failure.

It is the combination of symptoms obtained in a thorough review of systems and physical examination that narrows down the differential diagnoses. The most common cause of SVCS is malignant disease, with most patients having lung cancer. SVCS is considered a potentially life-threatening medical emergency (Sitton, 2000). These signs, coupled with history of tobacco use and weight loss, should point your physical examination toward assessing for a lung mass. *Answer 1:* **a.** *Answer 2:* **b.** *Answer 3:* **b.** *Answer 4:* **d.**

QUESTIONS

5. How can you explain why Mrs. Hogan did not have more severe distress?
  1. The obstruction grew slowly over time.
  2. Collaterals developed.
  3. The obstruction was so severe that she learned to accommodate.
  4. Being female, she minimized her symptoms.
     a. 1 & 2
     b. 2 & 3
     c. 1, 2, & 4
     d. All of these

6. What is a sign that Mrs. Hogan was in crisis, potentially threatening her life?

7. What is the initial step for treating Mrs. Hogan?

   a. Simulating immediate radiation
   b. Determining a definitive histopathologic diagnosis
   c. Performing bronchoscopy
   d. Admitting her to the intensive care unit

ANSWERS

5. The signs and symptoms of SVCS depend on the rate of development, the size of obstruction, and whether there has been sufficient time for collateral circulation to develop. If this had developed at a faster rate or had become more severe, Mrs. Hogan would have experienced respiratory distress with stridor because of laryngeal edema (Haapoja & Blendowski, 1999). *Answer 5:* **a.**

6-7. A chest radiograph shows a mass in the right side of the chest. The chest radiograph provides the clinician with a quick view of her lungs, which can reveal an enlarged heart in the case of cardiac tamponade or heart failure. It will also show any gross abnormalities, leading to more discriminating diagnostic tests. A CT scan of the thorax reveals pinpoint narrowing of the SVC at the level of the azygos arch, with preferential flow of contrast material into the azygos arch. There is a 4.0-by-3.4-cm mass at the right hilum and mediastinal lymphadenopathy in both the aortopulmonary and peritracheal regions. In the abdomen, there is a 2-by-2-cm mass on the right adrenal gland. Bronchoscopy is performed, and a needle biopsy shows small cell lung cancer. Before any treatment can occur, the tissue diagnosis of malignancy-induced SVCS needs to be made. Chemotherapy is initiated as soon as a tissue diagnosis is obtained. *Answer 6:* **See text.** *Answer 7:* **b.**

QUESTIONS ───────

8. What stage is Mrs. Hogan's lung cancer?

9. What chemotherapy agents are commonly used to treat small cell lung cancer?

ANSWERS

8. Most clinicians use a limited versus extensive staging system for small cell lung cancer, even though the American Joint Commission on Cancer advocates using the TNM staging system. *Limited stage* is defined as a tumor confined to one hemithorax, which may include regional lymph nodes that can be enclosed within one radiotherapy port without excessive toxicity to the patient.

Extensive stage is defined as disease existing beyond one radiation therapy port procedure (Hide, Pass, & Glatstein, 1997).

Because of the rapid growth rate in small cell lung cancer, procedures for staging may differ from those for NSCLC. The recommended staging examinations are as follows: history and physical examination, complete blood count, blood urea nitrogen, creatinine, liver function tests, chest radiograph, CT scan of the thorax (to include abdominal examination if liver function tests or abdominal examination is abnormal), and bone scan (if bone pain); follow-up plain films should also be obtained. A CT scan of the head should be included if the neurologic examination is abnormal. Other procedures, such as bone marrow biopsy, may be done depending on the individual practitioner's style or requirements for clinic trials (Hide, Pass, & Glatstein, 1997). *Answer 8:* **According to the limited versus extensive staging system, Mrs. Hogan would be classified as having extensive-stage small cell lung cancer because her CT scan showed bilateral pulmonary nodules and an adrenal mass, which is a common site for metastasis in lung cancer.**

9. Common chemotherapy regimens for small cell lung cancer include (1) etoposide and cisplatin (EP); (2) cyclophosphamide, doxorubicin, and vincristine (CAV); (3) cyclophosphamide, doxorubicin, and etoposide (CAE); and (4) etoposide and carboplatin (EC) (Ihde, 1992; Ingle, 2000). EP is currently the standard induction therapy for small cell lung cancer. Chemotherapy may be combined with radiotherapy in limited-stage small cell lung cancer, whereas chemotherapy alone is used in extensive-stage small cell lung cancer.

The treatment of SVCS is most often combination chemotherapy and/or radiation therapy. Combination chemotherapy and radiation therapy are both effective in treating SVCS caused by small cell lung cancer. Response rates for symptom improvement have been reported to be 93% after chemotherapy and 94% after mediastinal radiation therapy (Chan, Dar, Yu, et al., 1997). However, radiation therapy is the treatment of choice in SVCS caused by non–small cell lung cancer. Prompt therapy is critical to minimize respiratory and cerebral life-threatening complications associated with SVCS (Sitton, 2000). *Answer 9:* **See text.**

Case Study continued

Mrs. Hogan will receive treatment with EP. She reports to the thoracic oncology clinic for her first treatment. She confides that she is worried about the potential side effects because she had a friend who underwent chemotherapy and experienced multiple adverse side effects. In addition, she is concerned about the effect of her disease and treatment on her two teenage children and is not sure what she should tell them.

QUESTIONS

10. Given Mrs. Hogan's concerns, you would do all of the following *except:*
  a. Reassure her that the side effects associated with chemotherapy are temporary
  b. Tell her that teenagers may act out with anger during a parent's illness
  c. Suggest that she hold a family conference to discuss her illness and treatment and have the family prioritize expectations
  d. Discuss that she may want to relinquish some of her responsibilities so that she will have added energy for things that are important to her

11. What antinausea medication or medications are best to use for Mrs. Hogan?
  1. Ondansetron
  2. Dexamethasone
  3. Prochlorperazine
  4. Metoclopramide
    a. 1& 2
    b. 2 & 4
    c. 3 only
    d. 1, 2, & 3

12. All of the following are potential side effects of cisplatin *except:*
  a. Mucositis
  b. Ototoxicity
  c. Renal failure
  d. Hypomagnesemia, hypocalcemia

13. While reviewing the laboratory values before Mrs. Hogan's treatment, you note that her sodium is low at 125 mEq/L. You suspect that she may have SIADH. What additional studies would be ordered to confirm this diagnosis?
  1. Plasma osmolality
  2. Urine sodium
  3. Serum uric acid, phosphate, and calcium
  4. Serum and urinary potassium
    a. 1 & 2
    b. 1, 2, & 4
    c. 3 & 4
    d. None of these

14. What symptoms are associated with SIADH?
  1. Headaches
  2. Tenderness along the distal long bones
  3. Lethargy
  4. Paresthesias
    a. 1 only
    b. 1 & 4
    c. 1 & 3
    d. All of these

15. What is the most effective intervention for SIADH associated with small cell lung cancer?
  a. Fluid restriction
  b. Chemotherapy
  c. Demeclocycline
  d. Intravenous administration of hypertonic saline solution and furosemide

ANSWERS

10. Providing care to both the individual and family is considered part of the oncology APN's role. Families with school-age or teenage children face certain challenges when one of the adults is diagnosed with cancer. Children of this age are engaged in activities outside the house and are becoming more independent. Thus the diagnosis may result in family turmoil. Parents are often concerned about what to tell their children and need to understand normal developmental responses to illness (Hymovich, 1993). Open and honest communication is the best approach. Because the family's ability to collaboratively prioritize expectations and activities is a factor in promoting the family's ability to cope with illness, suggesting a family conference is a good idea. Although communication is essential during a parent's illness, it does not guarantee acceptance by children. Teenage children, in particular, may experience difficulty because they may perceive the illness as a threat to their independence. As a result, they may act out with angry behavior or act indifferent toward the sick parent (Loney, 1998). Honest and ongoing communication between the child and parent is essential to maintain the relationship. The nurse can suggest that Mrs. Hogan relinquish some of her responsibilities so that she will have energy for important things that she wants to do. Many adults try to maintain their preillness pace, but treatment-related fatigue might make this difficult. Giving adults "permission" to relinquish or delegate less important tasks may help them have the time and energy for quality family experiences (Barhamand, 1998).

The nurse would not reassure Mrs. Hogan that the side effects of chemotherapy are only temporary. Mrs. Hogan is concerned that she will have an experience similar to that of her friend who underwent chemotherapy. Therefore it is most appropriate to try to dispel her fears and any myths about treatment. It is important to tell her that everyone is unique and that response to treatment varies among individuals. The nurse should provide Mrs. Hogan with accurate information about potential side effects. *Answer 10:* **a.**

11. Nausea and vomiting can be a significant side effect associated with chemotherapy. Antiemetic treatment has improved significantly over the past 10 years to help control this problem. Patient assessment for patients receiving chemotherapy should include potential risk factors for emesis (Table 2-6). Antiemetic regimens are individualized and developed according to the emetic potential of the agent and expected duration of nausea and vomiting (Wickham, 1999).

Because cisplatin is a highly emetogenic chemotherapy agent at higher dosages, it requires combination antiemetic prophylaxis. Classes of antiemetics include serotonin ($5HT_3$) receptor antagonists (most often used during the first 2 days after chemotherapy) that act by blocking the $5HT_3$ receptors on vagal afferent fibers that relay sensory information to nausea/vomiting control centers in the brain. Phenothiazines (prochlorperazine and thiethylperazine) are oral dopamine antagonists that have both tranquilizing and antiemetic effects and are especially useful for the prevention of nausea and vomiting with mildly emetogenic chemotherapy. Because these medications act differently than $5HT_3$ receptor antagonists, they can be added to the regimen containing $5HT_3$ and are helpful in regimens to prevent delayed nausea and vomiting. Butyrophenones (haloperidol and droperidol) are major tranquilizers. They appear to be as effective as the phenothiazines but less effective than other antinausea medications. They can be used in combination with other medications. Metoclopramide is classified as a substituted benzamide and is

the most commonly used drug in this class for chemotherapy-related nausea and vomiting. However, therapeutic use of these drugs requires maintenance of an adequate plasma level. Diphenhydramine is added to the regimen to decrease extrapyramidal side effects. It can be used to prevent cisplatin-associated emesis, but it is not as effective as the $5HT_3$ receptor antagonists. Benzodiazepines can induce temporary amnesia and can be used to prevent anticipatory nausea and vomiting. Cannabinoids may be an option in patients who do not respond to conventional treatment. Corticosteroids are hypothesized to prohibit prostaglandin synthesis. The most commonly used corticosteroid is dexamethasone, which is often used in combination therapy to enhance the effect of $5HT_3$ receptor antagonists or metoclopramide. Because of the highly emetic nature of cisplatin, combination antiemetic agents should be chosen for Mrs. Hogan. Serotonin antagonists, such as ondansetron, are effective agents to use with cisplatin therapy. Combining serotonin antagonists with a corticosteroid enhances efficacy. In addition, because cisplatin may also cause delayed nausea and vomiting, a prescription for prochlorperazine would also be given so that Mrs. Hogan can continue her antiemetic treatment at home. *Answer 11:* **d.**

12. Cisplatin is an alkylating agent. Potential side effects of cisplatin are severe nausea and vomiting, nephrotoxicity, peripheral neuropathy, ototoxicity, electrolyte imbalances (hypokalemia, hypocalcemia, hypomagnesemia, hypophosphatemia), impaired fertility, and anaphylactic reactions (Berkery, Cleri, & Skarin, 1997). Although myelosuppression is mild with low to moderate dosages, more pronounced leukopenia and thrombocytopenia can occur with higher dosages. Pretreatment with antiemetic medication and hydration

TABLE 2-6	Risk Factors for Emesis with Chemotherapy
RISK FACTOR	**EFFECT**
Antineoplastic drug	Drugs with higher emetic potential are more likely to cause emesis (i.e., cisplatin has high emetic potential).
Gender	Women who are of menstrual age are more likely to experience poor emetic control compared with men or older women.
Age	Persons younger than 45-55 yr report more intense nausea than those who are older and are also more likely to develop anticipatory nausea and vomiting.
History of motion sickness	Persons with a history of motion sickness may be at greater risk for emesis compared with those who do not have this problem.
Alcohol intake	Persons with a history of chronic high alcohol intake may experience less nausea than those who do not report intake of alcohol.

Adapted from Wickham, R. (1999). Nausea and vomiting. In Yarbro, C. H., Frogge, M. H., & Goodman, M. (Eds.). *Cancer symptom management* (pp. 228-263). Boston: Jones and Bartlett.

should be administered to minimize gastrointestinal and nephrotoxicity. Mucositis is not a potential side effect of cisplatin. Mucositis is often associated with antimetabolite agents (e.g., cytarabine) and antitumor antibiotics (daunorubicin). *Answer 12:* **a.**

13. SIADH is a paraneoplastic syndrome resulting from nonphysiologic release of vasopressin from either the posterior pituitary gland or an ectopic source leading to impaired renal free-water excretion. Although rare, it is most commonly associated with small cell lung cancer and is often detected at diagnosis. SIADH consists of hyponatremia, decreased plasma osmolality, and inappropriately concentrated urine. Laboratory studies that are used to diagnose SIADH are serum osmolality (less than 275 mOsm/kg), urine sodium (greater than 25 mEq/L), and urine osmolality (urine osmolality greater than serum osmolality). In addition, renal, adrenal, and thyroid function are normal in SIADH (Haapoja, 2000). *Answer 13:* **a.**

14. Symptoms in SIADH, often vague and nonspecific, are related to the severity of hyponatremia and the rate at which it develops. Mild hyponatremia is considered 125 to 134 mEq/L, whereas moderate is 115 to 124 mEq/L and severe is less than 110 to 114 mEq/L. The most important symptoms to be aware of are changes in mental status, such as confusion, lethargy, combativeness, and seizures, because these may be related to brain cell edema. Other symptoms may include headaches, anorexia, muscle cramps, and weakness (Haapoja, 2000; Jones, 1999). Tenderness along the long bones is associated with hypertrophic pulmonary osteoarthropathy, which is a paraneoplastic syndrome occurring in primary or metastatic lung tumors. *Answer 14:* **c.**

15. The most effective treatment for SIADH is to treat the underlying disease. Therefore chemotherapy is the most effective intervention for small cell lung cancer. Standard first-line therapy for mild to moderate SIADH is 800 to 1000 ml/day water restriction. In some instances lithium and demeclocycline may be used to treat chronic mild to moderate hyponatremia. Severe, symptomatic hyponatremia is an oncologic emergency requiring rapid treatment. Administration of hypertonic saline solution is initiated to increase serum sodium. Intravenous furosemide may also be administered to facilitate water loss. Emergency treatment is given in a controlled, closely monitored setting such as an intensive care unit (Haapoja, 2000). *Answer 15:* **b.**

Case Study continued

Mrs. Hogan arrives at the clinic for her fourth cycle of EP. You begin preparation for her treatment and notice that she has a drooping right eyelid. On physical examination, her right eye deviates outward.

QUESTIONS

16. Which of the following clinical findings should you also expect to find on Mrs. Hogan's physical examination?
   a. Inability to shrug shoulders
   b. Loss of head rotation
   c. Difficulty swallowing
   d. Impaired extraocular movement of the right eye

ANSWERS

16. Ptosis and right eye deviation signal a third cranial nerve paralysis with the pulling of the eye outward by the sixth cranial nerve. The other abnormality noted with third cranial nerve paralysis is inability of the affected eye to perform upward, downward, and inward movements. With third cranial nerve paralysis evident on physical examination, she may have a metastatic brain tumor. A full assessment to determine the extent of cranial nerve involvement may also include examination of the visual acuity, visual fields, ocular fundi, pupillary reactions, corneal reflexes, facial sensation, and jaw movements (Bickley & Hoekelman, 1999). Table 2-7 provides information about the other cranial nerves. *Answer 16:* **d.**

Case Study continued

You discuss Mrs. Hogan's new physical examination findings with the thoracic oncology attending physician. An MRI of the brain is done, and multiple metastases are visualized. A team conference is held to discuss Mrs. Hogan's care. Radiation therapy and dexamethasone to minimize any cerebral swelling are identified as the best treatment options. The thoracic oncology attending meets with Mrs. Hogan and her husband and provides information about the results of the scan and that the goal for her care is palliation and symptom relief. Mrs. Hogan finishes her radiation therapy and comes to clinic for a follow-up appointment. During your visit with Mrs. Hogan, she tells you that she wants to be kept comfortable and be at home with her family as much as possible. She is worried about how her family will manage after her death.

| TABLE 2-7 | Summary of Cranial Nerves | |
CRANIAL NERVE	FUNCTION	EXAMINATION
I (olfactory nerves and tract)	Smell	• Test sense of smell by having patient close his or her eyes and smell something familiar.
II (optic nerve)	Vision	• Visual acuity • Visual fields • Ocular fundi
III (oculomotor nerve)	Constrict pupils Eye movement Elevate eye lid	• Pupillary reactions • Extraocular movements
IV (trochlear)	Eye movement	• Extraocular movements
V (trigeminal)	Sensation of face Corneal reflex Innervate muscles of mastication	• Corneal reflexes • Jaw movements • Light touch on face
VI (abducens)	Eye movement	• Extraocular movements
VII (facial)	Innervate facial muscles Buccinator Taste anterior tongue	• Facial movements
VIII (vestibulocochlear)	Equilibrium Hearing	• Hearing • Test lateralization (Weber's test*) • Compare air and bone conduction (Rinne test†)
IX (glossopharyngeal)	Taste Superior pharyngeal muscles	• Swallowing and rise of the palate • Gag reflex
X (vagus)	Innervate sensory portions of the viscera of pleura and abdomen Motor innervation of larynx and pharyngeal muscles Parasympathetic innervation to heart, lungs, and most of digestive tract	• Voice and speech
XI (accessory)	Innervate muscles of the neck, sternocleidomastoid, and trapezius	• Shoulder and neck movements
XII (hypoglossal)	Innervate muscles of the tongue	• Tongue symmetry and position

Adapted from Bickley, L. S., & Hoekelman, R. A. (1999). *Bate's guide to physical examination and history taking.* Philadelphia: JB Lippincott.
*Test for lateralization. Sensorineural loss causes lateralization to less affected ear and AC > BC.
†Test to compare air and bone conduction. Conduction loss causes lateralization to more affected ear and BC > AC.

QUESTIONS

17. Which of the following interventions is(are) appropriate to assist Mrs. Hogan in dealing with her impending death?
1. Initiating a referral to hospice
2. Scheduling a closure interview with Mrs. Hogan and her husband
3. Beginning to discuss how she wants to be remembered and how she wants to say good-bye to her husband and children
4. Assessing her social network size and availability of help
   a. 1 only
   b. 1 & 2
   c. 1, 3, & 4
   d. All of these

17. It is appropriate to initiate a referral to hospice. Hospice care is provided in the person's home and is appropriate when the prognosis is 6 months or less. An interdisciplinary approach to care is provided, and bereavement follow-up is often provided for family members. Because Mrs. Hogan has two children, ongoing care directed toward helping them with their grief will be an important aspect of care. The nurse can begin a discussion of how Mrs. Hogan wants to be remembered and how she wants to say good-bye to her husband and children. This will give her an opportunity to personalize how she wants to be remembered. For example, some parents may leave videos, audiotapes, and/or family albums for their children to remember them. Assessing Mrs.

Hogan's social network and availability of help is also essential. Hospice provides care that is based on the assumption that she has a primary caregiver who will be available. Her husband will most likely need assistance in providing care. Therefore identification of potential formal and informal support networks is necessary. Finally, it is recommended to schedule a closure interview with the patient, family, and staff. This meeting allows the patient and family members to ask any questions that they may have and to express any feelings that they have about the care that has been rendered; it also allows the staff to identify patient needs for hospice care (Goodman, 1999). In addition, this meeting allows the APN to promote a smooth transition among care settings (i.e., clinic, hospice, and patient's home). After the meeting, the APN can call the hospice and provide a report on the issues and anticipated needs of the patient and family. *Answer 17:* **d.**

REFERENCES

Agency for Health Care Policy and Research. (1994). *Clinical practice guideline: Management of cancer pain.* Rockville, MD: United States Department of Health and Human Services, Agency for Health Care Policy and Research Publication No. 94-0592.

Bach, P. B., Cramer, L. D., Warren, J. L., & Begg, C. B. (1999). Racial differences in the treatment of early-stage lung cancer. *N Engl J Med, 341,* pp. 1198-1205.

Barhamand, B. A. (1998). Coping with cancer: Family issues. In Burke, C. C. (Ed.). *Psychosocial dimensions of oncology nursing care* (pp. 28-52). Pittsburgh: Oncology Nursing Press.

Barron, A. M., & White, P. (1996). Consultation. In Hamric, A. B., Spross, J. A., & Hanson, C. M. (Eds.). *Advanced nursing practice: An integrative approach* (pp. 165-183). Philadelphia: WB Saunders.

Berkery, R., Cleri, L. B., & Skarin, A. T. (1997). *Oncology pocket guide to chemotherapy,* 3rd ed. London: Mosby.

Bickley, L. S., & Hoekelman, R. A. (1999). *Bates' guide to physical examination and history taking.* Philadelphia: JB Lippincott.

Caplan, G., & Caplan, R. (1993). *Mental health consultation and collaboration.* San Francisco: Jossey-Bass.

Cataldo, J. K., Cooley, M. E., & Giarelli, E. (2000). Smoking and cancer. In Jennings-Dozier, J. K., & Mahon, S. (Eds.). *Cancer prevention, detection, and control: A nursing perspective.* Pittsburgh: Oncology Nursing Press.

Chan, R. H., Dar, A. R., Yu, E., et al. (1997). Superior vena cava obstruction in small cell lung cancer. *Int J Radiat Oncol Biol Physics, 38,* pp. 513-520.

Cooley, M. E., & Jennings-Dozier, K. (1998). Lung cancer in African Americans: A call for action. *Cancer Pract, 6,* pp. 99-106.

Enck, R. E. (1994). *The medical care of terminally ill patients.* Baltimore: Johns Hopkins University Press.

Fontana, R. S., Sanderson, D. R., Woolner, L. B., et al. (1986). Lung cancer screening: The Mayo program. *J Occup Med, 28,* pp. 746-750.

Frank-Stromborg, M., & Cohen, R. F. (2000). Assessment and interventions for cancer detection. In Yarbro, C. H., Frogge, M. H., Goodman, M., & Groenwald, S. L. (Eds.). *Cancer nursing: Principles and practice* (p. 150). Boston: Jones and Bartlett.

Ginsberg, R. J., Vokes, E. E., & Raben, A. (1997). Non-small cell lung cancer. In Devita, V. T., Jr, Hellman, S., Rosenberg, S. A. (Eds.). *Cancer principles & practice of oncology,* 5th ed (pp. 858-911). Philadelphia: Lippincott-Raven.

Gobel, B. H., & Donovan, M. I. (1987). Depression and anxiety. *Semin Oncol Nurs, 3,* pp. 267-276.

Goodman, M. (1999). Saying good-bye. In Yarbro, C. H., Frogge, M. H., & Goodman, M. (Eds.). *Cancer symptom management* (pp. 627-642). Boston: Jones and Bartlett.

Haapoja, I. S. (2000). Syndrome of inappropriate antidiuretic hormone. In Yarbro, C. H., Frogge, M. H., Goodman, M., & Groenwald, S. L. (Eds.). *Cancer nursing: Principles and practice* (pp. 913-919). Boston: Jones and Bartlett.

Haapoja, I. S., & Blendowski, C. (1999). Superior vena cava syndrome. *Semin Oncol Nurs, 15*(3), pp. 183-189.

Harwood, K. V. (1999). Dyspnea. In Yarbro, C. H., Frogge, M. H., & Goodman, M. (Eds.). *Cancer symptom management* (pp. 45-57). Boston: Jones and Bartlett.

Henschke, C. I., McCauley, D. I., Yankelevitz, D. F., et al. (1999). Early lung cancer action project: Overall design and findings from baseline screening. *Lancet, 354,* pp. 99-105.

Hide, D. C., Pass, H. I., & Glatstein, E. (1997). Small cell lung cancer. In Devita, V. T., Jr, Hellman, S., Rosenberg, S. A. (Eds.). *Cancer principles & practice of oncology,* 5th ed. Philadelphia: Lippincott-Raven.

Hoffman, P. C., Mauer, A. M., & Vokes, E. E. (2000). Lung cancer. *Lancet, 355,* pp. 479-485.

Hymovich, D. P. (1993). Child rearing concerns of parents with cancer. *Oncol Nurs Forum, 20,* pp. 1355-1360.

Ihde, D. C. (1992). Chemotherapy of lung cancer. *N Engl J Med, 327,* pp. 1434-1441.

Ingle, R. J. (2000). Lung cancers. In Yarbro, C. H., Frogge, M. H., Goodman, M., & Groenwald, S. L. (Eds.). *Cancer nursing: Principles and practice* (pp. 1298-1328). Boston: Jones and Bartlett.

Janjan, N. A. (1997). Radiation for bone metastasis: conventional techniques and the role of systemic radiopharmaceuticals. *Cancer, 80,* pp. 1628-1645.

Jones, L. A. (1999). Electrolyte imbalance. In Yarbro, C. H., Frogge, M. H., & Goodman, M. (Eds.). *Cancer symptom management* (pp. 438-456). Boston: Jones and Bartlett.

Lin, E. (In Press). Constipation. In Yasko, J. M. (Ed.). *Nursing management of symptoms associated with chemotherapy.* Philadelphia: Meniscus Publications.

Loney, M. (1998). Death, dying, and grief in the face of cancer. In Burke, C. C. (Ed.). *Psychosocial dimensions of oncology nursing care* (pp. 152-179). Pittsburgh: Oncology Nursing Press.

Maher, K. E. (2000). Radiation therapy: Toxicities and management. In Yarbro, C. H., Frogge, M. H., Goodman, M., & Groenwald, S. L. (Eds.). *Cancer nursing: Principles and practice* (pp. 325-351). Boston: Jones and Bartlett.

Mayne, S. T., Janerich, D. T., Greenwald, P., et al. (1994). Dietary beta carotene and lung cancer risk in US nonsmokers. *J Natl Cancer Inst, 86*, pp. 33-38.

Mayne, S. T., Redlich, C. A., & Cullen, M. R. (1998). Dietary vitamin A and prevalence of bronchial metaplasia in asbestos-exposed workers. *Am J Clin Nutr, 68*, pp. 630-635.

Mountain, C. F. (1997). Revisions in the international system for staging lung cancer. *Chest., 111*, pp. 1710-1717.

Omenn, G. S., Goodman, G. E., Thornquist, M. D., et al. (1996). Effects of a combination of beta carotene and vitamin A on lung cancer and cardiovascular disease. *N Engl J Med, 334*, pp. 1150-1155.

Paice, J. (1999). Pain. In Yarbro, C. H., Frogge, M. H., & Goodman, M. (Eds.). *Cancer symptom management* (pp. 118-147). Boston: Jones and Bartlett.

Sitton, E. (2000). Superior vena cava syndrome. In Yarbro, C. H., Frogge, M. H., Goodman, M., & Groenwald, S. L. (Eds.). *Cancer nursing: Principles and practice* (pp. 900-912). Boston: Jones and Bartlett.

Sivesind, D. M., & Rohaly-Davis, J. A. (1998). Coping with cancer: Patient issues. In Burke, C. C. (Ed.). *Psychosocial dimensions of oncology nursing care* (pp. 4-26). Pittsburgh: Oncology Nursing Press.

Tobacco Use and Dependence Clinical Practice Guideline Panel. (2000). A clinical guideline for treating tobacco use and dependence, *JAMA, 283*, pp. 3244-3254.

U.S. Department of Health and Human Services. (2000). *Healthy people 2010: Conference edition.* Washington, DC: Author.

Wickham, R. (1999). Nausea and vomiting. In Yarbro, C. H., Frogge, M. H., & Goodman, M. (Eds.). *Cancer symptom management* (pp. 228-263). Boston: Jones and Bartlett.

Wingo, P. A., Giovino, G. A., Miller, D. S., et al. (1999). Annual report to the nation on the status of cancer, 1973-1996, with a special section on lung cancer and tobacco smoking. *J Natl Cancer Inst, 91*, pp. 675-690.

Wrede-Seaman, L. (1996). *Symptom management algorithms for palliative care.* Yakima, Washington: Janssen.

3 Colorectal Cancer

Nancy Jo Bush

CASE | STUDY

Mr. Smith is a 64-year-old African American man who presented to his primary physician with a history of blood in his stool for 2 months' duration. He initially suspected that his hemorrhoids caused the bleeding. Mr. Smith is reassured that the first step is to determine the exact cause of the blood in his stools and from that point the physician can discuss treatment.

QUESTIONS

1. The physician initially suspects a colorectal malignancy. In terms of causes of cancer deaths overall in the United States, how is colorectal cancer ranked?
- **a.** First
- **b.** Second
- **c.** Third
- **d.** Fourth

2. The incidence of colorectal malignancies increases significantly in which of the following age groups?
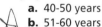
- **a.** 40-50 years
- **b.** 51-60 years
- **c.** 61-70 years
- **d.** 71 years or older

3. The mortality rates from colorectal cancer are increasing in which group?
- **a.** African Americans
- **b.** Hispanics
- **c.** Caucasians
- **d.** Asians

ANSWERS

1. The incidence and mortality from colorectal cancer for men and women in the United States is second only to lung cancer. It is the third leading cause of cancer deaths in the United States for men and women and the second leading cause of cancer deaths overall. Estimated new cases in the year 2000 are 131,200; 93,800 from colon cancer and 36,400 from rectal cancer. The annual death rate from colorectal cancer is 56,300—46,600 from colon cancer and 8300 from rectal cancer (American Cancer Society [ACS], 2000). *Answer 1:* **b.**

2. Colorectal cancer affects both genders equally, although rectal and anal cancer is seen more commonly in men than in woman. The incidence of colorectal cancer increases with age, with the risk beginning at age 40. The mean age at diagnosis is 60 to 65 years (Saddler & Ellis, 1999). *Answer 2:* **c.**

3. The mortality rates for both men and women have decreased in the past 20 years, reflecting decreasing incidence rates and earlier detection; an exception is that the incidence and mortality rates for African American men continues to rise (ACS, 2000). The differences in incidence and mortality rates attributable to race and ethnicity may be the result of socioeconomic factors (Saddler & Ellis, 1999). Colorectal cancer occurs most commonly in Western industrialized countries (Northern America, Northern Europe, and New Zealand); incidence is lowest in Third World countries. *Answer 3:* **a.**

Case Study continued

The initial assessment of Mr. Smith's history shows that he has always been in relatively good health. He smoked a pack of cigarettes a day for 20 years but stopped 10 years ago. He drinks socially (a few beers a week). Mr. Smith tried to eat a balanced diet, but states that during workdays he is prone to indulge in fast food. He has not really noticed any change in bowel habits, although he has been using laxatives as he gets older because it is harder to move his bowels. Even with laxative use, Mr. Smith notes more discomfort and constipation in recent months.

Mr. Smith is a poor historian but thought his father died of some sort of cancer, possibly colon or prostate. His mother died of breast cancer when she was in her early forties. Mr. Smith has two siblings and three children who are alive and well. He is currently a high school principal but plans to retire in 1 year.

QUESTIONS

4. What risk factors in Mr. Smith's health history relate to colorectal cancer?
   a. Age greater than 50 years, race, gender
   b. Age greater than 60 years, gender, cigarette history
   c. Age greater than 60 years, race, dietary habits
   d. Race, occupation, laxative use

5. You also know that several genetic premalignant polyposis syndromes are associated with an increased risk of colorectal cancer. These include all of the following *except:*
   a. Familial adenomatous polyposis (FAP) coli
   b. Huntington's chorea
   c. Hereditary nonpolyposis colorectal cancer (HNPCC)
   d. Lynch II syndrome

6. Which of the following chronic illnesses increases the risk of a person developing colorectal cancer?
   a. Diverticulitis
   b. Pancreatitis
   c. Cholecystitis
   d. Crohn's disease

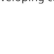

ANSWERS

4. The specific causes of colorectal cancers are not known, but research indicates that environment, nutrition, genetic factors, and predisposing illnesses such as bowel disorders may contribute (Murphy, 1997; Saddler & Ellis, 1999). Diet is an important factor to consider when evaluating the risks for colon cancer. Persons who migrate to the United States from low-incidence countries such as Asia assume the same colon cancer risk of their adoptive country if they assimilate diets rich in saturated animal fats and cholesterol. This supportive evidence suggests that diet and environment both play a role in colorectal cancer (Gold & Sakurai, 1996; Saddler & Ellis, 1999). Furthermore, diets that are also high in refined carbohydrates and low in fiber, vitamins (A, C, E), selenium, and calcium have demonstrated additional risk, especially in Western countries (Gold & Sakurai, 1996).

Carcinogens such as charbroiled meats, fish, and fried foods are also considered contributing factors. Fats and meat products may actually alter the normal concentration of cholesterol and bile salts, thus serving as cancer promoters by damaging the colonic epithelium and increasing the proliferation of the colonic epithelial cells. Reduced dietary fiber acts as a promoting factor by increasing the contact time between carcinogenic substances and the colonic mucosa, which increases the potential for mutagenic changes. *Answer 4:* **c.**

5. Family history and genetic factors also play a role in the development of colorectal cancer. Individuals with first-degree relatives who have had colorectal cancer have a threefold risk of having the disease (Murphy, 1997). This risk is greatest with two first-degree relatives having had colon cancer or if the colon cancer was diagnosed before the age of 50 years (Saddler & Ellis, 1999). Persons with a family history of genetic premalignant polyposis syndromes are at a greater risk. In Mr. Smith's case, he is unsure of his family history, but further questioning may help him identify specific familial patterns. Familial polyposis syndromes (FAP, Gardner's, Turcot, and Peutz-Jeghers) are autosomal dominant and manifested by thousands of colonic adenomas that have a high malignant potential. Any polyp more than 2 cm is considered high risk (Gold & Sakurai, 1996). In the case of FAP, thousands of polyps develop in the colon and rectum in late adolescence, and these individuals have a 100% risk of developing colon cancer (Saddler & Ellis, 1999).

HNPCC is another autosomal-dominant inherited condition. This disease is characterized by the development of one or multiple adenomatous polyps, but not polyposis as in the case of FAP. Patients with HNPCC develop colon cancer at the mean age of 45 years, and these cancers occur as two different types: (1) type A, Lynch type I, a familial, site-specific, nonpolyposis colon cancer, and (2) type B, Lynch type II, a nonpolyposis colon cancer associated with family cancer syndrome, which is an autosomal-dominant predisposition for adenocarcinomas of all types, especially colon, ovary, breast, and endometrium (Saddler & Ellis, 1999). In taking a family history, it is important to note a history of any member who has had ovarian, breast, or uterine cancer. A personal history of any of these cancers also increases the risk of developing a colorectal cancer. Other genetic abnormalities can also trigger chromosomal and oncogenic changes causing epithelial mutations that form malignant tumors in the colon. These include the adenomatous polyposis coli (APC) gene, K-ras oncogene, p53 suppressor gene, mutated in colon cancer (MCC) gene, and the deleted in colon cancer (DCC) gene (Workman, 1996). *Answer 5:* **b.**

6. Bowel disorders may also contribute to a risk for colorectal cancer. Polyposis adenomas, the most common type of bowel polyps (accounting for 80% of polyps), increase their malignant potential as they grow larger (over 10 to 15 years) and cellular changes occur (Murphy, 1997). Villous adenomas (which produce excessive mucus) are approximately 10 times more likely to become cancerous than polyps (Gold & Sakurai, 1996). Inflammatory bowel disorders (e.g., ulcerative colitis, Crohn's disease) are associated with dysplasia and malignant lesions—approximately a thirtyfold increase in risk, depending on the disease duration and involvement (Gold & Sakurai, 1996). Although chronic inflammatory bowel disease is present in only approximately 1% of patients with newly diagnosed colorectal cancer, it clearly defines a subgroup of patients at increased risk over the general population (Goosenberg, 1997). Finally, persons with a personal history of colorectal cancer are also at an increased risk for either a local recurrence at the site of the initial surgical anastomosis or a secondary primary malignancy of the colon (Saddler & Ellis, 1999). *Answer 6:* **d.**

Case Study continued

When taking Mr. Smith's medical history you notice that he appears anxious and uncomfortable. He admits that he rarely sought medical treatment and has not been to a doctor "in years." He expresses that although he has always been in good health, he has been feeling somewhat fatigued the last few months, and he has "lost a few pounds." He has never followed an exercise program and feels tired after a full day's work at the office.

QUESTIONS

7. Based on established guidelines, Mr. Smith should have had his first rectal examination for early detection of colorectal cancer at what age?
   a. 30
   b. 40
   c. 50
   d. 60

8. Screening of high-risk populations with a family history of colorectal cancer is considered which of the following?
   a. Primary prevention
   b. Secondary prevention
   c. Tertiary prevention
   d. High-risk prevention

9. Chemoprevention for colorectal cancer includes which of the following?
   a. Nonsteroidal antiinflammatory drugs (NSAIDs)
   b. Aspirin
   c. Calcium
   d. All of these

10. What explanation for performing a rectal examination do you give to Mr. Smith?
   a. Presence of stool confirms a functioning bowel
   b. Presence of cancer can be ruled out with a digital rectal examination (DRE)
   c. Blood in the stool can be detected with a DRE
   d. Chronic laxative use decreases rectal sphincter tone over time, contributing to constipation

ANSWERS

7. The ACS (2000) recommends that asymptomatic persons begin early detection screening beginning at age 50. *Answer 7:* **c.**

8. Primary prevention of colorectal cancers focuses on risks that can be minimized or controlled in an effort to prevent carcinogenic changes. A high-fiber, low-fat diet that includes cruciferous vegetables (e.g., broccoli, cabbage, brussel sprouts) has been the main focus of primary prevention for colorectal cancer. Adequate weight control and exercise are also important as a means of reducing body fat stores and decreasing risk. Mr. Smith's dietary habits (e.g., fast food) and his sedentary lifestyle are noted risk factors for colorectal cancer.

Secondary prevention focuses on identifying high-risk individuals, including those with a family history of colorectal cancer, hereditary syndromes, or precancerous conditions such as inflammatory bowel disease (Olson, Morrison, & Ashley, 1998a, 1998b). Dietary interventions aimed at preventing polyp production in patients identified at high risk are currently being investigated. Two recent studies showed no evidence that diet affects the growth of precancerous lesions in persons who had previous polyps removed. Follow-up in both studies and other studies are needed to determine whether dietary changes affect the molecular genetic characteristics of polyps. Even in light of this research, a high-fiber, low-fat diet consisting of fruits and vegetables is encouraged to improve overall health and prevent chronic disease (Studies investigate, 2000). *Answer 8:* **b.**

9. Chemoprevention is a new strategy that focuses on blocking the action of carcinogens at the cellular level before the appearance of cancer. Research trials have been under way to identify agents that interfere with carcinogen formation, that act by detoxifying carcinogens, or that directly inhibit or prevent the development of colorectal cancer (Gold & Sakurai, 1996).

Calcium carbonate is thought to bind endogenous bile acids in the intestines, preventing cytotoxic damage to the epithelial cells of the colon. NSAIDs and long-term low-dose aspirin are believed to prevent carcinogenesis by reducing proinflammatory prostaglandin production (COX-2 inhibitors, 2000; Saddler & Ellis, 1999). Multiple epidemiologic studies have demonstrated that people who have taken aspirin for at least 10 years have approximately a 50% reduction in their risk of colorectal cancer (COX-2 inhibitors). Celecoxib (Celebrex), a COX-2 inhibitor, was most recently approved by the U.S. Food and Drug Administration (FDA) for polyp reduction in patients with FAP (Celebrex is approved, 2000). Other preventive measures under investigation include reductions in smoking and alcohol consumption and the use of hormone replacement therapy in postmenopausal women (Saddler & Ellis, 1999). *Answer 9:* **d.**

10. Screening and early detection guidelines for colorectal cancer have been clearly defined (Table 3-1). The goal of screening for colorectal cancer is twofold: to detect early-stage adenocarcinomas and to detect and remove adenomatous polyps, which are precursors of cancerous lesions (Smith, Mettlin, Davis, & Eyre, 2000). The ACS (2000) recommends that asymptomatic persons begin early detection screening beginning at age 50. The ACS recommends three options for colorectal surveillance: the fecal occult blood test (FOBT), flexible sigmoidoscopy, and colonoscopy. A DRE should be done at age 50 and repeated thereafter at the same time as a sigmoidoscopy, colonoscopy, or double-contrast barium enema. Annual DRE alone is no longer recommended because of its low sensitivity (Smith, et al., 2000). People with a personal or strong family history of colorectal cancer or adenomatous polyps and people with a personal history of inflammatory bowel disease should begin colorectal screening earlier or undergo screening more often as determined by their primary health care practitioner (ACS, 2000). *Answer 10:* **c.**

| TABLE 3-1 | American Cancer Society Recommendations for the Early Detection of Colorectal Cancer in Average-Risk, Asymptomatic People, Age 50+ |||

TEST OR PROCEDURE	FREQUENCY	INDICATIONS
Digital rectal examination (DRE)	Beginning at age 50; thereafter, before FSIG, colonoscopy, or DCBE	Low in sensitivity; detects low rectal/anal lesions; limited to few centimeters
FOBT and FSIG	Annual FOBT and FSIG at age 50; thereafter, FOBT every year and FSIG every 5 yr	FOBT: inexpensive; easy to perform; false negatives; FSIG: visualizes to 60 cm; rectal and sigmoid colon. FOBT requires dietary preparation and serial specimens; positive FOBT must be followed up by additional testing; positive FSIG must be followed up with colonoscopy for biopsy
DCBE	*or* DCBE at age 50; thereafter every 5-10 yr	Diagnostic of lesions >5 mm and up to splenic flexure; more diagnostic than barium enema
Colonoscopy	*or* Colonoscopy at age 50; thereafter, every 10 yr	Visualizes into transverse colon; allows for biopsy of lesions, should be done on high-risk individuals

Adapted from Gold, S. C., & Sakurai, C. (1996). Colorectal cancer. In McCorkle, R., Grant, M., Frank-Stromberg, M., & Baird, S. B. (Eds.). *Cancer nursing: A comprehensive textbook*, 2nd ed (pp. 652-676). Philadelphia: WB Saunders; and Smith, R. A., Mettlin, Cl. J., Davis, K. J., & Eyre, H. (2000). American Cancer Society guidelines for the early detection of cancer. *CA Cancer J Clin, 50*, pp. 34-49.
DCBE, Double-contrast barium enema; *FOBT*, fecal occult blood test; *FSIG*, flexible sigmoidoscopy.
Note: The ACS recommends three options for colorectal surveillance beginning at age 50: FOBT and FSIG, with FOBT repeated annually and FSIG repeated every 5 years; or total colon examination with DCBE every 5-10 years; or colonoscopy every 10 years.

Case Study continued

Upon further inquiry, Mr. Smith states that he has been experiencing some abdominal bloating and heartburn, sometimes relieved by lansoprazole (Prevacid). He denies abdominal pain but states that constipation exacerbates the feelings of abdominal fullness and discomfort. You perform a thorough physical examination focusing upon the gastrointestinal (GI) system.

QUESTIONS

11. During palpation of the right upper quadrant, Mr. Smith pulls away slightly, appearing that he is guarding. What further examination should you carry out?

a. Percussion above and below the normal area of the liver to identify the size and span of the liver and the liver's edge

b. Ballottement for any suspected masses by thrusting the fingers of the right hand suddenly and forcefully into the area of the suspected mass

c. Assessment for the presence of rebound tenderness, which occurs after the sudden release of deep pressure on the abdomen

d. Determination of whether the patient feels pain when you press lightly or deeply into the abdomen

12. What abnormality might lead you to evaluate for peristaltic waves?

a. Pain on palpation

b. Abdominal distension

c. Hypoactive bowel sounds

d. Aortic bruit

13. Which physical assessment finding is suggestive of obstruction?

a. Abdominal muscle weakness

b. Palpated liver 2 cm below costal margin

c. High pitched bowel sounds in right upper quadrant

d. Rebound tenderness

14. Which of the following would you expect to find if Mr. Smith had a tumor in the ascending colon?

a. Bright red blood in the stool

b. Tenesmus

c. Gas pains

d. Palpable mass

15. Evaluating Mr. Smith's history and physical examination, you know that the clinical features of colorectal cancer are most directly related to which of the following?

a. Patient's dietary history

b. Patient's history of inflammatory bowel disease

c. Location of the tumor in the bowel

d. Patient's bowel habits

ANSWERS

11. Mr. Smith's tenderness upon palpation of the right upper quadrant may indicate liver metastases. Further examination should include palpation and percussion for the size and span of the liver and location of the liver's edge (Leasia & Monahan, 1997). *Answer 11:* **a.**

12. Mr. Smith's abdominal distension should lead you to evaluate for ascites by seeing whether you can elicit peristaltic waves. Ascites is a late symptom of colorectal cancer. Other signs of advanced malignancy include palpation of an abdominal mass, hepatomegaly, or splenomegaly. *Answer 12:* **b.**

13. The physical examination should include inspection, auscultation, and then palpation of the abdomen. Inspection may demonstrate abnormalities such as abdominal distension and peristaltic waves, whereas high-pitched or absent bowel sounds on auscultation may indicate obstruction. *Answer 13:* **c.**

14. A tumor in the ascending colon may present with a palpable abdominal mass. Any patient who presents with anemia must be worked up for occult GI bleeding related to the malignancy if hematologic causes are ruled out. The aim of the FOBT is to discover blood in the stool that occurs from colorectal cancer or commonly from polyps larger than 2 cm (Smith, et al., 2000). *Answer 14:* **d.**

15. The signs and symptoms of colorectal cancer are most directly related to the physiology of the bowel and the location of the tumor (Table 3-2). Most primary colonic lesions are located in the proximal bowel: sigmoid and descending colon (52%), transverse colon (16%), and cecum and ascending colon (32%) (Cameron, 1994). Symptoms may range from anorexia, weight loss, and vague abdominal pain to more evident symptoms such as constipation, blood in the stool, and a palpable mass. Signs strongly suggesting cancer include a palpable abdominal or rectal mass and blood in the feces. *Answer 15:* **c.**

TABLE 3-2	Signs and Symptoms of Colorectal Cancer
LOCATION	**CLINICAL FEATURES**
Ascending colon	Dull vague abdominal pain; may radiate to the back
	Dark or mahogany red blood in the stool
	Anemia as a result of bleeding
	Fatigue/malaise caused by anemia
	Anorexia and weight loss
	Rare obstruction
	Palpable abdominal mass
Transverse colon	Blood in stool
	Changes in bowel habits
	Potential bowel obstruction
Descending colon	Bright red bleeding mixed with stool
	Changes in bowel habits
	Colicky pain
	Anorexia; nausea and vomiting
	Decreased caliber of stool (pencil stools)
	Rectal pressure, incomplete evacuation of stool
	Constipation alternating with diarrhea
Rectum	Bright red bleeding coating the stool
	Changes in bowel habits; constipation or diarrhea
	Rectal urgency
	Tenesmus
	Sense of incomplete evacuation
	Perineal and buttock pain
Anus	Bleeding
	Pain on defecation
	Sensation of a mass
	Severe anal itching

Adapted from Nakagaki, D. K., & Hiromoto, B. M. (1997). Colorectal cancer. In Gates, R. A., & Fink, R. M. (Eds.). *Oncology nursing secrets* (pp. 150-156). Philadelphia: Hanley & Belfus; and Murphy, M. E. (1997). Colorectal cancers. In Otto, S. E. (Ed.). *Oncology nursing*, 3rd ed (pp. 124-139). St. Louis: Mosby.

Case Study continued

Assessment of Mr. Smith's GI system reveals the following:

- Tenderness to light palpation in the right upper quadrant
- Slightly distended abdomen
- Bowel sounds (BS) (+) × 4
- Negative peristalsis
- Negative bruit
- Negative hepatosplenomegaly (HSM)
- Negative costovertebral angle (CVA) tenderness

- Negative rebound tenderness
- Negative palpable mass

Findings also included hemoccult-positive stool and a hemoglobin level of 11 g/dl. Additional preliminary tests and a colonoscopy are ordered.

QUESTIONS

16. Which of the following is a major differential diagnosis that must be considered for right upper quadrant tenderness?
   a. Diverticulitis
   b. Cholecystitis
   c. Intestinal obstruction
   d. Peptic ulcer

17. In addition to a complete blood count, all of the following laboratory data would be pertinent to order for Mr. Smith *except*:
   a. Total iron-binding capacity
   b. AST *liver*
   c. Lactate dehydrogenase
   d. Blood urea nitrogen (BUN) *renal*

18. Which tumor marker should you order during the initial workup of Mr. Smith?
   a. AFP
   b. Human chorionic gonadotropin (HCG)
   c. Carcinoembryonic antigen (CEA)
   d. CA 19-9

19. Which of the following is another late symptom of colorectal cancer?
   a. A change in bowel habits
   b. Blood in the stool
   c. Weight loss
   d. Abdominal pain

ANSWER

16. Differential diagnosis of abdominal pain in adults involves ruling out common causes such as gastroenteritis, peptic ulcer disease, irritable bowel syndrome, appendicitis, cholecystitis, diverticulitis, and pancreatitis (Seller, 1996). All of these conditions can present with acute or sudden onset of abdominal pain or cause intermittent or recurrent abdominal pain, as in Mr. Smith's case. The finding of RUQ tenderness could indicate cholecystitis, whereas tenderness in the LLQ is suggestive of irritable colon or diverticulitis (Seller, 1996). Mr. Smith did not present with other symptoms related to cholecystitis (e.g., colicky pain, nausea, vomiting, dark urine, light stool, jaundice). Associated symptoms of a colonic tumor that are present include abdominal distension, anemia, constipation, decreased effectiveness of

TABLE 3-3 Diagnostic Testing for Colorectal Cancer	
DIAGNOSTIC TESTS	**INDICATIONS**
Complete blood count (CBC)	Check hemoglobin and hematocrit levels indicative of anemia/ blood loss
Alkaline phosphatase (ALP)	Ectopic production by neoplasm causes elevations
Aspartate aminotransferase (ASP)	Liver function
Blood urea nitrogen (BUN)	Renal function
Chest radiograph	Pulmonary status
Computed tomography (CT) scan of the abdomen and pelvis	Important for diagnostic workup; evaluates liver and periaortic nodes for metastases
Carcinoembryonic antigen (CEA)	Nonspecific tumor marker; not recommended for screening but helpful with other findings to indicate possibility of colon carcinoma; used to monitor treatment and recurrence

laxatives, weight loss, anorexia, and blood in the stool. Anorexia, weight loss, and anemia are often indicative of late-stage disease (Seller, 1996). *Answer 16:* **b.**

17. Diagnostic laboratory tests for Mr. Smith should include a complete blood count, liver (AST) and renal function (BUN) tests, and tumor markers such as alkaline phosphatase (ALP) and a baseline carcinoembryonic antigen (CEA) (Table 3-3). *Answer 17:* **a.**

18. Tumor markers are biochemical markers that can be detected in the bloodstream as tissue becomes abnormal (Gold & Sakurai, 1996). CEA is a nonspecific marker for colorectal cancer; normal CEA is less than 2.5 ng/ml for nonsmokers and less than 5.0 ng/ml for smokers. CEA is not recommended for screening because of its low sensitivity and specificity, especially in the early stages of disease. However, elevated serum levels can be used in conjunction with other findings to make the decision to perform diagnostic workup for colon carcinoma (Wallach, 1996). If the CEA is elevated before surgical resection and falls to normal postoperatively, it can be used as an indicator of tumor burden and to monitor recurrence. Antigens such as colon-specific antigen (CSA) and colon-specific antigen protein (CSAP) are currently being evaluated for their usefulness in the detection and monitoring of colorectal cancers (Murphy, 1997). Remaining diagnostic tests should include chest radiograph and computed tomography scan of the abdomen and pelvis. Definitive diagnosis of colorectal cancer is confirmed by tissue biopsy of the suspicious site after initial assessment and screening tests are carried out (Strohl, 1998). *Answer 18:* **c.**

19. Weight loss, anorexia, and anemia often indicate late-stage disease (Seller, 1996). *Answer 19:* **c.**

Case Study continued

Colonoscopy revealed a 6-cm villous lesion in the ascending colon. Mr. Smith underwent surgery. His cancer is staged as stage III, Duke's C2. Liver biopsies were negative for metastases, and his postoperative CEA was 0.6 ng/ml.

QUESTIONS

20. Which of the following levels of tumor penetration define a stage C2 diagnosis?
- **a.** Into the muscularis layer
- **b.** Through the muscularis into serosa or perirectal fat
- **c.** Into the muscularis with positive regional lymph nodes
- **d.** Into the serosa or perirectal fat with positive regional lymph nodes

21. What surgical procedure will Mr. Smith be advised to undergo?
- **a.** Hemicolectomy
- **b.** Colostomy
- **c.** Abdominoperineal resection
- **d.** None of these

22. What treatment will most likely be recommended for Mr. Smith postoperatively?
- **a.** Follow-up only
- **b.** 5-Fluoruracil–based chemotherapy
- **c.** 5-Flroruracil–based chemotherapy with radiation therapy
- **d.** Radiation therapy only

23. What drug is used in combination with fluorouracil as the standard care for locally advanced colorectal cancer?
- **a.** Levamisole
- **b.** Leucovorin
- **c.** Xeloda
- **d.** Irinotecan

20. Mr. Smith's stage III, Duke's C2 is based on the Astler-Collier modification of the Duke's staging system combined with the TNM system for colorectal carcinoma (Table 3-4). Mr. Smith's tumor has penetrated through the muscularis into the serosa, and his regional lymph nodes are positive. *Answer 20:* **d.**

21. The primary treatment for colorectal cancer is surgical resection. Even in late stage disease, surgery is often recommended to prevent the risk of bleeding or obstruction (Nakagaki & Hiromoto, 1997). The surgical procedure of choice for resectable disease is an en bloc resection of the colon, called a *hemicolectomy* (NCCN, 1996). Low anterior resection or abdominoperineal resections are indicated for rectal carcinomas, depending on the proximity of the tumor to the anal sphincter. Sphincter-sparing approaches include transanal resection, posterior proctectomy, and a coloanal pull-through (Cohn, 1994). Small tumors may be resected with an adequate margin so that a colostomy is not necessary; a permanent colostomy may be needed if the tumor is large, making end-to-end anastomosis impossible, or if the tumor is in the rectum or anus (Strohl, 1998). The principles of

surgical resection include (1) intraabdominal assessment, (2) confirmation of visceral metastases, (3) mesenteric and nodal dissection, (4) adequate margins of resection, and (5) anastomosis or the creation of a stoma when applicable (Greene, 1999). *Answer 21:* **a.**

22. Recommended treatment for patients with stage III carcinoma of the colon is 5-fluorouracil–based adjuvant chemotherapy (NCCN, 1996). Patients with stage III node-positive disease have a risk as high as 70% of recurrence and death during the 5 years following surgical resection (McDonald, 1999).

Radiation therapy would not be recommended for Mr. Smith at this time. Radiation therapy is a major part of treatment for rectal cancer (tumors below the peritoneal reflection) but is not used to treat colon cancer (McDonald, 1999). Radiation therapy is indicated preoperatively to reduce bulky rectal tumors, to improve the rate of surgical resectability, and to eradicate microscopic disease. In stage B or C rectal cancers, radiation may be used postoperatively to prevent local recurrence or to eliminate remaining disease in the case of positive surgical margins (Nakagaki & Hiromoto, 1997). The role of radiation therapy in colon cancer is treating metastatic disease to other organs (e.g., bladder, abdominal wall), as palliative treatment for painful metastases, or to prevent obstruction or control bleeding in inoperable patients (Nakagaki & Hiromoto, 1997). Innovative treatments for colorectal cancer include intraoperative radiation therapy and stereotactic radiation therapy (Iwamoto, 1999). *Answer 22:* **b.**

23. Adjuvant therapy of colon cancer was first recommended in 1990 based on the results of clinical trials showing survival benefits for stage III colon cancer with 5-Fluorouracil plus levamisole. Recent studies have shown that 5-fluorouracil plus leucovorin-based regimens for 6 months is equivalent to 5-fluorouracil plus levamisole for 12 months. Leucovorin is a vitamin that enhances the effectiveness of 5-fluorouracil. It is still unclear whether adjuvant therapy offers any significant survival benefit for patients with stage II colon cancer (McDonald, 1999). *Answer 23:* **b.**

Case Study continued

Following colon resection, Mr. Smith received 5-fluorouracil and leucovorin for 6 months. He tolerated the treatment well, with minimal adverse effects. He maintained his weight and appetite, and his CEA level remained normal.

TABLE **3-4** Staging Systems for Colorectal Cancer
ASTLER-COLLER MODIFICATION OF DUKE'S CLASSIFICATION
Stage A: tumor confined to the mucosa of the intestine
Stage B1: tumor penetrates into the muscularis layer of the intestine
Stage B2: tumor penetrates through the muscularis into serosa or perirectal fat
Stage C1: B1 with positive regional lymph nodes
Stage C2: B2 with positive regional lymph nodes
Stage D: Metastatic disease
STAGE GROUPINGS BASED ON TNM STAGING
Stage 0: T_{is}, N_0, M_0
Stage I: T_1 or T_2, N_0, M_0 (Duke's A)
Stage II: T_3 or T_4, N_0, M_0 (Duke's B)
Stage III: Any T; N_1, N_2, or N_3; M_0 (Duke's C)
Stage IV: Any T, any N, M+ (Duke's D)

Adapted from Nakagaki, D. K., & Hiromoto, B. M. (1997). Colorectal cancer. In Gates, R. A., & Fink, R. M. (Eds.). *Oncology nursing secrets* (pp. 150-156). Philadelphia: Hanley & Belfus.

QUESTIONS

24. Adverse effects of combination 5-fluorouracil and leucovorin include all of the following *except:*
- **a.** Anaphylaxis
- **b.** Myelosuppression
- **c.** Stomatitis
- **d.** Diarrhea

25. What is the most common site of colorectal metastases?
- **a.** Adrenal glands
- **b.** Liver
- **c.** Bone
- **d.** Brain

ANSWERS

24. Overall, the regimen of 5-fluorouracil and leucovorin is well tolerated by most patients. There are many different doses and schedules of this protocol (Cohen, 1999), and adverse reactions depend on specific drug administration (e.g., continuous infusion versus bolus) and individual patient tolerance. A common schedule of weekly boluses of 5-fluorouracil with leucovorin infusion may prevent side effects that can occur with 5-day courses of 5-fluorouracil (e.g., alopecia) or those that can occur with continuous infusions of high-dose 5-fluorouracil (e.g., phlebitis). The myelosuppressive effects of 5-fluorouracil are dose–related, and the toxicity is enhanced by the combination effect of leucovorin sodium (Wilkes, Ingwersen, & Barton-Burke, 2000). The nadir is 10 to 14 days after drug administration, with neutropenia and thrombocytopenia being the most likely result. Stomatitis is a severe adverse reaction that may herald severe bone marrow suppression; diarrhea may be a dose-limiting toxicity. Other common adverse reactions include changes in skin integrity and pigmentation, photosensitivity and photophobia, and dacryocystitis (an inflammation of the tear ducts and lacrimal gland). Neurologic effects (e.g., cerebellar ataxia, disorientation, euphoria, altered gait, nystagmus) are rare but may require discontinuation of treatment (Wilkes, Ingwersen, & Barton-Burke, 2000). *Answer 24:* **a.**

25. The most common site of metastases from colorectal cancer is the liver (Saddler & Ellis, 1999). This tendency to metastasize to the liver is because of the colon's venous drainage via the portal system (Nakagaki & Hiromoto, 1997; Saddler & Ellis, 1999). Liver metastases may also occur as a result of lymphatic spread, via the hepatic arterial circulation, or by direct tumor invasion (Saddler & Ellis, 1999). In contrast, rectal cancer has the

propensity to metastasize to the lungs because venous drainage is mainly via the middle and inferior hemorrhoidal veins to the vena cava. The peritoneum is another common site of disease spread. Colorectal cancer rarely spreads to the brain, bone, ovaries, or adrenal glands (Nakagaki & Hiromoto, 1997). *Answer 25:* **b.**

Case Study continued

At the time of a follow-up examination 1 year later, Mr. Smith's CEA is 7 ng/ml. Repeat staging examinations reveal a single 8-cm hepatic metastasis.

QUESTIONS

26. Mr. Smith and his wife are understandably distressed regarding the recurrence of his disease. They ask you if there is any hope for curative treatment. What is the best response?
- **a.** "Once the cancer has recurred, the only hope is for disease control."
- **b.** "There are possible treatments for liver metastases, but hope for cure is impossible."
- **c.** "Liver metastases is very serious, so you should just hope for as much time left as possible."
- **d.** "Treatments are available for liver metastases. Further evaluation is necessary, and you should discuss the possible treatment options with your physician."

27. Which of the following is a quality-of-life issue most relevant to patients with progressive colorectal cancer?
- **a.** Social functioning
- **b.** Financial impact of the disease
- **c.** Sexual functioning
- **d.** Nausea and vomiting

28. All of the following are emerging treatments for metastatic colorectal cancer *except:*
1. Irinotecan
2. Oxaliplatin
3. Capecitabine
4. Gemcitabine
   - **a.** 1, 2, & 3
   - **b.** 2, 3, & 4
   - **c.** 1, 3, & 4
   - **d.** All of these

ANSWERS

26. The impact of disease recurrence is overwhelming to the patient and family because in many cases, this means that the hope for cure is gone. When the patient and family are facing this realization, it is important to reframe their hopes within the possible treatment outcomes for disease control or remission. In the case of Mr. Smith, a hepatic lobectomy may be an option because there is only one single, solitary nodule. Unfortunately, in many cases surgical resection is not possible because multiple segments of the liver are involved (Saddler & Ellis, 1999). Newer techniques, such as hepatic cryosurgery and stereotactic radiation therapy, are showing promise in controlling unresectable hepatic metastases (Iwamoto, 1999; Saddler & Ellis, 1999). It is important that the available treatment options for Mr. Smith be investigated and discussed with his physician to provide him with both a realistic understanding of his disease status and to ensure that he and his wife regain feelings of control and emotional equilibrium. *Answer 26:* **d.**

27. Relatively little research has been published addressing the long-term quality of life for colorectal cancer patients (Grant, 1999). The surgical interventions and adjuvant treatments necessary for this disease challenge a patient's most intimate physical, social, and sexual well-being. Stoma patients are confronted with changes in body image, feelings of social stigma, and social isolation related to embarrassing bowel function. Both stoma and nonstoma patients may experience changes in sexual functioning related to surgical intervention (Grant, 1999). Men may have erectile and ejaculatory problems with the severing of nerves from an abdominoperineal resection. For women, surgical dissection, in which the vagina is separated from the rectum, may cause a decrease in the length of the vagina, a lack of lubrication, or discomfort with intercourse (Strohl, 1998). In several studies impaired sexual functioning has been shown to be more common for patients with stomas. However, sexuality is also challenged for patients who undergo sphincter-saving resection that results in changes in bowel patterns and rectal leakage (Grant, 1999). For patients like Mr. Smith, disease recurrence and further adjuvant treatment also affects quality of life. Adverse effects from chemotherapy or radiation will present specific physical challenges for the patient, and the necessity to adapt to the chronic nature of the illness will present psychologic and emotional challenges for both the patient and family. Nurses are in a unique position to provide the physical and emotional resources necessary to maintain and improve the quality of life for this special population (Grant, 1999). *Answer 27:* **c.**

28. Other therapies are emerging as effective treatments against metastatic or 5-fluorouracil–resistant colorectal cancer. Newer regimens consist of novel agents, such as irinotecan (CPT-11), approved by the FDA to be used alone or in combination with 5-fluorouracil and leucovorin (Viele, 1999). Several clinical trials are currently investigating the role of oxaliplatin, used alone or again in combination with 5-fluorouracil and leucovorin (Rothenberg, 2000). Two new oral agents, tegafur (investigational) and capecitabine (Xeloda) are also among the many new treatments on the horizon. These newer agents used alone or in combination with a 5-fluorouracil/leucovorin regimen may share common side effects (nausea and vomiting, mucositis, diarrhea, dehydration, and skin toxicity) that demand prompt nursing intervention. Specific agents such as CPT-11 also require advanced nursing knowledge and management of dose-limiting toxicities (e.g., secretory diarrhea) (Viele, 1999). *Answer 28:* **a.**

REFERENCES

American Cancer Society (ACS). (2000). *Cancer facts and figures 2000.* Atlanta: Author.

Cameron, R. B. (1994). Malignancies of the colon. In Cameron, R. B. (Ed.). *Practical oncology* (pp. 273-282). Norwalk, CT: Appleton and Lange.

Celebrex is approved for polyp reduction in FAP patients. *Oncol News Intl, 9*(1), pp. 1, 10, 41.

Cohen, A. M. (1999). Colorectal cancer: Evolving concepts in diagnosis, treatment, and prevention. *CA Cancer J Clin, 49*(3), pp. 199-201.

Cohn, A. L. (1994). Colorectal carcinoma. In Wood, M. E., & Bunn, P. A. (Eds.). *Hematology oncology secrets* (pp. 280-281). Philadelphia: Hanley & Belfus.

COX-2 inhibitors new prevention strategy for colon cancer. *Oncol News Intl, 9*(1), p. 11.

Gold, S. C., & Sakurai, C. (1996). Colorectal cancer. In McCorkle, R., Grant, M., Frank-Stromberg, M., & Baird, S. B. (Eds.). *Cancer nursing: A comprehensive textbook,* 2nd ed. (pp. 652- 676). Philadelphia: WB Saunders.

Goosenberg, E. B. (1997). Inflammatory bowel disease flare . . . or colon cancer? *Primary Care Cancer, 17*(8), pp. 26-28, 32.

Greene, F. L. (1999). Laparoscopic management of colorectal cancer. *CA Cancer J Clin, 49*, pp. 221-228.

Grant, M. M. (1999). Quality of life issues in colorectal cancer. *Dev Support Cancer Care, 3*(1), pp. 4-9.

Iwamoto, R. R. (1999). Emerging strategies using radiation therapy for colorectal cancer: Intraoperative radiation therapy and stereotactic radiation therapy. *Dev Support Cancer Care, 3*(1), pp. 10-12.

Leasia, M. S., & Monahan, F. D. (1997). *A practical guide to health assessment.* Philadelphia: WB Saunders.

McDonald, J. S. (1999). Adjuvant therapy of colon cancer. *CA Cancer J Clin, 49*, pp. 202-219.

Murphy, M. E. (1997). Colorectal cancers. In Otto, S. E. (Ed.). *Oncology nursing*, 3rd ed. (pp. 124-139). St. Louis: Mosby.

Nakagaki, D. K., & Hiromoto, B. M. (1997). Colorectal cancer. In Gates, R. A., & Fink, R. M. (Eds.). *Oncology nursing secrets* (pp. 150-156). Philadelphia: Hanley & Belfus.

NCCN. (1996). NCNN colorectal practice guidelines. *Oncology*, *10*(suppl 11), pp. 140-175.

Olson, S. J., Morrison, C. H., & Ashley, B. W. (1998a). Prevention of cancer. In Itano, J. K., & Taoka, K. N. (Eds.). *Core curriculum for oncology nursing*, 3rd ed. (pp. 681-694). Philadelphia: WB Saunders.

Olson, S. J., Morrison, C. H., & Ashley, B. W. (1998b). Screening and early detection of cancer. In Itano, J. K., & Taoka, K. N. (Eds.). *Core curriculum for oncology nursing*, 3rd ed. (pp. 695-710). Philadelphia: WB Saunders.

Rothenberg, M. L. (2000). New options for front-line treatment of metastatic colorectal cancer: A tale of two drugs. *Colorectal Cancer Index Rev*, *1*(2), pp. 4-7.

Saddler, D. A., & Ellis, C. (1999). Colorectal cancer. *Semin Oncol Nurs*, *15*, pp. 58-69.

Seller, R. H. (1996). *Differential diagnosis of common complaints*. Philadelphia: WB Saunders.

Smith, R. A., Mettlin, C. J., Davis, K. J., & Eyre, H. (2000). American Cancer Society guidelines for the early detection of cancer. *CA Cancer J Clin*, *50*, pp. 34-49.

Strohl, R. A. (1998). Nursing care of the client with cancer of the gastrointestinal tract. In Itano, J. K., & Taoka, K. N. (Eds.). *Core curriculum for oncology nursing*, 3rd ed. (pp. 459-483). Philadelphia: WB Saunders.

Studies investigate effects of diet on polyps. *ONS News*, *15*(6), p. 13.

Viele, C. S. (1999). New developments and side effect management for colorectal cancer. *Dev Support Cancer Care*, *3*(1), pp. 13-18.

Wallach, J. (1996). *Interpretation of diagnostic tests*. Boston: Little, Brown.

Wilkes, G. M., Ingwersen, K., & Barton-Burke, M. (2000). *Oncology nursing drug handbook*. Boston: Jones and Bartlett.

Workman, M. L. (1996). Gene therapy. In McCorkle, R., Grant, M., Frank-Stromberg, M., & Baird, S. B. (Eds.). *Cancer nursing: A comprehensive textbook*, 2nd ed. (pp. 458-469). Philadelphia: WB Saunders.

4 Prostate Cancer

Nancy Jo Bush

CASE | STUDY

Bob Gentleman, a 65-year-old African American male, presents to the urology clinic with symptoms of increasing urinary frequency and nocturia of 1 year's duration. He had a genitourinary workup 2 years ago, at which time he states that he was found to have an enlarged prostate. He did not follow up after this examination. He seeks attention now because he saw some blood in his urine stream. He has not had a routine physical examination nor does he recall the results of any blood tests done. "I only had that exam 2 years ago because it was required for my life insurance policy."

His past history is unremarkable except for borderline hypertension that has been treated by exercise and diet. Bob states that he generally feels well. His weight has remained stable, and he has not had any systemic manifestations such as fevers, chills, or night sweats. He denies a history of smoking and drinks beer in moderation. Bob's family history was remarkable in that his father died of "some type of cancer—maybe prostate" and his mother died of a heart attack. He has one sister, alive and well. Bob does not currently take medications, nor does he have known allergies. He works as a broker for an investment firm.

QUESTIONS

1. What two initial examinations are warranted?
   a. Complete blood count (CBC) with differential
   b. Digital rectal examination (DRE) and prostate-specific antigen (PSA)
   c. Ultrasound and flat-plate of the abdomen
   d. Retrograde pyelogram and cystogram

2. All of the following are true regarding DRE *except:*
   a. The median sulcus of the prostate can be felt between the two lateral lobes.
   b. Only the posterior surface of the prostate is palpable.

   c. Benign prostatic hypertrophy (BPH) feels similar to prostate cancer on DRE.
   d. Prostate cancer is associated with a hard, irregular, asymmetric nodule.

3. PSA is:
   a. Produced only by the prostate gland
   b. A nonspecific, nonsensitive assay of prostatic function
   c. Not influenced by patient age
   d. Not influenced by BPH

4. Common causes of PSA elevation include all of the following *except:*
   a. DREs
   b. Prostatitis
   c. BPH
   d. Needle biopsy of the prostate

ANSWERS

1. A thorough urologic examination is warranted and includes a DRE and PSA. Other diagnostics that may be needed include a urinalysis, creatinine level, cystoscopy or intravenous urography, and ultrasound for prostate size and residual volume if the DRE and PSA are inconclusive. *Answer 1:* **b.**

2. A DRE is a necessary component of the urologic assessment and allows for palpation of the prostate gland through the anterior wall of the rectum. On DRE the median sulcus of the prostate can be felt between the two lateral lobes and only the posterior surface of the prostate is palpable. DRE's effectiveness as a screening tool for prostate cancer is limited because only nodules on the posterior lobe may be detected (Lind, 1997). *Answer 2:* **c.**

3. The advent of the PSA blood assay has brought about one of the most significant advances in the management of prostate cancer (Brawer, 1999; Lind, 1997). Although clinical and legal issues abound regarding the use of PSA as a screening tool (Brawer, 1999; Gerard & Frank-Stromberg, 1998; Lind, 1997), this tumor marker is widely used

as a diagnostic tool for prostate cancer. The antigen is a glycoprotein produced only by prostate tissue, and it is therefore prostate specific; however, it increases with inflammation and benign growth, as well as from cancer (Lind, 1997). Common causes of PSA elevation include prostatitis; BPH; and manipulation of the gland with cystoscopy, needle biopsy, or transurethral resection of the prostate (TURP). DRE does not influence or raise the PSA levels causing false-positive results; therefore a DRE may be performed before ordering a PSA (Vestal & Glode, 1994). *Answer 3:* **a.**

4. A normal PSA range is 0 to 4 ng/ml. Elevations of PSA can be present up to 6 months before clinical evidence of disease (Miaskowski, 1999). The normal range of PSA value is influenced by both patient age and ethnicity. PSA values increase with age, and normal values are slightly higher in African American men (Table 4-1). Serum levels may also vary according to the differentiation of the tumor, the volume or bulk of the tumor, and the amount of BPH (Brawer, 1999; Miaskowski, 1999). False-positive PSA results can be both a financial and emotional burden to the patient. A borderline PSA result requires further investigation with transrectal ultrasound (TRUS) to calculate prostate density or to perform an ultrasound-

guided biopsy (Brawer, 1999; Lind, 1997). The patient and family will also experience fear and anxiety related to abnormal PSA results. These dilemmas make it imperative that you consider which recommendations to follow in counseling and managing both asymptomatic patients and those who are at risk (Gerard & Frank-Stromberg, 1998) (Table 4-2). *Answer 4:* **a.**

Case Study continued

On DRE an area of firmness is palpated on Bob's prostate. His PSA is greater than 30 ng/ml.

QUESTIONS

5. Which of the following is true regarding the incidence of prostate cancer?
   a. Incidence rates are now declining.
   b. With the advent of PSA testing, incidence rates climbed dramatically.
   c. Prostate cancer is the second leading cause of cancer death in men.
   d. All of these

6. Bob has all of the following risk factors for prostate cancer *except:*
   a. African American male
   b. Positive family history
   c. Increasing age
   d. BPH

7. Differential diagnosis for prostate cancer must include which of the following?
   a. Diabetic neuropathy
   b. Prostatitis
   c. Stress incontinence
   d. a and b only

ANSWERS

5. The American Cancer Society (ACS; 2000) estimates 180,400 new cases of prostate cancer in the United States during the year 2000. Prostate cancer rates are now declining, although earlier diagnosis in asymptomatic men by the use of PSA has

TABLE 4-1	Age-Specific Reference Ranges for Prostate-Specific Antigen (PSA) Test According to Race		
AGE (YR)	WHITES (NG/ML)	AFRICAN AMERICANS (NG/ML)	
40-49	0.0-2.5	0.0-2.0	
50-59	0.0-3.5	0.0-4.0	
60-69	0.0-3.5	0.0-4.5	
70-79	0.0-3.5	0.0-5.5	

From Morgan, T. A. (1996). Age-specific reference ranges for serum prostate-specific antigen in black men. *N Engl J Med, 335,* pp. 304-310.

TABLE 4-2	Guidelines for Follow-Up of Early Detection for Prostate Cancer with Digital Rectal Examination (DRE) and Serum Prostate-Specific Antigen (PSA)	
	PSA RESULTS	**DRE RESULTS**
	Positive	Negative
0.4 ng/ml	Transrectal ultrasound with biopsy	Follow, with yearly DRE and PSA, assessing rate of change
4-10 ng/ml	Transrectal ultrasound with biopsy	Follow, with yearly DRE and PSA, assessing rate of change; or use transrectal ultrasound to calculate PSA density; if elevated PSA density, biopsy
≥10 ng/ml	Transrectal ultrasound with biopsy	Transrectal ultrasound with biopsy

From Maxwell, M. B. (1993). Cancer of the prostate. *Semin Oncol Nurs, 9,* pp. 237-261.

contributed to a dramatic increase in incidence rates in the previous decade. This disease is the second leading cause of cancer death in men, with an estimated 31,900 deaths in the year 2000 (ACS, 2000). Except for skin cancers, prostate cancer has been said to be the most common malignant disease in humans (von Eschenabach, 1999). The biologic changes associated with prostate cancer are challenging medicine because the disease can remain latent in some men, progress slowly in others, and be virulent and fatal to those most unfortunate (von Eschenabach, 1999). *Answer 5:* **d.**

6. The strongest risk factors for prostate cancer are age, race, and family history (Cook, 1997). Most prostate cancers are diagnosed in men older than 65 years of age. African Americans have the highest incidence rates of prostate cancer in the world (ACS, 2000) and in comparison to white men, they develop the disease at a younger age, have more extensive disease at diagnosis, and have a mortality rate two times greater (Collins, 1997; Cook, 1997). The role of testosterone levels and gene expression for an enzyme called 5α-*reductase* as possible causes for the ethnic differences in prostate cancer are under investigation (Miaskowski, 1999). A positive family history of a first-degree relative, father or brother, also predisposes a man to prostate cancer at a rate two to three times higher than the general population. International studies have supported the possibility that diet, specifically in regard to fats and red meat, may contribute to prostate cancer, possibly by increasing the levels of sex steroid hormones or carcinogens released at time of cooking (ACS, 2000; Miaskowski, 1999). Occupational exposures to cadmium, farming, and rubber manufacturing continue to be investigated. The role of other possible causes, such as smoking and vasectomy, remains inconclusive (Cook, 1997; Miaskowski, 1999). *Answer 6:* **c.**

7. The differential diagnosis for prostate cancer must include BPH, prostatitis, and neurologic dysfunction. BPH is a progressive but benign overproduction of prostate tissue and is a common cause of bladder outlet obstruction in men older than 60 years of age. Presenting symptoms include nocturia, dysuria, frequency, urge incontinence, retention, and the sensation of a full bladder after voiding (Shuler & Knudtson, 1999). BPH can be differentiated from most prostate cancers on DRE. BPH presents as a firm, smooth, symmetric enlargement of the gland, in contrast to prostate cancer, which is associated with a hard, irregular, asymmetric gland that varies in consistency (Miaskowski, 1999). Microscopic or gross hematuria may occur from rupture of blood vessels over an enlarged prostate and can occur in patients with BPH. Infection, bladder carcinoma, and various neurologic diseases may also cause hematuria, so cystoscopy or intravenous pyelography (IVP) is necessary to rule out such possibilities as a stone or cancer. Bladder distension may be caused by a gradual obstruction from prostate enlargement or carcinoma causing overflow incontinence or nocturia (Seller, 1996). Prostatitis is an acute or chronic infection of the prostate gland with similar symptoms, such as nocturia, dysuria, and frequency. However, prostatitis is an infectious, versus obstructive, process and will therefore present with associated symptoms of infection, such as fever, chills, malaise, myalgias, and low back pain (Shuler & Knudtson, 1999). Finally, neurologic disorders such as diabetes and multiple sclerosis, which may have a negative effect on the genitourinary system, must also be ruled out (Seller, 1996). *Answer 7:* **d.**

Case Study continued

A TRUS-guided needle biopsy shows malignancy involving both lobes. Bob has a Gleason score of 6. Bob is informed that he has cancer of the prostate. You explain that before the best treatment can be chosen, a staging workup will need to be done.

QUESTIONS

8. A Gleason score is calculated based on which of the following?
   a. Patient's performance status
   b. Histologic grade of the tumor
   c. Presence of metastasis
   d. Need for further treatment

9. Signs and symptoms of early stage prostate carcinoma may include all of the following *except:*
   a. Hematuria
   b. Dysuria
   c. Bone pain
   d. Hydronephrosis

10. Which of the following laboratory tests is the most useful when staging prostate cancer?
   a. Blood urea nitrogen
   b. Serum acid phosphatase
   c. Urinalysis
   d. CBC

---

8. Histologic examination of tissue biopsy samples provides the definitive diagnosis of prostate cancer. Histopathology also determines the growth patterns and differentiation or grade of the tumor cells. In simplified form, prostate cancer can be graded on a scale of 1 to 3; grade 1 is well differentiated, grade 2 is moderately well differentiated, and grade 3 is poorly differentiated. Tumor growth rates are related to the degree of cellular differentiation; well-differentiated, or grade 1, tumors would predictably resemble normal glandular tissue and have a slower rate of proliferation (Lind, 1997). Because of a wide variability of growth patterns, cell types, and degree of anaplasia with prostate cancer, a Gleason score is calculated. It is considered more reliable and is now used as the standard to report the degree of prostate malignancy (Maxwell, 1993). The Gleason score is obtained by sampling two different sites for the degree of tissue differentiation and growth patterns. A histologic grade is assigned to the predominant (primary) cellular pattern of one site and to the lesser (secondary) cellular pattern at the second site. Each pattern is assigned a score of 1 to 5. These two scores are summed to obtain the Gleason score, which may range from 2 to 10. This score is indicative of prognosis: The lower the score, the less aggressive the tumor (Lind, 1997; Maxwell, 1993). *Answer 8:* **b.**

9. Following definitive diagnosis, it is also important to determine whether the patient is experiencing early or late signs and symptoms. Early-stage prostate cancer may be asymptomatic. As the tumor progresses, it causes urinary obstruction resulting from the location of the prostate (Figure 4-1) and the patient may complain of early symptoms similar to those Bob was experiencing. A palpable bladder also indicates urinary obstruction. The presence of palpable supraclavicular or inguinal lymph nodes may indicate metastatic disease, and unexplained weight loss is always an ominous sign of advanced disease (Miaskowski, 1999). Symptoms of late-stage prostate cancer are often associated with bone metastases, with pain being a common patient complaint (Cook, 1997). *Answer 9:* **c.**

10. An initial staging workup will determine the presence of bone or liver metastases. A bone scan should be obtained, and any suspicious areas on the bone scan should be further evaluated with skeletal radiographs (Maxwell, 1993; Miaskowski, 1999). In some instances an acid phosphatase is a good marker for extracapsular involvement (Maxwell, 1993); however, it is most often used to monitor future response to hormonal treatment of prostate cancer (Miaskowski, 1999). Staging for prostate cancer includes both the TNM (tumor, node, metastases) and American Urological Association staging systems (Table 4-3). *Answer 10:* **b.**

Case Study continued

Bob and his wife are extremely anxious about his diagnosis. Bob asks, "What if this is the cancer my dad died from?" He feels uninformed regarding possible treatments and outcomes.

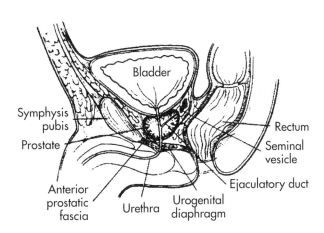

Figure 4-1 Diagrammatic representation of midsagittal section of the male pelvis showing the relationship of the prostate to nearby structures. (From Maxwell, M. B. [1993]. Cancer of the prostate. *Semin Oncol Nurs, 9*[4], pp. 237-251.)

TABLE 4-3	American Urological Association Staging System for Prostate Cancer
STAGE	DESCRIPTION
A	Clinically unsuspected disease
A1	Focal carcinoma, well differentiated
A2	Diffuse carcinoma, usually poorly differentiated
B	Tumor confined to prostate gland
B1	Small, discrete nodule of one lobe of gland
B2	Large or multiple nodules or areas of involvement
C	Tumor localized periprostatic area
C1	Tumor outside prostate capsule, estimated weight <70 g, seminal vesicles uninvolved
C2	Tumor outside prostate capsule, estimated weight >70 g, seminal vesicles involved
D	Metastatic prostate cancer
D1	Pelvic lymph node metastases or ureteral obstruction causing hydronephrosis or both
D2	Bone, soft tissue, organ, or distant lymph node metastases

QUESTIONS

11. What treatment modalities are available to patients with prostate cancer?
   a. Watchful waiting
   b. Radical prostatectomy
   c. Radiation therapy
   d. All of these

12. Which of the following patients would be a strong candidate for watchful waiting?
   a. A 60-year-old with a Gleason score of 9
   b. A 70-year-old with bone metastases
   c. A symptomatic 67-year-old with a PSA of 7 ng/ml
   d. An 82-year-old with a history of coronary artery bypass

13. Major complications of radical prostatectomy can include which of the following?
   a. Erectile dysfunction
   b. Hemorrhage
   c. Urinary incontinence
   d. All of these

14. When counseling a patient regarding proposed treatment for prostate cancer, which of the following is *least* important to ascertain?
   a. Knowledge about the range of treatment options

   b. Potential effect of treatment on sexual functioning
   c. Opinions of the patient's children regarding the best course of action
   d. Strength of the patient's desire to have treatment

ANSWERS

11-14. The Gleason score, stage of the disease, age and performance status of the patient, and patient choice determine treatment options for patients with prostate cancer. Treatment choices for all stages include radical prostatectomy, external or internal radiation, androgen ablation, cryotherapy, and watchful waiting (Lind, 1997). In general, surgery or radiation is the treatment of choice for localized tumors. Radical prostatectomy is a treatment option when the tumor is confined to the prostatic capsule. Carried out either by a perineal or retropubic approach, this major surgery removes the entire prostate and capsule in addition to the seminal vesicles and a portion of the bladder neck (Cook, 1997). Although advances in surgical technique and nerve-sparing approaches are being made, significant morbidity, such as stress incontinence and erectile dysfunction, may occur for many patients. Both of these side effects are influenced by the patient's age and presurgical performance.

Radiation therapy is used for disease that is clinically confined to the prostate or surrounding tissues. It may be used for any stage or for patients who are considered surgical risks. In the case of radiotherapy, lymph node dissection is optional (Maxwell, 1993). Complications of external beam radiation include acute cystitis, proctitis, diarrhea, tenesmus, and urinary frequency (Maxwell, 1993). Diminished sexual potency may also occur over time (Lind, 1997). Brachytherapy using substances such as iridium-192, gold-198, iodine-125, and palladium-103 inserted under TRUS, is also an option for localized prostate cancer (Vestal & Glode, 1994). This option is beneficial for older men (Lind, 1997), and new technologies related to brachytherapy appear to be as promising as radical prostatectomy (Abel, Blatt, Stipetich, et al., 1999).

Cryosurgery is another option for local treatment; however, long-term outcomes related to erectile dysfunction and survival are still uncertain (Lind, 1997). Comparison of survival statistics for radical prostatectomy versus local radiation continues. For clinically localized prostate cancer, it has been argued that radical prostatectomy is the only treatment that reliably ablates the prostate gland to provide a curative effect (Catalona, Ramos, & Carvalhal, 1999).

A final option for localized prostate cancer is watchful waiting. This approach is determined by the stage of the disease and the patient's age and comorbid status. Because of the variability of prostate cancer—latent, slow-growing, or aggressive tumors—watchful waiting may be an appropriate option for patients in advanced age or for those who have major concurrent illness (Maxwell, 1993). Also termed *expectant management,* this choice may also be appropriate for men older than 65 years of age who have low-grade disease and minimal tumor volume, as well as in men in their seventies with low- to moderate-grade disease who have a low probability of dying from prostate cancer (Miaskowski, 1999). These subgroups may choose conservative management by close follow-up in lieu of treatment-related morbidity. *Answer 11:* **d.** *Answer 12:* **d.** *Answer 13:* **d.** *Answer 14:* **d.**

Case Study continued

Bob and his wife are counseled regarding the treatment options. You are concerned that they are confused and need support in making a decision. You counsel them to take some time to sort through all of the options and make some specific recommendations regarding decision-making strategies.

QUESTIONS

15. Bob asks you, "Which is a better treatment: surgery or radiation?" What is the best response?
- **a.** "If I were you, surgery would be my choice because I would want to make sure it is out."
- **b.** "I think that radiation therapy is going to prove to be the best treatment in the long run with the least amount of side effects."
- **c.** "I know this is a difficult decision, but with all the necessary information, I am confident that you will make the right decision."
- **d.** "I don't think I could make such a hard decision with such limited choices."

16. What is the first step to take in advising Bob and his wife about how to make a decision?
- **a.** Providing them with a list of treatment options with pros and cons listed
- **b.** Asking Bob what kind of a death his father experienced
- **c.** Asking Bob if he prefers reading material or a video that explains all the options

- **d.** Walking Bob and his wife through a decision-making algorithm specifically designed for patients with a diagnosis of prostate cancer

ANSWERS

15. The emotional impact of the diagnosis of prostate cancer is a powerful one, and feelings of anxiety may be compounded by the dilemmas that each patient choosing treatment faces. The patient may become overwhelmed with treatment recommendations from different specialists (e.g., urologist, radiation oncologist, surgeon), each recommending their specialty treatment as the most logical choice (Lind, 1997). It is at this juncture that your psychosocial interventions are most crucial. The patient and family will need educational and emotional support to decipher and integrate information so that they can make informed choices. You must advocate for the patient and support each patient's individual choices for treatment. In addition, each treatment regimen for prostate cancer will be an assault on the man's sexuality and body image. Although survival is paramount, the treatment-related effects of incontinence and erectile dysfunction may be of the patient's utmost concern, and these sensitive issues must be addressed during informed consent for surgery or radiation therapy. Often, these quality-of-life issues are not addressed forthrightly because the professional may assume that they take a back seat to survival concerns. *Answer 15:* **c.**

16. Scheduling an appointment specifically to help a patient make a decision using a step-by-step algorithm may provide an opportunity both to assess the patients needs and desires and to progress through the decision-making process, answering questions as you go. In addition, patients can avail themselves of written, videotaped, or computerized material as they prefer. Groups such as Man-To-Man or US Too may be appropriate for some men. *Answer 16:* **d.**

Case Study continued

Bob has a radical prostatectomy. Surgery revealed microscopic invasion of the capsule and involvement of the right seminal vesicle, a stage C lesion. The lymph nodes were negative, and the staging workup was also negative at the time of surgery. Bob's initial postoperative PSA was 0.7 ng/ml. A repeat PSA done 4 months later was 1.2 ng/ml. Nine months after radical prostatectomy, Bob comes to medical oncology for consultation. His most recent PSA is 2.6 ng/ml, which is highly suspicious of microscopic recurrence. A bone scan and magnetic resonance imaging (MRI) of the abdomen and pelvis are negative. Androgen ablation with monthly leuprolide acetate (Lupron) depot injections is begun. He is asymptomatic but is extremely anxious and expresses that he feels powerless to keep the cancer at bay.

QUESTIONS

17. Androgen blockade can be achieved with which of the following?
- **a.** Luteinizing hormone-releasing hormone (LHRH) agonists
- **b.** Antiandrogens
- **c.** Combined Lupron and eulexin (flutamide)
- **d.** All of these

18. Why should an antiestrogen such as flutamide be administered before an agonist such as Lupron?
- **a.** To minimize the side effect of erectile dysfunction
- **b.** To reduce the initial LHRH flare
- **c.** To act as a test dose for Lupron
- **d.** To boost the effectiveness of Lupron

19. Side effects of hormonal therapies for prostate cancer include all of the following *except:*
- **a.** Decreased libido
- **b.** Erectile dysfunction
- **c.** Gynecomastia
- **d.** Loss of facial hair

20. What intervention is most appropriate in regard to the patient's anxiety and powerlessness?
- **a.** Referral to a support group
- **b.** Determination of the severity of the anxiety and discussion with the patient of possible remedies
- **c.** Consultation with the physician about starting a course of radiation therapy
- **d.** Prescribing anxiolytic drugs

ANSWERS

17. Most prostate tumors are hormone dependent. The goal of androgen ablation therapy is to reduce the circulating plasma testosterone to castration levels. This can be accomplished with the use of estrogen therapy, LHRH agonists, antiandrogens, and androgen synthesis inhibitors. Until the early 1990s, estrogens such as diethylstilbestrol (DES) were the primary agents used in the treatment for androgen ablation therapy. This synthetic, nonsteroidal estrogen acts by directly inhibiting the hypothalamic production of LHRH, resulting in the suppression of luteinizing hormone (LH) from the anterior pituitary with subsequent suppression of testosterone (Maxwell, 1993; Miaskowski, 1999). With the advent of newer agents and because of the significant side effects of DES (e.g., cardiotoxicity, thrombophlebitis), the drug is seldom used today except in rare cases of metastatic prostate management (Miaskowski, 1999). *Answer 17:* **d.**

18. The newer pharmacologic agents used for androgen ablation include the LHRH agonists (leuprolide, goserelin) and the antiandrogens (flutamide, bicalutamide). LHRH agonists are synthetic peptides administered by parenteral injection; they act by occupying the receptors for LHRH in the pituitary gland. When initially administered, the release of LH is increased, causing a rise in serum testosterone, or a "flare." With continuous treatment, the pituitary "burns out" and the LH and testosterone levels fall to castration levels (Maxwell, 1993; Saxman & Nichols, 1999). Side effects of LHRH agonists include sexual dysfunction with decreased libido and erectile dysfunction, hot flashes, and gynecomastia because of the estrogenic-like effects. *Answer 18:* **b.**

19. Antiestrogens such as flutamide exert their effect by blocking the action of testosterone at the androgen receptor, but they do not interfere with LH production; therefore patients maintain their potency and libido (Miaskowski, 1999). It was once thought that combined or total androgen blockade using both an LHRH agonist and flutamide delayed disease progression and improved survival (Miaskowski, 1999). Recent evidence does not support this finding. Because of this lack of a survival benefit and the added cost and toxicity of two drugs, combined therapy is no longer recommended (Saxman & Nichols, 1999). However, giving flutamide before the administration of LHRH agonists can prevent the testosterone "flare" reaction that can occur (Iwamoto, 1999), which if it occurs, may worsen symptoms in patients with metastatic disease. *Answer 19:* **d.**

20. Rising PSA levels or recurrent disease presents a new emotional challenge for the patient. When recurrence strikes, the hope for cure diminishes. Although Bob is asymptomatic at this time, his fear of disease recurrence is realized with the rising PSA level and a new medication order. Long-term effects of the radical prostatectomy, in addition to the side effects of Lupron therapy, mandate that you inquire about Bob's perception of his sexuality and body-image changes. Alternative methods of sexual expression should be encouraged, and referrals to appropriate agencies for sexual counseling should be provided (Miaskowski, 1999). The appropriateness of drug therapy or a support group will depend on the severity of the psychologic discomfort and the patient's coping style. *Answer 20:* **b.**

Case Study continued

After another year, Bob's PSA is 6.9 ng/ml. He complains of dull pain in his lower back, which is exacerbated by movement. A bone scan demonstrates an abnormality in the L3-L4 area. MRI confirms that the abnormality is consistent with malignancy. Computed tomography (CT) scans of the liver and pelvis are negative.

QUESTIONS

21. Treatment for Bob's bony metastases will most likely include which of the following?
   1. Continuance of Lupron therapy
   2. Local radiation therapy treatment
   3. Radiopharmaceuticals (e.g., strontium-89)
   4. Chemotherapy
      a. 1 & 2
      b. 1 & 3
      c. 2 & 4
      d. 2 & 3

22. Based on Bob's presentation, what oncologic emergency do you need to consider?
   a. Superior vena cava syndrome
   b. Spinal cord compression
   c. Hypercalcemia
   d. All of these

23. Bob and his wife should be taught that which of the following signs is indication of cord compression progression?
   a. Back pain that seems to radiate
   b. Tingling and weakness in the lower extremities
   c. Continued need for morphine for pain relief
   d. Headaches

ANSWERS

21. Initial physical assessment in Bob's case should include pain assessment: location, quality, and aggravating factors (e.g., spinal tenderness on palpation); sensory perception (to pain, pressure, and temperature); motor deficits (e.g., deep tendon reflexes, weakness, gait changes); and autonomic dysfunction (e.g., urinary/bowel retention or incontinence) (Forster, 1998). Pain without other symptoms is an early indicator of spinal cord compression (SCC). As the cord becomes further compressed, sensory and motor function will become altered. Treatment consists of corticosteroids, methylprednisolone, or dexamethasone to decrease spinal cord edema and local radiation therapy to the site of bony metastases. Bob's treatment would most likely be continuance of Lupron therapy with the addition of local radiation treatment to his bony metastases. Radiopharmaceuticals such as strontium-89 are effective in the treatment of widespread bony metastases with unrelenting pain when conventional therapies fail (Altman & Lee, 1996) but would not yet be used in Bob's case. In addition, strontium-89 can cause prolonged and sometimes irreversible myelosuppression, which might inhibit the use of chemotherapy and radiation. Bob's metastatic bone pain should be treated with nonsteroidal antiinflammatory drugs (NSAIDs). These agents relieve bone pain by decreasing subperiosteal swelling around nerve endings and by decreasing prostaglandin synthesis (Ruzicka, Gates, & Fink, 1997). *Answer 21:* **a.**

22-23. The major oncologic emergency associated with prostate cancer is epidural SCC (Miaskowski, 1999). This was not evident on Bob's MRI scan, but the possibility must always be considered. The mass effect of SCC is the result of tumor invasion with associated edema that compresses the cord, resulting in ischemia and neural damage (Peterson-Rivera & Watters, 1997). Back pain is the initial symptom in more than 95% of patients, and although the pain is most often localized, it may radiate or be radicular in nature (caused by nerve root compression). It may be sudden in onset and described as severe, dull, or aching (Forster, 1998). The pain is often exacerbated with recumbency or when the patient coughs, bears weight, or performs the Valsalva maneuver (Peterson-Rivera & Watters, 1997). Prompt intervention is mandatory to spare neurologic function. The primary prognostic factor related to functional outcome is detection and intervention within 24 hours of SCC (Forster, 1998). Progression of symptoms may begin with sensory deficits such as numbness on a continuum to motor weakness and autonomic dysfunction (Miaskowski, 1999). *Answer 22:* **b.** *Answer 23:* **b.**

Case Study continued

Combined androgen blockade with Lupron and flutamide is continued, and Bob's spinal metastases are treated with local radiation and NSAIDs. His condition remains stable for 8 months, when he begins to complain of increased generalized pain in his right hip and lower back; he also complains of fatigue and anorexia. His serial PSA levels rise to more than 200 ng/ml. A bone scan is positive for multiple metastatic sites. Bob's disease is deemed hormone refractory. Flutamide is discontinued, but Lupron is continued every month.

QUESTION

24. Why was flutamide therapy discontinued?
    a. Flutamide withdrawal has been shown to improve clinical symptoms and decrease PSA levels.
    b. Rising PSA levels prove that the hormonal therapy is no longer working.
    c. Flutamide may exacerbate bone pain.
    d. Flutamide suppresses the appetite.

25. How long does it usually take for a patient with metastatic prostate cancer to become refractory to hormone therapy?
    a. 6 to 12 months
    b. 18 to 24 months
    c. 25 to 36 months
    d. More than 3 years

26. All of the following are indications that prostate cancer has become refractory to hormone therapy except:
    a. Rising serial PSA levels
    b. Rising prostatic acid phophatase levels
    c. Decrease in hormone-related side effects
    d. Increasing symptoms despite continued therapy

27. Which of the following statements best describes the rationale for continuing Lupron therapy?
    a. Chemotherapy is not a viable option in the treatment of prostate cancer.
    b. Patients whose disease progresses while taking hormone therapy may have exacerbation of symptoms if testosterone levels are allowed to rise.
    c. Continuing Lupron is the only option available to treat metastatic prostate cancer.
    d. There is no role for Lupron therapy in hormone-resistant prostate cancer.

28. Bob's wife draws you aside and asks why you do not give Bob chemotherapy. Your answer is based on all of the following understandings except:
    a. External beam radiation therapy is effective in most patients with bone metastases.
    b. Effective chemotherapy regimens for bone metastases are still under investigation.
    c. A variety of hormonal regimens are available.
    d. Chemotherapy would be too debilitating given his physical status.

ANSWERS

24. Flutamide withdrawal has been shown to improve clinical symptoms and decrease PSA levels for a median of 3 to 4 months. The mechanism for symptomatic improvement with flutamide withdrawal syndrome is not clearly understood but may be the result of physiologic changes in the structure of the androgen receptor causing the antiandrogen to have an agonist effect versus an antagonist effect for a short period. Clinical improvement in the patient's pain depends on the half-life of the antiandrogen (Iwamoto, 1999; Miaskowski, 1999). Ketoconazole, an antifungal agent, blocks adrenal and testicular steroid synthesis and adrenal androgen production and has been used to treat patients who have failed combined hormone therapy and flutamide withdrawal. Because of the adrenal suppression, hydrocortisone replacement therapy is necessary (Iwamoto, 1999). *Answer 24:* **a.**

25-26. Indications of hormone-refractory prostate cancer usually occur 18 to 24 months after hormones are begun and include (1) rising PSA levels, (2) increasing symptoms while taking hormone therapy, (3) increased prostate acid phosphatase levels, (4) positive bone scans, and (5) CT evidence of progressive disease in the soft tissues (Iwamoto, 1999). *Answer 25:* **b.** *Answer 26:* **c.**

27. Bob was experiencing increasing generalized pain in addition to fatigue. Anorexia, weight loss, and decreasing performance status are additional symptoms of advancing prostate cancer. Positive bone scans demonstrating "hot spots," which are representative of metastases, and CT scans can confirm soft tissue involvement in the abdomen, pelvis, or other parts of the body (Iwamoto, 1999). With patients like Bob, whose disease progresses while he is taking hormone therapy, treatment is usually continued to prevent exacerbation of symptoms, especially pain caused by rising testosterone levels if the LHRH agonist is discontinued (Saxman & Nichols, 1999). Despite rising PSA levels,

continuing the Lupron therapy may also control the proliferation of a fraction of malignant cells in addition to preventing a flare of the disease if the therapy is stopped (Iwamoto, 1999). *Answer 27:* **b.**

28. Chemotherapy is often considered only for palliation because most agents have minimal response rates and have yet to demonstrate increased survival (Saxman & Nichols, 1999). Chemotherapeutic agents that have been used to treat metastatic prostate cancer include doxorubicin, cyclophosphamide, fluorouracil, methotrexate, cisplatin, mitoxantrone, and estramustine in combination with vinblastine. Most are administered as single agents. Patients treated with mitoxantrone and prednisone have improved pain control and a reduced need for analgesics when compared with patients treated with prednisone alone (Iwamoto, 1999; Saxman & Nichols, 1999. *Answer 28:* **d.**

References

Abel, L. J., Blatt, H. J., Stipetich, R. L., et al. (1999). Nursing management of patients receiving brachytherapy for early stage prostate cancer. *Clin J Oncol Nurs, 3,* pp. 7-15.

Altman, G. B., & Lee, C. A. (1996). Strontium-89 for treatment of painful bone metastasis from prostate cancer. *Oncol Nurs Forum, 23,* pp. 523-527.

American Cancer Society (ACS). (2000). *Cancer facts & figures 2000.* Atlanta: Author.

Brawer, M. K. (1999). Prostate-specific antigen: Current status. *CA Cancer J Clin, 49,* pp. 264-281.

Catalona, W. J., Ramos, C. G., & Carvalhal, G. F. (1999). Contemporary results of anatomic radical prostatectomy. *CA Cancer J Clin, 49,* pp. 282-296.

Collins, M. (1997). Increasing prostate cancer awareness in African American men. *Oncol Nurs Forum, 24,* pp. 91-93.

Cook, S. K. (1997). Prostate cancer. In Gates, R. A., & Fink, R. M. (Eds.). *Oncology nursing secrets* (pp. 202-208). Philadelphia: Hanley & Belfus.

Forster, D. A. (1998). Spinal cord compression. In Chernecky, C. C., & Berger, B. J. (Eds.). *Advanced and critical care oncology nursing* (pp. 566-577). Philadelphia: WB Saunders.

Gerard, M. J., & Frank-Stromberg, M. (1998). Screening for prostate cancer in asymptomatic men: Clinical, legal, and ethical implications. *Oncol Nurs Forum, 25,* pp. 1561-1569.

Iwamoto, R. R. (1999). *Hormone refractory prostate cancer: A case study and overview of nursing strategies for effective clinical practice.* Pittsburgh: Oncology Education Services.

Lind, J. M. (1997). The challenges of elevated prostate-specific antigen and early-stage prostate cancer. *Dev Support Cancer Care, 1,* pp. 61-65.

Maxwell, M. B. (1993). Cancer of the prostate. *Semin Oncol Nurs, 9,* pp. 237-261.

Miaskowski, C. (1999). Prostate cancer. In Miaskowski, C., & Buchsel, P. (Eds.). *Oncology nursing: Assessment and clinical care* (pp. 1471-1501). St Louis: Mosby.

Peterson-Rivera, L., & Watters, M. R. (1997). Spinal cord compression. In Gates, R. A., & Fink, R. M. (Eds.). *Oncology nursing secrets* (pp. 352-355). Philadelphia: Hanley & Belfus.

Ruzicka, D., Gates, R. A., & Fink, R. M. (1997). Pain management. In Gates, R. A., & Fink, R. M. (Eds.). *Oncology nursing secrets* (pp. 284-303). Philadelphia: Hanley & Belfus.

Saxman S. B., & Nichols, C. R. (1999). Urologic and male genital malignancies. In Skeel, R. T. (Ed.). *Handbook of cancer chemotherapy* (pp. 314-332). Philadelphia: Lippincott Williams & Wilkins.

Seller, R. H. (1996). Voiding disorders and incontinence. In Seller, R. H. (Ed.). *Differential diagnosis of common complaints,* 3rd ed. (pp. 371-378). Philadelphia: WB Saunders.

Shuler, P. A., & Knudtson, M. D. (1999). Genitourinary and gynecologic disorders. In Millonig, V. L., & Miller, S. K. (Eds.). *Adult nurse practitioner certification review guide* (pp. 373-449). Potomac, MD: Health Leadership Associates.

von Eschenbach, A. C. (1999). The challenge of prostate cancer. *CA Cancer J Clin, 49,* pp. 262-263.

Vestal, C., & Glode, L. M. (1994). Prostate cancer. In Wood, M. E., & Bunn, P. A. (Eds.). *Hematology oncology secrets* (pp. 308-312). Philadelphia: Hanley & Belfus.

5 Melanoma

Nancy Jo Bush

CASE STUDY

Cindy Dietzman is a 29-year-old white woman referred to the dermatologist by her primary care physician for changes in a mole in her right axilla. Cindy had thought that the recent bleeding from the mole might have been related to her accidentally nicking the mole when shaving. The dermatologist is suspicious of malignant melanoma and performs a biopsy on the mole. Before leaving the office, Cindy says to you, "It can't be anything serious. I haven't been in the sun for the past 3 years."

QUESTIONS

1. Your response to Cindy will be related to your understanding of all the following risk factors for melanoma *except:*
   a. How easily fair-skinned individuals sunburn
   b. History of basal cell carcinoma
   c. Family history of melanoma
   d. History of blistering sunburns

2. A new nurse in the clinic asks you what type of biopsy to anticipate. Your answer, based on your knowledge of optimal diagnostic technique for melanoma, is:
   a. Incisional
   b. Punch
   c. Excisional
   d. Needle

ANSWERS

1. Malignant melanoma is the most deadly form of skin cancer, and it is increasing at a faster rate than any other solid tumor (Gale & Richards, 1999). The American Cancer Society (ACS, 2000) estimates that melanoma will be diagnosed in approximately 47,700 persons in the United States in the year 2000. Since the early 1970s, the incidence of melanoma has increased significantly on an average of 4% per year (ACS, 2000), with estimates that 1 in 87 Americans may develop melanoma during their lifetime (Benson, 1999).

Melanoma occurs less often than the other two types of skin cancer—basal cell and squamous cell carcinoma—but it is more lethal because it has a high risk of metastases. Known risk factors for melanoma include fair-skinned individuals and those of northern European ancestry. Most likely, Cindy has blond or red hair and blue eyes, and she may report a history of the two most important risk factors: intense sun exposure with multiple, severe sunburns as a child or the presence of a large number of atypical nevi, also called *dysplastic nevi syndrome.* A personal or family history would also place Cindy in a higher risk group (Gale & Richards, 1999; Hoffman, 1994). Although melanoma occurs most often in individuals with fair skin, it can also occur in dark-skinned individuals; however, the presentation is different. Melanoma may appear on the palms, soles of the feet, nail beds, and mucous membranes of dark-skinned individuals (Gale & Richards, 1999). Although melanoma most commonly arises from preexisting nevi, it has been known to arise spontaneously.

Melanoma arises from melanocytes, the melanin-producing cells in the skin. Melanomas most commonly occur on the lower extremities in women and on the trunk in men, particularly on the back (Becker, 1997). The melanocytes responsible for melanoma may also migrate to the eye, respiratory tract, and gastrointestinal system (Hoffman, 1994). Unusual primary sites include the eyes, palate, gingiva, anus, vulva, and very rarely, the foregut or central nervous system (Wagner & Casciato, 1995).

Signs and symptoms of melanoma are organized according to the *ABCD* acronym that summarizes local manifestations or changes in a mole (Box 5-1 and Figure 5-1). Any change in the color, shape, border, or size of a mole can be indicative of malignancy. Variegated shades of red, white, blue, brown, or black may present with jagged, irregular borders (Cameron & Wong, 1994). Moles larger than 5 mm are also suspicious (Gale & Richards, 1999). Changes in surface characteristics, such as scaling, crusting, ulceration, or nodularity, must be noted. In Cindy's case,

BOX 5-1 An ABCD Approach to the Early Detection of Melanoma

A = Asymmetry: Melanoma lesions are typically irregular shaped.
B = Border: Melanoma lesions often have uneven, ragged, notched edges, or irregular borders.
C = Color: Melanoma lesions often contain varying shades of blacks and browns.
D = Diameter: Melanoma lesions are often larger than 6 mm (about the size of a pencil eraser).

From Miaskowski, C., & Buschel, P. (1999). *Oncology nursing: Assessment and clinical care.* St. Louis: Mosby.

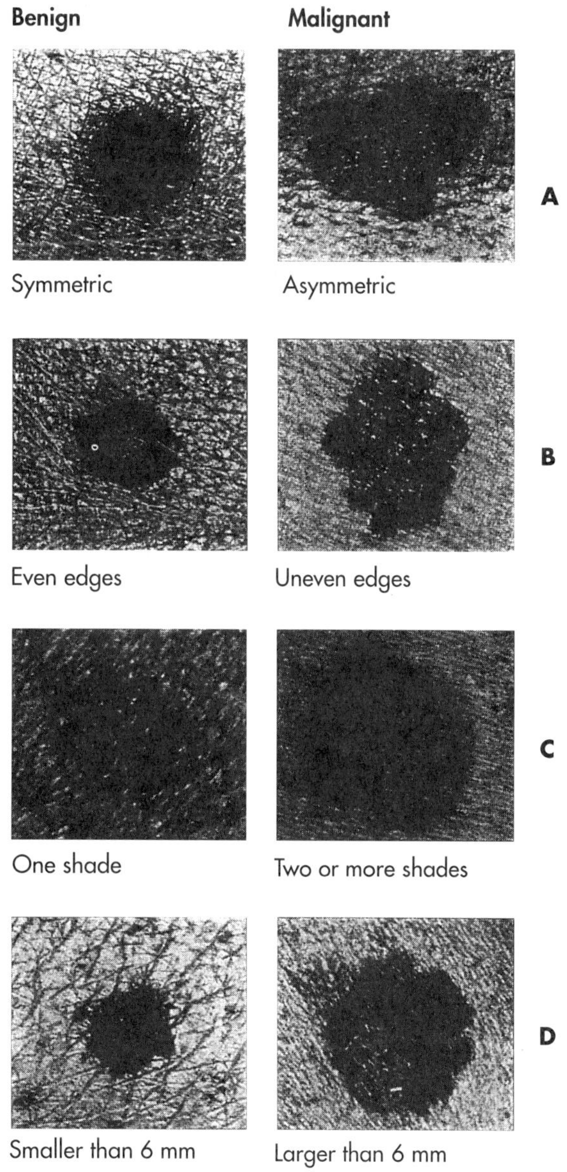

bleeding of the mole was the presenting sign that she observed. Additional signs, such as changes in sensation (e.g., itching, pain) or a sudden elevation of a macular nevus, must also be considered (Cameron & Wong, 1994). *Answer 1:* **b.**

2. The staging, prognosis, and treatment of melanoma depend on the results of an excisional biopsy. The excisional biopsy must go through the underlying fat to obtain an adequate tissue sample to determine tumor level and depth of invasion of the entire circumference of the mole (Becker, 1997). Incisional biopsies are recommended only for lesions more than 2 cm wide (Benson, 1999). *Answer 2:* **c.**

Case Study continued

Cindy's mole is diagnosed as a superficial spreading malignant melanoma, Clark's level IV, Breslow level 2.8.

QUESTIONS

3. Clark's level is a pathologic determination based on which of the following?
 a. Color variation in the mole
 b. Degree of differentiation of the cells
 c. Skin level penetrated by the melanoma cells
 d. Diameter of the original mole

4. Breslow's level is based on which of the following?
 a. Skin layer penetrated by the melanoma cells
 b. A measurement of the depth of the tumor
 c. Extent of the excisional biopsy
 d. Degree of differentiation of the cells

5. Both Clark's and Breslow's levels are important indicators of which of the following?
 a. Treatment and prognosis
 b. Length of time the mole has been present

Benign **Malignant**

Symmetric — Asymmetric — **A**
Even edges — Uneven edges — **B**
One shade — Two or more shades — **C**
Smaller than 6 mm — Larger than 6 mm — **D**

Figure 5-1 ABCDs of melanoma. **A,** Asymmetry; **B,** border; **C,** color; **D,** diameter. (From American Cancer Society, *Understanding melanoma.* Atlanta: American Cancer Society.)

 c. Differentiation of the tumor
 d. Lymph node status

6. All of the following are important diagnostic measures for Cindy at this time *except:*
 a. Chest radiograph
 b. Sentinel node mapping
 c. Blood chemistry panel
 d. Magnetic resonance imaging (MRI) scan of the brain

TABLE 5-1   Common Types of Cutaneous Melanoma

TYPE (%)	INCIDENCE	COLOR/CHARACTERISTICS	GROWTH	LOCATION
Superficial spreading (70%-75%)	Male:female 1:1 5th decade	Tan, brown Flat, crusty, irregular borders	Radial growth 1-5 yr; rapid vertical growth	Women: legs Men: back
Nodular (10%-15%)	Male:female 2:1 5th decade	Blue-black, blue-gray, red-blue Raised; bleeding may occur	No radial growth All vertical growth <1 yr; aggressive	Head, neck, and trunk
Acral lentiginous	Hispanic Oriental African American	Tan, brown, black	Radial growth; months to years	Palms, soles, subungual
Lentigo melanoma (5%)	Male:female 1:3 7th decade	Tan, brown Mottling, irregular	Radial growth: decades; slow growing	Head, neck, temple, cheeks, and hands

From Becker, M. (1997). Malignant melanoma. In Gates, R. A., & Fink, R. M. (Eds.) *Oncology nursing secrets* (pp. 196-201). Philadelphia: Hanley & Belfus.

ANSWERS

3-4. Most melanomas arise from the skin. Cutaneous melanomas are classified according to their growth patterns: superficial spreading melanoma (SSM), nodular melanoma (NM), lentigo maligna melanoma (LMM), and acral lentiginous melanoma (ALM). Melanoma has two growth patterns: horizontally on the surface of the skin and vertically into the epidermis and lower. Tumors discovered in the radial or horizontal growth phase carry a better prognosis because these tumors have not yet developed metastatic potential, unlike tumors in the vertical growth phase, which have invaded the dermis (Benson, 1999). SSM is the most common type of melanoma, accounting for 70% of cases. They most often arise in a preexisting mole and are most commonly found on the legs in women and on the back in men. SSM is characterized by a horizontal growth pattern on the surface of the skin that may progress slowly over 1 to 5 years. NMs account for 15% of melanomas; occur more often in men than in women; and are typically found on the head, neck, and trunk. NMs are more aggressive because these tumors grow rapidly and vertically from the onset. LMs, also called *Hutchinson's freckles,* carry the best prognosis of all melanomas because they have a slow, horizontal growth phase that can last up to 20 years. Typically, LMs occur in the elderly and can be found on the head, neck, cheek, temple, or hands. Last, ALMs arise quickly, over 3 to 36 months, and are most common in African Americans, Asians, and Hispanics. ALMs are known to appear on the palms; soles; subungual regions; and sometimes in the mucous membranes, anus, vagina, and conjunctiva (Benson, 1999; Wagner & Casciato, 1995) (Table 5-1). The staging of melanoma is determined based on two criteria: (1) the

BOX 5-2   Clark's Microstaging System

Clark's level I: melanoma in situ
Clark's level II: invading the papillary dermis
Clark's level III: invading the papillary-reticular dermal interface
Clark's level IV: invading the reticular dermis
Clark's level V: invading subcutaneous tissue

From Miaskowski, C., & Buschel, P. (1999). *Oncology nursing: Assessment and clinical care.* St. Louis: Mosby.

degree of tumor invasion into the skin, referred to as Clark's level (Box 5-2), and (2) the thickness of the tumor in millimeters or Breslow's level (Figure 5-2). *Answer 3:* **c.** *Answer 4:* **b.**

5. Cindy's melanoma is stage IIA. After the initial staging of melanoma, the possibility of metastatic disease must be assessed. Prognostic indicators include the depth of invasion, the presence of positive lymph nodes, and the presence of distant metastases. Tumors with less than 0.85 mm of invasion have a very low metastatic potential (Wagner & Casciato, 1995). Palpation of regional lymph nodes and biopsies of any suspicious nodes are both recommended. The role of elective lymph node dissection (ELND) remains controversial because it may not affect survival (Becker, 1997; Wagner & Casciato, 1995). Patients with thick (more than 4.0 mm) lesions have a high probability of systemic disease at diagnosis and would not benefit from ELND. Patients with melanomas of intermediate thickness (e.g., more than 0.75 but less than 4.0 mm) are at risk for metastatic disease, with the regional draining lymph nodes acting as sanctuaries for residual disease. Research data identifying a survival benefit of ELND in this

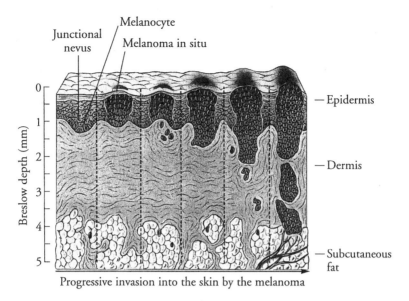

Figure 5-2 Progressive growth of melanoma. (From Miaskowski, C., Buschel, P. *Oncology nursing: Assessment and clinical care*, 1999, St. Louis, Mosby.)

selected group of patients are inconclusive to date. *Answer 5:* **a.**

6. Sentinel lymph node mapping and biopsy have helped in identifying patients who may benefit from node dissection (Morton, Wen, Wong, et al., 1992). A preoperative lymphoscintigraphy is performed to identify the regional lymph node basin; a radionucleotide dye such as isosulfan blue is then intraoperatively injected into the skin at the site of the primary melanoma. The first, or "sentinel," node that absorbs the dye is identified and removed for histologic analysis. If this node is negative for melanoma cells, there is a less than 5% chance that the remaining nodes are invaded. Sentinel lymph node mapping and biopsy techniques are proving to be both sensitive and specific measures to determine the optimal surgical and medical management of intermediate to high-risk melanomas such as Cindy's (Becker, 1997; Benson, 1999).

In Cindy's case, a metastatic workup should also include a chest radiograph and computed tomography (CT) scan of the abdomen and pelvis. Secondary sites for metastases are the lungs, necessitating a preoperative chest radiograph. Other metastatic sites for melanoma include the liver, brain, and bones. Therefore evaluation of serum liver chemistries is also important. Patients with stage III or IV melanoma require further metastatic workup. CT of the chest may be

indicated to evaluate possible lymph nodules more accurately, and any patient with palpable abdominal masses or complaints of gastrointestinal symptoms requires CT scanning of the abdomen and pelvis. Finally, magnetic resonance imaging (MRI) of the brain is necessary for any patient complaining of central nervous system symptoms such as headache or blurred vision (Becker, 1997; Hoffman, 1994). *Answer 6:* **d.**

Case Study continued

Cindy is distraught at the serious nature of the diagnosis, stating, "I wouldn't have even followed-up on this mole if it weren't for the concern of my primary physician. I can't believe I didn't take this seriously." She is scheduled for a wide excision.

QUESTIONS

7. What is the best response to Cindy's concern and guilt regarding the serious nature of her diagnosis?
  a. "I would not have been concerned about that mole either because it was in your axilla and constantly nicked by your razor."
  b. "I understand your concerns that you may have been unaware of the changes in your mole, but the most important issue now is to move forward with the necessary treatment."

   c. "In your case it would have not made a difference when you sought treatment."
   d. "You will constantly second-guess yourself and that is unhealthy."

8. The surgeon calls and asks you to visit Cindy. She is refusing to sign the informed consent and is upset, particularly about being asked to sign for a skin graft or surgical flap when she was only expecting a wide excision. What should you tell Cindy?
   a. "A skin graft or flap will be used only if the surgeon cannot bring the wound edges together."
   b. "You have not been paying close enough attention to the explanations that your doctor has given you, probably because this is all so upsetting."
   c. "I understand why you are upset; the consent form is too broad. I will ask the surgeon to redo the consent for a limited wide excision only."
   d. "Even if a skin graft or flap is needed to close the wound, it will have a minimal cosmetic effect."

ANSWERS

7. Addressing Cindy's emotional concerns and her reactions to the diagnosis are of utmost importance. The psychosocial effects and emotional reactions created by this disease are similar to those experienced by all patients with cancer, in addition to those unique to melanoma (Bush, 1999). Cindy is young and healthy, so undoubtedly she will experience shock and disbelief about the serious nature of her diagnosis. Emotional reactions such as anxiety and confusion are common and expected. Cindy may also have fears related to body-image changes that will occur with the wide excision and sentinel node biopsy. These surgical assaults may also cause her to feel vulnerable and helpless. Cindy's expression of guilt regarding a possible delay in diagnosis related to her lack of knowledge regarding the possibility that the change in her mole could be malignant is understandable. It is important that the you acknowledge these feelings while reinforcing her positive coping skills. You must also assess Cindy's need for emotional support and refer her to appropriate educational and psychosocial resources. Research has demonstrated that patients with melanoma who receive educational materials and emotional support at diagnosis and who then apply effective cognitive and behavioral coping skills have lower recurrence rates and improved survival (Blanchard, Albrecht, & Ruckdeschel, 1995;

| BOX **5-3** | **Psychosocial Nursing Interventions for Melanoma Patients** |

1. Identify current and past coping skills, and assess effective and ineffective strategies used by the patient and family.
2. Provide appropriate information to meet knowledge deficits regarding the disease, treatment, and follow-up care.
3. Include the family, significant others, and social support systems in the plan of care.
4. Promote continuity of care across all health care settings, with appropriate referral and follow-up.
5. Refer the patient and family to appropriate psychosocial support systems, such as I Can Cope.
6. Promote hopefulness and feelings of control through education regarding health promotion, sun protection, skin self-examination, nutrition, and exercise for immune function.

From Bush, N. J. (1999). Bringing home the daffodils: The psychosocial impact of melanoma. *Dev Support Care, 2,* pp. 126-132.

Fawzy, Fawzy, Hyun, & Wheeler, 1997). Psychosocial nursing interventions for patients with melanoma are provided in Box 5-3. *Answer 7:* **b.**

8. After the initial diagnosis, surgery is the primary treatment for melanoma. The width of surgical margins is guided by the depth of the primary melanoma. For melanomas less than 1 mm thick, a wide excision consisting of a 1- to 2-cm margin around the primary tumor is recommended; for primary lesions 1 to 3 mm thick, a 3-cm margin is recommended, and for lesions greater than 3.0 mm, a 3- to 5-cm margin is recommended (Cameron & Wong, 1994). Large incisions may require skin grafting or flaps, depending on the site of the primary tumor (e.g., forearm) when primary closure is not possible. Body-image changes may result because the patient is left with a constant reminder of the cancer diagnosis and treatment. Staging and treatment recommendations are further outlined in Table 5-2. *Answer 8:* **a.**

Case Study continued

Cindy's surgery is uneventful. Her excision site is closed primarily, and the sentinel node biopsy is negative for metastatic disease. Plans for Cindy's follow-up care must be discussed. She has numerous questions regarding necessary lifestyle changes, inquires about the risk that her family

TABLE 5-2	Staging and Treatment for Melanoma

STAGE	DESCRIPTION
0	Melanoma in situ
IA	Primary melanoma <0.75 mm or Clark's level II
IB	Primary melanoma 0.76-1.50 mm or Clark's level III
IIA	Primary melanoma 1.51-4.0 mm or Clark's level IV
IIB	Primary melanoma >4 mm or Clark's level V
III	Regional lymph nodes or in-transit metastases
IV	Systemic metastases
TREATMENT	
I and II	Surgical excision of the primary tumor
III	Surgical excision of the primary tumor with or without radical lymphadenectomy; with or without interferon therapy
IV	No standard treatment; clinical trials recommended.

From Becker, M. (1997). Malignant melanoma. In Gates, R. A., & Fink, R. M. (Eds.). *Oncology nursing secrets* (pp. 196-201). Philadelphia: Hanley & Belfus.

members have in regard to melanoma, and expresses the desire to get pregnant and start a family.

QUESTIONS

9. Which of the following is true regarding follow-up care for melanoma?
   a. Follow-up care will depend on the stage of disease and risk of recurrence.
   b. Early-stage disease requires only yearly follow-up.
   c. Follow-up care will include a physical examination and review of systems only.
   d. Once diagnosed with a melanoma, a patient does not need regular dermatologic examinations.

10. What should be included in patient education regarding melanoma but is often overlooked?
   a. Skin self-assessment
   b. ABCDs of melanoma detection
   c. Ultraviolet risks in winter months
   d. All of these

11. Which of the following statements best describes what you should say to Cindy regarding the familial risk of melanoma?

   a. "Your siblings are at no greater risk than the general population."
   b. "Because you have been diagnosed at a young age and your family may share your risk of sun exposure, they should be advised about early detection."
   c. "Genetic testing might be a good idea for your family members."
   d. "Your family members should be screened by a dermatologist every 6 months."

12. What is your advice to Cindy and her husband regarding her desire to get pregnant?
   a. "There is no risk with pregnancy and melanoma."
   b. "This is a serious disease and not a time to be thinking about having children."
   c. "Melanoma may be influenced by pregnancy, so I think that we should discuss the best plan for starting your family with your physician."
   d. "Why don't you wait and think about starting a family after you know whether your treatment has been curative."

ANSWERS

9. The stage of disease and risk of recurrence determine follow-up care for melanoma. At a minimum, even early-stage patients should be evaluated at least every 6 months for the first 2 years after diagnosis (Hoffman, 1994). Patients at a higher risk of recurrence should be seen every 3 months. Patients at higher risk include those with lymph node involvement, thick primary tumors, ulcerated tumors, or tumors of the head and neck. Follow-up examinations should include a complete dermatologic examination, physical examination, and review of systems, noting any unusual symptoms related to the gastrointestinal or central nervous systems. A thorough evaluation of the local surgical site and regional lymphatic drainage area are necessary. Chest x-ray studies and laboratory chemistries are recommended every 6 to 12 months (Hoffman, 1994). *Answer 9:* **a.**

10. Skin examination is an important part of follow-up for any melanoma patient. Patients with a history of melanoma are at a greater risk of developing a secondary melanoma, and the risk is greater for patients who have multiple dysplastic nevi or a family history of melanoma (Becker, 1997). Cindy should also be taught skin self-examination and the ABCDs of early detection. In addition to the benefit of early detection, skin self-assessment will increase Cindy's confidence

| BOX 5-4 | Patient Education Regarding Sun Protection |

1. Understand the risks of ultraviolet (UV) light exposure and melanoma.
2. Avoid sun exposure between the height of UV intensity from 10 AM to 3 PM.
3. Use protective equipment such as umbrellas and tents to prevent direct exposure.
4. Wear appropriate clothing such as wide-brimmed hats, long-sleeve shirts, and pants.
5. Use sunscreens with a skin protection factor (SPF) of 15 or higher on all exposed skin.
6. Replace sunscreen yearly to ensure adequate potency and freshness.
7. Apply sunscreen 30 minutes before exposure, and reapply every 2 hours, after swimming, or if perspiring.
8. Apply an adequate amount of sunscreen evenly over the body.
9. Do not use tanning beds or sun lamps.
10. UV risks are also present in winter months and protection is needed during sport activities such as skiing.

Adapted from Becker, M. (1997). Malignant melanoma. In Gates, R. A., & Fink, R. M. (Eds.). *Oncology nursing secrets* (pp. 196-201). Philadelphia: Hanley & Belfus.

and feelings of control over her disease process. Cindy must be counseled regarding her risk for a secondary melanoma and the importance of sun protection and the use of sunscreens, even in winter (Gupta & Davis, 1999). These strategies are outlined in Box 5-4. *Answer 10:* **c.**

11. It is also important to address Cindy's concerns regarding her family members and to educate her about their risk of developing melanoma (Loescher, 1999). There are differences in sporadic or nonfamilial versus familial melanoma. In familial melanoma the median age at diagnosis is 34 years, younger than patients who present with sporadic melanoma. The lesions in familiar melanoma are most often thinner, and the presence of dysplastic nevi is more common. Last, with familial melanoma the disease has a vertical transmission across two or more generations with one or more first-degree relatives diagnosed (Fraser, Goldstein, & Tucker, 1997). At present, there is no genetic test that can detect familial melanoma, but because family members often share environmental risks such as sun exposure and lifestyle, Cindy's relatives should be advised to perform skin self-examinations and appropriate dermatologic care, especially if dysplastic nevi syndrome is present. *Answer 11:* **b.**

12. In female patients who are diagnosed at a young age, family planning may be a concern. If the patient does not bring it up, it should be openly discussed as part of follow-up care. The relationship between melanoma and pregnancy remains uncertain (Becker, 1997). What is known is that hormonal changes during pregnancy accelerate the level of melanocyte-stimulating hormone and that nevi may show an increase in size and pigmentation as a result of these changes. Questions remain concerning the effect of pregnancy on the outcome of melanoma, and any decision to become pregnant should be discussed with the physician with these issues in mind. For patients who are pregnant at time of diagnosis, the influence of the pregnancy on the melanoma and the effects of the treatment on the pregnancy must also be discussed (Becker, 1997). *Answer 12:* **c.**

Case Study continued

After a 22-month disease-free interval, Cindy notes a painful mass in her right axilla. Fine-needle aspiration (FNA) is positive for malignant cells. A therapeutic lymph node dissection reveals malignant melanoma metastatic to the lymph nodes with extracapsular spread. Reevaluation with radiologic scans rule out chest or visceral metastases. Cindy is started on adjuvant treatment with interferon-alfa-2b therapy. Cindy and her husband are instructed regarding the treatment, administration, expected side effects, and implications of immunotherapy. Cindy copes with the news realistically and uses her available support systems. Her main concern is her ability to continue working as a sales representative because she finds her position stressful at times because of the frequent travel.

QUESTIONS

13. What is the role of interferon in the treatment of melanoma?
   a. Adjuvant interferon is indicated for patients with tumors more than 4 mm thick and after therapeutic lymph node dissection.
   b. Adjuvant interferon has proven to prolong relapse and increase overall survival in patients with high-risk melanoma and with metastatic disease.
   c. Adjuvant interferon is approved for patients who are disease free at the time of surgical excision but who are at high risk of systemic recurrence.
   d. All of these

14. Which of the following side effects of interferon therapy are most likely to interfere with Cindy's ability to perform her job?
   a. Fatigue and weakness
   b. Nausea and vomiting
   c. Myalgias and arthralgias
   d. Fever and chills

15. Psychosocial support for Cindy is imperative at this stage of her disease and treatment for which of the following reasons?
   a. Cindy's stage of disease is now terminal, and she must be prepared realistically for this outcome.
   b. Interferon therapy has been reported to cause or exacerbate depression.
   c. Cindy will need to quit her job during interferon therapy, and this may cause anxiety about finances.
   d. Side effects of interferon therapy include changes in sexuality and body image.

16. If Cindy's disease progresses while she is receiving interferon therapy, what treatment options will be considered?
   a. Single-agent chemotherapy
   b. Biochemotherapy
   c. Melanoma vaccine
   d. All of these

17. What role does radiation therapy play in the treatment of melanoma?
   a. Melanoma is considered a radiosensitive tumor.
   b. Radiation therapy is used for prophylactic treatment of regional lymph nodes.
   c. Radiation therapy is generally reserved for palliative treatment of certain metastatic sites.
   d. Radiation therapy can be used before wide excision to control local recurrence.

ANSWERS

13. Interferon is a form of immunotherapy. This drug appears to have direct antiproliferative action against tumor cells or viral cells. Although its direct mechanism of action is unknown, it is thought to be cytotoxic by inhibiting replication of tumor cells. It modulates host immune responses by enhancing the phagocytic activity of macrophages and augmenting specific cytotoxicity of lymphocytes for target cells (Springhouse, 1998). Results of a large, randomized, multicenter study in high-risk melanoma patients demonstrated significant improvements in relapse-free and overall patient survival with postoperative adjuvant interferon therapy (Donnelly, 1998; Gale & Kiley, 1998). Based on this trial, the U.S. Food and Drug Administration approved interferon-alfa 2-b therapy as an adjuvant treatment after surgical excision in patients free of disease but at high risk for systemic recurrence. Interferon also produces objective responses in patients with metastatic melanoma and is most effective in patients like Cindy who have small-volume, nonvisceral metastatic disease and a good performance status (Sondak & Margolin, 1998). Interferon for high-risk melanoma is administered intravenously 5 days per week for 4 weeks as induction treatment and followed by subcutaneous self-administration three times weekly for 48 weeks, unless the disease progresses or adverse reactions develop. Dosage modifications may be necessary, depending on side effects and patient tolerance. It is a long and challenging treatment regimen for patients, and nursing interventions are aimed at patient education regarding self-care in managing side effects and patient compliance (Donnelly, 1998). *Answer 13:* **d.**

14. Expert nursing care is required for managing the patient receiving adjuvant interferon (Kiley & Gale, 1998). Most side effects from interferon therapy are constitutional: fever and chills, nausea and anorexia, and myalgias and arthralgias. Overwhelming fatigue is the most distressing side effect and may progress with therapy and may be dose limiting. This side effect is likely to interfere with Cindy's ability to continue working and traveling at her previous level of performance. The flulike effects of interferon can be managed by the prophylactic use of analgesics such as acetaminophen or ibuprofen. Adequate hydration and small, frequent meals may help combat the nausea and anorexia associated with long-term treatment, as well as potentially lessen the symptoms of fatigue. Patient education regarding pacing activities and scheduling rest periods with exercise are important to meet the challenges of fatigue and weakness experienced by most patients. *Answer 14:* **a.**

15. Psychosocial support is very important for patients like Cindy because interferon has been reported to cause or exacerbate symptoms of depression (Donnelly, 1998). It will be important for you to differentiate symptoms of depression (e.g., anxiety, sadness) from other possible central nervous system effects of interferon (e.g., change in cognitive function, sedation, apathy, stupor). Ongoing neurologic assessments are imperative, and patients who are experiencing depression should be referred to appropriate supportive resources or for psychiatric care if needed (Donnelly, 1998). Patients must be monitored for abnormal clinical laboratory functions such as mild myelosuppression and elevations of serum transaminases (Sondak & Margolin, 1998). Assessment for hepatotoxicity should be ongoing. *Answer 15:* **b.**

16. If Cindy's disease progresses while she is taking interferon, other treatment options are available to her. However, there is no effective systemic therapy. Few durable remissions have been obtained, and there are considerable toxicities of available regimens (Sondak & Margolin, 1998). Interleukin-2 (IL-2, Proleukin) is the only other recombinant biologic agent that has demonstrated antitumor effect in melanoma. This is administered at high dosages and has serious multisystem toxicities. Multiagent systemic therapy for melanoma is presented in Table 5-3. Dacarbazine (DTIC) is the standard single agent choice for the treatment of melanoma, although nitrosoureas, platinum-containing drugs, and the taxanes are sometimes used. Multiagent chemotherapy has rarely provided a median survival time greater than 10 months and does not appear to effectively prevent or treat central nervous system metastases (Nathanson, 1999). No one program has proven effective for stage IV metastatic disease. Biochemotherapy (the use of chemother-

apy followed by biotherapy with both interferon and IL-2) has only shown a modest gain in survival duration compared with polychemotherapy regimens. In addition, biochemotherapy is a toxic and complex treatment course. Hormones such as tamoxifen and megestrol have shown some activity when combined with other chemotherapeutic agents, and new investigational drugs such as temozolomide demonstrate antimelanoma activity in addition to possible central nervous system metastases prevention potential (Nathanson, 1999). *Answer 16:* **d.**

17. The role of radiation therapy in melanoma is often limited to palliative treatment of metastases to the brain, spinal cord, or bones. The major oncologic emergency associated with melanoma is spinal cord compression, in which radiation therapy has a definitive role. Radiation therapy may sometimes be used for symptomatic nodal metastases in sites not accessible to surgical intervention (Benson, 1999). When patients are confronted with progressive disease and a median survival time of 6 to 12 months, the best option may be to encourage the patient to enroll in a clinical trial. If you work with melanoma patients, you will have to keep abreast of referral treatment centers that may provide the hope of the most effective individualized treatment and access to experimental drugs (Becker, 1997). Investigational trials in the area of melanoma research include numerous vaccine protocols and gene therapy. Participating in clinical trials may also provide patients with a sense of hope and altruism, believing that they are contributing to the progress of science and a possible cure for this disease. *Answer 17:* **c.**

TABLE **5-3** | **Systemic and Multiagent Therapy for Melanoma**

SINGLE AGENTS	MULTIAGENT REGIMENS
Dacarbazine	DBD:DTIC (dacarbazine)
Nitrosoureas (BCNU, CCNU)	BCNU (carmustine)
Cisplatin	DDP (cisplatin)
Carboplatin	
Paclitaxel	CVD:DDP (cisplatin)
Vinca alkaloids (VCR, VLB)	VLB (vinblastine)
Ifosfamide (with mesna)	DTIC (dacarbazine)
Procarbazine	
Dactinomycin	Biochemotherapy: CVD regimen as above
Biologics	Interleukin-2 Interferon-alfa
Interferon-alfa (2a or 2b)	Granulocyte colony-stimulating factor
Interleukin-2 (high dose)	

From Nathanson, l. (1999). Melanoma and other skin malignancies. In Skeel, R. T. (Ed.). *Handbook of cancer chemotherapy* (pp. 353-371). Philadelphia: Lippincott Williams & Wilkins.

REFERENCES

American Cancer Society (ACS). (2000). *Cancer facts & figures 2000.* Atlanta: Author.

Becker, M. (1997). Malignant melanoma. In Gates, R. A., & Fink, R. M. (Eds.). *Oncology nursing secrets* (pp. 196-201). Philadelphia: Hanley & Belfus.

Benson, L. (1999). Malignant melanoma. In Miaskowski, C., & Buchsel, P. (Eds.). *Oncology nursing: Assessment and clinical care* (pp. 1643-1678). St. Louis: Mosby.

Blanchard, C. G., Albrecht, T. L., & Ruckdeschel, J. C. (1995). The role of social support in adaptation to cancer and to survival. *J Psychosocial Oncol, 13,* pp. 75-95.

Bush, N. J. (1999). Bringing home the daffodils: The psychosocial impact of melanoma. *Dev Support Care, 2,* pp. 126-132.

Cameron, R. B., & Wong, J. (1994). Malignant melanoma. In Cameron, R. B. (Ed.). *Practical oncology* (pp. 118-132). Norwalk, CT: Appleton and Lange.

Donnelly, S. (1998). Patient management strategies for interferon alfa-2b as adjuvant therapy of high-risk melanoma. *Oncol Nurs Forum, 25*, pp. 921-927.

Fawzy, F. I., Fawzy, N. W., Hyun, C. S., & Wheeler, J. G. (1997). Brief, coping oriented therapy for patients with malignant melanoma. In Spira, J. L. (Ed.). *Group therapy for medically ill patients.* New York: Guilford Press.

Fraser, M. C., Goldstein, A. M., & Tucker, M. A (1997). The genetics of melanoma. *Semin Oncol Nurs, 13,* pp. 108-114.

Gale, D. M., & Kiley, K. E. (1998). Malignant melanoma and adjuvant alpha interferon-2b for patients at high risk of relapse. *Clin J Oncol Nurs, 2,* pp. 5-10.

Gale, D. M., & Richards, J. (1999). An overview of malignant melanoma. *Dev Support Care, 2*(4), pp. 113-118.

Gupta, S. M., & Davis, I. (1999). Sunscreens and melanoma prevention. *Dev Support Care, 2,* pp. 119-123.

Hoffman, S. L. (1994). Cutaneous melanoma. In Wood, M. E., & Bunn, P. A. (Eds.). *Hematology oncology secrets* (pp. 313-317). Philadelphia: Hanley & Belfus.

Kiley, K. E., & Gale, D. M. (1998). Nursing management of patients with malignant melanoma receiving adjuvant alpha interferon-2b. *Clin J Oncol Nurs, 2,* pp. 11-16.

Loescher, L. (1999). Familial cutaneous melanoma. *Dev Support Care, 2,* pp. 124-125.

Morton, D. L., Wen, D. R., Wong, J. H., et al. (1992). Technical details of intraoperative lymphatic mapping for early stage melanoma. *Arch Surg, 127,* pp. 392-399.

Nathanson, L. (1999). Melanoma and other skin malignancies. In Skeel, R. T. (Ed.). *Handbook of cancer chemotherapy* (pp. 353-371). Philadelphia: Lippincott Williams & Wilkins.

Sondak, V. K., & Margolin, K. A. (1998). Melanomas and other skin cancers. In Pazdur, R., Coia, L. R., Hoskins, W. J., & Wagman, L. D. (Eds.). *Cancer management: A multidisciplinary approach* (pp. 361-386). New York: PRR.

Springhouse. (1998). *Nurse practitioner's drug handbook.* Springhouse, PA: Author.

Wagner, R. F., & Casciato, D. A. (1995). Skin cancers. In Casciato, D. A., & Lowitz, B. B. (Eds.). *Manual of clinical oncology* (pp. 288-299). Boston: Little, Brown.

6 Surgical Therapy

Leslie Mathews

CASE 1 STUDY

John Stanford, a 60-year-old African American man, presents with complaints of vague abdominal pain and blood streaking his stool.

History of Present Illness
Reports general good health until about 3 months ago, when he started having abdominal cramping and increased constipation; little relief from laxatives. Denies change in diet; appetite somewhat lessened, with 18-pound weight loss (over 2 to 3 months).

Past Medical/Surgical History
Hypertension for 5 years; no history of excessive bleeding. Has never been hospitalized; has no past surgical history.

Medications
Takes a thiazide diuretic and one aspirin daily. No medication allergies.

Social History
Smoking history: 1 pack per day for 40 years (40 pack/years), alcohol use rare; married, works as a mail carrier.

Family History
Father died of colorectal cancer at age 72. Mother died of cardiac-related illness at age 76. Has three brothers, all alive; 64, 63, and 56 years. One brother has lung cancer, currently receiving therapy; one brother has hypertension and type II diabetes. Has three sons: 43, 42, and 40. All are alive and well. No other significant family history.

QUESTIONS

1. What is the most important component in evaluation of the surgical oncology patient?
   a. History and physical examination
   b. Metastatic workup
   c. Cardiac risk index
   d. Tolerance for anesthesia

ANSWERS

1. A detailed medical history and physical examination are the most important factors in the evaluation of the surgical patient. They constitute the best possible screening processes and provide nearly all the clinical data necessary for detection of diseases that may affect the surgical outcome. Additional preoperative tests should be obtained based on these clinical data and the nature of the surgical procedure. Although the metastatic workup is important for staging, it is guided by clinical information obtained in the history and physical examination. The cardiac risk and anesthesia tolerance are important for determining operative cardiac and pulmonary risk. The goal of the perioperative evaluation is to assess the patient's overall health, identify any undetected medical conditions, and correct any comorbid conditions (Carson & Eisenberg, 1994).

The patient's general state of health is considered when determining the role of surgery. Age alone is less likely to be a limiting factor. Other areas of concern are quality-of-life issues, general health habits, host resistance, nutritional status, and the extent of preexisting medical conditions. See Box 6-1, p. 79. *Answer 1:* **a.**

QUESTIONS

2. The information obtained in the history thus far is leading you to adapt a specific focus of systems assessment as you begin. In what areas do you need to focus?
   1. Gastrointestinal (GI)
   2. Urinary
   3. Respiratory
   4. Cardiovascular
      a. 1 & 2
      b. 1 & 3
      c. 2 & 3
      d. 3 & 4

ANSWERS

2. Although it is important to cover all areas in the review of systems, Mr. Stanford's information should guide you to ask particular questions regarding GI symptoms (e.g., bowel history, ab-

dominal symptoms) and respiratory symptoms (smoker). *Answer 2:* **b.**

QUESTIONS

3. What symptoms should you ask about when considering a diagnosis of colon cancer?
1. Increased laxative use
2. Productive cough
3. Thin stools
4. Urine color
5. Hemorrhoids
6. Melena
   a. 1, 2, 3, & 4
   b. 1, 2, 3, & 6
   c. 2, 4, 5, & 6
   d. 1, 3, 5, & 6

4. The clinical manifestations of colon cancer are related to the anatomic location of the tumor. Mr. Stanford's symptoms (constipation, abdominal pain, and melena) are most suggestive of a colon cancer in which part of the large intestine?
   a. Ascending colon
   b. Transverse colon
   c. Sigmoid colon
   d. Anus and rectum

ANSWERS

3. Tumors arising in the descending colon most often produce obstructive symptoms, which cause alterations in bowel habits. Vague abdominal pain and increased use of laxatives in older patients suggest cancer. Gas pain, decrease in stool caliber ("pencil stools"), hemorrhoids, and urgency to defecate on awakening suggest a distal lesion. The most common symptoms of a sigmoid lesion are abdominal pain and melena. *Answer 3:* **d.**

4. Masses in the ascending colon are more likely to be silent until they are large. Common symptoms include fatigue, iron deficiency anemia, and a palpable mass. Alterations in bowel habits are seldom seen because stool in the ascending colon is liquid and obstruction related to a tumor rarely occurs.

Lesions in the transverse colon manifest symptoms such as constipation alternating with diarrhea; rectal tumor symptoms include sensation of incomplete evacuation and bright red rectal bleeding. Symptoms generally correspond to sites involved, but nonspecific symptoms, such as weight loss, fatigue, and night sweats, may be the initial manifestations of any underlying malignancy. The aggressiveness of the cancer may be revealed by the duration and extent of symptoms; the degree of physical impairment also influences

treatment decisions regarding palliation (Hoebler, 1997). *Answer 4:* **c.**

QUESTIONS

5. What is the proper sequence for examination of the abdomen?
   a. Auscultation, percussion, inspection, palpation
   b. Auscultation, inspection, palpation, percussion
   c. Inspection, auscultation, percussion, palpation
   d. Inspection, percussion, palpation, auscultation

6. What is the span of the normal adult liver?
   a. 6 to 12 cm in the midclavicular line
   b. 2 to 4 cm in the midsternal line
   c. Undetectable in the midsternal line
   d. Greater in women than in men

ANSWERS

5. It is necessary to auscultate the abdomen before percussion and palpation because percussion may alter the frequency and intensity of bowel sounds. The absence of bowel sounds is not established unless no sounds are detected during 5 minutes of continuous auscultation. Percussion is an important means of assessing the size and density of abdominal organs, as well as detecting fluid or air in the abdomen. *Answer 5:* **c.**

6. The span of the normal liver is 6 to 12 cm in the midclavicular line; it is 4 to 8 cm in the midsternal line. It is usually greater in men than in women and greater in tall people compared with short people (Bates, 1995). Table 6-1 notes important factors to consider in the assessment of oncology patients who require surgery. *Answer 6:* **a.**

Case Study continued

Physical Examination

Weight, 170 pounds; height, 71 inches; blood pressure, 150/88 mm Hg; SKIN: anicteric without rash or bruises; HEENT: without thrush or mucositis; BACK: without spinal tenderness; CHEST: with coarse inspiratory crackles; CARDIAC: S_1/S_2, no murmurs or rubs; ABDOMEN: without palpable intraabdominal masses, ascites, or hepatosplenomegaly; EXTREMITIES: without edema; NEUROLOGIC: nonfocal examination.

The major role of surgery in cancer diagnosis is to procure tissue for evaluation. The diagnosis of cancer must be based on histologic confirmation. Common surgical techniques for obtaining a

TABLE **6-1** Factors to Consider in the Assessment of Oncology Patients Requiring Surgery		
AREA OF ASSESSMENT	**ENTITY**	**RISK**
Cardiovascular disease	Recent myocardial infarctions (<3 mo), severe cardiac ischemia, previous use of anthracycline chemotherapy (doxorubicin)	>30% risk of reinfarction, perioperative infarction, congestive heart failure, and pulmonary edema
Previous surgical procedures	Previous surgical experiences, response to anesthesia, and postoperative complications	Anesthesia reactions, malignant hyperthermia
Pulmonary disease	Smoking history; chronic obstructive pulmonary disease; emphysema; prior use of bleomycin, methotrexate, or busulfan; high concentrations of oxygen given to patients who have previously received bleomycin	Postoperative atelectasis, pneumonia, prolonged intubation, prolonged pulmonary toxicity and difficulty in efforts to wean from mechanical ventilation postoperatively, respiratory failure
Coagulopathy	Bleeding history, patient and family history, undetected inherited coagulopathies	Prolonged bleeding, hemorrhage, thromboembolism
Liver and kidney diseases	Renal or hepatic dysfunction, prior use of methotrexate	Problems managing hemostasis, intravascular volume, and electrolyte balance; hepatic fibrosis; both organs are important in the response to and clearance of anesthetics
Medications	Allergies; warfarin or aspirin must be stopped preoperatively, whereas others, such as steroids and insulin, must be continued	Prolonged bleeding, anaphylaxis
Prior cancer therapies	Bleomycin, doxorubicin, alkylating agents, and corticosteroids	Delayed wound healing, anesthesia risk
Prior radiation therapy	Particularly if the surgical incision is in the treatment field	Will affect healing and can contribute to fistula development, rejection of tissue grafts, anastomotic leaks, obstruction, and hemorrhage
Metabolic alterations	Diabetes, thyroid, syndrome of inappropriate antidiuretic hormone secretion, hypercalcemia	Delayed wound healing, infection, anesthesia risk
Neurologic deficits	Prior vincristine sulfate (Oncovin), cis-platinum; peripheral nerve dysfunction	May be incorrectly attributed to postanesthesia or intraoperative central nervous system events

tissue sample include needle aspiration, core-needle biopsy, and incisional and excisional biopsies. Mr. Stanford is scheduled for a biopsy.

QUESTIONS

7. An excisional biopsy includes removal of:
   a. A portion of tissue at the tissue margin
   b. Fluid or tissue via aspiration
   c. The complete tumor with little or no margin of surrounding tissue
   d. A wedge of tissue from a large tumor

8. Fine-needle aspiration (FNA) is the best approach to biopsy in which situation?
   a. Grading of solid tumors
   b. Establishment of types of lymphoma

   c. Accurate diagnosis after radiation
   d. Retrieval of cells instead of tissue

9. Regarding a core-needle biopsy, all of the following are true *except:*
   a. It can be done under local anesthesia.
   b. It necessitates a surgical scar.
   c. It can be performed in the outpatient area.
   d. It is adequate for tissue histology.

ANSWERS

7. Surgical diagnostic techniques include needle aspiration, incisional and excisional biopsies, and core-needle biopsies. When an accurate diagnosis of tumor type and grading is necessary, an incisional or excisional biopsy is required. A small

BOX **6-1** **Surgical Principles in Oncology:**
Initial Management

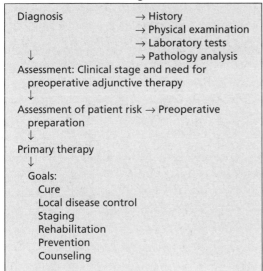

Diagnosis → History
→ Physical examination
→ Laboratory tests
↓ → Pathology analysis
Assessment: Clinical stage and need for
preoperative adjunctive therapy
↓
Assessment of patient risk → Preoperative
preparation
↓
Primary therapy
↓
Goals:
Cure
Local disease control
Staging
Rehabilitation
Prevention
Counseling

From Daly, J. M., Bertagnolli, M., DeCosse, J. J., & Morton, D. L. (1999). Oncology. In Schwartz, S. I. (Ed.). *Principles of surgery*, 7th ed. (pp. 297-364).

wedge of tissue from a larger tumor is removed for an incisional biopsy. This is particularly useful in sarcomas, large tumors, and unresectable tumors. Excisional biopsy is the total removal of all tissue with little or no margin of surrounding normal tissue. It is generally limited to use in the removal of small tumors (Frogge & Kalinowski, 1997; Rosenberg, 1997). Table 6-2 lists surgical biopsy techniques. *Answer 7:* **c.**

8. FNA involves using a fine needle guided into the questionable tissue and aspirating tissue fragments. There are associated false-negative results with this approach because there are inherent problems with cell analysis and the aspirate usually does not provide enough specimen for histologic diagnosis. *Answer 8:* **d.**

9. Core-needle biopsy is the retrieval of a small core of tissue using a specially designed needle. Ultrasound guidance enhances the accuracy in obtaining adequate tissue. The core sample is sufficient for diagnosis of most tumors and is convenient and relatively cost-effective. Advances in imaging techniques have vastly improved needle placement and guidance. This has ultimately improved the accuracy and safety of needle placement along the target path while avoiding injury to other structures. *Answer 9:* **b.**

QUESTIONS

10. Which of the following laboratory studies are crucial for Mr. Stanford before surgery?
  a. Complete blood count (CBC), electrolytes, liver function tests
  b. Carcinoembryonic antigen (CEA), electrolytes, prothrombin time/partial thromboplastin time (PT/PTT)
  c. CBC, liver function tests, CEA
  d. CBC, electrolytes, hepatitis screen

11. The preoperative laboratory studies required are for all of the following reasons *except:*
  a. To monitor preexisting conditions
  b. To identify anemia
  c. To perform routine screening
  d. To evaluate liver metastasis

12. What is the usefulness of the CEA in patients with colorectal cancer?
  a. Screening purposes
  b. Evaluation of residual or recurrent disease
  c. Guidance for preoperative management
  d. Determination of a complete response

ANSWERS

10-11. Laboratory studies performed before surgery evaluate important preoperative parameters and are used to monitor preexisting conditions. The hematocrit and hemoglobin are simple inexpensive tests that should be ordered for all patients undergoing surgery. The prevalence of anemia in asymptomatic patients is relatively high. Obtaining a PT/PTT is controversial as a preoperative screen for bleeding in those who do not have a personal or family history of excessive bleeding. Increases in both lactate dehydrogenase (LDH) and alkaline phosphatase are present in only about 15% of patients with liver metastasis (Carson & Eisenberg, 1994). *Answer 10:* **a.** *Answer 11:* **d.**

12. CEA is a glycoprotein present in GI mucosa. It is useful as a tumor marker for patients who have CEA-producing adenocarcinomas. However, colorectal cancers of all stages can be present in the face of a normal CEA. Elevations may be caused by hepatitis (both alcoholic and viral), cholelithiasis, pancreatitis, renal failure, diverticulitis, fibrocystic breast disease, and smoking. Therefore CEA levels are not used for routine screening, but rather for postoperative surveillance as a marker for tumor recurrence and in monitoring response to chemotherapy. CEA is associated with, but not the

TABLE 6-2 | Surgical Biopsy Techniques

TECHNIQUE	USES IN CANCER CARE	ADVANTAGES	DISADVANTAGES
Fine-needle aspiration 20-22 gauge	Retrieves cells vs. tissue Used when high suspicion for malignancy Used for solid, palpable lesions Examples: breast, thyroid, cervical adenopathy	Quick Avoid surgical scar Local anesthesia Outpatient	Need trained cytologist False-negative results Cannot be used to diagnose lymphoma, sarcoma
Percutaneous needle aspiration 20-23 gauge	Retrieves cells vs. tissue Used for solid, nonpalpable lesions Radiologic localization, CT, MRI, US, Mammogram Examples: lung, breast	May avoid need and cost of surgery Local anesthesia Outpatient	False-negative results Cannot be used to diagnose lymphoma, sarcoma Special stains procedures cannot be done
Core-needle biopsy 14-20 gauge Tru-cut automated biopsy gun	Retrieves tissue Used for both palpable and nonpalpable lesions through radiographic approach Examples: pancreas, liver, stereotactic breast biopsy, retroperitoneum	Avoids surgical scar Local anesthesia Outpatient	Need technically trained and skilled personnel Risk injury to adjacent structures Risk tumor cell seeding along biopsy tract
Incisional biopsy	Obtain wedge of tissue for solid, large mass Example: head and neck tumors, liver	Obtain tissue diagnosis when mass too large to easily remove surgically Local and/or IV sedation	Necessitates scar Requires OR time Bleeding at site Risk of infection
Excisional biopsy	Solid, palpable mass Removal of complete lump with little or no planned margin	Day surgery Remove all gross disease	Risk of infection Requires scar
Endoscopic biopsy	Used for solid mass in lumen Used to obtain cytologic brushings and/or tissue	Avoids surgical procedure Can place scar cosmetically Day surgery	Pain and trauma associated with scope
Laparoscopic biopsy	Used to sample tissue–abdomen, pelvis, lymphadenopathy, pancreas, liver	May avoid need for more major surgery Decreased length of stay	Decreased ability to assess complete abdomen

From McCurkle, R., Grant, M., Frank-Stromberg, M., & Baird, S. (1996). *Cancer nursing: A comprehensive textbook*, 2nd ed. Philadelphia: WB Saunders.
CT, Computed tomography; *IV*, intravenous; *MRI*, magnetic resonance imaging; *US*, ultrasound.

determinant of, a complete response. An elevated, sustained postoperative CEA is related to tumor recurrence in most patients. Rising CEA levels (serial changes greater than 35% of baseline) may indicate progression of disease. Its significance is more relative postoperatively. Recent studies have demonstrated that mass preoperative screening does not result in a change in operative planning in almost 99% of patients. Institutions establish their own policies for routine preoperative tests that should be ordered, and the patient's condition dictates the need for any additional testing (Daly, Bertagnolli, DeCosse, & Morton, 1999). *Answer 12:* **b.**

QUESTIONS

13. All of the following additional initial diagnostic tests might be recommended for Mr. Stanford because colon cancer is suspected, *except:*

   a. Abdominal computed tomography (CT) scan
   b. Barium enema
   c. Colonoscopy
   d. Sigmoidoscopy

ANSWERS

13. Patients suspected of having colon cancer must have the entire colon evaluated for multiple primary sites (synchronous lesions). Most colorectal cancers are diagnosed by the following examinations, to be performed in sequence until a diagnosis is reached: (1) rectal examination, (2) sigmoidoscopy with biopsy, and (3) colonoscopy with biopsy or double-contrast barium enema. The barium enema may reveal synchronous lesions in the right colon that may have been missed by colonoscopy. Although CT scans can be performed as part of the preoperative evaluation, their use is controversial. The primary role of the preoperative CT scan in tumors above the peritoneal reflection is to screen for hepatic metastasis; staging of hepatic lesions by CT alone is considered less accurate than pathologic staging done intraoperatively (Engstrom, Benson, & Cohen, 1996). *Answer 13:* **a.**

QUESTIONS

14. Mr. Stanford's daughter tells you that she is quite concerned about her dad's smoking and asks if there is any connection to smoking and colorectal cancer. Your answer incorporates your knowledge that smoking is known to be a risk factor for the increased incidence of all the following *except:*

   a. Peptic ulcer
   b. Colorectal cancer
   c. Laryngeal carcinoma
   d. Carcinoma of the bladder

ANSWERS

14. Some of the more common adverse effects of smoking are cancers of the lung, chronic obstructive pulmonary disease (COPD; e.g., chronic bronchitis, emphysema), myocardial infarction, and systemic atherosclerosis. Some of the less common adverse effects are peptic ulcer and cancer of the larynx, esophagus, kidney, pancreas, and bladder. There is no known association between cigarette smoking and colorectal cancer. *Answer 14:* **b.**

QUESTIONS

15. Mr. Stanford's wife voices concern about her husband undergoing surgery because he has smoked for so long. What of the following could *best* improve Mr. Stanford's pulmonary status preoperatively?

   a. Obtaining preoperative pulmonary function tests
   b. Initiating prophylactic bronchodilator therapy
   c. Providing instruction for deep-breathing exercises
   d. Advising Mr. Stanford to stop smoking at least 1 week before the scheduled surgery

ANSWERS

15. Smoking, even without chronic lung disease, is a risk factor for postoperative pulmonary complications. The value of preoperative pulmonary function testing (PFT) is controversial. It is agreed that patients who will be undergoing lung resection should have PFT to evaluate lung capacity and pulmonary reserve. However, these tests should be used selectively in patients scheduled for other surgical procedures. A review by Smetana (1999) found that the operative risk of pulmonary complications in smokers is lower in those who had stopped smoking at least 8 weeks before surgery than those who did not stop at all. Interestingly, there was a higher risk in those who had stopped smoking less than 8 weeks earlier. Preoperative instruction for deep-breathing and coughing exercises is generally regarded as standard practice (Schwartz, 2000). See Box 6-2. *Answer 15:* **c.**

Case Study continued

Mr. Stanford is scheduled for a low anterior resection. Certain preparations must be considered for all patients to minimize the risk of surgical complications. The following orders are written. Match the rationale for each order.

16. Ensure that aspirin has been discontinued 1 week before admission	a. Thrombosis risk
	b. Bleeding risk
	c. Infection risk
17. Discontinue diuretic on admission	d. Volume shifts
	e. Dehydration

18. Admit patient to hospital 1 day before surgery for bowel preparation:

   a. GoLYTELY 1 gallon
   b. Neomycin 1 g and erythromycin

| BOX 6-2 | Risk-Reduction Strategies |

PREOPERATIVE

Encourage cessation of cigarette smoking for at least 8 wk.

Treat airflow obstruction in patients with chronic obstructive pulmonary disease or asthma.

Administer antibiotics and delay surgery if respiratory infection is present.

Begin patient education regarding lung-expansion maneuvers.

INTRAOPERATIVE

Limit duration of surgery to less than 3 hr.

Use spinal or epidural anesthesia.*

Avoid use of pancuronium.

Use laparoscopic procedures when possible.

Substitute less ambitious procedure for upper abdominal or thoracic surgery when possible.

POSTOPERATIVE

Use deep-breathing exercises or incentive spirometry.

Use continuous positive airway pressure.

Use epidural analgesia.*

Use intercostal nerve blocks.*

From Smetana, G. W. (1999). Preoperative pulmonary evaluation. *N Engl J Med, 340*(12), pp. 937-943.
*This strategy is recommended, although variable efficacy has been reported in the literature.

     c. Base 500 mg at 1 PM, 2 PM, and 11 PM

19. Start intravenous hydration preoperatively; nothing by mouth (NPO) after midnight

20. Start external compression boots morning of surgery

21. Administer cefotetan 1 g 1 hour before surgery

———————————————— **ANSWERS**

16. The antiplatelet effect of aspirin may last for up to 1 week after a single dose and therefore should be discontinued before surgery. *Answer 16:* **b.**

17. Discontinuing diuretics contributes to maximizing the patient's volume status and blood pressure during surgery when blood loss is expected. It also reduces the chance of ion loss or shift, such as potassium. *Answer 17:* **d.**

18. Although there is some controversy over which particular bowel regimen is best, the data support that a mechanical preparation resulting in a stool-free colon and accompanied by oral antibiotics minimizes the incidence of postoperative wound infection. Neomycin and erythromycin reduce bacterial flora in the colon (Niederhuber, 2000). *Answer 18:* **c.**

19. The patient will be NPO for at least 8 hours before surgery. Therefore adequate hydration must be ensured, especially if the surgical procedure involves large volumes of fluid shifts. *Answer 19:* **d.**

20. Assessment of deep venous thrombosis (DVT) risk is very important. Coagulation abnormalities, both hemorrhagic and thrombotic, are well recognized in the cancer patient. Prophylaxis must begin before induction of general anesthesia. Types of prophylaxis include the following:

- External pneumatic compression stockings
- Heparin 5000 units subcutaneously 2 hours before and every 8 to 12 hours postoperatively until ambulation
- Low-molecular-weight heparin (LMWH) 5000 units subcutaneously starting the evening before surgery and every day for 5 to 10 days postoperatively

LMWH is heparin with antithrombotic properties that enhance inhibition of factor Xa and thrombin. Specific recommendations for DVT prophylaxis should be based on assessment of risk. *Answer 20:* **a.**

21. Intravenous antibiotics that effectively cover gram-negative bacilli and anaerobes, such as cefotetan and cefoxitin, are given just before the start of the operation as infection prophylaxis. Postoperative coverage is not generally necessary. *Answer 21:* **c.**

Case Study continued

Mr. Stanford underwent a low anterior resection with lymph node sampling. Pathology shows a poorly differentiated adenocarcinoma of the colon that extends into the muscularis propria; two pericolic lymph nodes of seven positive with clear margins.

QUESTIONS ————————————————

22. Pathologic staging can predict or determine which of the following?

    a. Disease responsiveness

    b. Local metastasis

c. Neoplasm's natural course
d. Clinical course

22. Pathologic staging gives insight into the nature of the course of the neoplasm, which is necessary to determine further treatment plans. The ability to resect is also determined by the tumor's relation to, and degree of invasion into and around, vital structures. Clinical staging includes findings acquired before definitive treatment: physical examination, imaging, biopsy, and some surgical exploration. Surgical evaluative and pathologic staging, as well as lymph node studies, are done after surgery (Frogge & Kalinowski, 1997; Rosenberg, 1997). *Answer 22:* **c.**

Case Study continued

Resection of colon cancer involves removal of the tumor, the tumor's blood supply, and the draining lymphatics. The remaining portions are then anastomosed. Match the surgical procedure with the correct anastomosis. Refer to Figure 6-1.

23. Right hemicolectomy

24. Extended right hemicolectomy

25. Total colectomy

26. Low anterior resection

a. Ileum to peritoneal reflection (above rectum)
b. Terminal ileum to proximal left colon
c. Descending colon to distal rectum
d. Terminal ileum to transverse colon

23. The right hemicolectomy is used for lesions involving the cecum, ascending colon, and hepatic flexure. *Answer 23:* **d.**

24. The extended right hemicolectomy is used for lesions in the right and transverse colon. It is the generally preferred procedure for transverse colon tumors. A transverse colectomy is rarely used because it requires an anastomosis between the ascending colon and the descending colon and it produces too much pull on remaining structures. *Answer 24:* **b.**

25. A total or subtotal colectomy involves removal of the bowel from the cecum to the peritoneal reflection. This results in chronic diarrhea postoperatively. It is indicated for multiple primary tumors and for hereditary nonpolyposis colon cancer (HNPCC). *Answer 25:* **a.**

26. The low anterior resection is used for lesions in the proximal one third to two thirds of the rectum and for tumors of the sigmoid colon. *Answer 26:* **c.**

Case Study continued

On the second postoperative day, Mr. Stanford develops a temperature of 100° F.

QUESTIONS

27. Which of the following questions can contribute the *most* helpful data in determining the source of Mr. Stanford's elevated temperature?
a. Is there any drainage from your incision?
b. Have you been performing coughing exercises?
c. Do you have suprapubic pain?
d. Are you drinking plenty of fluids?

28. On what assumption did you base your questions regarding the possibility of infection on the second postoperative day?
a. Because of altered skin integrity, incision sites are the most likely source for infection.
b. An indwelling Foley catheter has caused a urinary tract infection.
c. Dehydration is causing the fever.
d. Pneumonia is a common postoperative infection.

29. Mr. Stanford has not been performing coughing and deep-breathing exercises as ordered. He tells you that it hurts him to take deep breaths and that when he coughs, he feels like his incision will burst. In advising him, all of the following points should be considered *except:*
a. Pain medication should not be given before performing coughing and deep-breathing exercises because it can diminish respirations.
b. Splinting the incision with a pillow will help ease the discomfort of coughing.
c. Hypoventilation and retained secretions can lead to pneumonia.
d. Nebulizer treatments may facilitate loosening and removal of secretions.

27-28. The blood, lungs, and urinary tract are common sites of infection. All three sites require assessment yet the respiratory system is often the

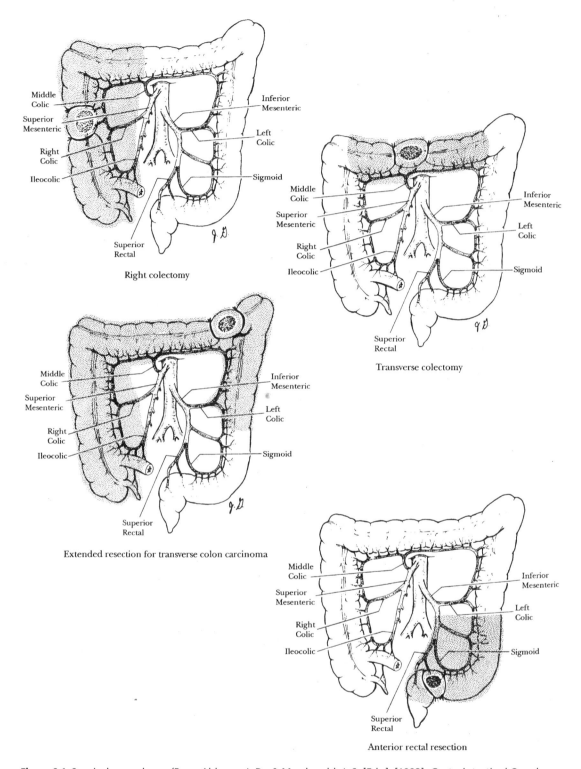

Figure 6-1 Surgical procedures. (From Ahlgren, J. D., & Macdonald, J. S. [Eds.]. [1992]. *Gastrointestinal Oncology.* Philadelphia: JB Lippincott.)

affected site. Incomplete lung expansion and retained secretions because of significant lack of movement, ambulation, and deep breaths often result in pneumonia. Many times, the chest radiograph ordered as part of the fever workup will reveal atelectasis and the beginnings of pneumonia. Negative blood cultures and urine samples sent at the same time rule out the other sites and assist in narrowing the antibiotic choice. Signs and symptoms more specific to a urinary tract infection include urine discoloration, hematuria, foul odor, and burning upon urination. Suprapubic pain is usually associated with bladder spasms where the Foley catheter is in place. Postoperative drainage is expected from the site and is not necessarily a sign of infection; localized erythema, increased tenderness/pain, and a foul odor suggest an infected incision site. Positive blood cultures, indicative of a systemic infection, can reflect seeding of an organism from a present or recently placed catheter and not necessarily an infected incision site.

Hospitalization allows close monitoring of fluid status. Unless Mr. Stanford has had excessive losses, either through emesis, diarrhea, or diuresis, the chance of him being volume depleted 2 days postoperatively is small. Rather, fluid overload is a more likely possibility. *Answer 27:* **b.** *Answer 28:* **d.**

29. Pain medication given 30 to 60 minutes before coughing and deep-breathing exercises or ambulation will lessen the amount of pain the patient experiences during these events, therefore allowing the patient to perform the exercises more efficiently. The other choices are all helpful in enhancing ventilation and removal of secretions. *Answer 29:* **a.**

QUESTIONS

30. In addition to a smoking history, what factors put a patient with cancer at particular risk for developing pneumonia?
1. Malnutrition
2. Altered immune function
3. Nosocomial organisms
4. Decreased mobility
   a. 1, 2, & 3
   b. 1, 2, & 4
   c. 1, 3, & 4
   d. 2, 3, & 4

ANSWERS

30. Cancer patients have a significantly increased risk of pneumonia developing. This may be because of altered immune function and local defense mechanisms in the lung from related therapies. Other factors such as decreased mobility

and cachexia-malnutrition syndromes also contribute. *Answer 30:* **b.**

Case Study continued

On the third postoperative day, Mr. Stanford's temperature rises to 102.1° F; his pulse is 110 beats/min; and he has shaking chills, chest pain, and a cough that is productive for purulent sputum.

QUESTIONS

31. A patient with pneumonia would most likely exhibit which of the following on physical examination?
   a. Decreased fremitus and hyperresonance to percussion
   b. Increased fremitus and dullness to percussion
   c. Increased fremitus and hyperresonance to percussion
   d. Decreased fremitus and dullness to percussion

32. Physical findings suggestive of pneumonia may include all of the following *except:*
   a. Productive cough
   b. Pleuritic chest pain
   c. Tympanic percussion
   d. Tachypnea

33. Which of the following findings on chest x-ray films confirms the diagnosis of pneumonia?
   a. Thickening of the pleura
   b. Diffuse patchy infiltrates
   c. Pulmonary fibrosis
   d. Blunting of the costophrenic angle

34. The following orders are written. Give a rationale for each order.
   a. Incentive spirometry: _____
   b. Antibiotic for gram-negative coverage: _____
   c. Stool cultures: _____
   d. Blood cultures: _____

ANSWERS

31. Incomplete lung expansion causes the distal alveoli to collapse, resulting in atelectasis. After surgery, this complication usually results from hypoventilation and excessive retained secretions, providing an excellent medium for bacterial growth, which causes stasis pneumonia. In this acute inflammation, the alveoli and bronchioles become plugged with a fibrous exudate, making them firm and inelastic. Bacteria, fungi, or viruses that cause pneumonia produce inflammatory exudates within the alveolar spaces (Weintraub & Neumark, 1996). This leads to consolidation of the lung parenchyma, which results in dyspnea, tachypnea, and rales. Decreased breath sounds, dullness to percussion, and increased fremitus are found over areas of consolidation. *Fremitus* (tactile fremitus) refers to vibrations that are perceived in a tactile, nonacoustic manner. *Answer 31:* **b.**

32. Pneumonia is characteristically accompanied by a cough with sputum production (productive cough), fever, chills, and pleuritic chest pain. Associated symptoms of headache, nausea and vomiting, anorexia, and lethargy may also be present. The signs of consolidation of the lung parenchyma include increased tactile and vocal fremitus, bronchophony, egophony, bronchial breath sounds, and possible fine rales over the consolidated area. These are often found with bacterial pneumonia, but the viral and mycoplasmal pneumonias characteristically show very few signs; often only rales are heard (Henkel & Fraser, 1995). *Answer 32:* **c.**

33. Patchy infiltrates and or areas of consolidation are associated with a diagnosis of pneumonia. Thickening of the pleura and pulmonary fibrosis are often related to findings of radiation-induced pulmonary complications; blunting of the costophrenic angle is most often associated with pleural effusions.

Pulmonary assessment is aimed at detecting atelectasis and pneumonia. Diminished breath sounds are auscultated, and flatness on percussion is noted. You should observe for decreased chest expansion and mediastinal shift toward the side of collapse. Also you should assess for fever; restlessness or confusion; worsening dyspnea; and elevated blood pressure, pulse rate, and respiratory rate.

To detect pneumonia, you should watch for the sudden onset of shaking chills with high fever and headache. Again, you should auscultate for diminished breath sounds or for telltale crackles over the affected lung area. The patient should be assessed for dyspnea, tachypnea, and sharp chest pain exacerbated by inspiration. A productive cough that has pink or rust-colored sputum may develop. You should observe for cyanosis and hypoxemia, confirmed by arterial blood gas measurement. Chest radiographs confirm the diagnosis and monitor infection progression. *Answer 33:* **b.**

34. Interventions: Order coughing and deep breathing exercises every 2 hours and incentive spirometry to facilitate complete lung expansion.

Administer antibiotics, often a second- or third-generation cephalosporin or beta-lactam.

Antimicrobials may cause diarrhea by causing nonspecific alteration of enteric flora or by causing pseudomembranous colitis (secondary to *Clostridium difficile*). *C. difficile* toxin–positive diarrhea as identified by stool cultures is treated with metronidazole 500 mg orally or intravenously three times daily for 7 to 14 days. Initial relapses are treated with longer courses of metronidazole, and refractory cases are treated with vancomycin 125 mg orally every 6 hours. Antimicrobial-associated diarrhea without evidence of pseudomembranous colitis usually responds to discontinuing the causative agent (Gross & Johnson, 1994; Henkel & Fraser, 1995).

Wound infection is the most common wound complication and the second most common nosocomial infection. It is also a major factor in wound dehiscence (the partial or total disruption of a surgical wound). Complete dehiscence leads to evisceration (the abrupt protrusion of wound contents). Abdominal wounds are more likely to dehisce and eviscerate than thoracic incisions. Copious serosanguinous drainage from the incision suggests wound dehiscence. The patient may also report a "popping sensation" after retching or coughing. Protruding contents is evidence of evisceration. When a lower abdominal wound eviscerates, coils of intestine may extrude from the abdomen.

Blood cultures rule out a concomitant bacteriemia, identify the organism, and with sensitivities, dictate the appropriate antibiotic. A leukocytosis supports the presence of an infection whether systemic or localized. Surgical incisions are assessed for increased tenderness, deep pain, and edema, especially from postoperative day 3 to day 5. You should monitor for increased pulse and temperature and an elevated white blood cell count.

Incisional site infections are usually caused by *Staphylococcus aureus*, coagulase-negative staphylococci, aerobic gram-negative bacilli, or enterococci. Obtaining a wound culture and sensitivities then results in vancomycin administration plus an aminoglycoside as initial therapy.

Incisional dehiscence or evisceration is treated by placing the patient in low Fowler's position with knees bent to decrease abdominal tension. The extruding contents are then covered with normal saline soaks. *Answer 34:* **See text.**

Case Study *continued*

Mr. Stanford comes to the emergency room months later complaining of abdominal pain, nausea, and vomiting for the past 24 hours.

QUESTIONS

35. Your differential diagnosis includes all of the following *except:*
- **a.** Paralytic ileus
- **b.** Appendicitis
- **c.** Bowel obstruction
- **d.** Anastomotic leak

ANSWERS

35. Sluggish peristalsis and paralytic ileus usually last 24 to 72 hours postoperatively and can cause abdominal distension. Nonabsorbable gas accumulates in the intestine and passes to the atonic portion of the bowel, remaining there until tone returns. A common acute postsurgical complication, paralytic ileus occurs whenever autonomic innervation of the GI tract is disrupted. Causes include intraoperative manipulation of intestinal organs; hypokalemia; wound infection; and medications, such as, codeine, morphine, and atropine (Fox, 1994; Frogge & Kalinowski, 1997). *Answer 35:* **a.**

Case Study continued

On physical examination of Mr. Stanford, you find the following:

- Temperature 98.9° F orally
- Abdominal distension with tenderness, negative peritoneal signs
- Rushes of high-pitched sounds on auscultation
- Negative rectal examination

QUESTIONS

36. A rectal examination can give you information about occult bleeding. What additional information does a rectal examination *not* give you?
- **a.** To monitor peristalsis
- **b.** To evaluate sphincter tone
- **c.** To determine whether there is fecal impaction
- **d.** To evaluate for hemorrhoids

ANSWERS

36. The rectal examination is an important part of the full GI evaluation of Mr. Stanford's abdominal distress. In addition to providing information of occult bleeding, a rectal examination is necessary to evaluate whether there is a mass in the anorectal region. This could be fecal impaction or progression of disease. Peristalsis cannot be evaluated by the digital rectal examination. *Answer 36:* **a.**

QUESTIONS

37. All of the following conditions are usually associated with the finding of decreased bowel sounds *except:*
- **a.** Advanced intestinal obstruction
- **b.** Peritonitis
- **c.** Paralytic ileus
- **d.** Brisk diarrhea

ANSWERS

37. Brisk diarrhea or early intestinal obstruction produces increased bowel sounds. Any condition that produces ileus (absence of peristalsis) will result in absent or decreased bowel sounds. This can occur with peritonitis, mesenteric thrombosis, pneumonia, myxedema, electrolyte abnormalities, and advanced intestinal obstruction. *Answer 37:* **d.**

Case Study continued

The signs of peritoneal irritation include rebound tenderness (Blumberg's sign), tenderness to light percussion of the abdomen, jar tenderness (Markel's sign), and guarding.

QUESTIONS

38. How is rebound tenderness evaluated?
- **a.** By pressing the right costal margin at the edge of the rectus muscle and asking the patient to take a deep breath
- **b.** By placing your straightened fingers on the abdomen and briefly jabbing them toward the back
- **c.** By pressing slowly on a tender area and then quickly withdrawing your hand
- **d.** By palpating all quadrants of the abdomen softly using the pads of your fingertips

ANSWERS

38. When a patient presents with intestinal obstruction, you should examine the patient for peritoneal signs. Voluntary rigidity, often accompanied by pulling away from the examiner, is a sign of resistance to palpation for reasons such as tense posture, a chilled external environment, cold hands of the examiner, or fear of pain or tickling. Involuntary guarding of abdominal muscles is caused by reflex muscle spasm from peritoneal irritation. Other signs of peritoneal irritation are rebound tenderness (Blumberg's sign), tenderness to palpation, and tenderness to vibration (Markel's sign), which can be tested by the heel jar test. Firmly and slowly pressing in, then quickly withdrawing your fingers performs rebound tenderness. The test is positive if pain is noted during the withdrawal maneuver. The other tests described are (a) Murphy's sign for cholecystitis, (b) ballottement, and (d) light palpation (Bates, 1995). *Answer 38:* **c.**

QUESTIONS

39. Common findings in intestinal obstruction include all of the following *except:*
- **a.** Ascites
- **b.** Distension
- **c.** Vomiting
- **d.** Pain

ANSWERS

39. The hallmarks of intestinal obstruction are abdominal pain, distension, vomiting, and obstipation. Symptoms vary in intensity, depending on the level of obstruction. An obstruction high in the small intestine commonly produces copious vomiting, whereas an obstruction in the colon may present with distension as the major symptom. On physical examination, the abdomen is usually distended and bowel sounds are typically high pitched and occur in rushes. In the late stages of obstruction, bowel sounds may be diminished or absent. Ascites is not commonly found in obstruction; it is usually associated with abnormal liver function or low plasma oncotic pressure. *Answer 39:* **a.**

Case Study continued

Abdominal films (flat and upright) are ordered and reveal a dilated and gas-filled colon without gas visualized in the colon distally. There is no free air under the diaphragm.

QUESTIONS

40. Your initial management includes all of the following *except:*
- **a.** Intravenous fluid
- **b.** Nasogastric (NG) tube
- **c.** Water-soluble barium enema
- **d.** CT scan of the abdomen and thorax

ANSWERS

40. An abdominal radiograph (flat and upright) will usually identify the site of obstruction. Management of bowel obstruction includes decompression of the bowel by placement of an NG tube. An NG tube decompresses the abdomen and may be sufficient to relieve obstruction in some cases. A water-soluble contrast enema will clarify the nature of the obstructing lesion, and the water-soluble contrast will be safe if there is a

perforation. The occurrence of free intestinal perforation is usually confirmed by free air under the diaphragm, which is taken in an upright or a left decubitus abdominal radiograph. A CT scan of the abdomen may be necessary to determine the extent of disease and involvement of surrounding structures. A CT scan of the thorax is not indicated at this time because the results will not alter the planned operative course.

Surgical intervention should be considered if the obstruction does not resolve after 4 to 5 days of decompression and if the patient's medical condition allows. Patients who have acute bowel obstruction usually require a three-stage operation. The first procedure involves decompression of the bowel through the creation of a diverting colostomy; the second stage is the complete evaluation of the bowel for synchronous lesions and definitive resection of the tumor. Closure of the colostomy, the third stage, is performed at a later date, usually at 12 weeks.

Other conditions that may cause bowel obstruction are diverticulitis, adhesions, acute pancreatitis, radiation injury, and vinca alkaloid neurotoxicity. *Answer 40:* **d.**

Case Study continued

Mr. Stanford is scheduled for a diverting sigmoid colostomy for obstructive, locally recurrent colon cancer. Mrs. Stanford tells you that they will never be able to manage that "bag-thing" at home. She does not believe she has the capability.

QUESTIONS

41. What considerations should you emphasize to address their concerns?
- **a.** The colostomy will be reversed in 3 months.
- **b.** Sigmoid colostomies can be regulated and controlled with irrigation.
- **c.** Output from Mr. Stanford's colostomy will be primarily liquid.
- **d.** Sigmoid colostomies do not require a bag.

ANSWERS

41. Diverting colostomies are usually temporary and are often reversed in 3 to 4 months. However, Mrs. Stanford's concern at this time is the maintenance of the colostomy itself, so these are the issues to be addressed. Patients with sigmoid colostomies can be instructed how to regulate the colostomy through irrigation. Once the colostomy is regulated (no leakage for 24 to 48 hours between irrigation), the stoma may be covered with a small, closed-ended pouch or gauze covering. Fecal output becomes softer and contains increased concentration of enzymes the higher up the bowel that the colostomy is located. The output will normally return to the normal preillness consistency (Gross & Johnson, 1994; Hoebler, 1997). *Answer 41:* **b.**

QUESTIONS

42. Your patient with a regulated sigmoid colostomy is about to start chemotherapy and radiation therapy. These therapies may cause diarrhea. Which statement would be the most helpful in minimizing the effects of the therapies?
   a. Irrigating with half the amount of water until treatment is concluded
   b. Switching to an open-ended appliance and emptying as needed
   c. Decreasing fluid intake during this time to decrease diarrheal output
   d. Starting prophylactic antidiarrheal agents to minimize output

ANSWERS

42. The recommendations are for the patient to stop irrigation until after treatment is completed and then switch to an open-ended appliance temporarily. Decreasing the fluid intake at this time will not reduce diarrhea and may cause dehydration if diarrhea occurs. On occasion, a formerly regulated patient will be unable to achieve beneficial results from irrigation after radiation therapy has ended. *Answer 42:* **b.**

Case Study continued

Mr. Stanford comes to the clinic complaining of right upper quadrant abdominal discomfort. He has had anorexia and weight loss but relates it to a virus he had a few weeks ago. A follow-up CT scan of the abdomen reveals a hypodense mass in the right lobe of the liver suspicious for metastatic cancer.

QUESTIONS

43. What is the predominant symptom of liver metastasis?
   a. Right upper quadrant pain
   b. A palpable liver nodule
   c. Abdominal ascites
   d. Presence of hepatitis B surface antigen

44. What results of blood work do not correlate with a suspicion of a hepatic metastasis?
   a. Elevated alkaline phosphatase
   b. Elevated white blood cell count with 65% lymphocytes

   c. Rising CEA (serial change greater than 35% of baseline)
   d. Normal SGPT

ANSWERS

43. Any combination of pain or discomfort in the right upper quadrant, weight loss, anorexia, fatigue, fever, or jaundice should raise the possibility of hepatic metastases; symptoms are present in 65% of patients. Although abdominal ascites, hepatomegaly, and palpable liver nodules may be present with hepatic metastases, the predominant symptom is right upper quadrant pain. High titers of hepatitis B surface antigen are found in the liver cells in 75% of patients with cirrhosis and primary liver cancer. Hepatitis markers are not correlated with liver metastasis. Approximately 25% of patients with colorectal carcinoma have liver metastases at the time of diagnosis. Eighty percent of patients presenting with recurrent colorectal cancer will have metastatic disease in the liver. *Answer 43:* **a.**

44. An elevation of the alkaline phosphatase level out of proportion to that of the transaminases suggests a mass lesion. The ALT/SGOT and LDH are elevated in more than two thirds of patients, but the SGPT/AST is commonly normal. A rising CEA may indicate progressive disease. Leukocytosis is not indicative of disease metastases (Lichtenstein & Haller, 1997). *Answer 44:* **b.**

QUESTIONS

45. Treatment for solitary hepatic metastases includes:
   1. Surgical resection
   2. Cryotherapy
   3. Hepatic intraarterial chemotherapy
   4. Systemic therapy
      a. 3 & 4
      b. 1 & 4
      c. All of these
      d. None of these

ANSWERS

45. Surgical resection of a liver metastasis should be considered when no extrahepatic metastatic disease is present and all of the apparent disease can be resected with free margins. A short disease-free interval between primary therapy and the development of metastasis may reflect the aggressiveness of the tumor but is not a contraindication to liver resection. Hepatic resection is accepted as the standard treatment for hepatic metastases because it provides the only opportunity for cure. A number of studies demonstrate overall survival of 65% at 2 years after resection and a 2-year disease-free survival of 25%. The use of hepatic artery chemotherapy is less clear. The rationale for this is that the liver has a dual blood supply. Normal hepatocytes receive most of their blood supply from the portal circulation, and hepatic metastases derive 80% of their supply from the hepatic artery. Therefore infusion of chemotherapy directly into the hepatic artery directly exposes the metastases to high concentrations while sparing the normal liver tissue. This suggests that there may be some benefit to an intrahepatic artery infusion; results of such trials are mostly controversial and not standard treatment at this time (Lichtenstein & Haller, 1997; Niederhuber, 2000; Rosenberg, 1997). *Answer 45:* **c.**

QUESTIONS

46. If Mr. Stanford had presented with a single pulmonary nodule on chest radiograph, without evidence of hepatic involvement, all of the following would be included in your differential diagnosis *except:*
  a. Pulmonary metastasis
  b. Primary lung cancer
  c. Lung abscess
  d. Pulmonary embolism

ANSWERS

46. Pulmonary metastases from colorectal carcinoma are discovered by routine chest radiograph or chest CT that was ordered on the basis of a rising CEA. Of patients with pulmonary involvement, 85% are asymptomatic. Radiologic imaging techniques of pulmonary metastases are inaccurate, partly because only 50% of pulmonary nodules occurring in patients with a history of colorectal cancer are pulmonary metastases. Mr. Stanford also has a smoking history, which increases the likelihood that this nodule is a primary lung cancer. Pulmonary emboli are generally too small to be evaluable on chest radiographs (Daly, Bertagnolli, DeCosse, & Morton, 1999; Lichtenstein & Haller, 1997). *Answer 46:* **d.**

QUESTIONS

47. In which of the following circumstances would palliative surgery be contraindicated?
  a. A large gastric cancer obstructing the gastroesophageal junction
  b. Breast carcinoma metastatic to the lungs that produces cough and shortness of breath
  c. A bleeding cecal cancer, 5 cm in diameter, with multiple liver and lung metastases

  d. Adenocarcinoma of the head of the pancreas with nodal involvement that produces jaundice

ANSWERS

47. All of these clinical scenarios represent disabling symptoms caused by incurable cancers. In many instances surgical resection may offer the best means of palliation for the patient. Consideration of surgery as a palliative measure depends on the mechanism of the symptom being produced, the likelihood that resection would be effective in alleviating the symptom, the rate of morbidity of the proposed surgical procedure, the availability of effective but less invasive palliative measures, and the life expectancy of the patient. Tumors with a hollow viscus generally produce symptoms by obstructing or bleeding. These are most effectively alleviated by resection or, in the case of obstruction, surgical bypass. The cases of gastroesophageal obstruction and of a bleeding cecal cancer are best managed by resection; biliary obstruction is managed with a biliary enteric anastomosis. The mechanism of pain in pancreatic cancer is ingrowth of tumor into the parietal nerves and somatic structures such that pain would not be relieved by pancreatectomy. The patient with breast cancer associated with shortness of breath likely has endobronchial metastases, lymphangitic spread, or associated pleural effusion and would not be appropriately treated with resection (Niederhuber, 2000; Rosenberg, 1997). *Answer 47:* **b.**

QUESTIONS

48. Prophylactic partial or complete resection of which of the following organs could be justified under certain conditions to prevent a future cancer?
  1. Testicle
  2. Colon
  3. Stomach
  4. Breast
  5. Gallbladder
  6. Pancreas
    a. 1, 2, & 4
    b. 4, 5, & 6
    c. 2, 4, & 5
    d. All of these

ANSWERS

48. Some diseases, conditions, and congenital or inherited genetic traits are associated with a high incidence of developing cancer. On occasion, the risk that a cancer will develop in an organ is sufficiently high that consideration is given to the prophylactic removal of part of or the entire organ. When these syndromes are present and cancers are likely to occur in nonvital organs, resection may prevent subsequent occurrence of a malignancy. Risk-benefit considerations include the likelihood that cancer will develop, the functional or cosmetic disability caused by loss of the organ, the morbidity of the surgical procedure itself, and the likelihood that the cancer will be disseminated and incurable if the organ is not prophylactically removed.

Undescended testicle (cryptorchidism) is associated with a higher incidence of testicular cancer, which is prevented by early prophylactic surgery. Surgical removal of the contralateral breast may be preventive in a patient with breast cancer who is at high risk for developing cancer in the other breast. Breast cancer is associated with a strong familial link in approximately 9% of the cases. As an alternative to observation, women with a very high risk may be candidates for prophylactic mastectomies to lower the risk of developing breast cancer. Patient education and genetic counseling should be prerequisites to this approach.

Familial polyposis of the colon is clearly an inherited condition that predisposes the individual to a higher risk for colon cancer. Prophylactic colectomy is usually advocated to prevent this cancer. Cholelithiasis and chronic cholecystitis are associated with the subsequent development of gallbladder cancer; however, the risk is not high enough to justify removal of the gallbladder in the asymptomatic patient. Although gastric and pancreatic tumors are highly aggressive and usually incurable, prophylactic resection of these organs is inappropriate (Niederhuber, 2000; Rosenberg, 1997). See Table 6-3. *Answer 48:* **a.**

QUESTIONS

49. Mr. Stanford's son is worried about his risk for developing colon cancer, especially with such a strong family history. What is the best response?
   a. "Having a first-degree relative increases your risk twofold compared with the general population."
   b. "With a family history of colon cancer, you should begin screening at age 45."
   c. "Because there is no hereditary familial syndrome, your risk is the same as that of the general population."
   d. "You and your brothers should be evaluated for familial adenomatous polyposis (FAP)."

TABLE 6-3	Common Predisposing Conditions and Their Associated Malignancies
CONDITION	**ASSOCIATED MALIGNANCY**
Cryptorchid testis	Testicular
Chronic ulcerative colitis	Colon
Familial adenomatous polyposis	Colon and rectum
Hereditary nonpolyposis colon cancer	Colon and rectum
Family history of colon cancer	Colon and rectum
Multiple endocrine neoplasia (types II and III)	Medullary cancer of the thyroid
Leukoplakia	Squamous
Family history of breast cancer	Breast and ovary
Family history of ovarian cancer	Ovary and breast

From Abeloff, M. D., Armitage, J. O., Lichter, A. S., & Niederhuber, J. E. (Eds.). (2000). *Clinical oncology*, 2nd ed. New York: Churchill Livingstone.

ANSWERS

49. In discussing risk for colorectal cancer, it is important to discuss two different groups: average-risk and high-risk individuals. Average-risk individuals are asymptomatic men and women age 50 years or older with no personal or family history of colorectal adenomatous polyps or cancer and no personal history of inflammatory bowel disease (e.g., ulcerative colitis, Crohn's disease). Those who have a first-degree relative with colorectal cancer have double the risk of developing adenomatous polyps (precursors of colorectal carcinoma) compared with the general population. Patients who are at high risk for colorectal cancer include those who have hereditary disorders, such as FAP or HNPCC.

A large, prospective study that looked at the incidence of colorectal cancer related to family history showed that those who had first-degree relatives with colorectal cancer had a 1.72 relative risk for its development. This was in comparison to those without a family history. Those who had two or more relatives with colorectal cancer had a relative risk of 2.75. The risk of colorectal cancer associated with a family history was greatest for younger patients (relative risk of 5.37 for those younger than age 45) and decreased progressively with advancing age. There was no difference between sex or tumor location.

Management of high-risk patients should include appropriate and aggressive surveillance or screening to help lower the risk for colorectal cancer. The patients should be given information and guidance so that they can make informed decisions regarding screening and prevention, not only for themselves but also for their families (Lichtenstein & Haller, 1997). *Answer 49:* **a.**

Case Study continued

The American Cancer Society and the National Cancer Institute recommend the following tests in screening asymptomatic individuals. Match the test with its recommended frequency.

50. Sigmoidoscopy

51. Stool guaiac test

52. Digital rectal examination

a. Every year after age 40

b. Every year after age 50

c. Every 3-5 years after age 50

Answer 50: **c.** *Answer 51:* **b.** *Answer 52:* **a.**

REFERENCES

Bates, B. (1995). *A guide to physical examination*, 2nd ed. Philadelphia: Lippincott.

Carson, J. L., & Eisenberg, J. M. (1994). The preoperative screening examination. In Goldmann, D. R., Brown, F. H., & Guarnieri, D. M. (Eds.). *Perioperative medicine: The medical care of the surgical patient*, 2nd ed. (pp. 15-23). New York: McGraw-Hill.

Daly, J. M., Bertagnolli, M., DeCosse, J. J., & Morton, D. L. (1999). Oncology. In Schwartz, S. I. (Ed.). *Principles of surgery*, 7th ed. (pp. 297-364). New York: McGraw-Hill.

Engstrom, P. F., Benson, A. B., & Cohen, A. (1996). NCCN colorectal cancer practice guidelines. *Oncology*, *10*(suppl), pp. 140-175.

Fox, K. R. (1994). Surgery in the patient with cancer. In Goldmann, D. R., Brown, F. H., & Guarnieri, D. M. (Eds.). *Perioperative medicine: The medical care of the surgical patient*, 2nd ed. (pp. 283-293). New York: McGraw-Hill.

Frogge, M. H., & Kalinowski, B. H. (1997). Surgical therapy. In Groenwald, S. L., Frogge, M. H., Goodman, M., & Yarbro, C. H. (Eds.). *Cancer nursing: Principles and practice*, 4th ed. (pp.229-246). Boston: Jones and Bartlett.

Gross, J., & Johnson, B. L. (1994). *Handbook of oncology nursing*, 2nd ed. Boston: Jones and Bartlett.

Henkel, T. J., & Fraser, V. J. (1995). Treatment of infectious diseases. In Ewald, G. A., & McKenzie, C. R. (Eds.). *The manual of medical therapeutics: The Washington manual*, 28th ed. (pp. 297-326). Boston: Little, Brown.

Hoebler, L. (1997). Colon and rectal cancer. In Groenwald, S. L., Frogge, M. H., Goodman, M., & Yarbro, C. H. (Eds.). *Cancer nursing: Principles and practice*, 4th ed. (pp. 1036-1054). Boston: Jones and Bartlett.

Lichtenstein, G. R., & Haller, D. G. (1997). *Hematology/ oncology clinics of North America: Colorectal cancer*. Philadelphia: WB Saunders.

Niederhuber, J. E. (2000). Surgical therapy. In Abeloff, M. D., Armitage, J. O., Lichter, A. S., & Niederhuber, J. E. (Eds.). *Clinical oncology*, 2nd ed. (pp. 471-481). New York: Churchill Livingstone.

Rosenberg, S. A. (1997). Principles of cancer management: Surgical oncology. In Devita, V. T., Hellman, S., & Rosenberg, S. (Eds.). *Cancer: Principles and practice of oncology*, 5th ed. (pp. 295-306). Philadelphia: Lippincott-Raven.

Schwartz, M. (2000). Care of the perioperative patient: A new dimension for advanced practice nurses. *J Am Acad Nurse Pract*, p. 81.

Smetana, G. W. (1999). Preoperative pulmonary evaluation. *N Engl J Med, 340*(12), pp. 937-943.

Weintraub, F. N., & Neumark, D. E. (1996). Surgical oncology. In McCorkle, R., Grant, M., Frank-Stromberg, M., & Baird, S. B. (Eds.). *Cancer nursing: A comprehensive textbook* (pp. 315-330). Philadelphia: WB Saunders.

7 Chemotherapy

Annette Wilkening Kuck

CASE STUDY

Sally Goldstein is a 43-year-old woman recently diagnosed with stage III breast cancer. A right-sided mastectomy with lymph node dissection was performed, and 8 of 20 nodes were positive for metastatic disease. The tumor was found to be estrogen and progesterone positive. Mrs. Goldstein's oncologist has recommended six cycles of docetaxel, doxorubicin, and cyclophosphamide. A left-sided venous access port is placed before her planned chemotherapy visit.

You have been asked to complete Mrs. Goldstein's admission history and review the treatment plan with her. When you enter the room, you notice that Mrs. Goldstein is crying. She is accompanied by a gentleman who appears supportive.

QUESTIONS

1. What should be your first step?
 a. Physical assessment
 b. Review of systems
 c. Psychosocial assessment
 d. Review of chemotherapy drugs

ANSWERS

1. Because Mrs. Goldstein is visibly upset, a review of systems, physical assessment, or immediate review of her chemotherapy treatment would be inappropriate. A psychosocial assessment will help determine the underlying cause of distress and respond to her needs at this time. *Answer 1:* **c.**

Case Study *continued*

Your psychosocial assessment reveals the information shown in Table 7-1. After your psychosocial assessment and discussion with Mr. and Mrs. Goldstein, you decide to provide them with written information and schedule another session to review the essential chemotherapy information. They agree and schedule another visit with you before her chemotherapy. When they return, you review the information on docetaxel, doxorubicin, and cyclophosphamide.

QUESTIONS

2. You teach Mrs. Goldstein about all of the following side effects of docetaxel *except:*
 a. Neutropenia
 b. Alopecia
 c. Diarrhea
 d. Hypersensitivity reactions

ANSWERS

2. Neutropenia is the most common dose-limiting side effect of docetaxel. It is reversible and noncumulative. The median time to nadir is 8 days. Severe neutropenia (absolute neutrophil count [ANC] of less than 500 cells/m^2) was reported in 76% of patients in docetaxel clinical trials (Cook & Troutner, 1996).

Mrs. Goldstein will need weekly complete blood counts (CBCs), differentials, and platelet counts to monitor for hematologic side effects. She will also need instruction on preventing infection and what signs and symptoms to report to her health care provider when her neutrophil count is low.

Mrs. Goldstein has already indicated that alopecia is of concern to her. In clinical trials alopecia occurred in 80% of patients (Cook & Troutner, 1996). She needs reassurance that the alopecia is reversible and needs to know what resources are available for wigs and head coverings. Hypersensitivity reactions rarely occur, but if they do, they generally occur shortly after initiation of the docetaxel infusion. Flushing and localized skin reactions do not require discontinuation of therapy. A severe reaction (e.g., severe bronchospasm, severe hypotension, diffuse urticaria) requires immediate discontinuation of docetaxel and aggressive treatment. Fluid retention has also been reported with the use of docetaxel. It is cumulative in incidence, generally not life-threatening, and slowly reversible after discontinuation of docetaxel therapy. It most commonly presents as edema but has been reported less commonly as pleural effusion, pericardial effusion, ascites, and weight gain. Diarrhea is not a common side effect of docetaxel. *Answer 2:* **c.**

TABLE 7-1 Psychosocial Assessment of Mrs. Goldstein	
PSYCHOSOCIAL ASSESSMENT	**YOUR FINDINGS**
Support systems	Married to Joseph. They have three children, ages 14, 10, and 7. She is active in her children's elementary school and feels that she has a strong circle of supportive friends. Her mother is alive but does not live nearby. Her two siblings, a brother and sister, live outside of the state.
Role relationships/domestic	Works full-time as an attorney, as does her husband. She has cleaning assistance for her home every 2 weeks.
Coping abilities	She has coped in the past by relying on friends and members of her religious community.
Psychologic status of spouse/ significant other; ability to serve as a support system	Spouse is very capable and supportive. Because of work constraints, he will be unable to come to all of the patient's office visits.
Communication patterns	Is very open about her feelings of anxiety about her upcoming treatment. Her husband acknowledges her fears and is trying to calm her.
Spirituality	Is very involved with her nonorthodox Jewish synagogue and draws a great deal of support from her synagogue and rabbi.

QUESTIONS

3. Which of the following medications helps prevent docetaxel hypersensitivity reactions and fluid retention?
  a. Dexamethasone
  b. Furosemide
  c. Allopurinol
  d. Ranitidine

ANSWERS

3. An oral corticosteroid regimen of dexamethasone 8 mg twice a day is started the day before docetaxel, the day of treatment, and the day after treatment. Furosemide and other oral diuretics may be indicated if fluid retention occurs. Allopurinol is used as prophylaxis for tumor lysis syndrome, which is rare in breast cancer. Ranitidine does not aid in the prevention of hypersensitivity reactions. *Answer 3:* **a.**

QUESTIONS

4. In addition to bone marrow suppression and alopecia, Mrs. Goldstein should be educated about all of the following side effects of doxorubicin *except:*
  a. Nausea and vomiting, mucositis, and diarrhea
  b. Purple urine
  c. Increased sensitivity to sun and tissue necrosis if extravasated
  d. Delayed cardiomyopathy

5. How often should you assess venous patency with doxorubicin administration?
  a. Before and after
  b. Before and during
  c. Before, during, and after
  d. During and after

6. What information does a MUGA scan provide?
  a. Ventricular muscle contraction strength
  b. Skeletal muscle strength
  c. Cardiac muscle ischemia
  d. Cardiac response to stress

ANSWERS

4. Purple urine is not associated with doxorubicin administration; red is. Patients should be informed that red-colored urine may last for 1 to 2 days after the dose of doxorubicin. Otherwise, patients may mistake the colored urine for hematuria.

Gastrointestinal side effects of doxorubicin include nausea and vomiting, which occurs 1 to 2 hours after administration; mucositis, which may occur 5 to 7 days after treatment; and diarrhea. Patients may find they have an increased sensitivity to sun exposure after doxorubicin treatment. They should be advised to avoid the sun and wear sun protection with a sun protection factor (SPF) greater than 15. The most critical dermatologic toxicity is extravasation, which can lead to tissue necrosis. Patients need to report pain or burning at the site of the intravenous infusion. *Answer 4:* **b.**

5. Assessment of venous patency is performed before, during, and after administration. *Answer 5:* **c.**

6. A dose-related effect on cardiac muscles can cause a delayed cardiomyopathy. Presenting symptoms similar to congestive heart failure may occur months to years after doxorubicin therapy. Assessment of the strength of left ventricular muscle contraction is indicated via a MUGA scan before treatment begins. Mrs. Goldstein's scan reveals an ejection fraction of 51%. *Answer 6:* **a.**

Case Study continued

Cyclophosphamide is a cell-cycle nonspecific alkylating agent whose mechanism of action is to cross-link DNA in tumor cells. It has some common side effects with docetaxel and doxorubicin, such as myelosuppression, alopecia, and nausea and vomiting.

QUESTIONS

7. Mrs. Goldstein should be taught about all of the following side effects of cyclophosphamide *except:*
   a. Hemorrhagic cystitis
   b. Amenorrhea
   c. Pulmonary toxicity
   d. Constipation

8. Mr. and Mrs. Goldstein seem to understand the information that you are relaying. At the end of the explanation, Mr. Goldstein says, "If each one of these drugs is so powerful, why use all three?" What is the best response?
   a. "Each drug has a different underlying mechanism of action, which increases the number of cancer cells killed with each cycle."
   b. "You will have to ask your doctor that question."
   c. "We get paid more the more drugs we give."
   d. "The drugs do not work if given individually."

ANSWERS

7. The risk of cystitis occurs because 5% to 25% of unchanged drug is excreted in the urine. Hemorrhagic cystitis can occur from 24 hours to several weeks following therapy. Patients are encouraged to force fluids to increase urinary frequency and output. Decreased estrogen and increased gonadotropin secretion develops in a significant number of women, causing amenorrhea, which may last up to 1 year. Cyclophosphamide has been associated with irreversible sterility in both sexes. Pulmonary toxicity is rare but can occur. It is characterized by pneumonitis. Constipation is not associated with the use of cyclophosphamide (Berkery, Cleri, & Skarin, 1997). *Answer 7:* **d.**

8. Combination chemotherapy is the use of two or more antineoplastic agents to produce additive or synergistic results against tumor cells. By combining agents with actions in different phases of the cell cycle, a larger number of cancer cells

are exposed to the cytotoxic effects during each treatment cycle. The goal is also to expose cells to the highest dosage of chemotherapy possible without life-threatening toxicity. Clinical studies have found that combining doxorubicin and cyclophosphamide reduce the incidence of recurrence in women with node-positive breast cancer (Groenwald, Frogge, Goodman, & Yarbro, 1997). The addition of a taxane can further reduce the risk of recurrence in this population (Henderson, Berry, Demetri, et al., 1998). *Answer 8:* **a.**

QUESTIONS

9. Mrs. Goldstein is now ready to undergo chemotherapy with docetaxel, doxorubicin, and cyclophosphamide. Mrs. Goldstein says, "Now I understand the chemotherapy drugs and the steroid, but what are all these other drugs for?" She hands you prescriptions for oral ondansetron, oral lorazepam, oral prochlorperazine, and rectal prochlorperazine. Your explanation could be summarized by which of the following statements?
   a. "Different antinausea medications have varying mechanisms of action and are helpful at different points of time during the chemotherapy cycle."
   b. "Just pick one and take it according to the package directions."
   c. "The rectal drug is longer acting than ondansetron."
   d. "Lorazepam is effective for only 3 days after your chemotherapy."

ANSWERS

9. Nausea and vomiting is often a great concern to patients undergoing chemotherapy for the first time. Patients often have never taken antinausea medications, and it can be confusing as to when to take the medication. A thorough explanation of the medications is warranted. (Table 7-2). *Answer 9:* **a.**

Case Study continued

Mrs. Goldstein undergoes her chemotherapy of docetaxel 120 mg, doxorubicin 80 mg, and cyclophosphamide 800 mg. Her baseline CBC, differential, and platelet count show a hemoglobin (Hgb) level of 11.7 g/dl; a white blood cell (WBC) count of 9.2 µ/L, with an ANC of 8.3 m/L; and platelets of 276,000 µ/L. One week later, she notifies the office that she is unable to eat or drink because of difficulty swallowing. She also notes that her tongue appears white.

TABLE 7-2 Antiemetic Therapy: Select Pharmacologic Agents for the Control of Chemotherapy-Induced Nausea and Vomiting

CLASSIFICATION	GENERIC NAME	TRADE NAME(S)	ROUTE	DOSAGE SCHEDULE	DURATION OF ACTION	ADVERSE EVENTS
Serotonin antagonist	Ondansetron	Zofran[a]	IV	0.15 mg/kg, q4h × 3 doses or 32 mg, 30 min before chemotherapy × 1	Half-life: 3-4 hr	Headache, diarrhea, constipation, fever, transient increases in serum SGOT/SGPT
			PO	8 mg bid × 3 days	PO bioavailability 60%	
	Granisetron	Kytril[b]	IV	10 μg/kg over 5 min, within 30 min of chemotherapy	Half-life: 8-10 hr	Headache, asthenia, diarrhea, constipation, fever, somnolence
			PO	1 mg bid		
	Dolasetron	Anzemet[c]	PO	100 mg, 1 hr before chemotherapy	Peak: 1 hr	Headache, diarrhea, dizziness, fatigue, abnormal liver functions
			IV	1.8 mg/kg, 30 min before chemotherapy, or fixed doses of 100 mg	Peak: 30 min	
Substituted benzamide	Metoclopramide	Reglan[d]	IV	2.0-4.0 mg/kg q2h × 4	Onset: 1-30 min; Half-life: 8-10 hr; Duration: 2 hr	Sedation, akathisia, acute dystonic reactions (increased incidence in patients <30 yr), diarrhea (high dosages), dry mouth
			PO	0.5-2.0 mg/kg q3-4 hr	Onset: 0.5-1 hr; Duration: 1-2 hr	
Phenothiazines	Prochlorperazine	Compazine[b]	IM	10 mg q3-4h	Onset: 10-20 min; Duration: 3-12 hr	Sedation, akathisia, extrapyramidal reactions, dry mouth, orthostatic hypotension, blurred vision
			IV	10-40 mg q3-4h	Onset: 10-20 min; Duration: 3-4 hr	
			PO	10 mg q4-6h	Onset: 30-40 min; Duration: 3-4 hr	
			Spansule	15-30 mg q12h	Onset: 30-40 min; Duration: 10-13 hr	
			PR	25 mg q4-6h	Onset: 60 min; Duration: 3-4 hr	
	Chlorpromazine	Thorazine[b]	IM	12.5-50 mg q4-6h	Onset: 15-30 min; Duration: 12 hr	Sedation, hypotension, dizziness, akathisia, extrapyramidal reactions, dry mouth
			IV	12.5-50 mg q4-6h	Onset: 5 min	
			PR	12.5-50 mg q4-6h	Onset: erratic	
	Perphenazine	Trilafon[e]	PO	4 mg q4-6h	Onset: erratic; Peak: 2-4 hr	Sedation, constipation, extrapyramidal reactions, dry mouth, rash
			IM	5 mg q4h	Onset: erratic; Duration: 6 hr	
			IV	5 mg q4h or 5 mg IVB followed by an infusion at 1 mg/hr for 10 hr: maximum dose 30 mg (inpatients) and 15 mg (outpatients) in 24 hr	Onset: 10 min; Duration: 6-24 hr	

	Generic	Brand	Route	Dose	Onset/Peak/Half-life	Duration	Side effects
	Thiethylperazine maleate	Torecan[f] Norzine[g]	IM PO PR	10 mg qd-tid 10 mg qd-tid 10 mg qd-tid	Onset: 30-60 min Onset: 45-60 min	Duration 3-4 hr	Drowsiness, extrapyramidal side effects (dystonia, torticollis, akathisia, gait disturbances), hypotension
Corticosteroids	Dexamethasone	Decadron[h]	IV	4-20 mg (10-20 mg given × 1, otherwise q4-6h)	Half-life: 3-4 hr	—	Dyspepsia, hiccups, increased appetite, euphoria, insomnia, fluid retention, hyperglycemia
	Prednisone	Hexadrol[i]	PO PO	4-8 mg q4h × 4 doses 2.5-15 mg q4-12h	Peak: 1-2 hr Peak: 1-2 hr	Duration: 2 days Duration: 1-1.5 days	Dyspepsia, hiccups, increased appetite, euphoria, insomnia, fluid retention, hyperglycemia
Butyrophenones	Haloperidol	Haldol[j]	IM PO	2-5 mg q2h × 3-4 doses 2-5 mg q2h × 3-4 doses	Onset: 15-30 min Onset: 40 min	Duration: 3-6 hr Duration: 4-6 hr	Sedation, akathisia, extrapyramidal reactions, orthostatic hypotension
	Droperidol	Inapsine[k]	IV IM IV	2 mg × 1 2-5 mg q4-6h 2-5 mg q4-6h or drip	Onset: 15-30 min Onset: 3-10 min	Duration: 3-6 hr Duration: 3-6 hr	Sedation, akathisia, extrapyramidal reactions, hypotension
Cannabinoids	Dronabinol	Marinol[f]	PO	2.5-10 mg 1-3 hr before chemotherapy, then q2h × 4-6 doses/day		—	Sedation, dry mouth, euphoria or dysphoria, dizziness, orthostatic hypotension
Drugs used to augment antiemetics	Diphenhydramine	Benadryl[l]	PO IM IV	25-50 mg q4h prn 25-50 mg q4h prn 25-50 mg q4h prn	Peak: 1-3 hr Onset: 30 min Onset: immediate	Duration: 4-7 hr Duration: 4-7 hr Duration: 4-7 hr	Sedation, dizziness, blurred vision/diplopia, dry mouth
	Lorazepam	Ativan[m]	IV PO SL	1-2 mg/m^2, not exceeding 3 mg 0.5-2 mg 0.5-2 mg	Peak 1-3 hr	Duration: 4-8 hr Duration 3-6 hr	Sedation, anterograde amnesia, dizziness, weakness, unsteadiness, disorientation, hypotension

Modified from Cleri, L.B. (1995). Serotonin antagonists: State of the art management of chemotherapy-induced emesis. *Oncol Nurs Treat Support*, 2(1), pp. 1-19. Copyright 1995 by Lippincott-Raven.

[a]Glaxo Wellcome Oncology/HIV, Inc., Research Triangle Park, NC; [b]SmithKline Beecham Pharmaceuticals, Philadelphia, PA; [c]Hoechst Marion Roussel, Kansas City, MO; [d]A.H. Robins Company, Inc., Richmond, VA; [e]Schering Corporation, Kenilworth, NJ; [f]Roxane Laboratories, Inc., Columbus, OH; [g]The Purdue Frederick Company, Norwalk, CT; [h]Merck & Co., Inc., West Point, PA; [i]Organon Inc., West Orange, NJ; [j]McNeil Pharmaceutical, Raritan, NJ; [k]Janssen Pharmaceutica, Titusville, NJ; [l]Warner Wellcome, Morris Plains, NJ; [m]Wyeth-Ayerst Laboratories, Philadelphia, PA.

QUESTIONS

10. Which of the following laboratory findings would be tied to the description of a white tongue?
  a. Platelets 165,000 mm^2
  b. Hgb 11.5/hematocrit 33
  c. Blood urea nitrogen (BUN) 35, creatinine 1.1
  d. WBC count 1.2 μ/L, ANC 500/ml

11. Mrs. Goldstein comes to the clinic for an urgent visit. What oral examination finding would you expect?
  a. White patches on the buccal mucosa and posterior pharynx
  b. Open ulcerated areas on her mucosa
  c. Vesicles on her upper lip
  d. Beefy, erythematous buccal mucosa

12. Which action should you take next?
  a. Recommend use of a saliva substitute
  b. Recommend removal of plaques with a soft toothbrush
  c. Recommend use of an ethanol-based mouthwash
  d. All of these

ANSWERS

10. The laboratory finding most closely linked with Mrs. Goldstein's description of a white tongue is that of her WBC count. She has a low ANC, which places her a higher risk for oral candidiasis. *Answer 10:* **d.**

11. The physical finding expected is white patches on the buccal mucosa and posterior pharynx. Although chemotherapy-induced mouth sores and herpes simplex are realistic possibilities, the presence of her white tongue leads you to suspect an oral candidal infection. Gently scraping the white patches away will also help confirm your diagnosis and promote patient comfort. *Answer 11:* **a.**

12. Artificial saliva is not warranted in this situation. Mouthwashes may be recommended, but without ethanol, because ethanol can be very drying to the oral mucosa. Antifungal treatment is indicated, along with comfort measures. Topical antifungal agents such as nystatin oral rinses or clotrimazole troches are typically used. Patients should be instructed to cleanse the mouth before administering the agent and not to eat or drink for at least 30 minutes after application. This promotes drug contact with the mucosal surfaces. Baking soda and/or salt rinses can be used to promote comfort and to cleanse the mouth.

Several combination mouth rinses are available through pharmacies, including nystatin, lidocaine, and Milk of Magnesia. Systemic treatment is also available via fluconazole and ketoconazole. Once-a-day dosing is an advantage but should be used with caution because fluconazole can be toxic to the liver. Carafate slurries can be used before meals and at bedtime to bind to the mucosa for pain relief and protection. *Answer 12:* **b.**

Case Study continued

Mrs. Goldstein notes minimal nausea and vomiting after her chemotherapy. Her temperature in the office is 98.6° F. She has been monitoring her temperature at home, with the highest value being 99.8° F.

QUESTIONS

13. Mrs. Goldstein should be counseled about infection prevention. Which of the following statements provides accurate information?
  1. "Take your temperature every day rectally."
  2. "Avoid close contact with anyone who has an upper respiratory infection."
  3. "Restrict your fluids to 1.5 L/day."
  4. "Wash your hands for 15 seconds after bathroom use and before preparing and eating food."
  5. "Do not share eating utensils with others."
  6. "Avoid direct pet care."
  7. "Avoid exercise."
    a. 1, 3, 4, & 6
    b. 2, 4, 5, & 6
    c. 1, 4, 5, & 7
    d. All of these

ANSWERS

13. Patients with known or anticipated granulocytopenia can help minimize their risk of infection by using common sense and good hygiene. The seven preceding statements represent the conceptual areas that should be covered in teaching. Mucosal integrity is disrupted by rectal temperatures, enemas, and straining to have a bowel movement and should be avoided. Appropriate monitoring of temperature orally or tympanically is recommended. The physician should be notified if her temperature rises above 101.5° F.

Other people can inadvertently share their bacteria and viruses. It is generally recommended that patients avoid crowds during this time. Family members should remain at least 3 feet away if they are feeling ill. Fluids should not be restricted, but rather encouraged to 2 to 3 L/day. Good handwashing is the single most effective tool in infection prevention, and patients should be taught the proper way to wash. Sharing eating utensils with others is not recommended. Patients can be exposed to clustered organisms with direct pet care; this is a job for helpful friends and family. Exercise appropriate to the patient's level of mobility improves oxygenation and decreases the risk for pulmonary infection. *Answer 13:* **b.**

Case Study *continued*

Mrs. Goldstein is given a patient information sheet detailing your explanation. She indicates understanding of the risk of infection and what to do if she develops a fever. Two days later, she contacts the office with a fever of 102° F and shaking chills. She is asked to come to the hospital immediately for evaluation. When she arrives, she indicates that she has developed a dry, unproductive cough but no other new symptoms. Her physical examination is unremarkable and does not show any signs of infection.

QUESTIONS

14. The following diagnostic examinations are indicated *except:*
   a. CBC, differential, platelets, creatinine, liver function tests
   b. Blood cultures
   c. Stool cultures
   d. Chest radiograph

ANSWERS

14. To evaluate her myelosuppression and metabolic state and to diagnose the underlying cause of her fever, additional testing needs to be performed. Mrs. Goldstein's CBC, differential, and platelet counts reveal an Hgb of 11.4 g/dl; WBC count of 1.0 µl, with ANC of 0.2/ml; and platelets of 162,000/µl. Her liver function tests and creatinine level were within normal limits. Blood cultures were negative after preliminary and final incubation. Urinalysis was unremarkable, and urinary culture was negative. The chest radiograph shows the venous access catheter in place and no evidence of infiltrates. Mrs. Goldstein does not have diarrhea at present, so a stool culture is not warranted in this situation. *Answer 14:* **c.**

Case Study *continued*

Figure 7-1 can be used to help determine how Mrs. Goldstein should be treated (Labovich, 1999).

QUESTIONS

15. Which type of therapy should be added to the next cycle of chemotherapy?
   a. Interleukin-11
   b. Granulocyte colony-stimulating factor (G-CSF) or granulocyte-macrophage colony-stimulating factor (GM-CSF)
   c. Erythropoietin
   d. Interleukin-6

ANSWERS

15. To prevent infectious complications from granulocytopenia with subsequent chemotherapy cycles, G-CSF or GM-CSF is indicated. These agents are given subcutaneously to stimulate the bone marrow to produce and differentiate neutrophils. They are indicated in the presence of chemotherapy-induced neutropenic fever and should be used in subsequent courses to prevent a recurrence of neutropenic fever. Interleukin-11 (oprelvekin) stimulates the proliferation of hematopoietic stem cells and megakaryocytic progenitor cells. This induces megakaryocytic maturation, resulting in increased platelet production. Erythropoietin stimulates red blood cell production, which then increases hemoglobin. Interleukin-6 is a recombinant product found in *Escherichia coli* and has been investigated in the treatment of cancer. *Answer 15:* **b.**

Case Study *continued*

After her third cycle of therapy, Mrs. Goldstein and the chemotherapy nurses noted that her venous access device is not drawing blood well. A catheter patency dye study was ordered. Mrs. Goldstein is found to have a fibrin sheath and is started on warfarin 1 mg/day orally. Just before her sixth cycle of chemotherapy, Mrs. Goldstein notices increased swelling with erythema of her left arm and presents to the emergency room.

QUESTIONS

16. What conditions should be included in a differential diagnosis?
   a. Thrombosis, lymphedema, cellulitis
   b. Extravasation, thrombosis, cellulitis
   c. Recurrent disease, cellulitis, lymphedema
   d. Thrombosis, lymphedema, extravasation

17. When you examine Mrs. Goldstein, you are reminded that her surgery was on the right side and that her catheter is on the left side. What physical findings on a focused physical assessment are consistent with a thrombosis?

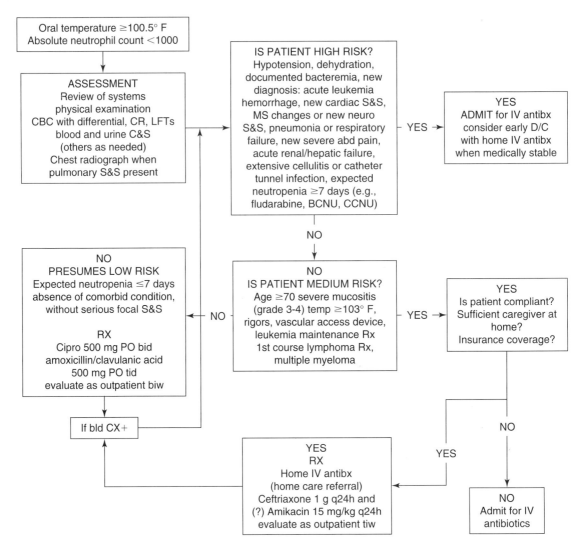

Figure 7-1 Evaluation and management of neutropenic fever. *CBC,* Complete blood count; *CR,* creatinine; *LFT,* liver function test; *C&S,* culture and sensitivity; *S&S,* signs and symptoms; *BCNU,* carmustine; *CCNU,* lomustine; *IV,* intravenous; *antibx;* antibiotics; *bld,* blood; *CX,* culture. (Courtesy D. Lovett, MD, and K. Dietz, RN.)

a. Unilateral swelling of left arm
b. Dusky, cyanotic appearance of left arm
c. Prominent superficial veins on left upper chest wall
d. All of these

18. Which diagnostic test is indicated to confirm the presence of a thrombosis?
a. Chest radiograph
b. Venous Doppler
c. Angiogram
d. Venogram via catheter

ANSWERS

16. Thrombosis needs to be included in a differential diagnosis of a swollen arm on the same side as

an implanted access device, because the presence of a foreign body increases the risk for clotting. Lymphedema should be considered if the patient has had a lymph node dissection or radiation therapy to the axilla. Cellulitis needs to be ruled out because the patient is describing erythema. *Answer 16:* **a.**

17. Physical findings include unilateral swelling as a result of decreased venous return. The decreased return may also contribute to a dusky, cyanotic appearance, which may be mistaken for erythema secondary to cellulitis. A prominent venous pattern may also be present because of decreased backflow through the veins. *Answer 17:* **d.**

18. Venous Doppler is indicated to assess for the presence of thrombosis. A chest radiograph assesses placement of the catheter but does not address the presence of a thrombus. In some scenarios a negative Doppler may need follow-up with a venogram if the patient's symptoms persist. *Answer 18:* **b.**

Case Study continued

Mrs. Goldstein's ultrasound reveals subclavian and internal jugular thrombosis. Therapeutic options include hospitalization for continuous infusion of heparin or outpatient management with low-molecular-weight heparin.

QUESTIONS

19. What factors should you assess before recommending a course of treatment?
 1. Manual dexterity
 2. Bleeding risk
 3. Location of thrombus
 4. Insurance coverage
   a. 1 & 2
   b. 1 & 3
   c. 2, 3, & 4
   d. All of these

ANSWERS

19. All of these factors are important areas to assess when determining treatment of deep vein thrombosis. Low-molecular-weight heparin is administered by subcutaneous injection and needs to be given by the patient or a family member. Mrs. Goldstein has already been giving herself G-CSF, so she would require little or no teaching on technique. Patients at high risk for bleeding need to be hospitalized for observation. Mrs. Goldstein is not currently at high risk. The location of the blood clot is also important. Management of pulmonary emboli or extensive clots requires close observation. Outpatient management is not recommended. Insurance coverage should be assessed and discussed with the patient because low-molecular-weight heparin may not be covered by insurance and can be a significant expense to the patient. *Answer 19:* **d.**

Case Study continued

After discussing it with Mrs. Goldstein and the oncologist, the decision is made to treat her as an outpatient using low-molecular-weight heparin. She is started on her injections and asked to start oral warfarin 24 hours later. A return office visit is scheduled in 3 days.

QUESTIONS

20. Which of the following assessments should be performed during the office visit?
   a. Physical examination of her right arm and upper chest wall
   b. International Normalized Ratio (INR)
   c. Neurologic examination
   d. Partial thromboplastin time (PTT)

ANSWERS

20. Once the patient is started on warfarin, the therapeutic dosage is determined by the INR value. The goal is to keep the patient's INR value between 2.0 and 3.0 or 2.5 and 3.5. Once the therapeutic range has been achieved, low-molecular-weight injections are discontinued. The patient's symptoms and venous access device are on the left side and need to be monitored. Neurologic examination is not indicated at this time. PTT is used as a screening test for coagulation disorders, not for the management of oral warfarin therapy. Mrs. Goldstein continues her injections for a week and then is maintained on oral warfarin. *Answer 20:* **b.**

Case Study continued

Mrs. Goldstein completes her therapy and tamoxifen is prescribed. She returns for her 1-year visit. Her major concern is that she stopped menstruating when chemotherapy started and has not resumed normal cycles. She has began having hot flashes, which are very uncomfortable for her. She is also concerned about the risk of cardiovascular disease because she has an extensive family history.

QUESTIONS

21. Additional evaluation may include all of the following *except:*
   a. Bone density examination
   b. Serum estrogen levels
   c. Lipid profile
   d. Serum calcium

ANSWERS

21. A bone density scan may be helpful to determine the patient's baseline and to determine whether additional pharmacologic interventions need to be taken to increase bone density. Serum estrogen levels will be decreased if the patient is in menopause. A lipid profile will identify the level of low-density lipoproteins (LDLs) and ratio to high-density lipoproteins (HDLs). Elevated levels of LDLs increase the risk for atherosclerotic disease. An abundance of HDLs will carry cholesterol from the peripheral tissues to the liver for excretion and reduce the risk of atherosclerotic disease. Serum calcium is not a true indicator of calcium absorption or storage in the bones. *Answer 21:* **b.**

Case Study continued

Mrs. Goldstein is interested in learning more about minimizing her risk of osteoporosis, cardiovascular disease, and genitourinary changes. Estrogen replacement therapy in patients with estrogen-positive tumors is controversial and generally not recommended.

QUESTIONS

22. Nonpharmacologic interventions for osteoporosis that can be recommended include all of the following *except:*
  a. Weight-bearing exercise
  b. Consumption of 1000 to 1500 mg of calcium per day
  c. High-fat, low-fiber diet
  d. Avoidance of excessive alcohol use and smoking

23. Pharmacologic interventions can help with the symptoms of menopause. Which of the following interventions is the best choice?
  a. Discontinuation of the tamoxifen
  b. Megestrol, venlafaxine, ergotamine, or clonidine
  c. Dong quai, ginseng, and vitamin E
  d. All of these

22. Decreased estrogen levels can put women at risk for osteoporosis and cardiovascular disease. Hot flashes can be disruptive and uncomfortable. Both pharmacologic and nonpharmacologic choices can help balance the symptoms and promote a healthy lifestyle. Weight-bearing exercise; adequate consumption of calcium; a low-fat, high-fiber diet; and avoidance of excessive alcohol can help minimize the risk. Exercise and relaxation techniques can help alleviate the vasomotor symptoms associated with hot flashes. *Answer 22:* **c.**

23. Discontinuation of the tamoxifen should not be done without extensive discussion between the oncologist and patient to ensure understanding of the risks and benefits of stopping tamoxifen before 5 years. Megestrol, venlafaxine, ergotamine, and clonidine have been used with success to minimize the discomfort and incidence of hot flashes. Dong quai, ginseng, and vitamin E are herbal/nutritional supplements that have been suggested as beneficial with hot flashes; however, scientific studies have not proven definite benefit (Oncology Nursing Society, 1999). *Answer 23:* **b.**

CASE 2 STUDY

Lena Benson is a married 81-year-old white woman with a history of breast cancer. She was diagnosed 4 years ago with a 1.5-cm, grade 3 infiltrating ductal tumor that was estrogen and progesterone positive. At the time of her right mastectomy and lymph node dissection, 1 of 11 lymph nodes was positive for tumor involvement. Adjuvant therapy of tamoxifen was ordered. She was last seen 3 months ago with no clinical evidence of recurrent disease. While spending the winter in Florida, she developed a productive cough of white phlegm. A chest radiograph showed some "congestion" according to her report. An antibiotic and cough syrup were prescribed, but her symptoms did not abate. She also noticed enlarging lumps under the skin in the sternal area and left upper back region. Around the same time, she developed intermittent, sharp upper abdominal pain, which was unrelated to activity, food intake, or bowel movements. She was seen by an oncologist in Florida and had further workup performed.

QUESTIONS

1. All of the following diagnostic tests are indicated *except:*
  a. Computed tomography (CT) scan of chest, abdomen, and pelvis
  b. Bone scan
  c. Lumbar puncture
  d. Fine-needle aspirate of subcutaneous lesions

1. Ms. Benson's symptoms and physical findings are suspicious for metastatic disease. Additional testing to determine the extent of disease, in the form of CT scans and a bone scan, should be done. Lung, liver, and bone are the most common sites for breast cancer metastases beyond the regional lymph nodes. Mrs. Benson's CT scan demonstrates multiple suspicious nodules in her lungs bilaterally, hepatomegaly with multiple masses throughout both lobes of the liver, and a subcutaneous mass in the right gluteal subcutaneous fat. Her bone scan shows multiple areas of increased uptake in the spine, skull, and pelvis compatible with metastatic disease. Degenerative changes are also noted in her right knee and left hip. The patient does not have neurologic symptoms to warrant a lumbar puncture. A fine-needle aspirate is indicated to determine the underlying histology of the lesions and do Her2-neu studies. *Answer 1:* **c.**

QUESTIONS

2. What is Her2-neu?
   a. A monoclonal antibody
   b. A growth factor found on breast cancer cells
   c. A serum tumor marker
   d. An oral chemotherapy agent

ANSWERS

2. Her2 is a *human* epidermal growth factor *receptor-2* that can be overexpressed or amplified on the cell surfaces of breast cancer tumors. It occurs in 25% to 30% of human breast cancers. Amplification and overexpression of Her2 have been associated with poor clinical outcome for women with breast cancer. In several studies patients with amplified Her2 exhibited decreased survival time and higher frequency for tumor recurrence (Preston & Cunningham, 1998). *Answer 2:* **b.**

Case Study continued

Mrs. Benson returns for further discussion of possible treatment options. Comparison of the specimen with the original breast cancer slides demonstrates that they are the same malignancy as in 1996. The tumor cells are 3+ for Her2. The patient, along with her husband and daughter, wishes to pursue treatment.

QUESTIONS

3. What is the goal of therapy?
   a. Curative
   b. Control
   c. Palliative
   d. Adjuvant

ANSWERS

3. Given the patient's widespread metastases, the goal of therapy is control of her disease and improvement in her respiratory and abdominal symptoms. Mrs. Benson has had very few health problems until recently. *Answer 3:* **b.**

QUESTIONS

4. The oncologist has determined that Mrs. Benson is eligible for a clinical research study using paclitaxel and trastuzumab. What is your primary role as an advanced practice nurse (APN) in this situation?
   a. To describe conventional treatment options that might be beneficial
   b. To educate the patient and family about the medications used in the clinical trial
   c. To conduct inpatient rounds while the physician explains the options
   d. To complete eligibility enrollment information for the clinical trial

ANSWERS

4. In the process of obtaining informed consent, the physician explains both the conventional treatment options and the clinical trial protocol. Risks and benefits should be covered. Additional education regarding the specific medications used in the trial may be one role for an APN in clinical trials. The other options do not use the APN skills in supporting the patient and the family. *Answer 4:* **b.**

Case Study continued

Mrs. Benson and her family have requested additional information regarding trastuzamab and paclitaxel and have scheduled a meeting with you. After assessing their baseline knowledge and learning needs, you find that they are well informed. They admit to being "information seekers" and are interested in learning more about trastuzamab. They are concerned about toxicities.

QUESTIONS

5. Given Mrs. Benson's age, which toxicity is she at greatest risk for?
   a. Pulmonary toxicity
   b. Hepatotoxicity
   c. Neurotoxicity
   d. Cardiac toxicity

6. What precautions can be taken to minimize her risk?
   a. Serial oxygen saturation readings during treatment
   b. Administration of amifostine at the first sign of neurologic toxicity
   c. Initiation of vitamin B_{12}
   d. Baseline cardiac assessment

7. What signs and symptoms will you counsel the primary nurses to assess for at each visit?
  a. Weight gain, fatigue, dyspnea
  b. Headache, paresthesias, constipation
  c. Dyspnea on exertion, tachycardia, chest pain
  d. Ascites, pedal edema, right upper quadrant abdominal pain

---

ANSWERS

5. Ventricular dysfunction and congestive heart failure have been reported with trastuzamab use. The risk of cardiac dysfunction may be increased in elderly patients. Mrs. Benson should undergo a baseline cardiac assessment, which includes a history and physical examination and one or more of the following: electrocardiogram, echocardiogram, or multigated angiography. *Answer 5:* **d.**

6. Oxygen saturation readings will not prevent cardiac or pulmonary toxicities from occurring. Amifostine is a cryoprotectant used to help prevent nephrotoxicity or neurotoxicity in certain patient populations but would not be helpful in this situation. Vitamin B_{12} is used to replace depleted stores in patients with anemia related to a low level of B_{12} (folate). *Answer 6:* **d.**

7. Cardiac toxicity is often manifested as congestive heart failure. Weight gain from fluid retention, fatigue, and dyspnea from weakened heart muscles may be found in patients with cardiac toxicity. *Answer 7:* **a.**

QUESTIONS

8. Paclitaxel is a member of the taxane class, which is a dipentene plant product derived from the needles and bark of the Western yew. What information is essential for Mrs. Benson and her family to understand before undergoing therapy?
  1. Dexamethasone is given before treatment to help prevent hypersensitivity reactions.
  2. Weekly blood draws are necessary to monitor for myelosuppression.
  3. Mucositis may occur during treatment.
  4. Arthralgia/myalgia occurs during the infusion.
  5. Paclitaxel is not irritating to the veins.
    a. 1, 2, & 3
    b. 2, 3, & 4
    c. 3, 4, & 5
    d. 1, 3, & 5

9. In addition to diphenhydramine, what other medication is used to help prevent hypersensitivity reactions?

  a. Allopurinol
  b. Cimetidine
  c. Acetaminophen
  d. Ibuprofen

ANSWERS

8. It is essential that Mrs. Benson be aware of side effects that can occur with paclitaxel infusion. Severe hypersensitivity reactions, myelosuppression, and mucositis can occur. *Answer 8:* **a.**

9. Dexamethasone 20 mg is given before the paclitaxel dose to help reduce the risk of severe hypersensitivity reaction. In addition, diphenhydramine 50 mg and cimetidine 300 mg are given 30 to 60 minutes before the paclitaxel dose. Reactions occur most commonly during the first 15 to 60 minutes of the infusion. Severe hypersensitivity reaction symptoms include dyspnea with bronchospasm, hypotension, chest pain, angioedema, and generalized urticaria. Minor manifestations include dyspnea, flushing, rash, skin reactions, tachycardia, and hypotension. Myelosuppression, including severe neutropenia and thrombocytopenia, has been associated with paclitaxel use. Mucositis is associated with higher dosages of paclitaxel. Arthralgias or myalgias occur 2 to 3 days after administration. Paclitaxel is a known irritant and has recently been reported as having vesicant potential. *Answer 9:* **b.**

Case Study continued

Mrs. Benson undergoes her first dose of trastuzumab and paclitaxel on separate days and tolerates both without incident. One week later, her daughter notifies the office that Mrs. Benson is having a great deal of body pain and is scheduled for a laboratory visit this morning. Arrangements are made for her to be seen.

QUESTIONS

10. Which symptom might you expect to find in Mrs. Benson's musculoskeletal review of systems?
  a. Severe joint pain, especially of her right knee and left hip
  b. Leg weakness
  c. Numbness of fingertips
  d. Ataxia

11. What would you expect to find on physical examination?
  1. Unilateral swelling of the right leg
  2. Pain noted on range of motion of the left leg
  3. Normal vibratory sensations

4. Positive Romberg test
   a. 1 & 2
   b. 2 & 3
   c. 2 & 4
   d. All of these

12. What accompanying sign would you expect with paclitaxel-related arthralgia?
   a. Erythema
   b. Swelling
   c. Joint changes
   d. Normal reflexes

────────────────────────────── **ANSWERS**

10. Your review of systems finds that Mrs. Benson is experiencing severe joint pain. Arthralgia/myalgia manifested as pain in the large joints of the arms and legs usually occurs in 2 to 3 days after paclitaxel administration. The duration of the pain varies with each patient but may last for 5 to 7 days. Reversible peripheral neuropathy can occur after several cycles of therapy. Numbness, tingling, and pain in the hands and feet are often the first symptoms to appear. *Answer 10:* **c.**

11. Mrs. Benson's physical examination reveals pain with range of motion and normal reflexes. It is important to assess the joints to determine the underlying cause of her new joint pain. Are they swollen, erythematous, or disfigured? Slight swelling of the joints is associated with osteoarthritis and may be present. *Answer 11:* **c.**

12. Paclitaxel-related arthralgia is not associated with erythema or joint changes. *Answer 12:* **d.**

QUESTIONS ──────────────────────────

13. What interventions would you recommend to Mrs. Benson to assist with management of her arthralgia?
   1. Minimization of movement of the most painful joints
   2. Heat/cold applications
   3. Nonsteroidal antiinflammatory drugs (NSAIDs)
   4. Massage therapy
   5. Sauna baths
      a. 1, 2, & 3
      b. 1, 3, & 5
      c. 2, 3, & 4
      d. All of these

────────────────────────────── **ANSWERS**

13. Applications of heat/cold, NSAIDs, and massage therapy have been recommended to help with pain management associated with chemotherapy-

induced arthralgia/myalgia. The goal is palliation of the symptoms. Heat and cold applications, massage therapy, and whirlpool baths may increase the patient's level of comfort. Regularly scheduled use of NSAIDs can help keep pain to a tolerable level. Patients may need encouragement to take pain medications regularly. Occasionally, patients require opioid narcotics to manage the arthralgia. In the long term, minimizing the patient's motion of the affected joints can lead to decreased range of motion and affect mobility. This intervention is not recommended. A sauna bath would not be beneficial in this situation. *Answer 13:* **c.**

QUESTIONS ──────────────────────────

14. It is anticipated that Mrs. Benson will be given six cycles of paclitaxel and 12 months of therapy with trastuzamab. Given her age and treatment plan, which of the following risk factors places Mrs. Benson at greatest risk for hematologic toxicity?
   a. Age
   b. Baseline CBC, platelet counts
   c. Renal dysfunction
   d. Cumulative effect of trastuzamab on hematopoiesis

────────────────────────────── **ANSWERS**

14. A degree of bone marrow suppression occurs as people age. Although overall myelosuppression can be problematic for patients receiving paclitaxel, Mrs. Benson is starting treatment with a low hemoglobin and red blood cell count. Continued monitoring of her blood counts and assessment of symptoms are necessary. *Answer 14:* **b.**

Case Study continued

Two weeks after her fourth cycle of paclitaxel, Mrs. Benson indicates to the chemotherapy nurses that she is extremely tired and has noticed increasing shortness of breath. When her weekly laboratory tests are completed, her Hgb is noted to be 8.0 g/dl.

QUESTIONS ──────────────────────────

15. What immediate corrective intervention is indicated?
   a. Chest radiograph to assess for cardiopulmonary changes
   b. MUGA scan to assess for cardiac ejection fraction
   c. Transfusion of 2 units of packed red blood cells
   d. Oxygen at 2 L/min via nasal cannula

15. A transfusion of packed red blood cells will help Mrs. Benson's symptoms of fatigue and dyspnea. Depending on the rest of your assessment, the chest radiograph and MUGA scan may be indicated after the transfusion and before her next chemotherapy treatment. The administration of oxygen is not warranted because there is no indication that Mrs. Benson's oxygen saturation on room air is low. *Answer 15:* **c.**

QUESTIONS

16. Because Mrs. Benson will need a type and crossmatch drawn, what other laboratory tests should you consider having done?
  a. Reticulocyte count
  b. Iron, ferritin, total iron-binding capacity (TIBC)
  c. Folate, vitamin B$_{12}$ level
  d. All of these

17. What medication could be beneficial for Mrs. Benson?
  a. Oprelvekin
  b. Epoetin alfa
  c. Sargramostim
  d. Filgrastim

16. All of the laboratory tests listed are appropriate to check. These tests are used to help differentiate the type of anemia that Mrs. Benson is experiencing. A reticulocyte level is usually decreased when the bone marrow is not producing enough athrocytes. An elevated reticulocyte count is often associated with anemia caused by hemorrhage. The iron studies will help determine whether Mrs. Benson has adequate iron stores and whether her anemia is related to iron deficiency. Pernicious anemia is related to decreased levels of folate and vitamin B$_{12}$. Mrs. Benson is found to have a decreased reticulocyte count but adequate iron and folate stores. A review of her CBC shows that her mean corpuscular volume (MCV) is within the normal range. *Answer 16:* **d.**

17. Epoetin alfa is a genetically engineered version of the body's natural hormone erythropoietin and is used to stimulate division and differentiation of committed erythroid progenitors in the bone marrow. Normal iron and folate stores are necessary, and if they are low, supplementation should occur simultaneously with epoetin alfa. It is approved for use in cancer patients with anemia who are undergoing chemotherapy. The starting dosage is 150 U/kg three times a week subcutaneously until target hemoglobin (12.0 g/dl) is reached. Some institutions have tried an alternative schedule of 40,000 units subcutaneously weekly. If hemoglobin has not increased more than 1 g/dl from baseline after 4 weeks, the dosage may be increased to 60,000 units weekly. Oprelvekin is a thrombopoietic growth factor used to stimulate platelet production. Sargramostim and filgrastim are used to stimulate WBC production (Albain, Hortobagyi, Ravdin, & Slamon, 1998). *Answer 17:* **b.**

Case Study conclusion

Four months after completion of paclitaxel, Mrs. Benson develops increasing abdominal pain and distension. A CT scan of her chest, abdomen, and pelvis reveals progressive disease. After extensive discussion with her family, Mrs. Benson elects to not undergo additional therapy and is placed on hospice care.

CASE 3 STUDY

Herschel Watson is a 77-year-old African American, married gentleman recently diagnosed with poorly differentiated lung carcinoma with both squamous cell and adenocarcinoma features. He began having respiratory difficulties approximately 1 year ago, when he was hospitalized for "chronic bronchitis and emphysema." Six months ago, he began having increasing shortness of breath and more frequent episodes of coughing, which were productive of brownish sputum. Three months ago, he was once again hospitalized and a repeat CT scan revealed evidence of a right lung mass and right hilar adenopathy. A CT-guided biopsy showed a non–small cell carcinoma.

QUESTIONS

1. Based on these findings, what oncologic emergency is Mr. Watson at most risk for?
  a. Sepsis
  b. Superior vena cava syndrome

c. Disseminated intravascular coagulation
d. Tumor lysis syndrome

───────── **ANSWERS**

1. Mr. Watson's right hilar adenopathy puts him at high risk for superior vena cava syndrome. The superior vena cava is located in the right anterior mediastinum and is surrounded by lymph nodes. Enlargement of these lymph nodes can compress the blood vessel and impair circulation. *Answer 1:* **b.**

Case Study continued

Mr Watson is seen in consultation by the oncologist, and the staging workup is completed. The results of his workup are as follows:

- CT scan of abdomen and pelvis: metastatic liver lesions as well as benign cysts
- Bone scan: increased activity in several posterior lateral ribs

Based on the underlying cancer diagnoses and the patient's extensive medical history, the physician recommends a trial of gemcitabine and vinorelbine tartrate every 3 weeks. Mr. Watson's medical history includes the following:

1. Chronic obstructive pulmonary disease (COPD) diagnosed 1 year ago
2. Pacemaker placed in 1995
3. Kidney stone removed in 1986
4. Microwave procedure for prostatic hypertrophy in 1998
5. Adult-onset diabetes mellitus, treated with glipizide
6. History of peripheral neuropathy in the hands and feet since 1990
7. Macular degeneration in his right eye

You have been asked to teach Mr. Watson about the recommended chemotherapy regimen and to review important side effects with him. Gemcitabine is a cell-cycle–specific antimetabolite.

QUESTIONS

2. As you review the information to give to Mr. Watson, you note that the major side effects of gemcitabine include which of the following?
1. Nausea and vomiting
2. Myelosuppression
3. Flulike symptoms
4. Injection site reaction
    a. 1 & 2
    b. 1 & 3

c. 1, 2, & 3
d. All of these

3. Vinorelbine tartrate, a member of the vinca alkaloid class, is a cell-cycle–specific agent inhibiting a cell's microtubule formation to create an antitumor effect. Important information for Mr. Watson and his wife includes which of the following statements regarding side effects?
1. Weekly blood counts are needed because of the possibility of leukopenia and granulocytopenia.
2. Abdominal cramping and diarrhea may occur during administration.
3. Erythema and tenderness at the site of the intravenous injection should be brought to the attention to the chemotherapy nurses.
4. Mr. Watson will be given a antiemetic before the chemotherapy. Prescriptions will be given to him to use for nausea, which may occur after his treatment.
    a. 1 & 2
    b. 1, 2, & 3
    c. 1, 3, & 4
    d. All of these

───────── **ANSWERS**

2. The major side effects of gemcitabine include nausea and vomiting, myelosuppression, and flu-like symptoms. Nausea and vomiting were reported in 69% of patients receiving single-agent gemcitabine for pancreatic cancer. It was usually of mild to moderate severity and well controlled with the use of antiemetics. Myelosuppression causing anemia, leukopenia, or thrombocytopenia can occur. However, the incidence of severe myelosuppression is rare and not found to be the reason for missed or reduced doses. A weekly CBC will help assess Mr. Watson's hematologic response to gemcitabine. Flulike symptoms such as headache, back pain, chills, myalgia, asthenia, and anorexia have been reported. Less commonly, cough, rhinitis, malaise, sweating, and insomnia were reported during clinical studies. The underlying mechanism of action for these symptoms is unknown. The symptoms were reported as mild and responded to acetaminophen 650 mg every 4 hours. Gemcitabine is not a vesicant or irritant and has not been associated with infusion site reactions if extravasated. Burning at the intravenous infusion site occurred initially and was reduced by diluting the infusion and slowing the administration rate. A maculopapular pruritic skin rash was observed in 30% of patients participating in clinical studies. The rash usually involved the trunk and extremities. The use of a topical corticosteroid improved or stabilized the rash through the continued gemcitabine course (Severance & Galassi, 1999). *Answer 2:* **c.**

3. Patient teaching regarding vinorelbine should cover myelosuppression, injection site reactions, and nausea and vomiting. Abdominal pain and cramping have not been associated with vinorelbine. In North American Studies of single-agent vinorelbine, overall incidence of leukopenia was found to be 92%. Granulocytopenias were found in 89% of patients. Weekly blood counts help assess the occurrence, grade, and duration of the bone marrow suppression. The onset of granulocytopenias was reported at 7 to 10 days, with nadir occurring at 14 days. Because 69% of the patients experienced severe to life-threatening granulocytopenias, Mr. Watson needs to be aware of the importance of the monitoring of his blood counts, the signs and symptoms of infection, and interventions aimed at preventing infection (Rieger, 1999).

Vinorelbine, a moderate vesicant, is known to cause venous irritation and phlebitis with site reactions, as reported in 28% of patients (Rieger, 1999). Signs and symptoms included erythema, vein discoloration, and tenderness over the length of the vein. Mr. Watson needs to inform the nurses if he experiences any discomfort because he currently does not have central venous access. Immediate notification will help minimize the severity of the irritation and possible extravasation. Nausea was reported by 43% of patients receiving single-agent vinorelbine (Rieger, 1999). It was most often rated as mild, and vomiting was not commonly associated with the occurrence of nausea. Antiemetics are commonly given intravenously before the administration of emetogenic chemotherapy. Regimens may vary by physician practice but may include a $5HT_3$ receptor antagonist and a steroid, such as dexamethasone. Mr. Watson and his wife need to be aware of the elevation in blood sugars, which can be created by the dexamethasone. Oral antiemetics are commonly used to treat nausea, which may occur in the days following chemotherapy. A review of the antiemetics prescribed is needed to ensure proper use by the patient. *Answer 3:* **c.**

Case Study continued

Mr. Watson has received two cycles of gemcitabine and vinorelbine, with the last cycle being 1 week ago. His wife notifies the office that Mr. Watson has developed severe weakness, loss of appetite, and constipation. An outpatient office visit is set up the same day for further evaluation.

Mr. Watson and his wife describe several concerns upon arrival. Over the weekend, the patient went to the garage to work on his snowblower. While bending over, he developed the sensation of inability to get up or down and needed to shout for a neighbor to help him up. Yesterday, his family notes that he got up to go to the bathroom, got confused, went to the laundry room, and was found passed out on the floor. The patient does not remember blacking out or any other details of the incident. His wife has noted a sharp decrease in his appetite. This morning, his fasting blood sugar was in the 500s. The patient has not had a bowel movement in 1 week. Medication review reveals the following:

- Digoxin 0.125 mg/day orally
- Lisinopril 5 mg orally every morning
- Metoprolol 1 tablet orally twice a day
- Warfarin 1 mg alternating with 2 mg orally daily
- Colchicine 0.6 mg/day orally
- Aspirin 325 mg/day orally
- Furosemide 20 mg/day orally
- Glipizide 10 mg/day orally
- Amitriptyline 50 mg orally at bedtime
- Baclofen 10 mg orally three times daily
- Multivitamin 1 tablet orally daily
- Albuterol inhaler 2 puffs four times daily
- Triamcinolone inhaler 2 puffs four times daily

A review of systems upon arrival reveals the following:

HEENT: Sore throat that has been present since before chemotherapy. No recent change in condition. No difficulty in swallowing noted. A marked decrease in appetite. No changes in taste or oral sensation.

Cardiovascular: Notes occasional midsternal chest pain upon deep inspiration. Reports increasing weakness and fatigue.

Respiratory: Notes no change in color, frequency, or nature of cough. On chronic oxygen at 2.5 L/min.

Gastrointestinal: Sharp decrease in appetite and fluid intake. No nausea or vomiting. No bowel movement in 1 week. Feels distended and uncomfortable.

Genitourinary: No burning, urgency, or frequency noted.

Extremities: Family notes increasing swelling of his feet bilaterally. Feels that his legs are weaker.

Neurologic: No other episodes of blackouts. Has noticed increased difficulty with dropping glasses. Notes no tingling or burning in lower extremities.

Musculoskeletal: Weakness as noted. No new myalgias or joint pain noted.

Hematologic: No bruising noted.

Upon physical examination, you find the following:

Vital signs: Temperature, 99.8° F orally; pulse, 108 beats/min; respirations, 20 breaths/min; blood pressure, 102/60 mm Hg; weight, 202 pounds (down 5 pounds since last visit).

General: Pale, elderly gentleman who appears anxious and debilitated and who is on nasal oxygen.

HEENT: Oral examination shows pink, moist mucosa without white patches or erythema.

Cardiovascular: Occasional irregularity with occasional skipped beats and occasional extra beat. Pacemaker generator is visible and palpable on the left infraclavicular region.

Respiratory: Lungs show decreased breath sounds bilaterally without adventitious sounds. On oxygen at 2.5L/min per nasal cannula. O_2 saturation is 92%. White sputum with blood flecks.

Abdomen: Bowel sounds present with slight distension. No tenderness, masses, or organomegaly noted.

Extremities: Lower extremities 1+ pitting edema bilaterally to his ankles.

Skin: Dry with multiple areas of open wounds and scratches. Left arm shows lower area is erythematous over vein without swelling or induration.

Neurologic: Patient is alert and oriented to person, place, and time. Reflexes are 1+ in all locations. Decreased muscle strength noted in lower extremities. No change in sensation found in lower extremities. Has decreased sensation in fingertips bilaterally.

QUESTIONS

4. Based on your physical examination, which laboratory tests should you order? Choose all that apply.
1. CBC, differential, and platelet count
2. Basic chemistries of electrolytes, BUN, creatinine, and glucose
3. PT/INR
4. Blood gases
   a. 1, 2, & 3
   b. 1, 2, & 4
   c. 1, 3, & 4
   d. All of these

ANSWERS

4. Mr. Watson could benefit from an evaluation of his CBC, basic chemistries, and coagulation status. It has been a week since Mr. Watson's last chemotherapy, and he may have developed leukopenia and granulocytopenia. His Hgb should be assessed and compared with previous values. This process can help determine the underlying cause of his weakness. A sudden drop in Hgb points to occult bleeding as a probable cause of the sudden onset of his weakness and fatigue. Thrombocytopenia may have also developed secondary to the myelosuppression of his chemotherapy regimen. His laboratory values are as follows: WBC count, 2.3 μl with an ANC of 1.7/ml, Hgb 10.7 g/dl (compared with 12.8 g/dl last week), and platelets 144,000/μL. A serum panel including basic chemistries, BUN, and creatinine can provide additional information regarding Mr. Watson's weakness. He is at risk for electrolyte abnormalities because he is elderly, which may decrease his renal function; existing cardiac disease, which predisposes him to congestive heart failure; and a diagnosis of lung cancer, which can cause the syndrome of inappropriate antidiuretic hormone secretion (SIADH). His glucose level should be tested regularly for treatment of his diabetes mellitus. His laboratory values are as follows: sodium, 128 mEq/L; potassium, 4.3 mEq/L; chloride, 90 mEq/L; CO_2, 27 mEq/L; BUN, 15 mg/dl; creatinine, 1.4 mg/dl; and glucose, 398 mg/dl. An INR is needed to determine whether Mr. Watson is currently receiving therapeutic doses of warfarin. He is receiving chronic warfarin therapy for his cardiac disease and pacemaker. Coagulation status is very sensitive to nutritional conditions. Mr. Watson's decreased appetite and food intake may have affected his anticoagulation status. An elevated INR would place him at greater risk for bleeding. The desired level of INR for a patient with a pacemaker is between 2.5 and 3.5. His INR is 1.4. Blood gases are not indicated at this time because he is not in respiratory distress. *Answer 4:* **a.**

QUESTIONS

5. What diagnostic examinations are indicated?
1. Head CT
2. Chest radiograph
3. MUGA scan
4. Pulmonary function tests

a. 1 & 2
b. 1 & 3
c. 2 & 3
d. 3 & 4

a. 1, 2, & 3
b. 1, 3, & 4
c. 2, 3, & 4
d. All of these

5. A CT of the head and chest radiograph are indicated. A CT scan of the head can identify tissue abnormalities by measuring increased or decreased density. Contrast substances will pass into abnormal brain tissue and help identify tumors, multiple sclerosis, aneurysms, or vascular abnormalities. Because Mr. Watson has been experiencing some neurologic changes, the underlying cause must be identified. One possible cause could be brain metastases from his non–small cell lung cancer. Given his significant cardiac history, age, and subtherapeutic coagulation, a cerebral accident is another possibility. His scan results are negative for metastases or infarct. A chest radiograph with anteroposterior (AP) and left lateral views can provide valuable information about the condition of the heart and lungs. Mr. Watson's chest radiograph shows the known right lower lobe lung mass with hilar enlargement and evidence of COPD. A MUGA scan and pulmonary function tests are not warranted at this time. A MUGA scan determines heart wall motion and ejection fraction. Anthracycline chemotherapy agents can decrease ejection fraction and alter cardiac status. Neither vinorelbine or gemcitabine are associated with this cardiac toxicity. If cardiac studies are indicated, Mr. Watson's cardiologist or internal medicine physician should be involved. At this time, Mr. Watson is not experiencing significant respiratory distress. He has undergone pulmonary function testing in the past. *Answer 5:* **a.**

Case Study continued

Based on your assessment, Mr. Watson will need to be hospitalized for observation and further diagnostic evaluation. His internal medicine physician and cardiologist are consulted to manage his diabetes mellitus, COPD, and cardiac disease. Mr. Watson's wife of 40 years notes that Mr. Watson has become increasingly anxious over the last few days.

QUESTIONS

6. Which of the following conditions may be causing anxiety?
1. Oversedation
2. Underlying COPD
3. Stress response to his medical condition
4. Abnormal metabolic state

6. Oversedation can make Mr. Watson lethargic. Withdrawal from sedatives could make Mr. Watson anxious. Other withdrawal states that can cause anxiety include alcohol, narcotics, cigarettes, or rebound from short-acting benzodiazepines. His anxiety may be caused by the other factors noted. Anxiety often accompanies a diagnosis of COPD resulting from the persistence of dyspnea and underlying hypoxia. Research studies have demonstrated increased levels of anxiety associated with the diagnosis of cancer. Mr. Watson's diagnosis was made recently, and he has just undergone chemotherapy. His recent change in medical status, which has not been diagnosed yet, is another stimulus for anxiety. Altered metabolic states such as pulmonary embolus, sepsis, and delirium can cause anxiety. Further assessment of Mr. Watson is needed to determine whether an altered metabolic state is contributing to his anxiety. *Answer 6:* **c.**

QUESTIONS

7. In meeting with Mr. Watson, you may recognize his anxiety by all of the following signs *except:*
    a. Restlessness, difficulty concentrating, wringing of hands
    b. Trembling, sense of doom, increased heart rate
    c. Cold, clammy hands; shortness of breath; increased perspiration
    d. Decreased heart rate, dilated pupils, calm appearance

7. Decreased heart rate, dilated pupils, and a calm appearance are not usually associated with anxiety. The sympathetic nervous system has been stimulated, which causes increased heart rate, increased blood pressure, and pupil constriction. Patients may manifest restlessness by pacing, wringing their hands, or not being able to remain seated. Trembling, hand tremors, or twitching may be noted by the examiner. Other extraneous movements such as foot shuffling or hand and arm movements may also be noted. Symptoms of autonomic hyperactivity, such as cold, clammy hands; paresthesias; gastrointestinal distress; hot-cold spells; tachypnea; and tachycardia, may be present. *Answer 7:* **d.**

QUESTIONS

8. Physical examination and laboratory results fail to find an organic explanation for Mr. Watson's anxiety. Appropriate interventions could include all of the following *except:*

    a. Providing adequate information and support

    b. Contacting Mr. Watson's pastor or hospital chaplain

    c. Instructing Mr. Watson to take buspirone on an as-needed basis

    d. Recommending lorazepam 0.5 mg to 1 mg every 4 to 6 hours as needed for anxiety

ANSWERS

8. Buspirone is a nonbenzodiazepine anxiolytic that must be taken regularly. The drug is started at a low dosage (15 mg/day) and increased by 5 mg/day at 3-day intervals. The optimal therapeutic response is not seen for 3 to 4 weeks. This pharmacologic intervention could be helpful to Mr. Watson, but only after physiologic causes have been ruled out. Information regarding his plan of care and environment may help allay some of his anxiety. Mr. Watson was becoming increasingly anxious at home and now will be entering the hospital. Diagnostic procedures should be explained carefully. Support for his wife and family is necessary. A social services or home health referral may be indicated to help them cope with Mr. Watson's medical needs at home. If Mr. Watson has a strong spiritual community or connection, it may help his anxiety to speak with his pastor or hospital chaplain. A short-acting, rapid-onset drug such as lorazepam or oxazepam may help allay acute anxiety if needed. A low dosage should be used because sedation, confusion, and motor incoordination may occur. Mr. Watson must be monitored carefully for these side effects. *Answer 8:* **c.**

QUESTIONS

9. Erythema of Mr. Watson's lower left arm is noted. The erythema is overlying the vein where he received his last dose of gemcitabine and vinorelbine. Appropriate interventions include which of the following?

    1. Hyaluronidase 150 units injected intradermally at the site of the erythema

    2. Warm compresses twice daily

    3. Avoidance of blood draws and intravenous infusions in his left arm

    4. Cold compresses

    a. 1 & 2

    b. 1 & 3

    c. 2 & 3

    d. 2 & 4

ANSWERS

9. Warm compresses and avoidance of blood draws are helpful interventions. Erythema and absorption may be aided by warm compresses. The primary goals are to facilitate skin integrity and to promote healing. Blood draws and intravenous infusions should be avoided in Mr. Watson's left arm until the erythema subsides. His veins and subcutaneous tissues are irritated and could break down more easily. Further problems can be prevented if Mr. Watson's arm is rested. Hyaluronidase should be injected intradermally at the time of a suspected extravasation to enhance systemic uptake of subcutaneous fluids by opening interstitial spaces. Too much time has passed since Mr. Watson's chemotherapy for hyaluronidase to be of benefit. Cold compresses have no therapeutic indication in this situation. *Answer 9:* **c.**

Case Study continued

You note that loss of appetite has been indicated as a problem by Mr. Watson and his wife. He has lost 5 pounds recently, but review of his records indicates that he has lost 20 pounds since his diagnosis of lung cancer. Multiple factors can contribute to anorexia in elderly patients with cancer.

QUESTIONS

10. Your assessment of Mr. Watson's anorexia needs to evaluate the effect of which of the following factors?

    1. Presence of taste alterations

    2. Fatigue

    3. Hyperglycemia

    4. Ill-fitting or uncomfortable dentures

    5. Continuation of smoking

    6. Basal metabolic rate

    a. 1, 2, 3, & 4

    b. 1, 2, 4, & 6

    c. 1, 2, 3, 4, & 5

    d. 1, 2, 4, 5, & 6

ANSWERS

10. Basal metabolic rate affects cachexia, not anorexia, which is defined as loss of appetite. Cachexia is a syndrome of progressive wasting that is associated with anorexia and metabolic alterations. Many factors can affect nutrition. Taste alterations can occur because of metabolic changes associated with malignancy and chemotherapy. Oral candidiasis can also cause taste changes. Mr. Watson's oral examination shows no evidence of oral candidiasis, but he does complain of food tasting different. Fatigue makes it difficult for patients to shop, prepare, and eat meals. Electrolyte abnormalities, such as hyperglycemia, can suppress appetite. Mr. Watson has a diagnosis of diabetes mellitus, and his blood sugars have been elevated at home. Other contributing factors include nausea and vomiting, stomatitis/mucositis, altered gastrointestinal motility, depression, altered mental status, and side effects of medications. Mr. Watson is extremely weak and lethargic, which is contributing to his decreased oral and food intake on admission. Environmental factors, such as difficulty in food preparation, can also contribute to loss of appetite and decreased food intake. Fortunately, Mr. Watson's wife is healthy and able to prepare food for Mr. Watson. For the elderly, dentition can also play a vital role in ability to eat. *Answer 10:* **c.**

QUESTIONS

11. To help treat Mr. Watson's anorexia, appropriate interventions could include all of the following *except:*
   a. Consultation with a dietitian
   b. Intravenous hydration
   c. Appetite stimulation with medication
   d. Consultation with a dentist

ANSWERS

11. Although many patients with hyperglycemia and anorexia may have accompanying dehydration, Mr. Watson does not appear dehydrated; his creatinine is 1.4 mg/dl, BUN is 15 mg/dl, and blood pressure is 102/60 mm Hg. Intravenous fluids would not help his anorexia or provide the adequate daily caloric intake he needs. Consultation with a dietitian will further assess Mr. Watson's nutritional status. The consultant can also help Mr. Watson and his wife develop nutritional strategies for improving his oral and food intake when he returns home. Several medications are available to stimulate appetite. These medications are indicated for cancer patients who are unable to maintain their weight because of poor food intake. A consultation with a dentist is appropriate if the patient is having difficulty with the teeth. Problems with missing teeth or ill-fitting dentures make it difficult for patients to chew. This problem can lead to a decreased desire to eat and weight loss. *Answer 11:* **b.**

QUESTIONS

12. Which of the following medications might be best as an appetite stimulant for Mr. Watson?
   a. Megestrol acetate oral suspension
   b. Dronabinol

   c. Low-dose prednisone
   d. Multivitamin with folate

ANSWERS

12. Megestrol acetate, a synthetic derivative of progesterone, has been used in hormonal treatment of advanced breast and prostate cancer. During its use, weight gain and increased appetite were found to be common side effects. It has been used to stimulate appetite and increase weight gain for other cancer patients. Dronabinol, an oral cannabinoid, has been used in patients with acquired immunodeficiency syndrome (AIDS) to stimulate appetite. Use as an appetite stimulant is being investigated in cancer patients. It would not be a good choice for Mr. Watson because of the reported side effects of anxiety/nervousness, confusion, and paranoid reaction (Genzar, 1998). Low-dose prednisone has also been used to stimulate appetite; however, the use of steroids could complicate Mr. Watson's diabetes mellitus. A multivitamin with folate would be helpful for Mr. Watson's nutritional status but would not increase his appetite. *Answer 12:* **a.**

Case Study continued

Mr. Watson has now been hospitalized for several days. His blood sugar levels have been normalized with the use of sliding-scale insulin. In addition, his cardiac status has been stabilized after it was discovered that his pacemaker generator was not functioning properly. Despite overall improved oral intake and increased activity, Mr. Watson has not had a bowel movement in 10 days.

QUESTIONS

13. Your physical assessment should include all of the following *except:*
   a. Auscultation of bowel sounds in all four quadrants
   b. Palpation of perirectal area and anal sphincter
   c. Percussion of the upper abdomen to determine the size of liver
   d. Palpation of the abdomen for tenderness, masses, or distension

ANSWERS

13. Percussion of the abdomen often includes assessment of liver size. However, your current assessment should focus on whether dull-sounding areas exist in normally tympanic areas. This can help identify any masses affecting Mr. Watson's bowel status. No areas of abnormality are found during your examination. Auscultation of bowel sounds helps determine whether the intestines are functioning. If bowel sounds are absent for 5 minutes, a bowel obstruction is suspected. Mr. Watson's bowel sounds are normal in all four quadrants. The perirectal area and anal sphincter need to be inspected and palpated for anal fissures, anorectal fissures, and hemorrhoids. These conditions make defecation painful and may make a patient suppress the urge to defecate. Your assessment finds Mr. Watson's perirectal area and anal sphincter intact. Palpation of the abdomen can help identify specific areas of tenderness, masses, or distension. Mr. Watson notes slight tenderness on palpation. Distension is present, but no abnormal masses are found. *Answer 13:* **c.**

Case Study continued

After an abdominal flat and upright radiograph determines that a bowel obstruction is not present, the diagnosis of constipation is made. Review of his medications shows that Mr. Watson does not take any regular bowel medications.

QUESTIONS

14. All of the following medications may be appropriate as an initial intervention *except:*

    a. Docusate sodium
    b. Castor oil
    c. Sennoside
    d. Sorbitol

ANSWERS

14. Castor oil is a strong stool stimulant acting primarily in the small intestine to promote peristalsis. It is not usually used for routine constipation, but rather for bowel evacuation before a bowel procedure. There are better choices for routine bowel care. Docusate sodium is a stool softener. It would be helpful for Mr. Watson to take it regularly. Because of his weakness and compromised respiratory status, Mr. Watson has significantly decreased his activity level. Increased immobility puts him at higher risk for chronic constipation. Senna-containing agents enhance intestinal fluid accumulation, which results in a softer, more liquid food bolus while also promoting peristalsis. Senna can be used regularly and titrated up for optimal bowel status. Senna should be prescribed at the initiation of an opioid regiment and continued until the analgesic is discontinued. Sorbitol is an osmotic laxative that is often used to stimulate initial bowel passage. It is less gas producing and less expensive than lactulose and may be helpful in Mr. Watson's situation to facilitate passage of hardened stool. It is most often used on an as-needed basis. In severe chronic constipation, it may be given on a frequent schedule. *Answer 14:* **c.**

Case Study conclusion

Mr. Watson's condition improves with the determination that the combination of his diabetes, cardiac condition, and postchemotherapy physical condition are the underlying causes of his increased weakness and altered neurologic status. Home health care is arranged so that he will have nursing visits, a home health aide, and a physical therapy assessment at home. Follow-up in the office is scheduled in 1 week with the oncologist to discuss further treatment.

CASE 4 STUDY

As an oncology clinical nurse specialist, you have been asked to assist a new staff nurse in the care for Sergio Markovitz, a 39-year-old, single Russian immigrant who has been admitted for his first cycle of EPOCH chemotherapy for recurrent lymphoma. The EPOCH treatment regimen is considered a dose-intensive chemotherapy regimen and contains etoposide, vincristine, doxorubicin, cyclophosphamide, and prednisone (Brogden & Nevidjon, 1995). Mr. Markovitz was diagnosed with non-Hodgkin's lymphoma 2 years ago, shortly after he immigrated to the United States. He has been treated with cyclophosphamide, doxorubicin, vincristine, and prednisone as an outpatient in the past. He completed chemotherapy and was found to be in complete remission. Recently, he developed back and right flank pain with some numbness and tingling in the right groin area. A CT scan showed evidence of a 6-cm mass in the right psoas area. He is now being admitted for treatment of his recurrent lymphoma. An implanted venous port was inserted this morning. Mr. Markovitz can speak some English.

QUESTIONS

1. Who would be the best person to assist with obtaining informed consent from Mr. Markovitz?
- **a.** His sister, who has been in United States for 15 years
- **b.** A community college Russian instructor
- **c.** The patient's wife, who immigrated to the United States at the same time
- **d.** A professional interpreter

1. A professional interpreter would be most beneficial to have at the time of informed consent. He or she can offer an unbiased transfer of information regarding treatment. A family member may be biased and misinterpret the explanation of treatment and the informed consent process. It is difficult to have an interpreter present 24 hours a day to aid communication. It would also be helpful to have the interpreter available for chemotherapy teaching. The hospital has agreed to support your request for interpretive services at admission and for teaching. *Answer 1:* **d.**

Case Study continued

The interpreter is present, and Mr. Markovitz would like to learn more about his chemotherapy. Because he has received doxorubicin, vincristine, prednisone, and cyclophosphamide previously, your learning assessment includes his baseline knowledge of those medications. He is interested in learning more about what different side effects he may experience with the increased dosage and continuous infusion.

QUESTIONS

2. Which of the following is the best response?
- **a.** "The side effects will be about the same."
- **b.** "With these higher dosages, the severity of the side effects may be greater. You may experience more mouth sores and low blood counts."
- **c.** "With the continuous infusions, the side effects diminish from the bolus injections given in the CHOP regimen."
- **d.** "You need to ask your physician about the side effects of treatment."

ANSWERS

2. Because higher dosages are given in dose-intense regimens, patients are at higher risk for severe toxicity. The underlying principle of dose-intensive treatment regimens is to treat the patient

with the highest dosage of chemotherapy for the greatest tumor response. A working knowledge of the acute and delayed toxicities is essential for nurses administering the chemotherapy and need not be deferred to the physician for teaching. To assist with accurate reporting/documentation of the toxicities, familiarity with the National Cancer Institute Common Toxicity Criteria is essential. Toxicities associated with EPOCH include neutropenia, febrile neutropenia, thrombocytopenia, vomiting, mucositis, constipation, central line complications, and peripheral neuropathy (Gemzar, 1998). *Answer 2:* **b.**

Case Study continued

Mr. Markovitz is curious about etoposide. The staff nurse you are orienting can explain that it is a chemotherapy agent that specifically targets cells during the growth phase of the cell's reproductive cycle.

QUESTIONS

3. The staff nurse asks you which specific side effects Mr. Markovitz should be educated about during his teaching session.
1. Myelosuppression
2. Nausea and vomiting
3. Arrhythmia
4. Alopecia
5. Mucositis
6. Constipation
- **a.** 1, 2, 3, & 4
- **b.** 1, 4, 5, & 6
- **c.** 1, 2, 4, & 5
- **d.** All of these

ANSWERS

3. Myelosuppression, nausea and vomiting, alopecia, and mucositis have been reported with the use of etoposide. In patients with preexisting cardiac disease, myocardial infarction and congestive heart failure have been reported. Patients are more likely to experience diarrhea as a gastrointestinal toxicity rather than constipation. *Answer 3:* **c.**

QUESTIONS

4. The chemotherapy has been prepared by the central pharmacy and has arrived on the floor. Before administering the chemotherapy, you review with the nurse that all of the following should be done *except:*
- **a.** Double-checking the physician orders for correct dose and schedule

b. Rechecking the patient's blood pressure
c. Assessing the venous access device for patency
d. Double-checking the chemotherapy for correct patient, drug, and dose

c. Enhancing the profession of oncology nursing)
d. Supporting the patient and nurse through a new experiences

————————————— **ANSWERS**

4. Avoidance of chemotherapy administration errors is critical. Drug doses and schedule should be determined by calculation of the patient's body surface area and the dose per meter squared. Mr. Markovitz will be receiving extravasating agents via continuous infusion, so venous patency is essential throughout the infusion. At the bedside, the chemotherapy should be double-checked for patient, drug, and dose accuracy. The patient's blood pressure, unless abnormal at last reading, is not relevant to the initiation of EPOCH chemotherapy treatment. *Answer 4:* **b.**

QUESTIONS

5. As the etopside is infusing, Mr. Markovitz grabs his chest, struggling to speak, and reports difficulty "getting his breath." What should you guide the staff nurse to do initially?
   a. Stop the infusion
   b. Continue infusion but administer epinephrine
   c. Do a stat electrocardiogram and hook up to cardiac monitor
   d. Call the physician to the unit stat

6. Lung auscultation reveals scattered high-pitched wheezes and upper airway coarse stridor sounds. What are possible causes for Mr. Markovitz's signs and symptoms?

7. What is the *most* likely cause?
   a. COPD
   b. Adult respiratory distress syndrome
   c. Bronchospasm
   d. Cardiogenic shock

8. What is the initial pharmacologic intervention?
   a. Epinephrine 0.5 mg subcutaneously
   b. Aminophylline intravenously
   c. Hydrocortisone 100 mg intravenously
   d. Lorazepam 5 mg intravenously

9. By educating the patient and staff nurse and by role modeling patient teaching and advocacy, you are doing all of the following *except:*
   a. Wasting your time
   b. Promoting patient safety and well-being during chemotherapy administration

————————————— **ANSWERS**

5. The bronchospasm Mr. Markovitz is experiencing is a sign of anaphylaxis to the etoposide. Immediate response should be discontinuation of the infusion and subcutaneous epinephrine. *Answer 5:* **a.**

6-7. Dyspnea, bronchospasm, and airway obstruction can be signs and symptoms of anaphylaxis to the chemotherapy. Almost all chemotherapeutic agents can cause an anaphylactic reaction, which usually occurs within the first few moments of an intravenous infusion (Von Honhen Leiten & Webster, 1998). Other signs and symptoms can include tachypnea, hypotension, tachycardia, chest tightness, dizziness, urticaria, pruritus, anxiety, restlessness, and feelings of impending doom. Possible differentials in this scenario include **bronchospasm secondary to anaphylaxis, cardiac angina or ischemia, and pulmonary embolus.** *Answer 6:* **See text.** *Answer 7:* **c.**

8. Failure to administer epinephrine early can negatively affect the patient's ultimate outcome. Epinephrine causes bronchodilation and also has chronotropic and inotropic effects, which enhance oxygenation and breathing ability while supporting hemodynamics (Kollef & Goodenberger, 1995; Labovich, 1999). Fluid replacement is indicated if the patient experiences hypotension and vascular collapse. If the bronchospasm persists, an aminophylline infusion can be instituted. Hydrocortisone, an adrenocorticoid, has a late onset but long duration and would not be a first-line drug. An anxiolytic drug such as lorazepam would add little, if anything, in this emergency situation. *Answer 8:* **a.**

9. Education and support are never a waste of time. By educating Mr. Markovitz, you help him take control of his health. Determining the barrier of his primary language and developing creative solutions to teach him will help him identify critical toxicities that need to be reported to his health care providers and help him cope with the side effects of treatment. Educating the staff nurse will help increase her efficacy and comfort with chemotherapy administration and care of oncology patients. *Answer 9:* **a.**

CASE 5 STUDY

Mr. Carl Monson is a 77-year-old married man with a history of Duke's BII colon carcinoma. He had no evidence of disease following hemicolectomy for 3 years until liver metastases were diagnosed 1 year ago. He was treated with seven cycles of 5-fluorouracil and leucovorin, with decreased size of the lesions noted on reevaluation. Four months after completing therapy, follow-up scans revealed increasing liver metastases. His oncologist has recommended irinotecan 350 mg/m^2 every 3 weeks. Mr. Monson has requested a meeting with you to discuss possible side effects of irinotecan. In the process of performing a learning assessment, you learn that Mr. Monson has a good grasp on the concept of what chemotherapy is and that he had very few side effects from his previous chemotherapy. He and his wife are very active and like to go skiing every winter. He is distressed about the progression of his recurrence and is quick to point out that his brother died in his sixties of colon cancer. A very talkative and direct person, he quickly starts asking questions regarding irinotecan.

QUESTIONS

1. Mr. Monson asks what the major side effects of irinotecan are. You reply that the four major toxicities include:
   1. Diarrhea
   2. Neutropenia
   3. Nausea and vomiting
   4. Stomatitis
   5. Abdominal cramping
   6. Metallic taste
      a. 1, 2, 3, & 4
      b. 1, 3, 4, & 5
      c. 2, 4, 5, & 6
      d. 1, 2, 3, & 5

2. What statement by Mr. Monson would indicate that he has a good understanding of irinotecan and its side effects?
   a. "After what I have been through, this will be a piece of cake."
   b. "I will have to eat and drink less."
   c. "I will need to watch my bowels for cramping and diarrhea."
   d. "This is too strong for me."

ANSWERS

1. The four major side effects of irinotecan are diarrhea, neutropenia, nausea and vomiting, and abdominal cramping during administration (Pharmacia Upjohn, 1997). Severe stomatitis was not common in early clinical trials. A metallic taste during administration has not been reported with irinotecan. Diarrhea may occur as either early on or late. Early-onset diarrhea occurs either during the infusion or within 24 hours after the treatment. Abdominal cramping may occur during the infusion, just before the development of diarrhea. Late-onset diarrhea occurs more than 24 hours after therapy and can be life-threatening. Neutropenia has been reported, requiring weekly monitoring. Nausea and vomiting can occur with the use of antiemetics recommended (Roxane Laboratories, 1996). *Answer 1:* **d.**

2. It is important to assess a patient's understanding of the chemotherapy regimen and side effects before treatment. Patients and families need to understand the critical side effects to watch for and to notify the health care providers about when they occur. Should diarrhea and neutropenia develop, Mr. Monson and his wife need to be aware of the management of diarrhea and the signs and symptoms of infection. *Answer 2:* **c.**

QUESTIONS

3. Mr. Monson and his wife arrive for his first dose of irinotecan. As the medication is infusing, Mr. Monson notes intense abdominal cramping. After assessing the cramping, you recommend that the primary nurse:
   a. Slow the infusion rate
   b. Stop the infusion
   c. Administer atropine 0.5 to 1.0 mg intravenously
   d. Administer hydrocortisone 100 mg intravenously

ANSWERS

3. Atropine is indicated for abdominal cramping. A sequence of associated symptoms, including abdominal cramping, diarrhea, diaphoresis, sense of warmth, flushing, vomiting, increased salivation, lacrimation, nasal congestion, and rhinorrhea, are caused by a cholinergic effect of irinotecan. Atropine as an anticholinergic medication can mediate these symptoms. Prompt administration of 0.5 mg of intravenous atropine relieves Mr. Monson's symptoms, and he tolerates the rest of the infusion without incident. Slowing or stopping the infusion has not been found to counter the cholinergic-induced symptoms. Hydrocortisone is not indicated in this situation. *Answer 3:* **c.**

Case Study continued

The following week, Mr. Monson comes in for his laboratory visit. He requests to be seen because of ongoing problems with diarrhea. He reports that he had one bout of diarrhea on the day of irinotecan therapy but that after one dose of loperamide, it resolved and he went 3 days without loose stools. Since Monday he has had two to three watery stools per day. The interval between stools is lengthened by the use of loperamide, but the diarrhea keeps returning. He has gone through three boxes of loperamide since his chemotherapy treatment.

QUESTIONS

4. In addition to fully reviewing the gastrointestinal system in your review of systems, what other areas should you focus on?
1. Respiratory
2. Hematologic
3. Neurologic
4. Cardiovascular
   a. 1 & 2
   b. 1 & 3
   c. 2 & 3
   d. 2 & 4

5. What diagnostic and laboratory tests should you order in addition to the weekly CBC, differential, and platelet count?
a. Electrolytes, BUN, creatinine
b. Stool culture and stool specimen of *Clostridium difficile*
c. Abdominal radiograph
d. All of these

6. Which physical finding would you expect on physical examination?
a. Dry skin with poor turgor, orthostasis
b. Enlarged lymph nodes, jaundice
c. Infrequent bowel sounds, pedal edema
d. Constricted pupils, positive Romberg

ANSWERS

4. In addition to focusing on Mr. Monson's gastrointestinal symptoms, which also include decreased appetite, further assessment is necessary regarding his hematologic and cardiovascular systems. He is 1 week postchemotherapy and is at risk for developing neutropenia; therefore it is essential to know if he has developed any fevers since receiving his chemotherapy. Because diarrhea can deplete the body's potassium level, cardiovascular symptoms such as slowed heart rate or irregular pulse should be identified in the review of systems. Mr. Monson denies any of these symptoms. His major complaint is that of fatigue. *Answer 4:* **d.**

5. Mr. Monson is at risk for hypokalemia and dehydration from prolonged diarrhea. His electrolytes and renal function should be assessed. His laboratory values reveal a WBC count of 1.5 µ/L with an ANC of 0.5/ml, Hgb of 12.3 g/dl, and platelets of 192,000/µl. His electrolyte panel demonstrates sodium of 137 mEq/L, potassium of 3.8 mEq/L, chloride of 103 mEq/L, CO_2 of 25 mEq/L, and creatinine of 0.6 mg/L. *Answer 5:* **d.**

6. Diarrhea often causes dehydration. An assessment of dry skin with poor turgor and orthostasis is consistent with dehydration. Enlarged lymph nodes and jaundice point toward progressive disease rather than dehydration. Bowel sounds are more likely to be active than infrequent. Pedal edema may be present but is not indicative of dehydration. *Answer 6:* **b.**

QUESTIONS

7. Possible management strategies for Mr. Monson include which of the following?
1. Alteration in diet to clear liquids for 24 hours, avoidance of dairy products, advancement to a bland diet
2. Recommendation for metoclopramide four times daily
3. Recommendation for atropine sulfate with diphenoxylate hydrochloride
4. Kaolin/pectin
   a. 1, 2, & 3
   b. 1, 3, & 4
   c. 2, 3, & 4
   d. All of these

ANSWERS

7. Dietary changes, an alternative antidiarrheal agent, and the use of kaolin/pectin can help manage Mr. Monson's diarrhea. Mr. Monson and his wife should be educated about dietary adjustments that can be made to help decrease the frequency of diarrhea. Written information can be used to reinforce the necessary dietary changes. Atropine sulfate with diphenoxylate hydrochloride is used to prolong gastrointestinal transit time. Kaolin/pectin helps add bulk to stools and decreases gastric motility and water content of stools. Metoclopramide is not indicated in diarrhea because its mechanism of action is to increase gastrointestinal motility. *Answer 7:* **b.**

Case Study conclusion

It is essential to instruct Mr. Monson and his wife about neutropenic precautions. Notification of his health care providers of a fever greater than 101.5° F should be stressed. With dietary changes and atropine sulfate with diphenoxylate hydrochloride on a scheduled basis for several days, Mr. Monson's diarrhea subsides. He is able to tolerate his second course of treatment without significant diarrhea. Follow-up CT scans show progression of his metastatic disease. Mr. Monson elects for no further treatment.

REFERENCES

Albain, K. S., Hortobagyi, G., Ravdin, P., & Slamon, D. (1998). *HER2 overexpression in breast cancer.* San Francisco: Genentech, Inc.

Berkery, R., Cleri, L. B., & Skarin, A. T. (1997). *Oncology pocket guide to chemotherapy,* 3rd ed. Baltimore: Mosby-Wolfe.

Brogden, J. M., & Nevidjon, B. (1995). Vinorelbine tartrate (Navelbine): Drug profile and nursing implication of a new vinca alkaloid. *Oncol Nurs Forum, 22*(4), pp. 635-646.

Cook, G. A., & Troutner, K. (1996). *Taxotere: An important advance in the treatment of metastatic breast cancer.* Collegeville, PA: Rhone-Poulenc Rorer.

Gemzar (gemcitabine HCl). (1998). *Drug package insert.* Indianapolis, IN: Eli Lily and Company.

Groenwald, S. L., Frogge, M. H., Goodman, M., & Yarbro, C. H. (1997). *Cancer nursing: Principles and practice,* 4th ed (pp. 958-952). Boston: Jones and Bartlett.

Henderson, I. C., Berry, D., Demetri, G., et al. (1998). Improved disease-free and overall survival from the addition of sequential paclitaxel but not from the escalation of doxorubicin dose level in the adjuvant chemotherapy of patients with node positive primary breast cancer. *Proc Am Soc Clin Oncol, 17,* p. 101a (Abstract 390A).

Kollef, M., & Goodenberger, D. (1995). Critical care and medical emergencies. In Ewald, G. A., & McKenzie, C. R. (Eds.). *The Washington manual* (pp. 184-232). Boston: Little, Brown.

Labovich, T. M. (1999). Acute hypersensitivity reactions to chemotherapy. *Semin Oncol Nurs, 15*(3), pp. 222-231.

Oncology Nursing Society. (1998). *Cancer chemotherapy guidelines and recommendations for practice.* Pittsburgh: Author.

Pharmacia Upjohn. (1997). *A question and answer guide to Camptosar injection,* p. 116.

Preston, F. A., & Cunningham, R. S. (1998). *Clinical guidelines for symptom management in oncology* (p. 267). New York: Clinical Insights Press.

Rieger, P. T. (June 1996). *Clinical handbook for biotherapy.* Boston: Jones and Bartlett.

Roxane Laboratories, Inc. (June 1996). Marinol drug insert.

Severance, S., & Galassi, A. (April 1999). Menopause in patients with cancer. *Am J Nurs, Suppl,* pp. 31-33.

8 Radiation Therapy

Esther Muscari Lin

Jack Carlson is a 62-year-old white man diagnosed with stage $T_{2(B)}$ prostate cancer, which was treated with prostatectomy 18 months ago while he was living in his retirement home in Florida. He presently has a rising prostate-specific antigen (PSA; 10 ng/ml) without clinical signs of disease, and he is referred by his urologist to the radiation therapy clinic of your teaching institution for a consultation. As you meet Mr. Carlson, he is quick to tell you that he is very familiar with the effects of radiation and knows what "he is getting into." As he hands you his pathology slides, scans, and paperwork, he tells you that he has everything under control. He asks that you proceed with your examination so that he can get to the golf course.

In the medical history, you note a 20-pack/year history of cigarette smoking and a diagnosis of a non–small cell lung cancer 18 months prior. In addition to chemotherapy, Mr. Carlson had thoracic radiotherapy for the non–small cell lung cancer. As you learn this, you make a mental note that this must have been what Mr. Carlson was referring to earlier.

Review of systems is negative, with the exception of "occasional" constipation and a long-standing history of hypertension controlled with β-blocker therapy. When asked about sexual function, Mr. Carlson waves his hand at you and tells you, "It is not an issue, and there is nothing to talk about."

Medications (as provided in a written list by Mrs. Carlson) include the following:

- Bicalutamide (Casodex) 50 mg/day orally
- Atenolol 50 mg/day
- Dulcolax suppositories 2 daily
- Metamucil daily

Mr. Carlson's social history includes living with wife of 40 years. He denies smoking, alcohol use, or drug use.

QUESTIONS

1. Upon your physical examination, what finding would surprise you given Mr. Carlson's history?
   a. Vital signs: temperature, 37.6° F; pulse, 110 beats/min; respiratory rate, 18 breaths/min; blood pressure, 120/80 mm Hg
   b. Skin: balding, thinning hair on arms and legs
   c. Lung sounds: inspiration equals expiration breath sounds
   d. Lower extremities: intact sensation and vibratory sensation

2. What lung and thorax characteristics are consistent with a cigarette smoking history?
   a. Tachypnea at rest
   b. Frequent cough with purulent mucus production
   c. Prolonged expiratory phase and decreased intensity
   d. Increased diaphragmatic excursion

3. Although Mr. Carlson's medical records indicate a negative digital rectal examination (DRE) and a previous prostatectomy, would a repeat examination be indicated and why?
   a. No, because the prostate has been removed, there would be nothing to palpate and recently done scans have been negative.
   b. No, recurrence, if suspected, is always at the site of the liver.
   c. Yes, because nerve-sparing prostatectomies place the patient at higher risk of recurrence at the site.
   d. Yes, residual disease can be at the previous site.

ANSWERS

1. Mr. Carlson's medical history warrants a thorough examination of almost every organ system.

Although the cardiac examination may be negative, the fact that his heart rate is elevated should raise a question in the examiner's mind. The antihypertensive action of atenolol is achieved by decreasing cardiac output and by suppressing renin release. The chronotropic effect is a decreased heart rate (Pearson, 2000). The increased heart rate should prompt further questioning if Mr. Carlson is taking this medication regularly, and if not, why. Is there a side effect that Mr. Carlson does not like? The other findings would be expected. The hair thinning patterns are consistent with increasing age. *Answer 1:* **a.**

2. Decreased breath sounds might be expected with a 20-pack/year history of smoking and chronic obstructive pulmonary disease (COPD). Prolonged expiration and decreased intensity would be accompanied by slight hyperresonance on percussion. Equal inspiration and expiration at a rate of 16 to 20 breaths/min is normal in the nonsmoker. In severe pulmonary fibrosis the patient is symptomatic and in distress, and the trachea can be shifted toward the affected side. Increased diaphragmatic excursion is predominantly noted with advanced pulmonary disease. A frequent and purulent cough is associated more with pneumonia and not necessarily a lengthy smoking history (Leasia & Monahan, 1997). *Answer 2:* **c.**

3. A DRE is still indicated especially because this is the first complete evaluation in the Radiation Therapy Clinic. Examination of the rectal vault, anus, and rectum provides a baseline evaluation before initiating therapy (Volpe, 1999). Although recurrence after prostatectomy tends to be via the lymphatic system to distant organs of lungs, liver, kidneys, and bone, residual disease and local recurrence is possible, especially if there had been positive margins or extracapsular extension. The standard of care includes the DRE. *Answer 3:* **d.**

QUESTIONS

4. What risk factors does Mr. Carlson have for sexual dysfunction?

ANSWERS

4. Men who are diagnosed with prostate cancer have a number of risk factors for sexual dysfunction. Sexual dysfunction includes decreased frequency and quality of erections, decreased morning erections, decreased intercourse, decreased ability to achieve sexual climax, changes in sexual desire, and change in orgasm (Helgason, Fredrikson, Adolfsson, & Steinbeck, 1995; Litwin, Hays,

Fink, et al., 1995). The diagnosis of cancer that involves the male sexual organ can assault a man's self-esteem and body image. Emotional and psychosocial reactions can interfere with desire as well as function. Although both radiotherapy and prostatectomy result in erectile dysfunction, post-prostatectomy patients have significantly worse sexual dysfunction than radiotherapy patients. Erectile dysfunction rates are higher in the radiotherapy groups that have larger pelvic field involvement. Despite higher rates of some type of remaining sexual functioning in patients receiving radiotherapy, patients report that in general there is a decline in the quality and frequency of sexual function (Helgason, Fredrikson, Adolfsson, & Steinbeck, 1995; Litwin, et al., 1995; Roach, Chinn, Holland, & Clark, 1996). Testosterone suppression from androgen ablative agents acts as medical castration and causes decreased libido and erectile dysfunction (Stempkowski, 1999). Some cardiac and antihypertensives can also interfere with erectile function. *Answer 4:* **prostatectomy, radiotherapy, hormonal manipulation, antihypertensives, and psychologic factors.**

QUESTIONS

5. Because there is no clinical evidence of disease, on what grounds would the radiation oncologist recommend a 5-week course of external beam radiation therapy followed by interstitial radioactive seed implants?
  a. Mr. Carlson is older than 60 years of age and is not expected to outlive the natural growth rate of prostate cancer.
  b. Mr. Carlson has been previously diagnosed and treated for prostate cancer and has a rising PSA within 2 years of diagnosis, which is a legitimate reason for treatment, despite the lack of pathologic evidence.
  c. Mr. Carlson is insistent on having some type of treatment.
  d. Mr. Carlson should have had adjuvant radiation therapy at his initial diagnosis.

6. The course of therapy recommended is 5 weeks of external beam radiotherapy followed by brachytherapy. What is the intent of this treatment plan?
  a. Curative
  b. Long-term local control
  c. Palliation
  d. None of these

ANSWERS

5. PSA is a sensitive and specific diagnostic aid. It is used in disease prognosis, as a marker of disease activity, and to detect recurrence in previously treated patients (American Society for Therapeutic Radiology and Oncology Consensus Panel, 1997; Takayama, Vessella, & Lange, 1994). Despite the fact that a rise in PSA levels after curative prostatectomy predicts localized residual or metastatic disease, Mr. Carlson's workup for distant metastasis has been negative. In patients who have a rising PSA 2 years after prostatectomy without evidence of disease, treatment includes hormonal agents and radioactive seed implants. *Answer 5:* **b.**

6. Because Mr. Carlson is relatively young and has no evidence of disease, the intent of therapy is curative (Anscher, Robertson, & Prosnitz, 1995). During palliative therapy, treatment courses are shorter, limited to the amount of radiation necessary to manage symptoms. Palliation radiotherapy seeks to avoid side effects of radiotherapy, resulting in lower radiation doses and shorter treatment courses. Planning for curative or long-term control of radiotherapy is complex and characterized by the willingness to risk short-term side effects (Hilderley, 1997). Curative therapy regimens are planned with the belief that the risk of microscopic metastasis is low, whereas long-term local control is designed with the belief that the local area can be controlled for any future disease; however, the risk of systemic spread still exists. *Answer 6:* **a.**

QUESTIONS

7. Which of the following pharmacologic interventions would you *most* likely see in Mr. Carlson's regimen?
   a. Immediate discontinuation of the bisacodyl and psyllium
   b. Increase in the atenolol dose to 100 mg/day
   c. Recommendation to taper and discontinue stool regimen by the end of the second week of radiation therapy
   d. Hold on the bicalutamide (Casodex) dose while Mr. Carlson receives external beam radiotherapy

8. As you speak with the couple about what they can expect with the course of radiation, what will be your first priority?
   a. Teaching about potential side effects and time of occurrence
   b. Learning more about Mr. Carlson's previous experience with radiotherapy
   c. Ascertaining what their communication and coping patterns have been
   d. Becoming certain that Mr. Carlson is fully informed for consent

ANSWERS

7. The localized side effects of radiation therapy will be from the organs within the pelvic radiation ports. Because radiation side effects are cumulative, skin erythema, diarrhea, possible cystitis, and proctitis are at risk for occurring in the third week of therapy. *Answer 7:* **c.**

8. Although education about side effects will support the care Mr. Carlson receives and the experience he has with 5 weeks of pelvic radiotherapy, learning about his previous experience is the first step. Most likely, he will be unable to believe what is told if he had a previous negative experience. It is possible that a distressing side effect or some other aspect of the previous treatment is cause for anxiety, fear, or depression. Learning his concerns first will help guide what additional information Mr. Carlson would benefit from as he is treated for a different cancer diagnosis as well as when to provide this information. *Answer 8:* **b.**

Case Study continued

Mr. Carlson has been coming for his daily radiation treatments for 3 weeks. He comes alone despite his wife's request to accompany him. Each day, he is quick to tell the receptionist upon his arrival that he is just fine, does not need to see anyone, and would appreciate her getting him in as quickly as possible. On Monday of the beginning of the fourth week, the nurse in radiation therapy pages you, requesting your assistance with Mr. Carlson. She reports over the telephone that he is quite agitated with her, complaining that "this is the absolute worst" he has ever been. He has never been treated this way and "demands" attention.

QUESTIONS

9. What two assumptions do you process as you head toward the clinic?
   1. _____
   2. _____

10. Provide two reasons why you will review Mr. Carlson's medication profile?
   1. _____
   2. _____

ANSWERS

Questions 7 through 10 are inquiring into the ability of the advanced practiced nurse (APN) to identify trends in patient responses and then use that information to educate patients and families, guide the care patients receive, and anticipate potential side effects or problems.

9. At approximately 3 weeks into radiotherapy of the pelvis, patients are at risk for the general side effect of fatigue and site-specific effects of diarrhea, rectal skin erythema and irritation, abdominal cramping, tenesmus, and occasionally hematochezia. Diarrhea, resulting from inflammation of the small and large bowel mucosa, is the most common acute side effect of radiotherapy. It can range from a few mild episodes (two to four) to severe (more than eight) watery, explosive episodes. Patients can become very upset because they have no control of when the episodes occur. As treatment continues, the severity of the diarrhea will worsen without intervention. Complicating Mr. Carlson's situation (and for many men receiving hormonal therapy), diarrhea can also be a side effect of the medication. The bowel regimen of a laxative and stool softener, common for many of the older generation, will also influence assessment and diarrheal management. Anticipating the intestinal responses to radiotherapy empowers the APN to taper the bowel regimen as the bowel side effect is expected. Hormonal manipulation is part of the treatment plan and should not be altered. The assumptions you process originate from your previous assessments and meetings with Mr. and Mrs. Carlson, along with the usual expected course of pelvic and abdominal radiotherapy. First, from your initial meetings with Mr. Carlson, it was made clear to you that controlling his care and environment is a strong and important need in his life. He wanted to be the one who made the final decisions in his care. Not only did he lose control with a cancer diagnosis, but he is unable to control the side effects of the therapy he is receiving. Control is crucial for this man's coping and lifestyle. Second, you consider what side effects a person receiving pelvic radiotherapy is at risk for at the fourth week. You know the effects of radiation therapy are cumulative and that pelvic radiation often results in profound diarrhea. If he has resisted decreasing his bowel regimen medications, then that combined with the expected diarrhea from pelvic radiation has probably resulted in episodes of diarrhea that could be explosive and uncontrollable. For a man who needs as much in control of his environment as Mr. Carlson, this could be devastating to him. Therefore, as you approach him, it will be with the understanding that this man could be feeling at a loss with the side effects and might in fact be in need of help. *Answer 9:* **See text.**

10. The medication profile, reviewed at each visit, assists in identifying drugs that could potentially influence side effects, whether prescriptive or over-the-counter. Casodex can result in diarrhea, but efforts to control diarrhea will be through addition of an antidiarrheal as opposed to hormonal adjustment. The bowel regimen Mr. Carlson has been on, if not stopped or adjusted at the onset of treatment as suggested, will contribute to the volume of diarrhea. Atenolol may occasionally cause diarrhea but usually at the onset of administration. It will be important to determine whether Mr. Carlson recently restarted the drug. *Answer 10:* **See text.**

QUESTIONS

11. What, if any, laboratory tests would you suggest?
  1. Complete blood count (CBC) with differential
  2. Electrolyte and renal panel
  3. Blood cultures
     a. 1 & 2
     b. 1 & 3
     c. 2 & 3
     d. All of these

12. On what organ systems will you focus your assessment? Why?
  a. Complete organ system assessment
  b. Cardiovascular, respiratory, integumentary
  c. Integumentary, gastrointestinal
  d. Cardiovascular, gastrointestinal, integumentary

ANSWERS

11. Blood cultures would be indicated if Mr. Carlson presented with or reported a temperature elevation. Electrolytes and renal function provide insight into fluid loss, dehydration, and hypokalemia. The CBC with differential, sometimes routinely done, may show the infection and anemia risk. Because significant anemia is not expected, lower-than-usual levels of hemoglobin and hematocrit should be evaluated for possible blood loss via the intestinal tract from possible mucosal ulceration. *Answer 11:* **d.**

12. Because Mr. Carlson is seen daily in the clinic and evaluated weekly, your assessment can be limited to the organ systems most affected by side effects of the radiation therapy. However, if other signs or symptoms are noted on examination, those organ systems should be assessed as well. Because the weekend has passed, it is possible that

Mr. Carlson has had significant diarrhea and volume loss to result in dehydration. Reports of dizziness, weakness, or syncope in conjunction with orthostatic vital signs will be critical in assessing volume status. A flat, soft, nontender abdomen with normal bowel sounds, although hyperactive, will contribute to your gastrointestinal assessment. Rectal skin examination without digital examination is indicated because interventions to promote skin integrity will be depend on skin condition, suspicion of superficial infection, and degree of discomfort. *Answer 12:* **d.**

QUESTIONS

13. What other possible symptoms might accompany the onset of diarrhea?
   a. Bleeding
   b. Cystitis
   c. Erectile dysfunction
   d. Nausea

ANSWERS

13. Diarrhea, rectal urgency, crampy abdominal pain, and bleeding associated with bowel movements are the problems patients report as bothersome and the ones that accompany the diarrhea that generally occurs at the end of the third week (Shrader-Bogen, Kjellberg, McPherson, & Murray, 1997). It is possible for bleeding to occur with even a few episodes of diarrhea because an erythematous reaction of the skin in the radiation field occurs, resulting in more friable skin, which is prone to easy breakdown and bleeding from repeated stool contact. Nausea is less likely to occur when the abdomen is not in the radiation field. Because Mr. Carlson has been taking Casodex, which suppresses testosterone production, erectile dysfunction has most likely already occurred. Although cystitis can occur 3 to 5 weeks into therapy, it is not in conjunction with the diarrhea. Cystitis is also associated with mucosal inflammation from the bladder being in the radiation field. Symptoms usually subside 2 to 8 weeks after treatment completion as mucosal healing occurs. *Answer 13:* **a.**

QUESTIONS

14. Which of the following bowel elimination characteristics would be *least* likely to accompany other reported characteristics in Mr. Carlson's fourth week of radiation?
   a. Has abnormal or "different" odor
   b. Increases in frequency after meals
   c. Limits social activities
   d. Causes incontinence at times

ANSWERS

14. Although infection must be ruled out in the person presenting with frequent, watery, and at times, explosive bouts of diarrhea, it is not in the forefront of possible causes of diarrhea in the person 4 weeks into radiation therapy. The ability to anticipate the occurrence and timing of side effects such as diarrhea is an asset of the APN. Although the presence of an abnormal odor will be asked, it is with the expectation that the practitioner will be able to rule it out and further narrow down the assessment. This knowledge enables the practitioner to complete a concise and appropriate assessment without obtaining a stool culture unless other signs and symptoms such as chills, fever, left shift, or hypotension are present. See Table 8-1. *Answer 14:* **a.**

QUESTIONS

15. Mr. Carlson's primary nurse points out that he has lost 3 pounds since his last weight a week ago and believes priority today should be given to nutritional counseling and dietary changes that will influence both diarrhea and his nutritional status. As the APN involved with Mr. Carlson's care, you believe a "higher" priority is diarrhea management. How will you achieve an optimal care plan for Mr. Carlson?
   a. Tell the nurse that diarrhea management needs to be prioritized over nutritional needs at this point but that nutritional counseling can occur later when side effects are under control.
   b. Suggest conducting an in-depth assessment of the diarrhea and corresponding symptoms together.
   c. Collaboratively, ask Mr. Carlson what he would prefer in terms of nutritional counseling and dietary management.
   d. Point out to the nurse that Mr. Carlson is at risk for dehydration and electrolyte imbalance, which could interfere with his schedule of radiation treatments.

ANSWERS

15. A successful working relationship among nursing colleagues requires respect of every participant's skills and contributions. Dictating care without collaboration will jeopardize the quality of relationships and sabotage the potential outcomes of people working together. It is insufficient to listen and disregard suggestions without taking the collaborator through the process of assessment and decision making. This

TABLE 8-1 | History Taking for Alteration in Bowel Elimination

HISTORY TAKING	QUESTIONS
Number of bowel movements/day	How frequent are your bowel movements? When was your last one? Do you have a feeling of urgency immediately before an episode?
Consistency	What change has occurred? Is it solid, semisolid, or all liquid?
Volume	How are you estimating the amount? small amounts, cup, prolonged bouts? Has there been any weight loss since it began?
Timing during day	Do you have an episode immediately after a meal? Are there any drinks or foods like dairy or fiber-filled foods that you associate with diarrhea? Does it occur more in the morning, middle of the day, evening, or night?
Associated symptoms	Do you have any cramping, bloating, or pain before and/or during an episode of diarrhea? Do you notice any change in color or odor? Have you seen blood or mucus in your stool? Do you have any rectal pain or feelings of incomplete evacuation after an episode?
Diet	What type of foods have you been eating—high in fiber, fat, or lactase?
Incontinence	Have you had any episodes of diarrhea when you were unable to get to a bathroom? Were these episodes preceded by anything different than the other episodes, such as sleeping, eating, exercising, and so on?
Medications	What over-the-counter medicines do you take? What herbal teas do you drink? What, if anything, do you do to help you sleep at night?
Perianal skin	Do you feel any burning, pain, or itching during or between bowel movements? Are you showering or bathing? Are you showering or bathing more, less, or with the same frequency? Have you tried any type of sitz bath? Have you used any ointment or lotion on your perianal area?

informal and "on-the-spot" consultation process educates the staff while strengthening collaboration and staff relationships. Although it can take more time and requires sensitivity on the part of the APN, the results are greater than the individual case because the nurse(s) involved will repeat the process in future similar situations. *Answer 15:* **b.**

Case Study continued

After conducting an in-depth assessment of Mr. Carlson's diarrhea, it is clear that he has moist desquamation of the perianal area accompanied by pain. The priority of care will be to decrease the diarrhea, institute a skin care protocol, and provide a pain relief regimen.

QUESTIONS

16. If you were teaching a colleague about your first option for pharmacologic intervention, how would you explain your choice?
   a. Aspirin because it reduces prostaglandin synthesis, increasing water and electrolyte absorption
   b. Codeine because it will provide relief while also acting as an antidiarrheal
   c. Diphenoxylate because it does not have significant opioid effects at antidiarrheal doses

   d. Loperamide because it can inhibit fluid and electrolyte secretion

ANSWERS

16. Loperamide (2-mg capsule; 1-mg/5 ml elixir) allows more tailoring of administrations to the frequency of the patient's diarrheal episodes. It can be titrated upward, having the highest antidiarrheal-to-analgesic ratio, and although chemically related to opiates, it does not have physical dependence characteristics. Patients can be instructed to take 4 mg initially and then 2 mg after each unformed stool until the diarrhea subsides, up to 16 mg/day. Patients can then take a maintenance dose (half the necessary dose divided between morning and evening administrations) if needed. The drug can be stopped promptly or adjusted as needed depending on the course of diarrhea. Codeine may occasionally be used as an antidiarrheal but is not often the first-line drug of choice. Diphenoxylate is limited in its ability to be titrated upward (Pearson, 2000). *Answer 16:* **d.**

Case Study continued

The skin care protocol agreed on between the primary nurse and yourself is to cleanse the area with one-third-strength hydrogen peroxide after each bowel movement and apply a hydrogel dressing to the affected area.

QUESTIONS

17. On what criteria did you base this strategy?
   a. This is the most cost-effective and standard regimen for typical and expected radiation therapy reactions.
   b. Ointments are better tolerated on inflamed skin than creams.
   c. Reepithelialization requires clean areas free of crusting.
   d. Because the hydrogel dressings are free of alcohol, they do not need to be removed during the radiation treatment.

ANSWERS

17. Skin care recommendations differ for the different types of radiation reactions. Erythematous reactions require interventions aimed at minimizing symptoms, maintaining skin integrity, and preventing infection. Dry desquamation can include hydrophilic topical ointments because they relieve dryness and are comforting. Moist desquamation requires interventions that promote reepithelialization and healing. Therefore cleansing without interfering with epithelial proliferation requires occlusive dressings containing hydrogels or hydrocolloids. These occlusive dressings promote healing by absorbing fluid to reduce the chance of maceration. They also contain the natural cells necessary for digestion of necrotic debris and help prevent infection and promote comfort. These types of dressings do need to be

removed before each radiation treatment (Gallagher, 1995). Moisture-vapor-permeable (MVP) dressings do not need to be removed because they are thin and do not act as a bolus material. However, MVP dressings allow fluid to accumulate because they are nonabsorbent and thus can lead to maceration (Dunne-Daly, 1995). See Table 8-2. *Answer 17:* **c.**

TABLE 8-2 Recommendations for Skin Care
ERYTHEMA
Skin care lotions, creams, gels, or ointments without alcohol, menthol, and other chemical irritants
1% hydrocortisone ointment
DRY DESQUAMATION
Same as for erythema
Cornstarch in dry areas only
MOIST DESQUAMATION
Dressings (e.g., hydrogel, hydrocolloid, polyurethane film)
Cleanse with ⅓ strength hydrogen peroxide, normal saline, or a wound cleanser
Silver sulfadiazine

From Sitton, E. (1997). Managing side effects of skin changes and fatigue. In Dow, K. H., Bucholtz, J. D., Iwamoto, R., Fieler, V., & Hilderley, L. (Eds.). *Nursing care in radiation oncology*, 2nd ed (pp. 79-100). Philadelphia: WB Saunders.

CASE 2 STUDY

You are asked to provide a lecture on radiation therapy to nursing students in a basic oncology course. As you are lecturing, a student asks about when people with cancer receiving radiation therapy lose their hair.

QUESTIONS

1. What is the knowledge that is lacking to prompt this question?
   a. Radiation side effects are cumulative; therefore alopecia is usually experienced in the third week of therapy.
   b. Alopecia is actually more distressing to women than to men.
   c. Alopecia is a localized, site-specific result of radiation therapy.
   d. The combination of chemotherapy and radiation therapy results in alopecia.

2. What is the most common general side effect of radiation therapy?
   a. Faint nausea
   b. Depression
   c. Skin reactions
   d. Fatigue

ANSWERS

1. The assumption that hair loss is an expected side effect of radiation therapy exists among the lay population. The knowledge lacking is that radiation side effects are site specific. The specific side effects are related to the tissues in the radiation field. *Answer 1:* **c.**

2. The most common general side effect experienced by people undergoing radiotherapy is fatigue. Although there are numerous influencing factors and the pathophysiology is unknown, it can affect quality of life and other symptoms experienced. Nausea is a site-specific response to abdominal radiotherapy. Although localized skin effects are common and a very mild erythema may occur within the first week of treatment, more pronounced inflammation and erythema with dry desquamation occurs later and is not as common as fatigue. Explaining the difference between general and site-specific information is often an introduction into the specific events or symptoms the patient may have. An in-depth explanation includes what to expect from radiation to the affected body area and a timeline of when to expect the specific symptoms. *Answer 2:* **d.**

QUESTIONS

3. What is the rationale for fractionated radiation doses?
  a. Toxicities are less severe.
  b. More patients can be treated per day.
  c. Higher therapeutic doses can be given in shorter periods.
  d. Radiation therapy no longer requires a hospital admission.

4. What is *simulation* and why is it performed?

5. How will you explain the difference between a linear accelerator and a cobalt machine for therapeutic radiation therapy?
  a. Both linear accelerators and cobalt machines are deeply penetrating and skin sparing, but cobalt machines require longer treatment times.
  b. Cobalt machines are used for superficial lesions.
  c. Linear accelerators have limited use because of poor skin tolerance.
  d. Cobalt machines are more commonly found in community settings as opposed to academic tertiary care centers because of their cost.

ANSWERS

3-4. When planning the dose, field, fractionation, and schedule for therapy, the radiation oncologist considers the histology, tumor size, stage of disease and prognosis, general health of the patient, and available equipment. *Simulation* defines the treatment field with radiographs and fluoroscopy, reproducing the target area for the treatment beam. Fractionation, or the determined

total dose to treat the cancer, is divided into smaller daily doses to maximize the tumor kill while preserving healthy tissue. *Answer 3:* **a.** *Answer 4:* **See text.**

5. Cobalt equipment is deeply penetrating and skin sparing. It is used for deep-seated tumors, but because of a slower dose rate, it requires longer treatment times. Linear accelerators are also deeply penetrating and skin sparing, which is good for deep-seated tumors; however, these accelerators can have a higher dose rate with shorter treatment times. Superficial lesions such as skin cancers can be treated with kilovoltage/x-ray machines (Hilderley, 1997). *Answer 5:* **a.**

QUESTIONS

6. A student in the class shares the story of her aunt who had "internal radiotherapy." The student is interested in knowing about the nursing care limitations. What is the most vital piece of information you need before you can answer this?
  a. Tumor site location
  b. Type of brachytherapy
  c. Inpatient or outpatient status
  d. Length of insertion time

7. Inpatient nursing care of the woman with a cervical implant includes all of the following *except:*
  a. Foley catheter insertion
  b. High-fluid, low-residue diet
  c. Head of the bed elevation to 15 degrees
  d. Usual self-care activities

ANSWERS

6. Intracavitary implants can be used for gynecologic cancers. For inpatients with implants, precautionary measures are taken to prevent displacement of the radioactive source while limiting the exposure to health care members. Bed rest, head of the bed elevation, anxiety, and pain relief measures are offered to maintain comfort and minimize movement. Knowing what type of brachytherapy for intracavitary or interstitial implants is necessary for designing nursing care. There are new delivery systems that eliminate an inpatient stay, pose less risk to personnel, and require shorter treatment times. Because bed rest is necessary in the inpatient setting to minimize the risk of displacement, the patient is unable to get out of bed, take a shower, or use the bathroom. *Answer 6:* **b.**

7. All activities are aimed at minimizing displacement. A urinary catheter keeps the bladder constantly drained, the diet minimizes diarrhea and bowel activity, and the bed elevation is limited to only 15 degrees for the patient to eat; any additional movement is discouraged. *Answer 7:* **d.**

Case Study continued

The student continues to say that her aunt's 42-year marriage has become strained since the radiotherapy for the cervical cancer. The aunt has voiced her fears that her husband is no longer interested in her sexually. The student asks you if there is anything associated with radiotherapy that may have contributed to this problem because her aunt feels so strongly that the radiotherapy is "at the root of the problem."

QUESTIONS

8. Recognizing certain trends in people's knowledge base and reactions to radiation therapy, the first possibility that needs clarifying is:
  a. Does a misperception exist about having residual radiation or being radioactive?
  b. There is a history of good communication in this relationship, and it has become problematic only with the cancer diagnosis.
  c. The wife actually has a poor prognosis, and the husband is trying to protect her.
  d. This student, the niece, is interfering and should refer the couple for a psychosocial referral.

ANSWERS

8. It is impossible to make an evaluation without an assessment. The first step in an oncology nursing assessment is learning about the aunt and uncle's perceptions and communication patterns. The most obvious recommendation would be that the patient speak with an oncology nurse familiar with her and her husband. There is no information given in this case about the patient and her husband's past communication patterns, the disease prognosis, other relationship factors, or physiologic changes (e.g., vaginal dryness dyspareunia) that may be contributing to the problem. A lack of communication, even minor, can lead to misperceptions. The first step in any evaluation is to learn people's perceptions, understandings, and fears. There are still beliefs that radiation, no matter what the dose or form, leaves a person radioactive. *Answer 8:* **a.**

Case Study continued

After treatment is completed, the aunt will have various needs and will be at risk for certain problems.

QUESTIONS

9. As you work with the nursing staff to plan long-term care for her, what two major pieces of information do you need?
  a. Follow-up visit schedule and maintenance therapy plan
  b. Disease prognosis and potential long-term side effects of radiotherapy
  c. Disease prognosis and available support systems
  d. Maintenance therapy plan and available support systems

10. What is the *most* likely long-term side effect the student's aunt is at risk for?
  a. Fatigue
  b. Skin erythema
  c. Vaginal stenosis
  d. Urinary incontinence

ANSWERS

9. The APN needs to identify trends in patient responses and the expected long-term side effects. Planning care requires a sense of what the disease prognosis and patterns of metastasis are. If the risk for metastasis is high, there will be a heightened awareness of presenting signs or symptoms during future encounters. At the time of discharge, the APN must consider what treatment the patient has had in order to teach about long-term side effects and what signs and symptoms should be reported. *Answer 9:* **b.**

10. As tissue healing occurs in the weeks and months after treatment completion, progressive fibrosis occurs, characterized by induration and thickening of the dermis and subcutaneous tissues. The loss of elasticity of the vaginal tissues, or vaginal stenosis, is noted by the woman during times of sexual activity and pelvic examinations. Repeated and ongoing dilation of the vagina with a dilator or through sexual intercourse is necessary to maintain the vaginal canal. *Answer 10:* **c.**

CASE 3 STUDY

Marvin Howard is referred to the nutritional support clinic for routine evaluation 6 weeks after an esophagogastrectomy, during which time a jejunostomy tube was placed prophylactically. He is 10% below his ideal body weight, his partner reports an intake reflective of anorexia, and he takes in most of his calories through supplements. Marvin is anticipating removal of the feeding tube. He has had 13 radiation treatments with limits of the field 2 inches above and below the nipple line and is planned for 12 more radiation sessions. He is receiving "sandwich" chemotherapy. He was hospitalized for the first week of radiotherapy treatment and will be hospitalized during the last 5 days of radiation treatments to receive continuous 5-fluorouracil (5-FU) administration.

QUESTIONS

1. Based on the information presented, what might be wrong with Marvin? Specify all possible problems.
   1. Esophageal stricture
   2. Taste alterations
   3. Xerostomia
   4. Oral stomatitis
      a. 1 & 2
      b. 1, 2, & 3
      c. 2, 3, & 4
      d. All of these

ANSWERS

1. The radiation field for esophageal cancer may include a boost to the tumor site area or at the anastomotic level. Strictures are common after esophageal resection and stomach pull-up. The erythema and edema that can result from radiation treatments can decrease the lumen opening, making it more difficult for food to pass. Dilation of the lumen is necessary to maintain patency and allow the patient to continue to eat. As fibrosis occurs in the weeks and months after radiation completion, repeated episodes of esophageal strictures can occur, requiring dilation. Stomatitis as a side effect of 5-FU may alter the mucous membranes and could be contributing to dysphagia. Mucositis of the esophagus or "esophagitis" as a result of radiation therapy can result when the neck, chest, or upper back is irradiated. Stomatitis or mucositis can effect the person's oral intake because of pain. Taste alterations that accompany 5-FU administration will also affect a person's

willingness to eat. Therefore the combination of 5-FU side effects and the surgical intervention greatly affect Marvin's potential to take in an adequate amount of calories orally. Xerostomia would have more risk of occurring if the salivary glands were in the radiation field, which they are not. *Answer 1:* **c.**

Case Study continued

Weekly examination of Marvin's mouth in the radiation clinic is as follows: Marvin is asked to remove any dental appliance, open his mouth while a flashlight is used to highlight the oral cavity, and a rating of stomatitis severity is written in his chart.

QUESTIONS

2. Considering this description of an oral assessment, what other behavior(s) is(are) indicated that could result in a more comprehensive oral assessment?
   1. The patient is instructed to keep a weekly diary.
   2. Assessment is performed daily rather than weekly.
   3. A gloved finger displaces the tongue and buccal mucosa.
   4. An oral assessment tool is placed inside the patient's infusion therapy chart.
      a. 2 & 4
      b. 1 & 4
      c. 2, 3, & 4
      d. All of these

ANSWERS

2. The oral mucositis that Marvin is experiencing is a result of the 5-FU and not the radiation therapy because the mouth is not being irradiated. Mucositis, which includes mild erythema, edema, sensations of dryness, or burning, occurs quickly because of the rapid turnover rate of epithelial cells. Mucositis usually presents within 10 days of drug administration and begins to resolve within 2 weeks. Therefore daily as opposed to weekly inspection to capture changes is indicated. Chemotherapy is administered only during the first and last week of radiation therapy; therefore side effects will be missed unless Marvin returns to the infusion or medical oncology clinic. Because he is being followed daily in the radiation therapy clinic, monitoring his chemotherapy-induced mucositis can be done at the same time. This gives the clinician in the radiation clinic information regard-

ing mucosal changes of the esophagus, which is being irradiated. An oral assessment tool should include descriptors for voice, swallowing, saliva, buccal mucosa, lips, tongue, gingiva, and teeth. Use of standardized measurement tools among clinicians is useful for comparison and evaluation of interventions. Taping the tool inside the patient's chart will promote a higher quality of assessment among care providers. In this case this patient is being followed closer in the radiation therapy clinic and should have a tool in that chart.

A gloved finger is a must in oral assessment because careful, in-depth evaluation requires exposing all areas of the oral cavity and cannot be done by simply having the patient open his or her mouth. The tongue needs to be gently displaced, and the cheek needs to be pulled away from the dentition. Although a daily diary can give patient's a sense of control, it could also detract from their energy reserves without providing much additional information. Most oral assessment data are obtained from careful inspection. *Answer 2:* **c.**

QUESTIONS

3. What diagnostic study would be best to evaluate Marvin's persistent dysphagia?
   a. Barium swallow
   b. Esophageal manometry
   c. Arteriography
   d. Endoscopic retrograde cholangiopancreatography (ERCP)

ANSWERS

3. Oral barium is observed as it passes through the reconstructed digestive tract. Spot radiographs are taken as the fluid passes through. Esophageal manometry measures esophageal sphincter pressure and peristaltic contractions. It is used to evaluate dysphagia, but only after barium swallow or esophagoscopy are normal because it detects motility disorders. An ERCP is indicated for endoscopic and radiographic examination of the biliary pancreatic ducts. *Answer 3:* **a.**

QUESTIONS

4. What is the least amount of additional information that you need to collect before being able to intervene with Marvin about his nutritional status?
   a. Human immunodeficiency virus (HIV) status, anthropometrics, ideal body weight
   b. Total iron-binding capacity (TIBC), albumin, ideal body weight
   c. Weight loss, prealbumin, transferrin
   d. Nitrogen balance, resting energy expenditure, goal weight

ANSWERS

4. Although anthropometrics contribute to an appreciation of muscle and fat mass, they are not an absolute when diagnosing nutritional abnormalities and creating a plan of care. TIBC in conjunction with serum iron and transferrin is needed to adequately diagnose iron deficiency. Transferrin, of which iron is coupled, is a transport protein. Albumin, prealbumin, and transferrin are all circulating proteins that fluctuate with body water changes and are generally used in standard laboratory tests for nutritional assessment. Because albumin has a long half-life (approximately 3 weeks), prealbumin and transferrin, which have shorter half lives (3 and 8 days, respectively), may be more helpful for this snapshot analysis of Marvin's true nutritional state, especially when considered in combination with how much weight he has lost. Nitrogen balance, calculated by measuring the urinary urea nitrogen in a 24-hour urine collection, is the most accurate measure of protein catabolism. The resting energy expenditure also estimates energy utilization and provides the information for the nutritional support prescription; however, it is not available in every center. The goal weight does not lend insight into the patient's actual status but rather what the weight should be for that patient's height and weight; this is not always realistic and in alignment with the individual patient. *Answer 4:* **c.**

Case Study continued

The dietitian and pharmacist are members of the nutritional support team and have not yet met with Marvin. After your review of the cancer treatment plan, nutritional laboratory results, and Marvin's goals with the collaborating physician and leader of the team, the physician comments that it is quite clear what needs to be done for Marvin. The clinic is full, with more patients to be seen and inpatient rounds still need to be made. It could be much more efficient to present the plan to Marvin and let him leave.

5. What would be the rationale for taking the time and having the previously mentioned team members meet with the patient and his partner? Choose all that apply.
   1. Marvin has been referred for a complete nutritional assessment and is paying one lump sum for the entire consultation; therefore he should have the experience of meeting with them.

2. Insights and observations from the other two members could compliment your assessment.
3. The two team members tend to be vocal when not included in patient rounds and could make for an uncomfortable situation.
4. Team building and maintenance require equal respect and consideration of everyone's contributions.
5. Marvin is having his jejunostomy tube removed and needs dietary counseling in anticipation of this.
6. Marvin's partner has vital information to share with the dietitian.
   a. 1, 3, 4, & 5
   b. 4 & 5
   c. 2 & 4
   d. 1, 2, 4, 5, & 6

5. One of the hallmark characteristics of a multidisciplinary team is respect and consideration of every team members' contributions. Each person comes to the team with a different specialty and skill, that when combined, contributes to a high-quality care plan. For example, the dietitian will capture information about eating habits and food choices that might be manipulated to maximize oral intake. This is useful immediately as well as in anticipation of the jejunostomy tube removal. The drug profile the pharmacist obtains contributes to drugs and side effects that hinder appetite or intake, as well as other observations possibly made during the history. A patient who is in the middle of a medical treatment that is causing decreased oral intake, weight loss, and possible malnutrition would most likely not receive the recommendations to have an indwelling feeding tube removed. It is more prudent to remove the tube only after oral intake is consistently adequate to maintain adequate protein and calorie nutrition. *Answer 5:* **c.**

Case Study continued

Marvin continues to lose weight. His oral mucositis worsens in pain intensity and saliva production, but he is close to completing the radiation treatment plan. The radiation oncologist suggests that Marvin just "wait it out" rather than begin some type of nutritional support.

QUESTIONS

6. What is the most likely rationale for the radiation oncologist's recommendation?

a. Within 2 weeks of treatment completion, the stomatitis will resolve and his oral intake will return.
b. Topical anesthetics can be used to help him gain relief and be able to ingest liquid supplements into his body until treatment is completed.
c. Nutritional support requires close monitoring and care that is too much for Marvin at this time.
d. Parenteral nutrition would be the best option for Marvin at this point, but the intravenous access it would require is an unnecessary risk.

7. What piece of information is missing that might influence the recommendation to Marvin?

6. The high turnover rate of the epithelial cells (10 to 14 days) results in quick recovery from the symptoms of stomatitis (Iwamoto, 1997). It is likely that this would be behind the radiation oncologist's thought processes. *Answer 6:* **a.**

7. However, the information that is missing is that Marvin is receiving sandwich chemotherapy and is scheduled to receive continuous 5-FU, a known insult to the mucous membranes. He has already experienced this effect. The combination now of more than 3 weeks of radiotherapy inducing stomatitis and the possible further insult of 5-FU place Marvin at a much higher risk of continued stomatitis, well beyond the normal recovery time expected at the completion of radiation therapy. The intensity of Marvin's stomatitis has been severe enough to substantially inhibit adequate oral intake and is an indicator that topical agents are insufficient pain relievers. This intensity of side effect requires a systemic and potent analgesic for relief. Although nutritional support requires monitoring, the amount and frequency necessary for enteral feedings are considerably less than for parenteral nutrition. Patients can be advanced in their enteral prescriptions at home by reporting their gastrointestinal responses to the nurse via the telephone. Parenteral nutrition is usually begun in the hospital and requires daily electrolyte panels, intensive patient/family education, and central venous access. The rule of thumb when considering nutritional support for a patient is to use the "gut" (gastrointestinal system) if it works, before ever considering the parenteral route. Also, for expected short-term (6 to 8 weeks) use, the enteral route is the choice of feeding route. *Answer 7:* **Stomatitis is the**

most common side effect of the chemotherapy planned, 5-FU.

Case Study continued

Marvin agrees to a course of enteral nutrition via his jejunostomy tube, which lasts 4 weeks. By the time the feeding tube is removed, he is eating 100% of his daily requirements to maintain protein-calorie nutrition. At 3 months after his tube removal, he has regained his weight, is enjoying a renewed appetite, and returns to work. At his 6-month follow-up in the oncology clinic, Marvin complains of chest tightness, as if food gets "stuck," and points to the middle of his chest. He is frightened because the feeling reminds him of his presenting symptoms for esophageal cancer. His weight is stable, nutritional laboratory values are within normal limits, and his physical examination is negative.

QUESTIONS

8. What diagnosis differential would be *least* considered at this point based on the provided information?
  a. Esophageal recurrence
  b. Esophageal stricture
  c. Esophageal fistula
  d. Peptic ulcer disease

9. Altering Marvin's diet to minimize alcohol, chocolate, fatty foods, and caffeine would be directed at treating what condition?
  a. Reflux esophagitis
  b. Pulmonary aspiration
  c. Premature satiety
  d. Candidal esophagitis

ANSWERS

8. Because of Marvin's cancer history, a recurrence is always considered. Reflux esophagitis, a result of lower esophageal sphincter pressure, has symptoms of heartburn, dysphagia, and chest pain, as well as other ear, nose, and throat symptoms. Peptic ulcer disease, or ulceration of the gastroduodenal mucosa, is a possible result of prolonged and severe stomatitis/mucositis. Because of the esophagogastrectomy, the stomach is most likely pulled up and "higher" in the patient's chest, thereby possibly confusing the clinical picture as the patient points to an area high on the chest. Answers a, b, and d all share similar symptoms as those presented in the case scenario. Commonly associated presenting signs of an esophageal fistula are infection, sepsis, and bleeding. Fistulas

can occur in the immediate postoperative period as well as be late effects of radiation fibrosis. An esophageal stricture is the most likely cause of Marvin's symptoms because 6 months is a common time of onset for radiation fibrosis, especially after a person has had esophageal surgery. *Answer 8:* **c.**

9. The lifestyle modifications of bed blocks, altered diet, and decreased alcohol and cigarettes are first-line interventions for reflux esophagitis, as well as adjuncts to pharmacologic therapy (H_2-receptors antagonists, metoclopramide, omeprazole, and cisapride). Pulmonary aspiration, Barrett's esophagus, bleeding, and esophageal strictures are all possible complications of reflux esophagitis (Woodley & Rubin, 1995). *Answer 9:* **a.**

QUESTIONS

10. What would be the first-line approach to managing an esophageal stricture in a patient such as Marvin?
  a. Endoscopic dilation
  b. Changing to a soft and liquid diet
  c. Surgical resection
  d. Increased hydration and use of artificial saliva

ANSWERS

10. With endoscopy, a balloon at the end of the scope is passed into the esophagus and is able to gradually inflate, pushing against the esophagogastric junction, manually stretching the tissue, and enlarging the lumen. Esophageal strictures resulting from tissue scarring from surgery and/or radiation therapy often require repeated dilations to maintain patency. Hesitating to dilate can result in progressive fibrosis and potential inability to dilate the lumen at all as time passes, thus placing the patient at risk for potential surgery to correct the problem. Dietary changes do not correct the problem of an esophageal stricture but only accommodate the inability to swallow solid foods. Surgery is often reserved until conservative interventions have been attempted. See Figure 8-1. *Answer 10:* **a.**

QUESTIONS

11. During the informed consent with the radiologist, Marvin refuses the dilation when he is told the risk of potential rupture from the balloon inflating against fibrotic tissue. You are paged to talk with Marvin about his refusal. What considerations would you include in your discussion with Marvin?

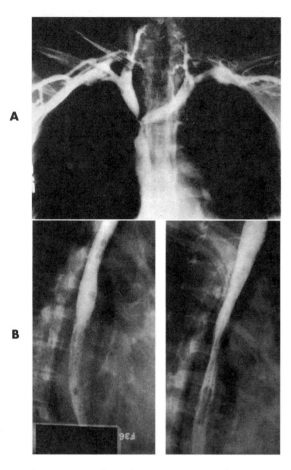

Figure 8-1 Esophageal stricture. **A,** Frontal view. **B,** Profile view.

1. The true risk of a rupture complication is small but is listed on the informed consent because any and all complications are included.
2. Radiated tissue has decreased elasticity, tends to be thinner in structure, and is more friable than healthy tissue.

3. Oral intake will continue to decrease, with progressive weight loss and most likely malnutrition because the lumen will continue to decrease as fibrosis progresses.
4. Marvin's other option is enteral nutrition, which could meet his entire protein and calorie nutritional requirements if he should choose to not have the endoscopy with balloon dilation.
   a. 1 & 2
   b. 1 & 4
   c. 2 & 3
   d. All of these

ANSWERS

11. Although the risk of esophageal rupture is low, minimizing the risk to the patient could lead the patient to think that *his or her* risk of rupture is close to nonexistent. The patient should be given the facts and allowed to interpret the meaning and risk to themselves within their own context of understanding. The APN can often be the patient's strongest advocate by virtue of the independence inherent in the role and the number of different settings the APN crosses to create, maintain, and enhance continuity of care. The tissue that will be pressed on with the inflated balloon is friable and at higher risk than healthy tissue to tear and bleed. Fibrosis is progressive, and there is no way to know how much the lumen diameter will decrease. The chance is real for it to actually close. As the lumen diameter decreases, the types of food able to pass will also decrease; in addition, the feelings of almost choking will interfere with the patient's attempts to eat. Weight loss and protein-calorie malnutrition will occur, at which point the patient might require surgery or long-term parenteral nutrition. Enteral nutrition is not an option for Marvin because of the esophagogastrectomy. The anatomy has changed and is no longer capable of hosting a feeding tube—gastrostomy, jejunostomy, or nasoduodenal. *Answer 11:* **c.**

CASE 4 STUDY

Millie, a 53-year-old white woman, recently underwent a head and neck resection for squamous cell carcinoma. She is an inpatient on the surgical oncology floor, and the staff has "concerns" about her ability to comply with the treatment plan. They have requested a consultation from you.

QUESTIONS

1. What is the rationale for asking the following questions before seeing Millie? What is the treatment plan? What behaviors have been exhibited by Millie that make the staff think she will have difficulty complying? What are the staffs'

concerns? What does the staff expect from you the APN?

1. Who is initiating the consult affects the extent of your involvement.
2. You might assess and recommend a treatment plan for something different than the staff identified problem.
3. You are seeking to see whether the staff members have "labeled" Millie.
4. Millie is most likely unable to provide a history.
5. The staff members routinely refer when they have a "noncompliant" patient.
   a. 1 only
   b. 2 & 4
   c. 1, 2, & 3
   d. 3 & 5

ANSWERS

1. Millie is not under your direct care; therefore your consultation will be in response to the staff's needs. Without learning who has initiated the consult influences your involvement. Your recommendations may be directly to the staff to guide them in their care of Millie. If there is a problem affecting Millie's care and comfort, recommendations may be made toward the entire team. Identifying the physicians responsible for her care also provides you with information from past experiences of how they perceive or welcome your input. Without gathering this information, the possibility exists for the APN to conduct an assessment on Millie without knowing what the potential problem or problems are. The information the staff provides is part of the history taking but does not imply that Millie is unable or unwilling to provide it. Frustration can lead anyone to perceive behavior in only one manner; therefore caution is warranted to not make conclusions about Millie's past behaviors and risk of noncompliance until your assessment is complete. *Answer 1:* **c.**

Case Study continued

Social History
Never married.
Lives alone, in back room of a tavern. Brother lives 5 minutes away and they see each other daily.
45-pack/year history of cigarette smoking; presently "down to" half a pack per day.
Regular alcohol use (daily beer intake).
Works as waitress in the tavern.
Occasional marijuana smoker 10 years ago.
Denies other substance abuse.

QUESTIONS

2. Before beginning to plan lifestyle changes for health promotion, what is the first factor that must be assessed ?
   a. Millie's understanding of the connection between cigarettes, alcohol, and head and neck cancers
   b. What financial resources are available to Millie
   c. Millie's satisfaction with her quality of life
   d. The brother's role and influence in Millie's life

ANSWERS

2. All of these points contribute to a thorough assessment and eventual plan of care, but the first thing to assess is Millie's comprehension of her disease. Because the cause of squamous cell cancer of the head and neck is most likely correlated to cigarette and alcohol abuse, no lifestyle changes can even be considered until Millie learns about the disease and the role her lifestyle may have had on the disease occurrence. *Answer 2:* **a.**

QUESTIONS

3. Once Millie understands the cause of squamous cell cancer, what concept needs to be explored as health-promotion plans are designed?
   a. Self-efficacy
   b. Self-value
   c. Self-determination
   d. Self-blame

ANSWERS

3. Self-efficacy, or the belief one holds about his or her abilities to change and incorporate health-promoting behaviors, plays an important role in the plan of care. Possibly in the exploration of this aspect, the nurse may encounter feelings of guilt, blame, and low self-esteem as the person struggles with beliefs of their abilities. *Answer 3:* **a.**

Case Study continued

Upon meeting Millie, you are struck by her tiny, almost emaciated and unkept appearance. Despite her size, she is quite loud in her speech and ideas. The meeting begins with hearing her story about the finding and diagnosis of the cancer for which she has had surgery. She noticed a bad odor in her mouth for some months and a sore along her gum that would not heal, but she did not think much of it, until bleeding from the sore became almost constant. She reports an uneventful medical health history, has no allergies, and has not seen a health care provider since visiting an emergency room 15 years ago for a sprained ankle, after slipping in the tavern.

She is not shy about her thoughts and shares her views that although the nurses have been nice to her while in the hospital, they just do not understand that she needs to get back to work because "unlike most women, she doesn't have someone to support her." She is aware that the doctors have told her she "needs" radiation therapy for her jaw and neck area, but she does not understand why because they also told her that they got "everything" when they operated. She expresses fears that her limited education causes her to be viewed as unintelligent and spoken down to. She worries that she is not being told everything. As you are talking, Millie is told over the intercom by the unit secretary that Dental Medicine is ready for her and transportation is on their way to take her in a wheelchair.

QUESTIONS

4. Because Millie is looking totally bewildered, what would your options be at this point?
   a. Explain the value of the dental consult to Millie and help her into the wheelchair for transportation.
   b. Cancel the dental appointment.
   c. Provide Millie with the next available appointment, the purpose of a dental consult, and allow her to make the decision.
   d. After explaining to her nurse what Millie has shared with you, together you discuss what to do about the impending dental appointment.

5. A dental assessment before head and neck radiotherapy, total body irradiation, or even prolonged chemotherapy is in anticipation and prophylaxis against which complication?
   a. Dental caries
   b. Osteoradionecrosis
   c. Trismus
   d. Xerostomia

6. In addition to the planned radiotherapy, what potential risk factors does Millie have for moderate to severe stomatitis? Choose all that apply.
   1. Oral intake less than body requirements
   2. Alcohol use
   3. Cigarette use
   4. A broken tooth

   a. 1 & 2
   b. 2 & 3
   c. 1, 2, & 3
   d. All of these

ANSWERS

4. Even though the APN is aware of the importance of a pretreatment dental consultation, patient autonomy is interfered with when a patriarchal or dominating approach is taken with patients. Millie should be the sole decision maker after being provided with all the necessary information to make an informed decision. Although it can be a great challenge to get patients into necessary appointments in a timely manner, postponing or going to an appointment needs to be in the patient's control. Otherwise, patients can allow others to take the responsibilities as well as the blame during times of crisis or critical points along the decision-making process. Explaining to Millie the value of a dental consult while the dental team waits for her places undue pressure on her and can result in her making a decision she really is not ready for. In addition, the APN was called in on the case as a consultant and not a direct caregiver. Any decisions that affect the patient while under the nurse's care should be in conjunction with the nurse. The best option would be to make Millie's nurse aware of all the facts, and then make a plan that includes Millie's wishes. *Answer 4:* **c.**

5. Dental carries can occur 3 to 12 months after oral irradiation and are considered a late effect of radiation therapy. Saliva contains electrolytes and a pH balance that protects against plaque formation and buffers the tooth enamel. Decreased saliva or xerostomia is characterized by a more acidic, thick mixture that promotes plaque, gingival inflammation, and gum recession. The lost buffering capacity can result in a demineralization of the tooth enamel and can lead to the formation of dental caries. A dental diagnostic evaluation with radiography and restorative therapy before radiation therapy is crucial for minimizing the chances of dental caries. Teeth that are unhealthy and that pose an added risk of infection during cancer treatment can be repaired or pulled. In addition, recommendations for the possible use of fluoride or saliva substitutes can be made at the time of the pretreatment dental consultation. Osteoradionecrosis is a result of radiation damage to the bones of the maxilla or mandible and occurs in approximately 20% of patients. Devascularization, fibrosis, and fatty degeneration of the bone occur, leaving the patient susceptible to infections and poor wound healing (Iwamoto, 1997). Patients with osteoradionecrosis present with persistent tooth or jaw pain and possibly nonhealing ulcers along the mucosa or gums. Trismus, also a late effect of radiation therapy to the head and neck, is tonic contractions of mastication muscles. It is seen more often in patients who have had surgery before radiotherapy, and the scar sites on the mastication muscles are the affected areas contracting. *Answer 5:* **a.**

6. Inadequate nutrition slows wound healing. Prolonged reepithelialization and healing of the mucous membranes can contribute to a prolonged episode of stomatitis. Alcohol and tobacco use contribute to the risk of dental caries, significant stomatitis, and osteoradionecrosis. A broken tooth can disrupt the integrity of the tongue, gums, or mucous membranes, establishing an environment for infection and contributing to the stomatitis experience. *Answer 6:* **d.**

References

American Society for Therapeutic Radiology and Oncology Consensus Panel. (1997). Consensus statement: Guidelines for PSA following radiation therapy. *Int J Radiat Oncol Bio Phys, 37,* pp. 1035-1041.

Anscher, M. S., Robertson, C. N., & Prosnitz, L. R. (1995). Adjuvant radiotherapy for pathologic stage T3/4 adenocarcinoma of the prostate: Ten-year update. *Int J Radiat Oncol Biol Phys, 33,* pp. 37-43.

Dunne-Daly, C. F. (1995). Skin and wound care in radiation oncology. *Can Nurs, 18,* pp. 144-162.

Gallagher, J. (1995). Management of cutaneous symptoms. *Semin Oncol Nurs, 11,* pp. 239-247.

Helgason, A., Fredrickson, M., Adolfsson, J., & Steinbeck, G. (1995). Decreased sexual capacity after external radiation therapy for prostate cancer impairs quality of life. *Int J Radiat Oncol Biol Phys, 32,* pp. 33-39.

Hilderley, L. J. (1997). Radiotherapy. In Groenwald, S. L., Frogge, M. H., Goodman, M., & Yarbro, C. H. (Eds.). *Cancer nursing principles and practice,* 4th ed (pp. 247-282). Boston: Jones and Bartlett.

Iwamoto, R. R. (1997). Cancers of the head and neck. In Dow, K. H., Bucholtz, J. D., Iwamoto, R., Fieler, V., & Hilderley, L. (Eds.). *Nursing care in radiation oncology,* 2nd ed (pp. 239-260). Philadelphia: WB Saunders.

Leasia, M. S., & Monahan, F. D. (1997). *A practical guide to health assessment.* Philadelphia: WB Saunders.

Litwin, M. S., Hays, R. O., Fink, A., et al. (1995). Quality of life outcomes in men treated for localized prostate cancer. *JAMA, 273,* pp. 129-135.

Pearson, L. J. (2000). *Nurse practitioner's drug handbook* (pp. 81-82). Springhouse, PA: Springhouse Publishing.

Roach, M., Chinn, D. M., Holland, J., & Clark, M. (1996). A pilot survey of sexual function and quality of life following 3D conformal radiotherapy for clinically localized prostate cancer. *Int J Radiat Oncol Biol Phys, 35,* pp. 869-874.

Shrader-Bogen, C. L., Kjellberg, J. L., McPherson, C. P., Murray, C. L. (1997). Quality of life and treatment outcomes: prostate carcinoma patients' perspectives after prostatectomy or radiation therapy. *Cancer, 79,* pp. 1979-1986.

Sitton, E. (1997). Managing side effects of skin changes and fatigue. In Dow, K. H., Bucholtz, J. D., Iwamoto, R., Fieler, V., & Hilderley, L. (Eds.). *Nursing care in radiation oncology,* 2nd ed (pp. 79-100). Philadelphia: WB Saunders.

Stempkowski, L. (2000). Hormonal therapy. In Held-Warmkessel, J. (Ed.). *Contemporary issues in prostate cancer. A nursing prospective* (pp. 170-194). Boston: Jones and Bartlett.

Takayama, T. K., Vessella, R. L., & Lange, P. H. (1994). Newer applications of serum prostate-specific antigen in the management of prostate cancer. *Semin Oncol, 21,* pp. 542-553.

Volpe, H. M. (2000). Radiation therapy. In Held-Warmkessel, J. (Ed.). *Contemporary issues in prostate cancer. A nursing prospective* (pp. 137-169). Boston: Jones and Bartlett.

Woodley, M. C., & Rubin, D. C. (1995). Gastroenterologic diseases. In Ewald, G. A., & McKenzie, C. R. (Eds.). *Manual of medical therapeutics,* 28th ed (pp. 336-363). New York: Little, Brown.

9 Biotherapy

Jeanne Erickson
Annette Wilkening Kuck

CASE 1 STUDY

Mary Johnson is 27 years old, is single, and attends graduate school for an advanced art degree. She is referred for treatment recommendations for newly diagnosed melanoma. After surgery for a right thigh lesion of 3 mm in thickness, lymph node resection revealed that three of five lymph nodes were positive for melanoma. With no evidence of metastatic disease, Ms. Johnson had stage III disease. She has recovered from surgery without complications, returning to her usual level of energy, activity, and weight.

Adjuvant therapy is recommended for Ms. Johnson. In discussing various treatment options, Ms. Johnson states that she is willing to tolerate significant side effects from the therapy that offers the best response. She agrees to begin outpatient treatment with interferon-a2b 20×10^6 U/m^2 intravenously five times weekly for 4 weeks, then 10×10^6 U/m^2 three times weekly for 48 weeks.

QUESTIONS

1. What factors contribute to the need for adjuvant therapy?
  1. Depth of invasion of primary lesion
  2. Presence of positive lymph nodes
  3. Patient age
  4. Number of primary lesions
  a. 1 & 2
  b. 1, 2, & 3
  c. 1, 2, & 4
  d. All of these

2. In explaining the rationale for the use of biotherapy as adjuvant treatment for melanoma, you explain that:
  1. Because melanoma is associated with spontaneous regressions, an immune mechanism is thought to be a significant factor in tumor growth.

2. Biotherapy is used to stimulate the person's own immune response against malignant cells.
3. Adjuvant chemotherapy has not shown a significant effect on disease-free survival for melanoma.
4. Melanoma can metastasize early, even with superficial lesions; therefore adjuvant therapy is recommended.
  a. 1 only
  b. 1, 2, & 4
  c. 1 & 3
  d. All of these

3. Interferon is a type of biotherapy classified as a:
  a. Monoclonal antibody, which will link to a specific antigen on the melanoma cell, causing cell lysis
  b. Cytokine, a protein molecule secreted by immune cells, which will regulate the immune response to destroy malignant cells
  c. Macrophage, which has phagocytic properties to digest malignant cells and activate lymphocytes to recognize other malignant cells
  d. Killer cell, which has direct cytotoxic activity against malignant cells

ANSWERS

1-2. Melanoma is associated with a high incidence of metastases and high mortality. Depth of invasion, presence of positive lymph nodes, and presence of distant metastases affect prognosis. The use of adjuvant chemotherapy has not been shown to improve disease-free survival, and melanoma is resistant to all but a few chemotherapy agents. Because melanoma is associated with spontaneous regressions, immune therapy and combined chemoimmunotherapy seem to hold the most promise (Atkins, 1997; Loescher & Ketcham,

1997). The 5-year survival with adjuvant interferon therapy was 46% (Kirkwood, Resnick, & Cole, 1997). *Answer 1:* **a.** *Answer 2:* **d.**

3. Interferons are classified as cytokines, soluble protein molecules secreted by T lymphocytes as part of the cell-mediated immune response. Cytokines are called the hormones of the immune system because they provide communication and coordination among a variety of diverse immune cells. During the immune response, cytokines act as signals between cells to stimulate growth, differentiation, and activation processes. Interleukins and hematopoietic growth factors are also cytokines (Wheeler, 1997). *Answer 3:* **b.**

QUESTIONS

4. Ms. Johnson completes the pretherapy assessment. Which of the following test results is a relative contraindication to beginning interferon therapy?
   a. MUGA scan with ejection fraction of 63%
   b. FEV_1 of 80% of predicted on pulmonary function tests (PFTs)
   c. Thyroid-stimulating hormone (TSH) of 20 μIU/ml
   d. White blood cell (WBC) count of $5.5 \times 10^3/mm^3$

ANSWERS

4. Patients should receive pretherapy assessment to diagnose any contraindications to interferon therapy. Interferon should be used with caution with patients who have cardiovascular, pulmonary, endocrine, and psychiatric diseases. In this pretreatment assessment, the results of the MUGA scan, PFTs, and WBC count are normal, but TSH is elevated, suggesting hypothyroidism (Pagana & Pagana, 2000). *Answer 4:* **c.**

Case Study continued

You teach Ms. Johnson that flulike side effects, including fever, chills, mild nausea, myalgias, and malaise, are common for most patients receiving biologic agents. Flulike symptoms are the predominant side effect of interferon therapy, but other organ toxicity may occur. Patients should be monitored for myelosuppression, hepatotoxicity, and central nervous system toxicity, such as depression and confusion. Gastrointestinal toxicity is dose related, causing anorexia, nausea, and weight loss. Cardiovascular side effects are uncommon with low-dose interferon (Rieger, 1999). Fevers related to interferon can be predicted and

successfully managed, and you review measures to manage fever related to interferon therapy.

QUESTIONS

5. With interferon, what is the pattern of fever expected to be?
   a. Onset of fever in 4 to 6 hours, duration of 24 hours
   b. Onset of fever in 12 hours, duration of 24 hours
   c. Onset of fever in 2 to 4 hours, duration of 4 to 8 hours
   d. Onset of fever in 24 hours, duration of 24 hours

6. Your written instructions to help Ms. Johnson manage fever related to the initiation of interferon therapy should include which of the following?
   a. Take acetaminophen 650 mg orally 1 hour before the first dose of interferon, then every 4 to 6 hours as needed to relieve fever
   b. Call whenever the fever is greater than 38° C because an evaluation for infection will need to be done
   c. Do not premedicate with acetaminophen; however, the medication can be used as needed for fevers after interferon administration
   d. Maintain fluid intake of 500 ml/day

7. Because you will be expecting Ms. Johnson to have a fever from the interferon, how will you tell her to monitor and report symptoms so that you can differentiate from an infectious etiology?

8. What pharmacologic and nonpharmacologic measures can you recommend to Ms. Johnson for relief of myalgias?

ANSWERS

5-6. Fever is common and expected with interferon, especially with the first doses. Fever usually begins 2 to 4 hours after injection and lasts up to 8 hours (Rieger, 1999). Premedication and subsequent doses of an antipyretic agent can block the pyrogenic activity of the cytokines on the hypothalamus and relieve the fever. *Answer 5:* **c.** *Answer 6:* **a.**

7. Distinguishing between an agent-associated fever and a fever caused by infection can be a challenge. Nurses should monitor for other signs and symptoms of infection, such as redness, swelling, tenderness, and drainage, as well as productive cough or painful, odorous urination. Patients can record a daily fever diary to identify fevers that occur outside the predictable pattern for interferon-related fever. Fevers that persist for more than 10 to 12 hours past a dose of interferon or a fever that is accompanied by hypotension would be suspect for an infectious etiology. *Answer 7:* **See text.**

8. If acetaminophen does not relieve the myalgias, nonsteroidal antiinflammatory drugs (NSAIDs) or narcotics may be tried. Nonpharmacologic measures, such as application of heat, relaxation, or distraction, may be helpful. Administration of the interferon injection closer to bedtime may improve tolerance to the flulike symptoms (Shelton & Turnbough, 1999; Viele & Moran, 1993). *Answer 8:* **See text.**

Case Study continued

Ms. Johnson completes the first 2 weeks of interferon therapy without complications. She tolerates moderate flulike symptoms with fevers up to 39° C. She manages her fatigue by "taking it easy" and has moved back in with her parents. Her blood counts and chemistry panel have remained within normal limits, her spirits are good, and she has experienced only mild nausea with a 3-pound weight loss in 2 weeks.

QUESTIONS

9. Ms. Johnson is thinking about having friends plan a visit at the end of these 4 weeks. She asks what the fevers and myalgias will be like then. Is it wise for her to plan this trip? Based on your knowledge and experience, what should you tell her?
- **a.** High fevers will probably continue for the first month of therapy.
- **b.** The fevers, chills, and myalgias will subside after 2 to 3 weeks of therapy.
- **c.** The fevers, chills, and myalgias will subside after 2 to 3 months of therapy.
- **d.** The flulike symptoms will occur unpredictably during the first few months of therapy.

ANSWERS

9. The development of tolerance to the acute flulike symptoms related to interferon usually develops within a few weeks of therapy. This phenomenon is called *tachyphylaxis.* It is likely that Mary will not have fevers, chills, and myalgias after 2 to 3 weeks of therapy (Shelton & Turnbough, 1999). A diary of fever curve and a record of the

severity of symptoms may be helpful to document the development of tolerance. *Answer 9:* **b.**

Case Study continued

During the fourth week of therapy, Ms. Johnson has elevated liver function tests; her alkaline phosphatase (ALT) is 80 IU/L, and her aspartate aminotransferase (AST) is 10 IU/L.

QUESTIONS

10. What liver function test (LFT)-associated symptoms, will you assess for?
- **1.** Nausea
- **2.** Indigestion
- **3.** Right upper quadrant pain
- **4.** Diarrhea
  - **a.** 1 & 2
  - **b.** 1, 2, & 3
  - **c.** 3 & 4
  - **d.** All of these

11. Which of the following abdominal examination findings suggests an enlarged liver?
- **a.** Interstitial retractions on inspection
- **b.** 6 cm of dullness on percussion over the liver
- **c.** Liver edge palpated 2 cm below right costal margin
- **d.** Decreased bowel sounds on auscultation

12. You consult with the physician regarding the treatment plan. Together you decide to:
- **a.** Continue on with treatment as planned
- **b.** Hold therapy and have Ms. Johnson return in 3 to 4 days for repeat LFTs
- **c.** Hold therapy and have Ms. Johnson return in 2 weeks for repeat LFTs
- **d.** Schedule a liver scan to evaluate for metastatic disease

ANSWERS

10. ALT and AST found in liver cells can be increased because of cancer, cirrhosis, viral hepatitis, and drug hepatotoxicity. Interferon can cause transient increases in LFTs, often with high dosages of the drug (Kirkwood, Resnick, & Cole, 1997). Therefore liver toxicity should be considered before imaging for liver metastases. Symptoms associated with elevated LFTs may include nausea, indigestion, and if the liver is enlarged, abdominal pain. *Answer 10:* **a.**

11. Physical findings that confirm an enlarged liver include palpation of a liver edge below the costal margin or percussion of a liver greater than 8 cm (Seidel, Ball, Dains, & Benedict, 1999). *Answer 11:* **c.**

12. Because the half-life of interferon is less than 10 hours, it is reasonable to recheck the LFTs again in 3 to 4 days (Rieger, 1999). The changes are reversible, and therapy may be resumed possibly at a lower dosage. If repeated hepatotoxicity occurs despite dosage delays and reductions, therapy may be discontinued. *Answer 12:* **b.**

Case Study continued

It is 7 days before Ms. Johnson's liver enzymes return within a normal range. Mary reports improved energy, appetite, and well-being while the interferon was held during this period, and she had her friends visit during this break in therapy. The interferon therapy will be resumed today at a decreased dosage.

QUESTIONS

13. What information is important to share with Ms. Johnson at today's visit?
  1. Flulike symptoms are likely to return because the therapy was stopped and restarted. Acetaminophen should be taken as previously scheduled at the start of therapy.
  2. She should still have a tolerance to the flulike symptoms.
  3. She should abstain from drinking beer and wine.
  4. She should not use any NSAIDs.
    a. 1 & 3
    b. 2 & 3
    c. 1, 3, & 4
    d. 2, 3, & 4

ANSWERS

13. Flulike symptoms do return when interferon therapy is stopped and restarted (Wheeler, 1997). Therefore Ms. Johnson should expect a fever today and plan measures to prevent and manage the other flulike symptoms. Mary should avoid excessive alcohol intake, which could contribute to hepatotoxicity, but she does not need to abstain from the use of NSAIDs because hepatotoxicity is not related to NSAID use (Shannon, Wilson, & Stang, 2000). *Answer 13:* **a.**

Case Study continued

During the sixth month of interferon therapy, Ms. Johnson registers to attend one class at school to resume work on her advanced art degree. After 3 weeks, however, she feels that the fatigue is

overwhelming and decides to take an incomplete. She feels bored and unproductive. She is tearful and discouraged during her monthly visit with you.

QUESTIONS

14. What potential contributing factors for the fatigue need to be evaluated?
  1. Sleep pattern and quality
  2. Nutritional and fluid status
  3. Hemoglobin and hematocrit values
  4. Quality and quantity of social activities
    a. 1 & 2
    b. 1, 3, & 4
    c. 1, 2, & 3
    d. All of these

15. Which of the following assessment data suggests a possible contributing cause of Mary's fatigue?
    a. High-normal mean corpuscular value (MCV)
    b. Albumin 3.4 g/dl, eating 2 meals a day
    c. Sleeping 7 hours at night, napping 2 hours in the afternoon
    d. Calling friends and planning weekly social outings

16. Which interventions might you suggest when you counsel Ms. Johnson?
  1. Suggesting adding an art project that would be a more relaxing, energy-restoring activity than going to class
  2. Identifying a physical exercise that Ms. Johnson could incorporate into her day
  3. Reassuring Ms. Johnson that most people receiving interferon will also develop a tolerance to fatigue and that she is likely to feel more energy, not less, as she continues therapy
  4. Suggesting that Ms. Johnson try to prioritize and limit involvement to necessary activities
    a. 1 & 2
    b. 1, 2, & 3
    c. 1, 2, & 4
    d. All of these

17. What are options for evaluating the success of your interventions to help Ms. Johnson manage her fatigue?

ANSWERS

14. Fatigue caused by biotherapy is likely to be more severe than that caused by other cancer treatments (Nail, 1997). Fatigue during interferon therapy is not likely to decrease over time but may persist and worsen (Wheeler, 1997). Other symptoms, such as sleep disturbances, poor nutrition, anemia, and depression, may contribute to fatigue (Winningham, 1999). *Answer 14:* **d.**

15. Mary's assessment reveals normal hematologic parameters, ruling out anemia as a contributing cause. Her albumin level, although slightly low, is insufficient to diagnose hypoproteinemia alone. Although she is eating only two meals a day, further analysis would be necessary to determine whether she is meeting her caloric requirements. Other nutritional parameters such as prealbumin, total iron-binding capacity (TIBC), and nitrogen balance need to be evaluated for a diagnosis of protein-calorie malnutrition. Because she is initiating and maintaining interest in social contacts, the presence of depression can probably be ruled out. Mary's 2-hour nap in the afternoon, however, may be contributing to her fatigue. Short naps (1 hour

or less) are recommended to promote rest, but longer naps may disrupt the quality and quantity of night-time sleep and result in more fatigue (Winningham, 1999). *Answer 15:* **c.**

16. Once other contributing factors are managed, your interventions should help Ms. Johnson maintain activities that are important to her and balance her activities with rest and relaxation (Winningham, et al., 1994). A manageable exercise program and activities that can relieve attentional deficit fatigue, such as art, music, and gardening, can be recommended as interventions for fatigue. *Answer 16:* **c.**

17. Strategies to evaluate the success of interventions to relieve fatigue may include a journal in which the patient records daily ratings of energy level, weekly measures of walking speed in a self-paced walking program, or daily records of hours slept or napped. *Answer 17:* **See text.**

CASE 2 STUDY

Matt Stanley is a 48-year-old store manager who recently underwent a surgical excision of a melanoma from his left chest. He had palpable lymphadenopathy in bilateral inguinal nodes, and a liver scan revealed two metastatic lesions. He has a good performance status and has complete healing after his surgery. He has agreed to receive combination chemotherapy and biotherapy with the following regimen:

- Cisplatin 200 mg/m^2 intravenously on day 1
- Interferon-a2b 10×10^6 U/m^2 intravenously every day for 5 days, beginning 6 hours after cisplatin
- Interleukin-2 18×10^6 U/m^2 intravenously over 6 hours on day 3, then
  - 18×10^6 U/m^2 intravenously over 12 hours, then
  - 18×10^6 U/m^2 intravenously over 24 hours, then
  - 1.13×10^6 U/m^2 intravenously over 24 hours for 3 days (days 5, 6, and 7)

This regimen is to be repeated every 4 weeks for two cycles; then Mr. Stanley's response should be evaluated.

QUESTIONS

1. On day 1, your assessment and interventions will be focused on the prevention and management of what acute toxicity?

1. Nephrotoxicity
2. Severe nausea and vomiting
3. Flulike symptoms
4. Cardiac dysfunction
5. Neurologic side effects
   a. 1, 2, & 3
   b. 1, 2, 4, & 5
   c. 2, 3, & 4
   d. All of these

2. Which of the following factors contributes to the risk of nephrotoxicity?
1. Concurrent use of aminoglycosides
2. Concurrent use of 5HT$_3$ antagonists
3. Preexisting cardiac disease
4. Preexisting renal disease
   a. 1 & 2
   b. 2, 3, & 4
   c. 2 & 4
   d. 1, 3, & 4

3. What other pharmacologic interventions should accompany the regimen on day 1 to prevent toxicity?
1. D$_5$1/2NS at 250 ml/hr
2. Furosemide 10 mg intravenously every 4 hours as needed to maintain urine output at more than 100 ml/hr
3. Mesna 1600-mg intravenous infusion over 24 hours

4. Ondansetron 24 mg orally before the cisplatin, then 8 mg orally every 8 hours for 24 hours
  a. 1 & 4
  b. 1, 2, & 3
  c. 2 & 4
  d. 1, 2, & 4

--- **ANSWERS**

1. On day 1, the patient will receive cisplatin and the first dose of interferon. The acute toxicity related to cisplatin includes nephrotoxicity and severe nausea and vomiting (Perry, Anderson, Door, & Wilkes, 1999 Wickham, 1999). Immediate side effects of interferon, also scheduled for day 1, are flulike symptoms. Neurologic and cardiac side effects may be delayed toxicities from interferon and are also associated with interleukin, scheduled for later in his therapy. *Answer 1:* **a.**

2. Concurrent use of aminoglycosides and preexisting renal disease would put the patient at a higher risk for nephrotoxicity. *Answer 2:* **d.**

3. To prevent nephrotoxicity, aggressive hydration and diuresis to maintain urine output at more than 100 ml/hr is recommended (Camp-Sorrell, 1997). Ondansetron is effective to prevent and manage the nausea related to cisplatin (Gandara, Roila, Warr, et al., 1998). *Answer 3:* **d.**

Case Study continued

During daily patient care rounds, the staff nurse indicates that Mr. Stanley is doing well on day 3 of his therapy except for a weight gain of 3 pounds in 24 hours and some mild pedal edema.

QUESTIONS

4. You suspect that Mr. Stanley is experiencing volume excess. What other assessment data could support your suspicion?
  1. Intake and output (I&O) records indicating intake exceeded output by 1200 ml in 24 hours
  2. Creatinine 1.3 mg/dl (1.0 yesterday), blood urea nitrogen (BUN) 28 mg/dl (23 yesterday)
  3. Rales on pulmonary examination
  4. Decreased pulse and blood pressure
    a. 1 & 3
    b. 2 & 4
    c. 1, 2, & 3
    d. All of these

5. You review Mr. Stanley's medication record to determine what additional medications might contribute to renal insufficiency. You identify the following medication with potential renal complications:
  a. Ibuprofen
  b. Loperamide hydrochloride
  c. Cimetidine
  d. Ondansetron

6. What interventions would be reasonable at this time to manage the fluid volume excess?
  1. Administration of furosemide 20 mg intravenously to encourage diuresis
  2. Administration of a fluid bolus of 500 ml of normal saline to increase urine output
  3. Discontinuation of the ibuprofen that he has been receiving to manage his myalgias
  4. Consideration of dialysis
    a. 1 & 3
    b. 2 & 4
    c. 1, 2, & 3
    d. All of these

--- **ANSWERS**

4. Renal toxicity in this protocol may be associated with the cisplatin that was administered on day 1 or the interleukin that began on day 3 (Caliendo, Joyce, & Altmiller, 1993). Patients with renal insufficiency may demonstrate signs and symptoms of fluid volume excess, such as peripheral and pulmonary edema, decreased urine output, and increased pulse and blood pressure. Laboratory values may demonstrate increased BUN and creatinine values (Camp-Sorrell, 1997). *Answer 4:* **c.**

5. Ibuprofen, an NSAID, may contribute to renal toxicity (Shannon, Wilson, & Stang, 2000). It should be discontinued and another analgesic substituted if necessary. *Answer 5:* **a.**

6. Additional fluids would not be warranted in a patient with renal insufficiency, and the insufficiency is not severe enough to warrant dialysis. It is reasonable to continue the interleukin at this time, promoting diuresis and observing for improvement once off the NSAID. Renal dysfunction is usually reversible once the interleukin is discontinued. *Answer 6:* **a.**

Case Study continued

On day 3, Mr. Stanley receives some oral premedications at 10:15, and he begins his interleukin infusion at 10:30. He vomits at 10:35. One hour later, his temperature rises to 39.6° C with slight chills. He feels nauseated. His pulse is 96 beats/min, and his blood pressure is 148/86 mm Hg, slightly above his baseline. His oxygen saturation is 96%. His nurse contacts you for guidance on assessing for capillary leak syndrome.

QUESTIONS

7. What physical finding on a pulmonary assessment is consistent with pulmonary edema related to capillary leak syndrome or volume excess?
- **a.** e to a changes at bases bilaterally
- **b.** Rales at bases bilaterally
- **c.** Localized wheezes in right lobe
- **d.** Decreased breath sounds in right base

8. Mr. Stanley has clear lung sounds and is not dyspneic. He is alert and oriented and has adequate urine output. He just complains of feeling hot and nauseated. Why is it appropriate to suggest administering a dose of acetaminophen with another antiemetic?
- **a.** The acetaminophen was probably not adequately absorbed.
- **b.** His liver is not yet compromised.
- **c.** An antipyretic could be effective to control his fever and nausea.
- **d.** He does not exhibit signs of acetaminophen toxicity.

9. What action would you take now?
- **a.** Recommend stopping the interleukin infusion until his symptoms are controlled and his vital signs return to baseline.
- **b.** Recommend the addition of dexamethasone to his antiemetic regimen.
- **c.** Recommend the addition of prochlorperazine.
- **d.** Recommend administration of a diuretic to prevent capillary leak syndrome.

ANSWERS

7. Flulike symptoms and capillary leak syndrome leading to pulmonary edema are potential complications of interleukin therapy (Sharp, 1993). Capillary leak syndrome may begin immediately after the administration of interleukin or at any time during the infusion and results from the extravasation of plasma proteins and fluid into extravascular space. As intravascular volume decreases, organ perfusion decreases, which can lead to organ dysfunction. Decreased blood pressure, renal insufficiency, edema, diarrhea, and weight gain may result (Caliendo, Joyce, & Altmiller, 1993; Reiger, 1999).

Pulmonary assessment should monitor for dyspnea, tachypnea, sputum production, cough, and breath sounds. Oxygen saturation, arterial blood

gases, and chest radiographs should be obtained as necessary. The pulmonary assessment finding consistent with pulmonary edema is bilateral rales in lung bases (Flick, 1988). *Answer 7:* **b.**

8-9. Mr. Stanley most likely spiked a fever because he did not absorb the acetaminophen. His fever is associated with uncontrolled flulike symptoms. His present condition does not warrant discontinuing the interleukin infusion, but close observation is warranted. Steroids are contraindicated during cytokine administration because steroids can alter the immune response and interfere with cytokine activity (Rieger, 1999). *Answer 8:* **a.** *Answer 9:* **c.**

Case Study continued

Mr. Stanley completed his treatment regimen and was discharged from the hospital on day 9, ambulatory, afebrile, and tolerating a regular diet. Five days later, however, you receive a call from Mr. Stanley. He has been unable to sleep more than 2 to 3 hours each night since his hospital discharge. He feels nervous and is unable to relax. He feels like he is "at the end of his rope," and he says, "This is too much for everyone. Maybe I should just stop this treatment and check out."

QUESTIONS

10. What are possible causes of Mr. Stanley's restlessness and insomnia 5 days after his chemobiotherapy?
- **a.** Hypercalcemia
- **b.** Hyperglycemia
- **c.** Steroid withdrawal
- **d.** Neurotoxicity

11. Mrs. Stanley calls you with her concerns that her husband talks about having "no hope." You make arrangements for Mr. Stanley to come to the clinic. What descriptions form Mrs. Stanley correlate with depression?
1. Weight gain
2. Weight loss
3. Agitation
4. Aggressive behavior
   - **a.** 1 & 3
   - **b.** 2 & 4
   - **c.** 1, 2, & 3
   - **d.** All of these

12. Mr. and Mrs. Stanley come to see you. Your assessment supports the diagnosis of depression, and you must assess his risk of harm to himself and others. Which of the following

behaviors suggests that Mr. Stanley requires protective steps against suicide?
   a. He has his daughter bring her children to visit him only once a week.
   b. His alcohol intake consists of three 6-ounce cocktails each night.
   c. He talks about dying but denies having a plan for his death.
   d. He is sleeping until 1 PM every day.

13. If Mr. Stanley is not a significant risk to himself or others, what is the most appropriate intervention?
   a. A trial of an antidepressant and anxiolytic is appropriate.
   b. Tolerance to this neurologic side effect does occur, and these symptoms will likely resolve within the next week. You suggest an anxiolytic.
   c. Depression is unlikely to be related to the interferon and interleukin 5 days after treatment. You refer him to a psychiatrist for evaluation.
   d. You encourage activity and socialization.

--- **ANSWERS**

10. Neurologic side effects, including sleep disturbances, depression, mood changes, and cognitive dysfunction, are possible with interferon and interleukin therapy (Kirkwood, Resnick, & Cole, 1997; Wheeler, 1997). Hypercalcemia and hyperglycemia are not likely to be problems following biotherapy, and steroids would be contraindicated for this patient receiving biotherapy. *Answer 10:* **d.**

11. Assessment findings significant for depression include significant weight loss or gain, sleep disturbances, psychomotor agitation or retardation, fatigue, feelings of worthlessness, diminished ability to concentrate, and recurrent thoughts of death or suicidal ideations (McDaniel, Musselman, Porter, et al., 1995; Much & Barsevick, 1997). *Answer 11:* **c.**

12. Assessment of suicidal risk is important in patients with depression. Preexisting psychopathology, an individual or family history of suicide, drug or alcohol use, severe physical symptoms, such as pain, and specific plans about death would raise an individual's risk of suicide. *Answer 12:* **b.**

13. Tolerance to neurotoxicity related to biotherapy does not occur. Antidepressants can be prescribed, but in some patients dosage reduction or discontinuation of therapy is necessary. Most of the neurologic side effects are reversible, although it may take months (Rieger, 1999). *Answer 13:* **a.**

CASE 3 STUDY

Teri Lee is a 55-year-old mother referred to your clinic with a recent diagnosis of metastatic melanoma. At her clinic visit today, you and the physician meet with Mrs. Lee and her husband to discuss treatment options, including her participation in a clinical trial.

QUESTIONS

1. During the discussion, the physician explains that Mrs. Lee is eligible to participate in a clinical trial comparing the effectiveness of two combination chemotherapy and biotherapy regimens. This is an example of what type of clinical trial?
   a. Phase I
   b. Phase II
   c. Phase III
   d. Phase IV

2. Mrs. Lee states she is interested in participating in the clinical trial. Which of the following elements are critical for you to include in the informed consent process?
   1. A discussion about appropriate alternative treatments besides the clinical trial, including the option for no treatment
   2. Reassurance that participation in the trial is voluntary and that the decision to participate will not jeopardize the quality of her care
   3. A description of how research findings will be presented and disseminated
   4. Identification of a time frame for which condition of patient confidentiality will be maintained
   a. 1 & 2
   b. 1, 2, & 4
   c. 2, 3, & 4
   d. All of these

--- **ANSWERS**

1. Many nurses participate in the care of patients receiving treatment in clinical research trials,

TABLE 9-1	Different Phases of Clinical Trials Conducted in the United States	
PHASE	PURPOSE	COMMENT
I	Determines maximum tolerated dose and describes pharmacology and pharmacokinetics in humans	Dosing starts at 10% of the LD_{10} in mice. Determine safe dose and schedule for phase II
II	Determines drug activity in specific tumors	Also determines administration schedule, toxicity, supportive care
III	New drug or drug combinations are compared against the standard therapy	Objective criteria: response rate, duration of response, survival, toxicity, and quality of life
IV	Role of drug in adjuvant/curative setting	Determines other uses, doses, schedules, and combination regimens

From Yarbro, C. H., Frogge, M. H., Goodman, M., & Groenwald, S. L. (2000). *Cancer nursing: Principles and practice,* 5th ed. Boston: Jones and Bartlett.

which help provide answers to questions about the best ways to prevent and treat cancer. Four sequential phases of clinical study are indicated when developing a new agent to provide information about the agent's toxicity, pharmacokinetics, and antitumor effectiveness (Table 9-1). *Answer 1:* **c.**

2. Nurses assume many roles in the clinical trials research process, such as data manager, patient recruiter, and patient educator. Nurses who assist with educating patients during the informed consent process need to be informed themselves about the essential components of informed consent. Box 9-1 lists eight elements of informed consent, as outlined by the National Cancer Institute. The treatment's risks and benefits and alternative treatments as well as issues related to confidentiality and compensation for injury must be included. Although patients may request information about research findings and study results, this information is not regarded as a critical element of the informed consent process. *Answer 2:* **b.**

Case Study continued

Mrs. Lee is admitted to the hospital for her first treatment with combination chemotherapy and biotherapy for stage IV melanoma. You review with her the chemotherapy protocol she will receive:

- Cisplatin 20 mg/m^2 intravenously over 30 minutes daily on days 1 to 4
- Vinblastine 1.2 mg/m^2 intravenously daily on days 1 to 4
- Dacarbazine 800 mg/m^2 intravenously over 1 hour on day 1 only

BOX 9-1	Eight Elements of Informed Consent

Study background
Risks and discomforts
Description of benefits
Alternative therapies
Confidentiality
Injury compensation
Contact referral
Voluntary participation/consent withdrawal

From Rosse, P. A., & Krebs, L. U. (1999). The nurse's role in the informed consent process. *Semin Oncol Nurs, 15*(2), pp. 116-123.

- Interleukin-2 9 MIU/m^2/day by central intravenous administration (CIV) on days 1 to 4 (96 hours)
- Interferon-a2b 5 MU/m^2 subcutaneously on days 1 to 5, 8, 10, and 12
- Granulocyte colony-stimulating factor (G-CSF) 5 µg/kg subcutaneously daily on days 7 to 16

Mrs. Lee begins her chemotherapy early on day 1. Six hours after beginning the interleukin infusion, the staff nurse calls you to see the patient. The patient's temperature is 38° C, pulse is 112 beats/min, respirations are 28 breaths/min, and blood pressure is 88/46 mm Hg. She has rigors and complains of mild dyspnea.

QUESTIONS

3. Which of the following physical findings is not associated with sepsis or complications of interleukin-2?
   a. Fever
   b. Hypotension

c. Distended neck veins

d. Dyspnea

4. All of the following interventions are appropriate measures at this time *except:*

   a. Obtaining blood and urine cultures and a chest radiograph

   b. Giving a 500-ml fluid bolus over 15 minutes

   c. Stopping the interleukin infusion

   d. Administering meperidine (Demerol) 25 mg intravenously to relieve the rigors

5. After your chosen interventions, Mrs. Lee remains hypotensive with a blood pressure of 80/46 mm Hg. You discuss possible treatment options with her nurse. What interventions do you choose now?

   1. Repeat a fluid bolus

   2. Begin dopamine infusion

   3. Prescribe a transfusion of 2 units of packed red blood cells (PRBCs)

   4. Consider antibiotic therapy

      a. 1 & 2

      b. 1, 2, & 4

      c. 2 & 4

      d. All of these

6. Twenty minutes later, Mrs. Lee's blood pressure remains 80/40 mm Hg. Her physical examination shows pulmonary rales, intake greater than output, and weight gain of 2.2 kg in 16 hours. She remains dyspneic, has no chest pain, and has no jugular venous distension. The most likely explanation for her continued hypotension is:

   a. Intravascular fluid volume excess

   b. Noncardiogenic edema

   c. Cardiogenic edema

   d. Pulmonary hemorrhage

7. What is your next step to relieve her hypotension?

   a. Start antibiotics

   b. Begin diuresis

   c. Increase the rate of the dopamine infusion

   d. Consider plasmapheresis

3. Hypotension may be caused by decreased vascular resistance and decreased vascular volume related to capillary leak syndrome. Patients may also be hypotensive from decreased fluid intake secondary to stomatitis and nausea and/or increased fluid losses secondary to diarrhea, emesis, and fevers. Infection must also be considered with fever and hypotension (Viele & Moran, 1993; Wheeler, 1997).

Flulike symptoms, including fever, chills, rigors, and headache are the most common side effects of interleukin therapy (Rieger, 1999). Fever is usually most severe after the first dose and occurs within 2 to 8 hours of administration. Distended jugular veins can be diagnostic of excess intravascular volume, not associated with either sepsis or interleukin toxicity. *Answer 3:* **c.**

4-5. An initial response to this patient's hypotension is to give fluid boluses to support intravascular volume. Vasopressors, such as dopamine, may be necessary to maintain adequate blood pressure. Interruption and dosage reduction of interleukin infusions may also be necessary in cases of persistent hypotension. Administration of meperidine to control the rigors, however, may complicate hypotension and is not recommended in the setting of decreased blood pressure (Caliendo, Joyce, & Altmiller, 1993; Sharp, 1993; Wheeler, 1997). *Answer 4:* **b.** *Answer 5:* **b.**

6-7. Fluid volume excess is a concern in a patient who demonstrates weight gain, fluid imbalance with intake greater than output, and pulmonary rales. The absence of jugular venous distension, however, suggests excess fluid is interstitial rather than intravascular. The use of diuretics to remove excess fluid at this time is not recommended because it may further contribute to depletion of intravascular volume. When fluid boluses are not effective at restoring blood pressure, increasing the dopamine infusion is a reasonable intervention. *Answer 6:* **b.** *Answer 7:* **c.**

CASE 4 STUDY

Sheryl Thomson is a 56-year-old woman receiving paclitaxel every 3 weeks for metastatic breast cancer. She has been receiving paclitaxel as second-line treatment for 11 months and shows no evidence of disease progression. However, she has become symptomatic from a hemoglobin ranging from 7.5 to 9 g/dl and a hematocrit ranging from 23% to 26%. Today you will discuss the evaluation and possible treatment for her anemia.

QUESTIONS

1. What symptoms of anemia is Ms. Thomson likely to describe?

2. What type of deficiency is the most likely cause of Ms. Thomson's anemia?
   a. Iron
   b. Folate
   c. B_{12}
   d. Chronic disease

3. Erythropoietin is most likely to benefit patients with which type of anemia?
   a. Iron deficiency anemia
   b. Folate deficiency anemia
   c. Myelosuppression
   d. Hemolytic anemia

4. What laboratory values would support a trial of erythropoietin in this patient?
   a. Low B_{12} levels
   b. Schistocytes on peripheral blood smear
   c. Low folate level
   d. Low reticulocyte count

5. Erythropoietin will be effective only if the patient has:
   a. Normal iron stores or receives replacement
   b. Normal renal function or is receiving dialysis therapy
   c. Normal liver function
   d. Normal vitamin D levels or receives replacement

6. In what time frame should you look for Ms. Thomson to respond to erythropoietin therapy?
   a. Hours
   b. Days
   c. Weeks
   d. Months

ANSWERS

1. Anemia is the most common hematologic abnormality in persons with cancer (Koeller, 1998).

Symptoms of anemia can include fatigue, shortness of breath, cold and exercise intolerance, anorexia, chest pain, headache, and inability to concentrate. In addition, patients may look pale and have tachycardia (Rieger & Haeuber, 1995). *Answer 1:* **See text.**

2. Anemia can result from multiple causes in the person with cancer, but bone marrow suppression from the disease and/or cancer treatment are the most common causes (Koeller, 1998). Iron deficiency anemia can result from blood loss, particularly in patients with known gastrointestinal tract malignancies and increased risk of bleeding. Anemia from nutritional deficiencies, such as folic acid deficiency or B_{12} (cobalamin) deficiency, may also be a factor. *Answer 2:* **d.**

3-4. Erythropoietin is a hematopoietic growth factor that stimulates red blood cell (RBC) precursors in the bone marrow to proliferate, differentiate, and mature. Erythropoietin is likely to benefit patients who demonstrate anemia from decreased production of RBCs secondary to cancer and cancer therapy, such as anemia of chronic disease and anemia related to myelosuppression. These anemias are evidenced by a low reticulocyte count, erythroid hypoplasia of the bone marrow, and decreased hemoglobin and hematocrit values (Koeller, 1998). *Answer 3:* **c.** *Answer 4:* **d.**

5. Before beginning erythropoietin therapy, it is important to treat other deficiencies that may contribute to anemia. The patient should have adequate iron stores or receive iron supplementation to support RBC production. *Answer 5:* **a.**

6. Patients respond to erythropoietin therapy first with an increase in reticulocyte count, followed by an increase in hematocrit. These increases may begin as early as 2 weeks but may take up to 4 weeks. If desirable increases in the hemoglobin and hematocrit values are not seen at 8 weeks, the dosage may be increased (Reiger, 1999). *Answer 6:* **c.**

CASE 5 STUDY

Ann Page is a 68-year-old white woman with a history of low-grade non-Hodgkin's lymphoma. She was originally diagnosed with bone marrow involvement (stage IV), presenting with back discomfort related to retroperitoneal lymphade-nopathy. After treatment with five cycles of 2-CDA, she had an excellent response to therapy but developed significant pancytopenia. A follow-up bone marrow biopsy showed minimal residual lymphoma and hypercellular marrow.

She has been followed in clinic and has been doing well for the last few years.

Ms. Page's visit today is prompted by increased back discomfort, similar to the pain she experienced at diagnosis. She has also had intermittent night sweats in recent months. Her appetite and weight have been stable. She has been treated with antiviral medications recently for herpes zoster of the left leg, associated with minimal cutaneous dissemination. Her physical examination is negative for adenopathy. A computed tomography (CT) scan of the chest, abdomen, and pelvis is completed, which reveals an increase in the size and number of retroperitoneal periaortic nodes. There is also minimal prominence of the mediastinal lymph nodes compared with her last CT scan.

On her visit, the oncologist discusses further treatment with rituximab, a monoclonal antibody.

QUESTIONS

1. You understand that this treatment decision is based on the following:
   1. Underlying diagnosis of B-cell low-grade non-Hodgkin's lymphoma
   2. An increased CD20 cell count at diagnosis
   3. Presence of night sweats
   4. Age
      a. 1 & 2
      b. 2 & 3
      c. 2 & 4
      d. 1, 2, & 3

ANSWERS

1. Rituximab is a genetically engineered chimeric human/murine monoclonal antibody. The antibody targets the CD20 antigen found on the surface of normal pre-B and B cells, including the malignant B cells found in B-cell non-Hodgkin's lymphoma. It may then induce antibody-dependent cell-mediated cytotoxicity and complement-dependent cytotoxicity (Rieger, 1999). Because the CD20 antigen is not found in the bone marrow, this mechanism of action does not cause significant myelosuppression. Because Ms. Page has continued problems with pancytopenia, this is an important consideration. The presence of CD20 antigen is determined during the diagnosis of non-Hodgkin's lymphoma. Rituximab targets the CD20 antigen, so it needs to be present for the treatment to be effective.

Ms. Page's increasing back pain, the radiologic

evidence of recurrence, and the recurrence of the night sweats suggest that treatment of her low-grade lymphoma is indicated at this time. *Answer 1:* **d.**

QUESTIONS

2. You plan to teach Ms. Page and her housemate about her proposed treatment with rituximab. Your discussion should include which of the following?
   1. A review of her current medications
   2. Her level of understanding about the treatment
   3. How the treatments will be scheduled
   4. Management of alopecia and increased infections
      a. 1 & 3
      b. 2 & 4
      c. 1, 2, & 3
      d. All of these

3. Following Ms. Page's review of the general chemotherapy booklets in the waiting area, all of the following statements demonstrate that she understands the side effects to report to her nurse *except:*
   a. "I need to tell the nurse if I feel chilled, feverish, or shaky."
   b. "I should report feeling sick to my stomach, stuffed up, or having diarrhea."
   c. "I need to call immediately if I have trouble breathing, feel flushed, or have a tickle in my throat."
   d. "This drug may cause numbness and tingling in my fingers and toes."

ANSWERS

2. When teaching about a new therapy, the patient needs information about how, when, and why the therapy will be administered. A review of current medications can identify potential drug interactions. Because rituximab is a prolonged infusion, patients need instructions on how to handle their routine medications. Because hypotension may occur during rituximab infusions, antihypertensive medications may be held 12 hours before therapy (Rieger, 1999). Medication review should also include a review of drug allergies and intolerances. Rituximab is contraindicated for patients with hypersensitivity or anaphylactic reactions to murine proteins or any component of the product. Sensitivities to acetaminophen and diphenhydramine may also alter the treatment plan because they are routinely used as premedications for rituximab.

It is important to determine Ms. Page's level of

understanding about her treatment before proceeding with teaching. A basic explanation of monoclonal antibody therapy helps patients differentiate this treatment from chemotherapy. Patients who are familiar with chemotherapy side effects, for example, can be reassured that myelosuppression and alopecia are not associated with rituximab. Because rituximab is given over several hours on a weekly basis for 4 consecutive weeks, the patient will need to make arrangements for travel. Patients are encouraged to bring snacks and diversions because the infusion is long. *Answer 2:* **c.**

3. Ms. Page needs to understand symptoms of infusion-related side effects and anaphylaxis. Symptoms such as chills, rigors, fevers (greater than 38° C), myalgias/arthralgias, urticaria, nausea, diarrhea, and mucosal congestion have been observed during the infusion of rituximab (Kosits & Callaghan, 2000). These symptoms need to be reported immediately to the nurse for immediate intervention. Because peripheral neuropathy is not associated with rituximab, statements about this side effect would not indicate effective teaching. *Answer 3:* **d.**

QUESTIONS

4. Ms. Page has a high circulating B-cell count. When initiating rituximab therapy, this finding puts her at high risk for which of the following complications?
- **a.** Syndrome of inappropriate antidiuretic hormone secretion (SIADH)
- **b.** Hypokalemia
- **c.** Disseminated intravascular coagulation
- **d.** Tumor lysis syndrome

5. What medication would be contraindicated for Ms. Page at this time?
- **a.** Hydrochlorothiazide
- **b.** Allopurinol
- **c.** Aldactone
- **d.** Leucovorin

ANSWERS

4. Because rituximab's mechanism of action is aimed at circulating B cells, patients with high B-cell counts may be at risk for electrolyte abnormalities from acute tumor lysis syndrome (Kosits & Callaghan, 2000). Tumor lysis syndrome is associated with hyperkalemia, hyperphosphatemia, and hypocalcemia. In addition, released nucleic acids are converted to uric acid. Acute renal failure can occur if uric acid or calcium phosphate crystallizes in the renal tubules. *Answer 4:* **d.**

5. Allopurinol is used to interfere with uric acid production and decrease the risk of tumor lysis syndrome. This medication should be initiated at least 12 hours before antitumor treatment (Camp-Sorrell, 1997). Thiazides are contraindicated when tumor lysis syndrome is likely because they acidify the urine, increasing the process of uric acid crystallization. *Answer 5:* **a.**

Case Study continued

Ms. Page returns to the office for her first dose of rituximab. Her assigned treatment nurse is relatively new and stops you in the hall to say, "I'm ready to begin Ms. Page's treatment, but I'm really nervous about giving this first dose." You discuss the orders for premedication and administration of rituximab with the nurse.

QUESTIONS

6. Which premedications are recommended before the administration of rituximab?
- **a.** Acetaminophen 650 mg orally and cimetidine 300 mg orally
- **b.** Acetaminophen 650 mg orally and diphenhydramine 50 mg intravenously
- **c.** Diphenhydramine 50 mg intravenously and ondansetron 16 mg intravenously
- **d.** Prochlorperazine 15 mg orally

7. Which of the following statements is true regarding the administration of the first dose of rituximab?
- **a.** Rituximab is given as a 12-hour infusion.
- **b.** Rituximab can be safely mixed with the premedications.
- **c.** Rituximab is infused slowly at 50 mg/hr with gradual rate escalations to a maximum rate of 400 mg/hr.
- **d.** Rituximab is infused slowly at 50 mg/hr with no rate escalations.

ANSWERS

6. The advanced practice nurse (APN) may recommend and help develop a rituximab infusion protocol as an educational and quality control tool for the staff. Routine premedication with acetaminophen and diphenhydramine is recommended to attenuate infusion-related symptoms (Kosits & Callaghan, 2000; Rieger, 1999). *Answer 6:* **b.**

7. A flulike infusion-related set of symptoms has been reported to occur predominantly within the first 3 hours of the first infusion. For this reason, the first dose of rituximab is started at 50 mg/hr and slowly escalated while assessing the patient every 15 minutes for the first hour and then every hour. Subsequent infusions may be started at 100 mg/hr and increased at 100-mg/hr increments every 30 minutes as tolerated, to a maximum of 400 mg/hr, if the patient tolerated the first infusion without difficulty. *Answer 7:* **c.**

Case Study continued

After reviewing the rituximab protocol with you, the nurse indicates that she feels more prepared to administer the rituximab treatment. You reassure her that you will stop by frequently during the infusion. Ms. Page tolerates the first 90 minutes of the infusion without difficulty and is currently receiving rituximab at a rate of 150 mg/hr. As you stop to speak with Ms. Page, she appears red in the face to you.

QUESTIONS

8. How do you differentiate between an infusion-related flulike side effect and anaphylaxis? What is your first response?

9. Ms. Page's symptoms appear to be flulike infusion-related symptoms, and with your interventions, her symptoms are controlled within 30 minutes. What is an appropriate intervention at this time?
- **a.** Restarting the infusion at the previous rate
- **b.** Restarting the infusion at half of the previous rate
- **c.** Discontinuing the infusion for the rest of the day
- **d.** Planning a hospital admission for more intensive monitoring for the remainder of her infusion

ANSWERS

8. Infusion-related side effects are most likely to occur within the first 3 hours of the first infusion and are generally mild to moderate. Anaphylactic reactions have not been reported with rituximab infusions, but patients should be assessed carefully for this complication (Kosits & Callaghan, 2000). Vital signs should be measured to assess for hypotension, fever, tachypnea, and bradycardia. Table 9-2 differentiates between the signs and symptoms associated with a flulike infusion-related reaction and anaphylaxis. *Answer 8:* **See Table 9-2 and text.**

9. For either an infusion-related side effect or anaphylaxis, your first response is to stop the infusion of rituximab immediately. Normal saline should be infused at a rate needed to support the

TABLE 9-2	Assessment of Flulike Symptoms versus Anaphylaxis		
SIGN/SYMPTOM	**RITUXIMAB**	**ANAPHYLAXIS**
Abdominal pain/ cramping	+	+
Bronchospasm	+	+
Chills	+	+
Hypotension	+	+
Nausea	+	+
Pruritus	+	+
Urticaria	+	+
Diarrhea	+	−
Fever	+	−
Mucosal congestion	+	−
Myalgia/arthralgia	+	−
Respiratory secretions	+	−
Anxiety/sense of impending doom	−	+
Cyanosis	−	+

patient's blood pressure, and additional medications may be given to relieve symptoms (e.g., diphenhydramine for a rash and repeated doses of acetaminophen for fever). Vital signs should be assessed every 5 minutes, and the patient should be placed in Trendelenburg position if significant hypotension develops.

Infusion-related side effects usually resolve within 30 minutes. Rituximab infusions may then be restarted at half the previous infusion rate. Side effects typically do not recur (Kosits & Callaghan, 2000). *Answer 9:* **b.**

Case Study continued

Ms. Page completes her course of rituximab infusions. Six weeks later, follow-up scans show regression of her lymph nodes.

QUESTIONS

10. What data would you monitor at her follow-up clinic visit and subsequent visits?
- **1.** Location and severity of back pain
- **2.** Skin rash
- **3.** Complete blood count with differential
- **4.** Uric acid level
  - **a.** 1 & 3
  - **b.** 2 & 4
  - **c.** 1, 2, & 3
  - **d.** All of these

ANSWERS

10. Your assessment on the follow-up examination needs to focus on areas of high risk and concern for Ms. Page. Because back discomfort was present at the time of recurrence, it is important to monitor for its presence. Skin assessment is also recommended because Ms. Page had an outbreak of herpes zoster. Although rituximab is not associated with significant hematologic side effects, Ms. Page has a history of pancytopenia, which needs to be monitored.

Serum uric acid level can be followed to assess for tumor lysis syndrome. However, tumor lysis syndrome is most likely to occur as treatment is initiated and usually responds to treatment and resolves within 7 to 10 days (Camp-Sorrell, 1997). Therefore assessment of uric acid levels 6 weeks after completion of rituximab therapy is not appropriate. *Answer 10:* **c.**

REFERENCES

Atkins, M. B. (1997). The treatment of metastatic melanoma with chemotherapy and biologics. *Curr Opin Oncol, 9,* pp. 205-213.

Caliendo, G., Joyce, D., & Altmiller, M. (1993). Nursing guidelines and discharge planning for patients receiving recombinant interleukin-2. *Semin Oncol Nurs, 9*(Suppl), pp. 25-31.

Camp-Sorrell, D. (1997). Chemotherapy: Toxicity management. In Groenwald, S. L., Frogge, M. H., Goodman, M., & Yarbro, C. H. (Eds.). *Cancer nursing: Principles and practice,* 4th ed. (pp. 385-425). Boston: Jones and Bartlett.

Flick, M. R. (1988). Pulmonary edema and acute lung injury. In Murray, J. F., & Nadel, J. A. (Eds.). *Textbook of respiratory medicine* (pp. 1359-1409). Philadelphia: Saunders.

Gandara, D. R., Roila, F., Warr, D., et al. (1998). Consensus proposal for 5HT3 antagonists in the prevention of acute emesis related to highly emetogenic chemotherapy. *Support Care Cancer, 6,* pp. 237-243.

Kirkwood, J. M., Resnick, G. D., & Cole, B. F. (1997). Efficacy, safety, and risk-benefit analysis of adjuvant interferon alfa-2b in melanoma. *Semin Oncol, 24*(Suppl 4), pp. 16-23.

Koeller, J. M. (1998). Clinical guidelines for the treatment of cancer-related anemia. *Pharmacotherapy, 18,* pp. 156-169.

Kosits, C., & Callaghan, M. (2000). Rituximab: A new monoclonal antibody therapy for non-Hodgkin's lymphoma. *Oncol Nurs Forum, 27*(1), pp. 51-59.

Loescher, L. J., & Ketcham, M. A. (1997). Skin cancers. In Groenwald, S. L., Frogge, M. H., Goodman, M., & Yarbro, C. H. (Eds.). *Cancer nursing: Principles and practice,* 4th ed. (pp. 1355-1373). Boston: Jones and Bartlett.

McDaniel, L. S., Musselman, D. L., Porter, M. R., et al. (1995). Depression in patients with cancer. *Arch Gen Psychiatry, 52,* pp. 89-99.

Much, J. K. & Barsevick, A. M. (1999). Depression. In Yarbro, C. H., Frogge, M. H., & Goodman, M. (Eds.). *Cancer symptom management,* 2nd ed. (pp. 594-617). Boston: Jones and Bartlett.

Nail, L. M. (1997). Fatigue. In Groenwald, S. L., Frogge, M. H., Goodman, M., & Yarbro, C. H. (Eds.). *Cancer nursing: Principles and practice,* 4th ed. (pp. 428-453). Boston: Jones and Bartlett.

Pagana, K. D., & Pagana, T. J. (2000). *Mosby's rapid reference to diagnostic & laboratory tests.* St. Louis: Mosby.

Perry, M. C., Anderson, C. M., Door, V. J., & Wilkes, J. D. (1999). *The chemotherapy sourcebook.* Baltimore: Williams & Wilkins.

Rieger, P. T. (1999). *Clinical handbook for biotherapy.* Boston: Jones and Bartlett.

Rieger, P. T., & Haeuber, D. (1995). A new approach to managing chemotherapy-related anemia: Nursing implications of epoetin alfa. *Oncol Nurs Forum, 22,* pp. 71-81.

Rosse, P. A., & Krebs, L. U. (1999). The nurse's role in the informed consent process. *Semin Oncol Nurs, 15*(2), pp. 116-123.

Seidel, H. M., Ball, J. W., Dains, J. E., & Benedict, G. W. (1999). *Mosby's guide to physical examination,* 4th ed. St. Louis: Mosby.

Shannon, M. T., Wilson, B. A., & Stang, C. L. (2000). *Health professionals drug guide 2000.* Stamford, CT: Appleton and Lange.

Sharp, E. (1993). Case management of the hospitalized patient receiving interleukin-2. *Semin Oncol Nurs, 9*(Suppl), pp. 14-19.

Shelton, B. K., & Turnbough, L. (1999). Flulike syndrome. In Yarbo, C. H., Frogge, M. H., & Goodman, M. (Eds.). *Cancer symptom management,* 2nd ed. (pp. 77-94). Boston: Jones and Bartlett.

Viele, C. S., & Moran, T. S. (1993). Nursing management of the nonhospitalized patient receiving recombinant interleukin-2. *Semin Oncol Nurs, 9*(Suppl), pp. 20-24.

Wheeler, V. S. (1997). Biotherapy. In Groenwald, S. L., Frogge, M. H., Goodman, M., & Yarbro, C. H. (Eds.). *Cancer nursing: Principles and practice,* 4th ed. (pp. 428-453). Boston: Jones and Bartlett.

Wickham, R. (1999). Nausea and vomiting. In Yarbro, C. H., Frogge, M. H., & Goodman, M. (Eds.). *Cancer symptom management,* 2nd ed. (pp. 228-253). Boston: Jones and Bartlett.

Winningham, M. L. (1999). Fatigue. In Yarbro, C. H., Frogge, M. H., & Goodman, M. (Eds.). *Cancer symptom management,* 2nd ed. (pp. 228-253). Boston: Jones and Bartlett.

Winningham, M. L., et al. (1994). Fatigue and the cancer experience: The state of the knowledge. *Oncol Nurs Forum, 21,* pp. 23-36.

CHAPTER

10 Hematopoietic Stem Cell Transplantation

Sandra A. Mitchell

Over the past 20 years, hematopoietic stem cell transplantation (HSCT) has evolved from an experimental treatment for patients with advanced acute leukemia, to being a therapeutically effective modality that is now standard therapy for selected diseases. HSCT permits treatment with intensive chemoradiotherapy, which is not possible without stem cell rescue; however, there can be significant complications, including toxicity from the conditioning regimen, complications that result from pancytopenia, immunologic complications in the case of allogeneic transplantation, and recurrent malignancy.

QUESTIONS

1. All of the following statements contain components of the rationale for HSCT *except:*

  a. Dose-intensive therapy may cure or offer quality life years for patients with selected malignant and hematologic diseases, with the antitumor effect thought to be proportional to the dose intensity.

  b. Hematopoietic cell transplantation offers a rescue to the patient from all of the dose-limiting toxicities of high-dose chemotherapy and radiation therapy used to destroy the tumor.

  c. Autologous transplants are mainly used to restore hematopoietic function in patients receiving high-dose chemotherapy, thus rescuing them from the lethal effects of the high-dose regimen.

  d. Allogeneic transplants offer the opportunity to replace abnormal or malignant hematopoietic or immune systems with normal hematologic and immune cells from a healthy donor. The associated allogeneic immune response between donor and recipient is also responsible for a beneficial antitumor effect.

ANSWERS

1. Transplantation is used to rescue the patient from the hematopoietic toxicity of the high-dose therapy; however, high-dose chemotherapy and radiation therapy have dose-limiting toxicities to the heart, lungs, kidney, and liver. These toxicities are responsible for some of the early and late complications experienced after the transplant. *Answer 1:* **b.**

QUESTIONS

2. Which of the following statements regarding sources of hematopoietic stem cells for transplantation is *incorrect*?

  a. The use of hematopoietic stem cells from sources other than marrow has resulted in the shift in terminology from *bone marrow transplantation* (BMT) to *stem cell transplantation* (SCT).

  b. Umbilical cord blood hematopoietic stem cells are an increasingly viable source of progenitor cells for transplantation.

  c. In the autologous transplant setting, bone marrow is used more than mobilized peripheral blood stem cells as the source of hematopoietic stem cells.

  d. Related allogeneic donors are preferred to unrelated donors because HLA matching is closer, with resultant lower incident of severe graft-versus-host disease (GVHD), and because they are more likely to be accessible for further donations of blood products and additional hematopoietic stem cells, if necessary.

ANSWERS

2. In both autologous and related allogeneic transplantation, peripheral blood stem cells have become the preferred source of hematopoietic stem cells for grafting. This is a result of the ease of harvesting, the ability to perform multiple collections, and the more rapid recovery of neutrophil and platelet counts seen in patients who receive grafts of peripheral blood stem cells rather than bone marrow (Wagner & Quinones, 1998). For autologous transplants, the additional advantages of using peripheral blood stem cells include the use of chemotherapy and growth factors for harvesting and the possibility of less tumor contamination in stem cells. *Answer 2:* **c.**

QUESTIONS

3. High-dose therapy with stem cell rescue is part of the standard consolidation or salvage treatment for which of the following malignancies?
   1. Multiple myeloma
   2. Acute leukemia
   3. Chronic leukemia
   4. Hodgkin's disease
   5. Non-Hodgkin's lymphoma
   6. Neuroblastoma
   7. Ewing's sarcoma
   8. Germ cell tumors
   9. Immunodeficiency diseases
   10. Ovarian cancer
   11. Metastatic breast cancer
      a. 2, 3, 4, 5, & 9
      b. All of these except 10 & 11
      c. All of these except 1, 8, 10, & 11
      d. All of these

ANSWERS

3. At present, the use of high-dose chemotherapy with SCT in the treatment of metastatic breast and ovarian tumors outside the context of large, controlled clinical trials is controversial (Williams & McCarthy, 2000). Further large, randomized trials comparing high-dose therapy with stem cell rescue versus the best available standard therapy for breast or ovarian cancer are urgently needed to define the role of high-dose therapy in these malignancies. *Answer 3:* **b.**

CASE I STUDY

Charles Jones is a 56-year-old man with chronic myelogenous leukemia (CML) in accelerated phase, initially treated with hydroxyurea. He is seen in consultation at your center regarding SCT. His medical history is significant for hypertension and type 2 diabetes. He is married and works as a supervisor in an accounting firm. He has two children, ages 26 and 30. He has two sisters. He is blood type A+, cytomegalovirus (CMV) positive.

> **Medications**
> Hydroxyurea 1 g orally daily
> Procardia XL 30 mg orally daily
> Glyburide 5 mg orally daily

QUESTIONS

1. In performing your initial assessment of Mr. Jones, which of the following components should have the greatest emphasis?
   a. Current laboratory data, including complete blood count (CBC) with differential, liver function tests (LFTs), and chemistries
   b. Detailed medical history, including childhood illnesses and usual weight and nutritional status
   c. Current disease status and history of patient's previous treatment, including total dosages and duration of therapy, prior transfusion history, and complications such as infections or hospitalizations
   d. Type of insurance coverage and psychosocial status

ANSWERS

1. Although all of the aforementioned elements may be important in the assessment of patient eligibility for transplantation, the most important elements are a determination of the patient's current disease status (in the case of a patient with CML, the CBC with differential and the bone marrow aspirate and biopsy, including cytogenetics and molecular diagnostics) and the history of the patient's previous treatment of the malignancy, including his disease response and associated complications. This information determines whether transplantation is indicated in this patient at this time in the natural history of the disease and whether it is the treatment of choice (Kapustay & Buchsel, 2000). The detailed medical history, nutritional assessment, and type of insurance and psychosocial status would be reviewed as the eligibility assessment process unfolds. *Answer 1:* **c.**

QUESTIONS

2. Possible sources of donor stem cells for Mr. Jones include any of the following *except:*
   a. Matched sibling
   b. Matched unrelated
   c. Syngeneic
   d. Autologous

2. All of these, except syngeneic, could be possible sources of stem cells for Mr. Jones. A syngeneic transplant involves the use of stem cells collected from an identical twin. Mr. Jones has no twin; therefore syngeneic transplant is not an option for him. Table 10-1 presents a comparison of autologous and allogeneic SCT. *Answer 2:* **c.**

Case Study *continued*

Mr. Jones has had a rather strained relationship with his sisters and is somewhat reluctant to approach them regarding serving as a donor. He asks whether it would simply be better to undergo unrelated SCT and avoid the need to use one of his sisters as a donor. You respond that that the donor of choice for an allogeneic transplant is currently an HLA-matched sibling.

QUESTIONS

3. What is the rationale for your response?
   a. Unrelated donor transplant is associated with increased risks of primary nonengraftment, graft rejection, GVHD, and rejection.
   b. The risk of developing infections such as

hepatitis in the posttransplant period is greater with unrelated donor transplants.
   c. Either autologous, related, or unrelated transplantation would be of equal effectiveness in this situation. The selection of a donor should be based on convenience, ease of access to the donor, and the patient's preferences for source of stem cells.
   d. The search for an unrelated donor will unnecessarily delay the patient from proceeding to transplant immediately.

3. Although the donor search and procurement process may take as long as 6 months, the primary rationale for the selection of an HLA-matched related donor is that unrelated donor transplant carries a greater risk of morbidity and procedure-related mortality (Gajewski & Champlin, 1998). The donor of choice for an allogeneic transplant in the treatment of selected hematologic malignancies, bone marrow failure syndromes, and congenital disorders of the hematopoietic system or inborn errors of metabolism is an HLA-identical, unaffected sibling. Autologous transplantation in the setting of CML in the accelerated phase cannot offer a cure but may extend survival and offer an

TABLE 10-1 Comparison of Autologous and Allogeneic Stem Cell Transplantation		
PARAMETER	**AUTOLOGOUS**	**ALLOGENEIC**
Indications	Hematologic malignancies and solid tumors; possible role in autoimmune disorders; future role in combination with gene therapy to treat genetic disorders, HIV, etc.	Hematologic malignancies, aplastic anemia, congenital bone marrow disorders, immune deficiency states, some inborn errors of metabolism
Source of stem cells	Autologous marrow or peripheral blood cells	Marrow, peripheral blood, cord blood, family donors, unrelated donors, HLA-matched or partially matched
Preparative regimen	Primarily designed to provide intensive myeloablative treatment to eradicate malignant disease	Required to provide immunosuppression to allow engraftment; intensive therapy for malignant disease; makes "space" for incoming stem cells
Posttransplant treatment	Supportive care, transfusions, growth factors, immune manipulation	Supportive care, transfusions, growth factors, immune manipulation, prophylaxis of GVHD
Infectious complication risk	Low—mainly in the early posttransplant period	High—sustained risk of infection for months or years
Major complications	Preparative regimen toxicity; disease recurrence/progression; treatment-related mortality usually <5%	Preparative regimen toxicity; disease recurrence/progression; GVHD; immune deficiency; treatment-related mortality 5%-35% depending on many patient, donor, and disease-related factors

From Treleaven, J., & Barrett, J. (1999). Introduction. In Barrett, J., & Treleaven, J. (Eds.). *The clinical practice of stem cell transplantation* (p. 6). Oxford: Isis Medical Media.
HIV, Human immunodeficiency virus; *GVHD*, graft-versus-host disease.

advantage over standard treatments, especially in patients not eligible for allogeneic transplantation because of their age, comorbidity, or the lack of availability of a related or unrelated hematopoietic cell donor (Cornish, Goulden, & Potter, 1998; Williams & McCarthy, 2000). *Answer 3:* **b.**

Case Study continued

Mr. Jones and his wife agree with his physician's recommendation that he consider allogeneic SCT.

QUESTIONS

4. Which of the following tests is Mr. Jones likely to undergo as part of his pretransplant eligibility evaluation?
   a. Two-dimensional echo, MUGA scan, dobutamine stress testing, pulmonary function tests (PFTs) with DLco
   b. 24-hour urine for creatinine clearance, MUGA scan, PFTs, and bone marrow aspirate and biopsy
   c. 24-hour urine for creatinine clearance, PFTs, cytogenetics for Philadelphia chromosome
   d. Psychologic evaluation, dobutamine stress

testing, electrocardiogram (ECG), infectious disease serologies

ANSWERS

4. Pretransplant eligibility testing is focused on the reevaluation of the disease process and the assessment of the functioning in major organ systems. Two-dimensional echocardiogram is a less sensitive measure of ejection fraction than MUGA scan, and dobutamine stress testing would be indicated only if the patient had a history of coronary artery disease, angina, or other symptomatology. The presence of the Philadelphia chromosome has already been established with the diagnosis of CML. Psychologic evaluation, although important to determining ways of supporting the patient through the transplant process, is not used to determine a patient's eligibility to proceed with transplantation. See Box 10-1. *Answer 4:* **b.**

QUESTIONS

5. In addition to an overview of the transplant process and a discussion of the preparative regimen and its immediate side effects, which

---

BOX **10-1**   **Pretransplant Evaluation of the Patient**

Pretreatment testing and evaluation of the patient undergoing hematopoietic stem cell transplantation includes the following:
- History of present illness, including presenting signs and symptoms, previous therapies, initial diagnosis, pathology and staging, complications, relapses or progressions, current disease status, transfusion history
- Medical history, including major illnesses, chronic illnesses, recurring illnesses, surgical history, childhood illnesses, and infectious disease exposure; for women, should also include menarche, onset of menopause or date of last menstrual period, pregnancies and outcomes
- Current medications
- Allergies
- Social and family history
- Performance status
- Current laboratory studies, including liver function tests, renal function, complete blood count
- Infectious disease serologies, including HIV, hepatitis B and C, cytomegalovirus, herpes simplex virus, HTLV-1, Epstein-Barr virus, toxoplasma titer, ABO and Rh typing

- HLA typing and DNA procurement for future engraftment studies (allogeneic transplant patients only)
- Chest radiograph
- Electrocardiogram
- MUGA scan
- Pulmonary function tests, including DLco
- 24-hour urine for creatinine clearance
- CT scans of chest and sinuses, if there are symptoms or a history of repeated infections
- Disease restaging, including CT scans, nuclear medicine scans, bone marrow aspirate and biopsy, cytogenetics, molecular diagnostics, and measures of minimal residual disease
- Dental evaluation, including full-mouth radiographs and cleaning
- Sperm/fertilized embryo banking
- Autologous stem cell backup if undergoing unrelated or mismatched transplantation
- Informed consent for treatment, transfusion support, clinical trials
- Nutritional evaluation, if appropriate
- Consultations with radiation therapy, infectious disease, pulmonary, cardiology, or renal services, if clinically indicated
- Financial screening
- Psychosocial evaluation

HIV, Human immunodeficiency virus; *HTLV,* human T-lymphotropic virus; *CT,* computed tomography.

of the following patient and family teaching points regarding HSCT is the highest priority to address with Mr. and Mrs. Jones in the initial teaching session?

a. Early and late complications, blood transfusion support, expected length of stay in hospital and the need to stay in close proximity of the treatment center discharge, usual process of recovery and rehabilitation

b. Infusion of peripheral blood stem cells and side effects, engraftment, common neutropenic infections, antibiotic support, blood transfusion support

c. Tissue typing, the names and side effects of commonly used medications, early complications of SCT, resources available for patient and family support

d. Signs and symptoms to report to the health care team; monitoring temperature, heart rate, respiratory rate, and blood pressure; central venous catheter care

ANSWERS

5. Although all of the topics listed are important for the patient and family to ultimately know, inclusion of all or most of these topics in the initial teaching session would be overwhelming. Furthermore, some of the information, such as central venous catheter care, names and side effects of commonly used medications, and precautions during periods of neutropenia and thrombocytopenia, is so detail-oriented that its inclusion would make it difficult for the patient to absorb information about the process, risks and benefits, and expected side effects of transplantation. In providing patient education about transplantation, it is important to take a longitudinal approach to ascertaining the priorities for learning and to take into account the information needs of the patient and family. The use of patient education checklists as a documentation tool will allow multiple providers to have input into the provision of education and helps ensure that all of the necessary points of patient education are ultimately provided. Written and audiovisual learning materials can be used to supplement and reinforce instruction provided in face-to-face sessions. *Answer 5:* **a.**

Case Study continued

A staff nurse approaches you with a concern that Mrs. Jones seems to ask so many questions of staff out in the hallway or by telephone to the nurse coordinator. However, when in face-to-face consultations with the patient, his wife, and the

physician team, neither Mr. nor Mrs. Jones asks very many questions. The clinic nurse expresses concern to you regarding the degree of informed consent this patient has for the upcoming treatment.

QUESTIONS

6. You can best help the staff nurse determine that informed consent has been obtained by:

a. Reviewing the chart together with the staff nurse to ascertain whether the consent form for transplant has been signed

b. Reviewing with the staff nurse what patient education has been provided during the informed consent process to determine whether the information provided was sufficiently comprehensive and detailed

c. Meeting together with the nurse and Mr. and Mrs. Jones to explore what they currently know about the proposed treatment, including risks, benefits, and alternatives; to determine additional learning needs; and to review his decision about consenting to the treatment

d. Reviewing with the staff nurse the principles underlying informed consent, including autonomy, self-determination, truth telling, and fidelity

ANSWERS

6. Informed consent is a process of shared decision making between the health care professional and the patient. Informed consent includes four components: (1) voluntary nature of consent; (2) thorough provision of information, including side effects, risks, benefits, and alternatives; (3) comprehension of information; and (4) competency of the person to make a decision (Ford, 1990).

Merely reviewing what information has been provided to the patient does not address the degree to which the patient has comprehended the information. In addition, there may be barriers to informed consent, such as communication difficulties; inadequate comprehension of the information presented; and lack of readiness to learn because of stress, pain, anxiety, or other factors. A signed consent form does not guarantee that the principles of informed consent have been met. Although written consent is required, its mere presence does not guarantee that the patient fully comprehends the implications of the chosen treatment.

It may be that either Mr. or Mrs. Jones feels somewhat intimidated or fearful when meeting with you or the physician team, or it may be that they have different information needs. Further exploration with Mrs. Jones of her perceptions and concerns could help elucidate her preference to discuss questions and issues separate from her husband.

Through this process, the staff nurse and the advanced practice nurse (APN) can assess the patient's comprehension of the information already provided and determine whether there is a need for information to be reviewed again or presented in a different manner, and evaluate any barriers to informed consent.

The issues of informed consent for SCT are similar to those of other technologically advanced therapies. However, because SCT is used in diseases that are incurable or fatal without transplant, the associated mortality of the treatment approach and the numerous long-term complications of the procedure (e.g., GVHD, pulmonary complications, infections) add a layer of complexity to the decision-making process for patients and families (Kletzel, Morgan, & Frader, 1998). In their quest for a cure, it may be difficult for patients to understand the ramifications of transplant-related morbidity and mortality (Kapustay & Buchsel, 2000), and patients or families may eventually come to feel that they never really had a sufficient appreciation of the physical or emotional burdens of SCT. The scientific complexity of the transplant process, our inability to make accurate predictions about the course and outcome of treatment in individual cases, and the narrow risk:benefit ratio add to the challenges of informed consent in SCT (Kletzel, Morgan, & Frader, 1998). In the final analysis, many patients or family members still feel an understandable human desire to attempt radical measures in desperate circumstances, even when they entirely understand the unpredictable nature of the outcome and the burdens inherent in the treatment. Our role is to ensure that the patient has been provided with complete and understandable information about the proposed treatment and that there has been no coercion that influences his or her subsequent decision about whether to undertake the treatment. *Answer 6:* **c.**

QUESTIONS

7. Both of Mr. Jones's sisters are identified as HLA matched. From the data given here, which of the two donors is most likely to be selected for Mr. Jones, who is blood type A+, CMV positive?
   a. Elizabeth, 43 years old, CMV negative, blood type O+, para 1, gravida 1, no comorbid health problems

   b. Elaine, 41 years old, CMV positive, blood type AB, para 0, gravida 0, no comorbid health problems

ANSWERS

7. Elaine would most likely be selected as the stem cell donor. If several sibling donors are available and are all equally good HLA matches, donors of the same sex, blood type, and CMV status as the patient are preferred. Donors who have never had blood product transfusions or been pregnant are also preferred. Comorbid health problems in the donor are also considered in the selection. Although Elaine is CMV positive, this is less important in donor selection given that Mr. Jones is CMV positive. The relevant factor here in donor selection is ABO mismatching. With type O+ blood, Elizabeth produces antibodies to A and B antigens. This may produce immediate as well as delayed hemolysis (Fox, 1998). Elaine, with blood type AB, would place the patient at minimal risk for either immediate or delayed hemolysis. See Box 10-2. *Answer 7:* **b.**

BOX **10-2** Evaluation of the Hematopoietic Stem Cell Donor

Pretreatment testing and evaluation of the hematopoietic stem cell donor usually includes the following:
- History and physical examination, noting history of serious or chronic illnesses, history of hematologic problems (including bleeding tendencies, cancer history, and transfusion history), current medications, allergies, and pregnancy history for females
- The presence of any risk factors for HIV or viral hepatitis infection are noted
- Physical examination for any abnormalities and an assessment of the adequacy of peripheral veins
- Complete blood count with differential, chemistries, liver and renal function tests, coagulation studies, ABO and Rh typing, pregnancy test
- Confirmatory HLA typing; DNA procurement for future engraftment studies (allogeneic donors only)
- Infectious disease serologies, including VDRL, HIV, hepatitis B and C, cytomegalovirus, herpes simplex virus, HTLV-1, Epstein-Barr virus, toxoplasma titer

HIV, Human immunodeficiency virus; *HTLV,* human T-lymphotropic virus.

QUESTIONS

8. Which of the following best explains the term *stem cell mobilization*?

  a. Mobilization is a process of stimulating the bone marrow, resulting in the proliferation of pluripotent stem cells in the marrow and their subsequent rapid release into the peripheral circulation.
  b. Mobilization is the collection of peripheral blood stem cells for subsequent transplantation.
  c. Mobilization is the method for stem cell procurement using commercial cell separators that are programmed to collect either lymphocytes or low-density leukocytes.
  d. Mobilization is the process of obtaining autologous bone marrow.

ANSWERS

8. Stem cells for subsequent transplantation may be collected from either the peripheral blood or directly from the bone marrow spaces. Peripheral blood stem cells are collected by mobilization and apheresis, whereas bone marrow is collected by bone marrow harvest, requiring direct aspiration of progenitor cells via multiple punctures of the posterior iliac crest. Mobilization is the process of stimulating the bone marrow, using either chemotherapy, cytokines (e.g., granulocyte colony-stimulating factor [G-CSF], granulocyte-macrophage colony-stimulating factor [GM-CSF]), or both to increase the numbers of progenitor cells in the peripheral circulation, resulting in a high yield of collected stem cells. Apheresis is the method of collecting stem cells from the peripheral blood, using commercial cells separators. *Answer 8:* **a.**

QUESTIONS

9. Elaine asks why she would be asked to donate peripheral blood stem cells rather than bone marrow. Your answer incorporates all of the following concepts regarding peripheral blood stem cells *except:*

  a. Engraftment of peripheral blood stem cells occurs at an accelerated rate compared with bone marrow.
  b. Use of peripheral blood stem cells decreases the discomfort and risks associated with bone marrow harvesting.
  c. Use of peripheral blood stem cells permits the collection of cells in an outpatient setting without the need for general anesthesia or inpatient hospitalization.

  d. Peripheral blood stem cells are less likely to be contaminated with tumor cells.

ANSWERS

9. Harvesting or collecting peripheral blood stem cells from healthy donors offers several advantages over bone marrow harvesting (Wagner & Quinones, 1998). Peripheral blood stem cells can be collected in an outpatient setting, without the need for general anesthesia or inpatient hospitalization. Peripheral blood stem cell collection methods decrease the risks associated with general anesthesia and avoid the discomfort of multiple punctures through the posterior iliac crests for bone marrow harvesting. Patients receiving peripheral blood stem cells have more rapid engraftment. This shorter duration of pancytopenia decreases the length of hospitalization, reduces the incidence of complications such as infection and hemorrhage, and reduces the need for prolonged transfusion support. Peripheral blood stem cells or bone marrow from a related sibling donor will not be contaminated with tumor cells. *Answer 9:* **d.**

QUESTIONS

10. Which of the following agents is Elaine most likely to receive to mobilize her peripheral blood stem cells before apheresis?

  a. GM-CSF
  b. G-CSF
  c. Cyclophosphamide
  d. Epogen

ANSWERS

10. The growth factor of choice for stem cell mobilization in the allogeneic donor is currently G-CSF (Russell & Miflin, 1998). As part of investigational protocols, other cytokines alone or in combination may also be used for allogeneic stem cell mobilization. Chemotherapy is never given to a healthy sibling donor, although it is used to mobilize stem cells in patients undergoing autologous transplantation. *Answer 10:* **b.**

QUESTIONS

11. In relation to the mobilization and collection of peripheral blood stem cells, which of the following aspects of teaching would not be provided to Elaine, who is an allogeneic donor?

  a. Self-care during periods of neutropenia and thrombocytopenia
  b. Reassurance that although no data on long-term effects of cytokines exist, few long-term adverse effects have been noted

c. Symptom management strategies for the side effects related to cytokine injections
d. Reassurance that the side effects of G-CSF are temporary and resolve within 1 to 2 days after discontinuing the cytokine

11. Allogeneic donors do not receive chemotherapy for mobilization of stem cells and thus would not be expected to develop neutropenia or thrombocytopenia. *Answer 11:* **a.**

CASE 2 STUDY

Jim Dunstan is a 19-year-old patient with relapsed Hodgkin's disease. He is undergoing stem cell mobilization with cyclophosphamide 3 g/m² and G-CSF 10 µg/kg/day.

QUESTIONS

1. A staff nurse new to the transplant area asks why Jim will be receiving chemotherapy and cytokine for stem cell mobilization while Elaine, her previous donor, was receiving only cytokine. Your response incorporates knowledge of which of the following concepts:

a. The chemotherapy agents used to mobilize stem cells for an autologous transplant contribute to decreasing tumor load.
b. Peripheral blood stem cells mobilized using chemotherapy and cytokines produce improved engraftment and more durable disease response.
c. Autologous peripheral blood stem cells are more efficiently and effectively mobilized into the peripheral bloodstream with chemotherapy and cytokine than with the use of cytokines alone.
d. With the combined use of chemotherapy and growth factors, the timing for release of progenitor cells into the peripheral blood is more predictable, with the result that the scheduling of stem cell collection is more precisely controlled.

ANSWERS

1. The use of chemotherapy and cytokine improves the likelihood of collecting an adequate number of progenitor cells to permit autologous transplantation and subsequent restoration of hematopoiesis (Walker, Roethke, & Martin, 1994). An additional advantage of using chemotherapy in the mobilization regimen is that it may further enhance tumor cytoreduction before the high-dose chemotherapy procedure itself. The advantages of using both chemotherapy and cytokine to mobilize stem cells into the peripheral blood is outweighed by the one disadvantage of using both chemotherapy and cytokine, namely that

with the use of chemotherapy and cytokine together, the timing of collection can be a little more difficult to predict, especially in heavily pretreated patients. *Answer 1:* **c.**

Case Study continued

In reviewing Jim's social history, you note that he is single and works full-time with a trucking company. He plans to continue working full-time if possible throughout his mobilization treatment so that he can have more time off from work during and following his transplant. In talking with Jim, he mentions that he feels somewhat overwhelmed with the treatment process and sheepishly admits that he sometimes misses appointments or does not follow through with recommendations. He lives more than 2 hours from the transplant center and comes to visits alone or with a buddy.

QUESTIONS

2. In assisting the staff to plan care for Jim, which of the following strategies can you implement with the staff to ensure coordination of care during the mobilization process?

a. Reduce the complexity of Jim's care by eliminating the need for laboratory draws until the day of stem cell collection
b. Instruct Jim to get in touch with his referring physician in his home community to see whether chemotherapy administration, office visits, and laboratory draws can be done at his office, which is located close to where Jim works
c. Reassure Jim that staff only expect him to do his best to adhere to the planned treatment schedule and that they understand he will need to make changes in his schedule of visits for laboratory and clinic evaluations to accommodate his work obligations
d. Develop a written calendar of events that must occur across the transplant process, including chemotherapy doses, dates for administration, dates to begin cyto-

kine, dates for laboratory draws, expected nadir, potential recovery, and potential dates for collection.

ANSWERS

2. Coordination of care during peripheral blood stem cell mobilization is critical to the ultimate success of the process. A written calendar of events helps explain the process to the patient and can serve as a valuable tool for coordinating the efforts and clarifying responsibilities of the transplant center, referring physician's office, home care staff, and the patient and family themselves. Blood work must be obtained at regular intervals to monitor the patient through the nadir of counts following chemotherapy and to coordinate the administration of transfusion support with platelets and packed red blood cells as required. The transplant center, the referring physician's clinic or office, or home care personnel can coordinate arrangements for the transfusion of irradiated blood products. Blood work at regular intervals also helps the transplant center identify the pace of white blood cell (WBC) count recovery. The initial recovery of the WBC count also indicates the point at which the transplant center should begin monitoring the number of peripheral blood progenitor cells, also known as *CD 34+ cells,* in the peripheral bloodstream. These blood tests are usually available only at laboratories capable of cellular immunology testing, which are usually located at larger hospitals or academic institutions. In addition, vascular access with a double-lumen apheresis catheter may need to be established immediately before stem cell collection, and this is usually inserted at the transplant center. For these reasons, patients who live a fair distance from the transplant center must be supported to make necessary arrangements for transportation and even overnight accommodations nearby the transplant center so that they can be nearby as their counts recover.

Communication with the referring physician and his or her office staff regarding patient care needs during the mobilization process can be invaluable to achieving the goal of keeping as much care as possible centralized in the patient's home community. However, the complexity of the process and the need for the transplant center to provide the overall coordination, with involvement of the referring physician and home care agency, dictates that the transplant center should initiate discussions with the referring physician regarding patient care needs and roles and responsibilities during the mobilization process. *Answer 2:* **d.**

QUESTIONS

3. Components of patient teaching provided to Jim include all of the following *except:*
  a. How to access 24-hour emergency care if needed for the development of complication
  b. The possible need for hospital admission for neutropenic fever secondary to chemotherapy administration and the need for the patient to be transferred to the transplant center for the imitation of apheresis when indicated
  c. The need to notify the health care team immediately in the event of catheter occlusion or development of fever; chills; bleeding; or tenderness, discharge, or induration at the central venous catheter exit site
  d. The scheduled day for stem cell collection to occur after the administration of mobilizing chemotherapy and cytokine

---

ANSWERS

3. When mobilization of peripheral blood stem cells is attempted with chemotherapy and cytokine, the timing of apheresis is determined by the recovery of blood counts rather than a scheduled day after administration of the mobilizing agent. Patients must be monitored closely by either the recovery of the WBC count following myelosuppression and/or by the measurement of peripheral blood CD 34+ cell count. Patient teaching must include the importance of frequent blood tests to determine the nadir following chemotherapy and to monitor the pace of WBC recovery so that the timing of collection is optimized. Self-care requirements during periods of neutropenia and thrombocytopenia and the need to notify the health care team immediately should signs or symptoms of bleeding or infection develop should also be reviewed (Burns, Tierney, Long, et al., 1995). *Answer 3:* **d.**

QUESTIONS

4. Preparation of the autologous or allogeneic donor to undergo apheresis for the collection of peripheral blood stem cells includes all of the following *except:*
  a. Avoidance of dairy products and calcium supplements for 3 weeks before apheresis
  b. Sensory expectations during the apheresis procedure, including timing and duration
  c. Explanations that hypovolemia may occur during collection, resulting in lightheadedness, vertigo, and hypotension

d. Avoidance of large amounts of fluid immediately before apheresis to reduce the need for the patient to urinate during procedure

---
ANSWERS

4. Donors should be instructed to increase their calcium intake (e.g., dairy products, calcium supplement, calcium-based antacids) 2 to 3 days before apheresis and through the completion of apheresis. This intervention may minimize the hypocalcemia that can occur as a result of the anticoagulant citrate dextrose (ACD) used to prevent the blood from clotting in the apheresis machine during the collection procedure. *Answer 4:* **a.**

QUESTIONS

5. Which of the following are possible side effects of the apheresis process?
   1. Thrombocytopenia
   2. Anemia
   3. Hypovolemia
   4. Bleeding
      a. 1, 2, & 3
      b. 3 only
      c. None of these
      d. All of these

ANSWERS

5. Thrombocytopenia and anemia can occur when there is inadvertent removal of platelets and red blood cells during the apheresis process. Hypovolemia can occur as a result of fluctuations in the circulating blood volume during apheresis. The citrate used as an anticoagulant during the processing of blood in the course of apheresis can result in minor bleeding, especially if the patient is severely thrombocytopenic. *Answer 5:* **d.**

QUESTIONS

6. Which of the following are principles of designing a regimen for transplant conditioning chemotherapy?
   1. High-dose treatment is based on the hypothesis that increasing the dose or dose rate will increase tumor cell kills, resulting in improved response and survival rates.
   2. High-dose regimens often use multiple agents, and the sequence of the drugs may be important with respect to pharmacokinetic and pharmacodynamic interactions and both toxicity and cell kill.
   3. Drugs with different nonhematologic dose-limiting toxicities should be combined in maximal doses.
   4. Treatment of early-stage disease will lessen the likelihood of developing either biochemical or physical resistance to therapy.
      a. 1, 2, & 3
      b. 1 & 3
      c. 1, 2, & 4
      d. All of these

ANSWERS

6. All of these are principles applied in selecting the composition, dose, and schedule of high-dose conditioning regimens (Petros & Gilbert, 1998; Rees, Beale, & Judson, 1998). *Answer 6:* **d.**

CASE 3 STUDY

David Hartman is receiving high-dose conditioning therapy consisting of total body irradiation 1125 cGy and cyclophosphamide 60 mg/kg for 2 days. His antiemetic regimen consists of the following:

- Dexamethasone 40 mg/day orally
- Kytril 1 mg/day intravenously
- Compazine 10 mg orally or intravenously every 4 hours as needed for nausea
- Ativan 1 mg orally or intravenously every 4 hours as needed for nausea

QUESTIONS

1. Which of the following side effects would you *least* expect to see in David with this regimen?
   a. Parotitis
   b. ECG abnormalities
   c. Fever
   d. Hypoglycemia

ANSWERS

1. Hypoglycemia is unlikely to occur in a patient who is receiving steroids. Parotitis and fever can occur as a result of the total body irradiation, although usually the steroids administered as antiemetics will also assist with the management of these symptoms. ECG abnormalities, including sinus tachycardia and arrhythmias, can occur in association with the administration of high-dose cyclophosphamide. The common adverse effects of individual agents commonly used in combination as part of the transplant conditioning regimen are depicted in Table 10-2. *Answer 1:* **d.**

TABLE **10-2** Nonhematologic Adverse Effects of High-Dose Therapy Regimens

AGENT	ADVERSE EFFECTS
Busulfan	Interstitial pulmonary fibrosis, hepatic dysfunction (including venoocclusive disease), acute cholecystitis, generalized seizures, mucositis, skin (hyperpigmentation, desquamation, acral erythema), nausea and vomiting
Carmustine (BCNU)	Hepatic, pulmonary, central nervous system, cardiac (arrhythmias, hypotension), nausea and vomiting
Cytosine arabinoside (Ara-C)	Cerebellar toxicity, encephalopathy, seizures, conjunctivitis, skin (rash, acral erythema), nausea and vomiting, diarrhea, renal insufficiency, liver function abnormalities, pancreatitis, noncardiogenic pulmonary edema, fever, arthralgias
Cyclophosphamide	Cardiac (cardiomyopathy, congestive heart failure, hemorrhagic cardiac necrosis, pericardial effusion, electrocardiographic abnormalities), interstitial pulmonary fibrosis, hemorrhagic cystitis, elevation in liver enzymes, nausea and vomiting, metabolic (syndrome of inappropriate antidiuretic hormone secretion)
Carboplatin	Nausea and vomiting, nephrotoxicity, liver function abnormalities (including venoocclusive disease), ototoxicity
Cisplatinum	Nausea and vomiting, neurotoxicity (peripheral neuropathy, ataxia, visual disturbances), ototoxicity, renal
Etoposide	Hypersensitivity reactions, hypotension, liver function abnormalities and chemical hepatitis, renal dysfunction, nausea and vomiting, metabolic (metabolic acidosis), mucositis, stomatitis; painful skin rash on the palms, soles, and periorbital area
Ifosfamide	Hemorrhagic cystitis
Melphalan	Acute hypersensitivity, renal, mucositis, nausea and vomiting, hepatic toxicity (including venoocclusive disease)
Thiotepa	Hyperpigmentation, acute erythroderma, dry desquamation, liver function abnormalities (including venoocclusive disease), mucositis, esophagitis, dysuria, hypersensitivity reactions
Total body irradiation	Nausea, vomiting, diarrhea, parotitis, xerostomia, stomatitis, erythema, pneumonitis, venoocclusive disease

Based on information from Chan (2000); Gupta-Burt & Okunieff (1998); Petros & Gilbert (1998); Rees, Beale, & Judson (1998); and Solimando, 1998.

QUESTIONS

2. David is scheduled to receive his allogeneic peripheral blood SCT. In precepting a new staff nurse providing care to David on day 0, you will include which of the following concepts?

  a. Stem cell infusion should be performed using an intravenous infusion pump to ensure a precise rate of administration; only normal saline is infused to prime and flush the tubing for stem cell administration.

  b. Complications of allogeneic stem cell infusion can include pulmonary edema, hemolysis, infection, and anaphylaxis.

  c. David should be informed that he may experience a garlicky odor or taste during and immediately after stem cell infusion.

  d. Vital signs and cardiac monitoring are required every hour after the stem cell infusion.

ANSWERS

2. Stem cells are a blood product and can precipitate reactions like any other transfusion product. Complications of allogeneic stem cell infusion can include pulmonary edema, hemolysis, infection, and anaphylaxis, although these are rare. Premedication with Tylenol and Benadryl is usually recommended, as is monitoring of vital signs and pulse oximetry before, during, and at intervals after stem cell infusion. Cardiac monitoring is often unnecessary. Normal saline is used to prime and flush the tubing for stem cell administration, but an intravenous infusion pump should never be used to administer stem cells. The garlicky odor or taste is created by the excretion in the breath of dimethylsufoxide (DMSO), the cryoprotective agent used in freezing autologous stem cells. David is receiving allogeneic stem cells, and these are not frozen; rather, they are administered immediately after collection and processing. *Answer 2:* **b.**

Case Study continued

David is day +2, status post allogeneic transplant after conditioning with total body irradiation, thiotepa, and cyclophosphamide. His CBC reveals a WBC count of 0.1%, a hemoglobulin (Hgb) of

8.2 g/dl, a hematocrit (Hct) of 24.6%, and platelets of 17,000/mm^3. His sodium is 126 mEq/L; potassium, 3.0 mEq/L; chloride, 98 mEq/L; CO_2, 18 mEq/L; blood urea nitrogen (BUN), 11 mg/dl; and creatinine, 0.6 mg/dl. His vital signs are temperature, 36.7° C; pulse, 100 beats/min; respirations, 22 breaths/min; and blood pressure, 108/55 mm Hg. The 24-hour fluid balance shows intake of 5600 and output of 2105. He is complaining of nausea, vomiting, diarrhea, and abdominal pain.

QUESTIONS

3. Based on your knowledge of the conditioning regimen and the preceding data, which of the following physical findings would be most likely on physical examination?
   a. Rales, peripheral edema, jugular venous distension
   b. Firm abdomen with absent bowel sounds and rebound tenderness, cardiac gallop (S$_3$), skin rash
   c. Skin pallor, rales, and peripheral edema, tenderness of the right upper quadrant
   d. Erythema or shallow ulcerations of the oral cavity, weakness, erythema of the skin, conjunctival pallor, petechial skin rash

4. In addition to pancytopenia and gastrointestinal (GI) toxicity, David demonstrates which of the following acute complications of high-dose therapy?
   a. Syndrome of inappropriate antidiuretic hormone secretion (SIADH)
   b. Venoocclusive disease of the liver
   c. Renal insufficiency
   d. Sepsis

ANSWERS

3-4. On day +2 following an allogeneic transplant, after conditioning with total body irradiation and cyclophosphamide, one would expect physical findings consistent with pancytopenia, including petechiae and pallor of the skin and mucous membranes. Erythema or shallow ulcerations of the oral cavity might also be present. Total body irradiation causes a generalized erythema of the skin. The patient has an intake greater than output for a 24-hour period, with an extremely low sodium level. The decreased urine output and hyponatremia suggest SIADH, probably as a result of high-dose cyclophosphamide. Additional studies should include a high urine osmolality and decreased serum osmolality. Congestive heart

failure (CHF) or renal failure are therefore unlikely causes for the decreased urine output; thus signs of CHF, such as rales, peripheral edema, jugular venous distension, and an S$_3$, would not be expected. There is no evidence of sepsis such as fever or mental status changes. Although the urine output is reduced, there is no evidence of renal insufficiency because the BUN and creatinine are within normal limits. Right upper quadrant tenderness suggests venoocclusive disease of the liver. Although David is at risk for venoocclusive disease of the liver at this stage posttransplant and the positive 24-hour fluid balance suggests weight gain, without LFTs, an assessment of the abdomen that demonstrates hepatomegaly or ascites, not right upper quadrant tenderness alone, and an abdominal ultrasound, it is unclear whether this patient is developing venoocclusive disease. *Answer 3:* **d**. *Answer 4:* **a**.

QUESTIONS

5. Which of the following statements about the development of hyponatremia in the patient with SIADH is correct?
   a. Hyponatremia develops because the amount of antidiuretic hormone (ADH) present in the body results in renal sodium wasting.
   b. Hyponatremia is unusual unless sodium is restricted in the diet.
   c. Hyponatremia results from an increase in total body water and sodium, the amount of water retained being greater than the amount of sodium.
   d. Hyponatremia occurs because water reabsorption by the kidney is increased, resulting in a decreased serum sodium and reduced plasma osmolality.

ANSWERS

5. The normal function of ADH is to promote reabsorption of water from the distal tubule of the kidney. SIADH occurs because there is increased secretion of ADH from the posterior pituitary gland, resulting in increased water retention by the kidney, increased total body water, and moderate expansion of plasma volume. The syndrome is characterized by weight gain, decreased urinary output with high urine osmolality, and decreased serum osmolality with low serum sodium (Singer, 1998). Sodium excretion, retention, and ingestion are not related to the action of ADH or SIADH. Chemotherapy agents associated with hyponatremia include high-dose cyclophosphamide, ifosfamide, and vincristine (Carlson & Casciato, 1995). *Answer 5:* **d**.

QUESTIONS

6. All of the following are treatments for SIADH *except:*

    a. D$_5$W at 100 ml/hr

    b. Oral fluid restriction and concentration of all intravenous medications in minimal volumes

    c. Demeclocycline 200 mg orally three times daily

    d. Hypertonic saline followed by furosemide

ANSWERS

6. The cornerstones of treatment for SIADH are restriction of free water in the intravenous fluids (avoidance of D$_5$W), oral fluid restriction, and concentration of all intravenous medications in minimal volumes (Carlson & Casciato, 1995). The treatment of SIADH is determined by the rate of development of hyponatremia and by the presence of neurologic sequelae. If feasible, fluid restriction to 800 to 1000 ml/24 hr is effective in slowly raising serum osmolality over 3 to 5 days. Demeclocycline induces renal resistance to ADH and facilitates free water excretion. It is given at a dosage of 150 to 300 mg orally three times daily; it is nephrotoxic with chronic use. If neurologic symptoms of hyponatremia (confusion, seizures, or coma) are present or if the serum sodium declines to less than 110 mEq/L, intravenous administration of 3% saline at a rate of 1000 ml every 8 hours, along with furosemide 40 to 80 mg intravenously, may be necessary (Carlson & Casciato, 1995). *Answer 6:* **a.**

QUESTIONS

7. You are paged later in the day by the nurse who reports the onset of fever, tachycardia, and tea-colored urine. Based on this report, you anticipate which of the following laboratory studies to be ordered for this patient?

    a. Urinalysis with microscopic examination, blood cultures, urine cultures, chest radiograph, CBC, and prothrombin time (PT), partial thromboplastin time (PTT), fibrinogen and International Normalized Ratio (INR)

    b. Urinalysis with microscopic examination, urine cultures, PT, PTT, and INR

    c. Blood cultures; surveillance cultures of throat, nose, and stool; and chest radiograph

    d. Blood cultures, urine cultures, chest radiograph, cross, and type

8. Your differential diagnoses for the hematuria include which of the following?

    a. Hemolysis secondary to transplantation, nephrolithiasis, urinary tract infection

    b. Hemorrhagic cystitis, coagulopathy, renal failure, malignancy

    c. Hemorrhagic cystitis, coagulopathy, urinary tract infection

    d. Hemolysis, urethral trauma, coagulopathy

ANSWERS

7. In further assessing the preceding signs and symptoms, it is important to recognize that the fever may or may not be related to the development of the hematuria and that it may in fact represent a separate process of neutropenic fever. The fever requires evaluation in and of itself with cultures of blood and urine and a surveillance chest radiograph. A CBC should be obtained both to gauge the degree of blood loss with resultant anemia and to determine the severity of thrombocytopenia. Coagulation studies with a PT, PTT, INR, and fibrinogen level will help gauge whether a coagulopathy is present. *Answer 7:* **a.**

8. The most likely differential diagnoses for the hematuria include hemorrhagic cystitis, coagulopathy, and urinary tract infection. Hemolysis is unlikely because it would be manifested as free hemoglobin in the urine rather than frank hematuria. Hemolysis is also unlikely because the patient received his transplant from an ABO-matched donor. Malignancy is unlikely in this scenario. *Answer 28:* **c.**

Case Study continued

David becomes progressively more oliguric and reports increasing abdominal pain. On examination he has suprapubic tenderness and costovertebral angle (CVA) tenderness. His urine remains tea-colored, and he is passing small clots. His coagulation studies reveal a PT of 16.1 seconds, PTT of 34 seconds, INR of 1.5, and fibrinogen of 344 mg/dl.

QUESTIONS

9. You would anticipate orders for:

    a. Vitamin K 10 mEq subcutaneously or intravenously daily for 3 days

    b. 1 unit of single-donor platelets

    c. Desmopressin 25 µg intravenously

    d. Cryoprecipitate

    e. 6 units of fresh frozen plasma

ANSWERS

9. Vitamin K replacement is appropriate treatment of David's prolonged PT. Cephalosporin antibiotics can interfere with vitamin K synthesis, as can prolonged periods of malnutrition, malabsorption states, and liver dysfunction (Graubert, 1998). Desmopressin works to control bleeding by increasing factor VIII and von Willebrand factor levels, as well as by improving platelet function therapy to control bleeding. It might be indicated for the correction of life-threatening hemorrhage and if no response is seen with other efforts to correct the underlying coagulopathy and thrombocytopenia, if present. Fresh frozen plasma is appropriate if the coagulopathy worsens or if David must undergo an invasive procedure with a high likelihood of bleeding (e.g., lung biopsy). Cryoprecipitate is not indicated because David is not hypofibrinogenemic. *Answer 9:* **a.**

Case Study continued

David's coagulopathy has been corrected through appropriate intervention; however, his platelet count is decreased to 19,000/mm³.

QUESTIONS

10. In addition to transfusing platelets, you anticipate all of the following *except:*
- **a.** Inserting a Foley catheter and beginning bladder irrigation
- **b.** Starting a 24-hour urine for creatinine clearance
- **c.** Obtaining a renal ultrasound
- **d.** Increasing fluids to 125 ml/hr

11. In addition, you are concerned about the development of which of the following types of renal failure?
- **a.** Intrarenal renal failure
- **b.** Postrenal renal failure
- **c.** Acute tubular necrosis
- **d.** Renal failure is not a concern; this patient has hemorrhagic cystitis

---
ANSWERS

10. Hemorrhagic cystitis is caused by urinary excretion of toxic metabolites of cyclophosphamide or ifosfamide, and it occurs in up to 35% of patients, even with appropriate prophylaxis (Long, 1998). The complication is most common after high-dose ifosfamide or cyclophosphamide therapy, but other agents, such as busulfan, etoposide irradiation, and viruses (e.g., CMV, adenovirus, and BK virus), have been implicated (Long, 1998).

Prophylactic measures are required to prevent hemorrhagic cystitis after high-dose therapy. The most commonly used approach is hyperhydration with the infusion of at least 3 L/m²/day beginning

before cyclophosphamide and continuing for at least 24 hours after its administration. Catheterization and continuous bladder irrigation have also been shown to be effective. MESNA (2-mercaptoethane sodium sulfonate) binds to acrolein, the toxic metabolite of cyclophosphamide, in the urine and prevents damage to the urinary tract. MESNA is generally dosed at 100% to 160% of the dose of cyclophosphamide and administered by either continuous infusion or in divided doses beginning at the initiation of cyclophosphamide and continuing after its completion.

The onset of oliguria in the adult merits insertion of a Foley catheter to establish whether urinary tract obstruction, in this case likely with clots, is responsible for the oliguria. A renal ultrasound may also be helpful to evaluate for hydronephrosis, given the abdominal pain, tenderness at the CVA, and oliguria. A recheck of the BUN and creatinine is also indicated; however, a 24-hour urine for creatinine clearance will not provide immediate data to direct your plan of care. *Answer 10:* **a.**

11. Ureter or urethral clotting from hemorrhagic cystitis can cause postrenal renal failure as a consequence of obstruction of outflow (Philpott & Kanfer, 1998). In the setting of fever and with tachycardia, a prerenal cause such as hypovolemia may also be a contributing factor. Intrarenal renal failure or acute tubular necrosis are less likely in this case study. *Answer 11:* **b.**

QUESTIONS

12. Your treatment of the febrile neutropenia is based on the knowledge that what type of infections are the most commonly encountered infections in the first week after transplantation?
- **a.** Bacterial
- **b.** Viral
- **c.** Fungal
- **d.** Protozoan

ANSWERS

12. Bacterial infection is the most commonly encountered infection in the first week after transplantation (Burt & Walsh, 1998). The relationship between the time of allogeneic HSCT and the organisms causing infections following transplantation is portrayed in Table 10-3. *Answer 12:* **a.**

QUESTIONS

13. Which of the following is *least* likely to be ordered as an empiric antimicrobial regimen for febrile neutropenia?
- **a.** Vancomycin, levofloxacin, famciclovir
- **b.** Imipenem, vancomycin, famciclovir

TABLE 10-3 Infections Following Allogeneic Hematopoietic Stem Cell Transplantation

PERIOD OF NEUTROPENIA (DAYS 0-30)	PERIOD OF ACUTE GVHD (DAYS 30-100)	PERIOD OF CHRONIC GVHD (DAY >100)
Gram-negative bacteria	Gram-negative bacteria	Encapsulated bacteria
Gram-positive bacteria	Gram-positive bacteria	Varicella-zoster
Herpes simplex	Cytomegalovirus	Cytomegalovirus
Candida species	BK virus	*Pneumocystis carinii*
Aspergillus species	Adenovirus	*Aspergillus* species
	Varicella-zoster	
	Candida species	
	Aspergillus species	
	Pneumocystis carinii	
	Toxoplasma gondii	

Adapted from Burt, R. K., & Walsh, T. (1998). Infection prophylaxis in bone marrow transplant recipients—Myths, legends, and microbes. In Burt, R. K., Deeg, H. J., Lothian, S., & Santos, G. W. (Eds.). *Bone marrow transplantation* (pp. 438-451). Austin: Landes Bioscience.
GVHD, Graft-versus-host disease.

c. Piperacillin, tobramycin, metronidazole
d. Cefepime, famciclovir

ANSWERS

13. Empiric initial therapy for a patient with an absolute neutrophil count (ANC) of less than 500/μl and a fever greater than 38.0° C or in whom infection is suspected without an obvious source is broad-spectrum empiric antibiotic coverage (Burt & Walsh, 1998). Although it is generally agreed that many antibiotic regimens are effective in the management of neutropenic fever and infections, careful selection of the initial antibiotic regimen may enhance efficacy and minimize adverse effects. Factors to be considered include the potential sites of infection, antimicrobial susceptibilities of local pathogens, institutional pathogens, and agents that have broad-spectrum antibacterial activity. Preexisting organ dysfunction and patient medication allergies may also shape the selection of one agent over another.

All regimens, except choice a, could provide adequate antibacterial coverage, although the regimen in choice c does not provide for prophylaxis against herpes simplex virus infection. The regimen in choice a provides inadequate coverage for gram-negative organisms. Different antibiotic regimens may be chosen, and the approach usually depends on institutional preference and history of prior unit/institution infections.

The initial evaluation should focus on determining the causative organism or organisms and potential sites of infection and on assessing the patient's risk for infection-associated comorbid medical disease. A rapid site-specific history and physical examination should be performed. The common sites of infection for patients with fever and neutropenia (e.g., alimentary tract, skin, lungs, sinus, intravascular access device sites) should be assessed thoroughly.

Initial laboratory evaluation should include a CBC, liver and renal function tests, oxygen saturation, and urinalysis. Chest radiographs should be obtained routinely but may have no or minimal findings in neutropenic patients who have a pulmonary infection. This baseline laboratory information is critical for developing a supportive care plan, assessing the patient's risk of infection, and monitoring for future treatment- and infection-associated toxicity.

Patients in whom fever persists beyond 4 days of initial antimicrobial therapy and in whom a site or source of infection has not been identified should undergo reassessment of their antimicrobial therapy. The need for a change in therapy should be based on the patient's clinical status and likelihood of early marrow recovery. Although fever resolution may be slow, persistent fever may suggest a nonbacterial infection, a bacterial infection that is resistant to the empiric antibiotic, the emergence of a secondary infection, a venous access or closed space infection, inadequate antimicrobial serum levels, or drug fever. The management of such patients may be complicated, and in some circumstances, serial antimicrobial changes will be necessary. Persistent fever after 4 days without a source is usually an indication for empiric therapy with amphotericin (National Comprehensive Cancer Center Network, 1999). *Answer 13:* **a.**

QUESTIONS

14. Which of the following statements best explains the rationale for intravenous immunoglobulin (IVIG) in patients undergoing an allogeneic SCT?

a. Hypergammaglobulinemia is a common finding in allogeneic transplant patients with GVHD.

b. Fungal infection is reduced in patients with adequate IgG levels.

c. Administration of IVIG is associated with a reduced rate of viral infection and GVHD in patients undergoing allogeneic transplantation.

d. There are no data to support the administration of IVIG in the allogeneic post-transplant patient; it is indicated only in the management of certain viral infections.

_____ **ANSWERS**

14. Hypogammaglobulinemia rather than hypergammaglobulinemia is a common finding in patients with GVHD (Chao, 1998). In addition, IVIG administration is associated with a reduced rate of viral infection and GVHD in patients undergoing allogeneic transplantation. Institutional protocols vary; however, IVIG is usually given at a dosage of 250 to 500 mg/kg at intervals as frequently weekly for the first 100 days (Abdel-Mageed, Graham-Pole, Del Rosario, et al., 1999; Chao, 1998). In the setting of chronic GVHD, immunoglobulin levels are monitored, and patients with hypogammaglobulinemia are supplemented appropriately (Seber & Vogelsang, 1998). Data do not suggest that fungal infections are reduced in patients with adequate IgG levels. _Answer 14:_ **c.**

Case Study continued

The hemorrhagic cystitis has diminished in response to your interventions. However, on day +5, David develops worsening mucositis, with increased odynophagia and severe oral pain. In addition, he remains febrile and is showing signs of liver dysfunction.

QUESTIONS _____

15. Based on this assessment, the safest, most effective choice(s) for symptom relief is(are) probably:

a. Percodan

b. Fentanyl 25-μg patch

c. Patient-controlled analgesia (PCA) with parenteral morphine, hydromorphone, or fentanyl

d. Intravenous meperidine

_____ **ANSWERS**

15. Use of the fentanyl patch during episodes of fever may result in inadvertent excess absorption of medication with subsequent signs of narcotic tox-

icity. Acetaminophen, which is a portion of Percodan, should be avoided in patients with evidence of liver dysfunction. In addition, in patients with febrile neutropenia, its use may mask fever. Furthermore, oral therapy is impractical given the patient's odynophagia. Meperidine is an inappropriate choice in a clinical situation because with longer-term use or in patients with renal compromise, there can be hazardous accumulation of the meperidine metabolite normeperidine (Buckley, 1998). The use of meperidine in the hematocrit (HCT) setting should be reserved for low-dose treatment. _Answer 15:_ **c.**

QUESTIONS _____

16. Which of the following findings suggests the diagnosis of venoocclusive disease in David, who is 6 days following matched, related SCT after conditioning with total body irradiation, thiotepa, and cyclophosphamide?

a. Fever, weight loss, increased bilirubin, jaundice, elevated creatinine

b. Weight gain, elevated bilirubin, right upper quadrant pain, hepatosplenomegaly

c. Weight gain, elevated transaminases, renal failure

d. Weight gain, jaundice, elevated bilirubin, fever

17. All of the following are components of the anticipated management plan for venoocclusive disease of the liver _except:_

a. Vigorous hydration with normal saline

b. Intake and output, daily weights, central venous pressure monitoring

c. Regular measurement of abdominal girth, assessment for the presence and progression of hepatomegaly and ascites

d. Dosage adjustments for medications based on renal and hepatic function

_____ **ANSWERS**

16. Venoocclusive disease of the liver is a potentially fatal liver disease that occurs in 15% to 20% of SCT recipients. Venoocclusive disease occurs when fibrous material accumulates, resulting in obstruction of small venules in the liver. Subsequently, there is acute liver congestion, with back-flow of blood and fluid loss from the hepatic vessels into the peritoneal cavity. In addition, renal blood flow decreases, causing further water and sodium retention.

Clinical manifestations of venoocclusive disease begin during the first 2 weeks after the transplant and are characterized by rapid weight gain, ascites, right upper quadrant pain, hepatomegaly, splenomegaly, and jaundice (Gluckman, 1994). Fever and elevated transaminases are not classic signs of venooclusive disease. *Answer 16:* **b.**

17. The approach to fluid management in the patient with venooclusive disease consists of fluid and sodium restriction and concentration of all medications in minimal intravenous fluids. Attempts are made to maintain intravascular volume and renal perfusion while monitoring for extravascular fluid accumulation. This may require central venous pressure monitoring. Other supportive strategies may include renal dose dopamine infusion, avoidance of diuretics that depleted intravascular volume, and chest physiotherapy to prevent pulmonary atelectasis (Gluckman, 1994). Strategies to prevent venooclusive disease of the liver are currently undergoing investigation and may include anticoagulation with heparin, fibrinolytics such as tissue plasminogen activator (tPA), prostaglandin E, and ursodeoxycholic acid (Actigall) (Bearman, 1995; McDonald, 1994). *Answer 17:* **a.**

Case Study continued

On days +7 through +9, David's creatinine is noted to be rising steadily, reaching a level of 2.1 mg/dl; his BUN is 62 mg/dl.

QUESTIONS

18. All of the following are causes of prerenal renal failure *except:*
  a. Hemorrhage
  b. Venooclusive disease of the liver, with hepatorenal syndrome
  c. Cardiomyopathy with CHF
  d. Ureter or urethral clotting from hemorrhagic cystitis

ANSWERS

18. Renal failure occurs when there is a decrease in renal function with a resultant retention of urea nitrogen and creatinine in the blood. Renal failure can result from prerenal, renal, and postrenal causes. Differentiating the suspected cause of renal failure helps the APN to select the most efficacious strategies for assessment and management.

Renal failure secondary to prerenal causes includes a functional decrease in renal blood flow and glomerular filtration rate (GFR) from a decrease in intravascular volume, low cardiac output states, third spacing of fluid, capillary leak, or renal vasoconstriction (Kaplan & Mujais, 1998). Ureter or urethral clotting from hemorrhagic cystitis is a cause of postrenal renal failure, resulting as a consequence of obstruction of outflow. *Answer 18:* **d.**

QUESTIONS

19. Which of the following maneuvers would distinguish prerenal renal failure from intrarenal renal failure?
  a. 24-hour fluid restriction
  b. Renal ultrasound
  c. Foley catheterization
  d. Check of urine sodium, urine osmolality, and fractional excretion of sodium

20. All of the following laboratory or physical findings suggest an intrarenal cause for David's renal failure *except:*
  a. High urine sodium (greater than 40 mEq/L), high fractional excretion of sodium (greater than 1%)
  b. Low urine sodium (less than 20 mEq/L), low fractional excretion of sodium (less than 1%)
  c. Urine eosinophils on urinalysis with microscopy
  d. Reduced urine osmolality

ANSWERS

19. In evaluating renal failure and determining the likely cause, a urine sodium, urine osmolality, and fractional excretion of sodium should be obtained simultaneously, before using a fluid challenge or diuretic. Obtaining these data after a fluid challenge or diuretic administration makes them much less meaningful. *Answer 19:* **a.**

20. In prerenal states, the kidney avidly retains sodium, usually resulting in a low urine sodium (less than 20 mEq/L), a fractional excretion of sodium of less than 1%, and a urine osmolality of more than 500 mOsm/kg/H_2O. With intrinsic renal failure, the urine sodium is more than 40 mEq/24 hr, with a fractional excretion of sodium of more than 1% and a low urine osmolality of less than 350 mOsm/kg/H_2O (Coyne, 1998).

Intrarenal or intrinsic etiologies of renal failure result from a variety of injuries to the renal blood vessels, glomeruli, tubules, or interstitia. These insults may be toxic (hepatotoxicity from aminoglycosides, intravenous contrast agents), immunologic (i.e., allergic interstitial nephritis secondary to penicillins or imipenem), or idiopathic (Coyne, 1998; Kaplan & Mujais, 1998; Powers & Lam, 1999). Eosinophils in the urine, along with the classic signs of fever rash and renal dysfunction, suggest a diagnosis of allergic interstitial nephritis (Coyne, 1998). Fluid restriction will not help clarify the cause of renal failure; however, a fluid challenge of 500 to 1000 ml infused over 30 to 60 minutes may help distinguish prerenal from intrarenal causes of renal failure, although some cases of intrinsic renal failure also may respond with increased urine output. A renal ultrasound and Foley catheterization will help identify lower tract obstruction and upper tract obstruction, respectively, but will not necessarily help distinguish prerenal from intrarenal causes of the renal failure. *Answer 20:* **b.**

QUESTIONS

21. What is the primary concern in the management of a patient with prerenal renal failure?
   a. Correction of hypoperfusion of the kidney
   b. Correction of mechanical or functional urine flow obstruction
   c. Urine alkalinization
   d. Immediate hemodialysis

22. All of the following are intervention strategies to reverse or correct specific prerenal causes of renal failure *except:*
   a. Hydralazine, digoxin, nitroglycerine, and nifedipine to manage CHF
   b. Volume replacement
   c. Dopamine drip at 3 µg/kg/min
   d. Short course of steroids

ANSWERS

21-22. The primary concern in the management of a patient with prerenal causes for renal failure is to correct hypoperfusion of the kidney (Kaplan & Mujais, 1998). This is usually accomplished by volume replacement using normal saline and/or packed red blood cells. Medications such as hydralazine, digoxin, nitroglycerine, and nifedipine may be used to help manage CHF by improving pump function, increasing preload, and decreasing afterload. Dopamine in vasodilator doses of 3 to 5 µg/kg/min may be administered in an attempt to improve renal blood flow (Coyne, 1998). Steroids are not used to treat prerenal causes but may have a role in allergic interstitial nephritis, an intrarenal cause for renal failure (Coyne, 1998). *Answer 21:* **a.** *Answer 22:* **d.**

QUESTIONS

23. Which of the following fluid, electrolyte, acid-base disorders would you also expect to see with acute renal failure?
   a. Metabolic acidosis, hypophosphatemia
   b. Metabolic acidosis, hyperkalemia, hyperphosphatemia
   c. Respiratory acidosis, metabolic acidosis, hypokalemia
   d. Respiratory alkalosis, hyperkalemia, hyperphosphatemia

21. Acute renal failure is usually accompanied by hyperkalemia, hyperphosphatemia, and hypocalcemia (Coyne, 1998). Metabolic acidosis also accompanies renal failure and may at times be severe or life-threatening (Kaplan & Mujais, 1998). *Answer 23:* **b.**

QUESTIONS

24. Which two tests are required to evaluate acid-base balance?
   a. Arterial blood gases (ABGs) and pulse oximetry
   b. ABGs and serum electrolytes
   c. ABGs and creatinine clearance
   d. Serum electrolytes and pulse oximetry

ANSWERS

22. The body's mechanisms for maintaining a balance of hydrogen ion to bicarbonate ion include the buffer systems in the blood fluids, the respiratory system, and the renal system. To adequately assess a patient's acid-base balance, arterial pH, $Paco_2$, and serum bicarbonate are required. Konick-McMahon (1998) provides helpful tips for interpreting ABGs. She suggests the following questions to guide the analysis:

1. Is the pH normal? Higher than 7.45 is alkalosis; lower than 7.35 is acidosis.
2. Is the Pco_2 normal? Higher than 45 mm Hg is indicative of acidosis because the respiratory system retains CO_2; lower than 35 mm Hg indicates an alkalosis because the lung blows off CO_2.
3. Is the HCO_3 normal? An HCO_3 above 28 mEq/L indicates kidney saving of bicarbonate, whereas a value below 22 mEq/L shows kidney wasting of bicarbonate or use of bicarbonate to buffer acid.
4. Which value, Pco_2 or HCO_3, corresponds to the pH? If the pH is acidotic (below 7.35), is the $Paco_2$ increased (respiratory) or is there a decreased bicarbonate (metabolic)? This is the primary disturbance. *Answer 24:* **b.**

QUESTIONS

25. Which of the following would be relatively contraindicated in a patient with a serum creatinine of 2.5 mg/dl and an estimated creatinine clearance of 35 ml/min?
   a. Computed tomography (CT) scan of the abdomen with contrast
   b. Inhaled pentamidine
   c. Amphotericin B
   d. Vancomycin

ANSWERS

25. CT of the abdomen with contrast is contraindicated. Intervenous contrast dyes can cause damage to tubular cells, especially in patients who are diabetic, are severely dehydrated, or have underling renal insufficiency (Powers & Lam, 1999). Contrast dyes that cause acute tubular necrosis include those used in intravenous pyelograms, CT scans, and coronary angiography. The intravenous contrast material used in ventilation/perfusion scans ($\dot{V}/\dot{Q}$ scans) or magnetic resonance imaging (MRI) does not cause renal tubular damage. Vancomycin should be dosed according to levels, and the interval for amphotericin B should be adjusted appropriately based on the estimated creatinine clearance. Inhaled pentamidine does not require dosage adjustment for renal dysfunction. *Answer 25:* **a.**

QUESTIONS

26. All of the following are true with regard to drug dosing and renal insufficiency in the SCT patient *except:*

a. The dosing and interval for administration of drugs that have predominant elimination via the kidney will be affected most by changes in renal function.

b. Methods of determining the GFR include a calculated estimate of the creatinine clearance and the 24-hour urine for creatinine clearance.

c. The calculated creatinine clearance is the most accurate way to estimate GFR when there is wide variability in the serum creatinine from day to day.

d. Cyclosporine, tacrolimus, gentamycin, phenytoin, tobramycin, amikacin, and lithium require monitoring of serum or whole blood levels to make appropriate decisions regarding dosage.

27. Which of the following groups of therapies all require adjustment for renal insufficiency?

a. Compazine, vancomycin, ganciclovir, cyclosporine

b. G-CSF, tobramycin, imipenem, acyclovir

c. Ondansetron, gentamycin, tacrolimus, total parenteral nutrition

d. Vancomycin, acyclovir, ceftazidime, fluconazole

ANSWERS

26. Renal impairment can affect both the clearance and action of many drugs. The dosing and interval for administration of drugs that have predominant elimination via the kidney will be most affected by changes in renal function. Two methods of determining the GFR are an estimated creatinine clearance and a 24-hour urine for creatinine clearance. When there is wide variability in the serum creatinine from day to day, a 24-hour urine for creatinine clearance is the most accurate method to gauge glomerular filtration. *Answer 26:* **c.**

27. With renal insufficiency, nonessential medications should be discontinued or held. Commonly used medications in SCT that require dose adjustment for renal dysfunction are presented in Table 10-4. Some centers adjust Prograf

TABLE **10-4** | **Supportive Care Medications Commonly Used in Hematopoietic Stem Cell Transplantation Requiring a Dosage and/or Interval Adjustment for Renal Dysfunction**

ANTIMICROBIALS	GASTROINTESTINAL	MISCELLANEOUS
Acyclovir	Cimetidine	Opioid analgesics, including codeine,
Aminoglycosides	Ranitidine	morphine, and meperidine
Amphotericin	Metoclopramide	Allopurinol
Cefepime		
Ceftazidime		
Ciprofloxacin		
Fluconazole		
Foscarnet		
Ganciclovir		
Imipenem		
Levofloxacin		
Vancomycin		

Adapted from Kaplan, B., & Mujais, S. (1998). Disorders of renal function and electrolytes. In Burt, R. K., Deeg, H. J., Lothian, S. & Santos, G. W. (Eds.). *Bone marrow transplantation* (pp. 408-422). Austin: Landes Bioscience; and Huey, W. Y. & Coyne, D. W. (1998). Dosage adjustments of drugs in renal failure. In Carey, C., Lee, H. & Woeltje, K. F. (Eds.). *The Washington manual of medical therapeutics*, 29th ed. (pp. 549-555). Philadelphia: Williams & Wilkins.

(FK 506) and cyclosporine dosages based on renal function, but usually, dosage adjustments are based on monitoring levels at frequent intervals. Compazine, ondansetron, and G-CSF do not require dosage adjustment for renal insufficiency because they are not primarily metabolized by the kidney (Kaplan & Mujais, 1998). *Answer 27:* **d.**

CASE 4 STUDY

Chris Mackie is now day +4 following autologous SCT for relapsed stage IV Hodgkin's disease. His medical history is significant for severe cardiomyopathy as a result of the aggressiveness of his previous chemotherapy regimens, with a cumulative anthracycline dose in excess of 500 mg/m^2. His pretransplant left ventricular ejection fraction was 49%. His morning CBC reveals a WBC of 0.3/mm^3, Hgb of 7.8 g/dl, Hct of 22%, and platelets of 11,000/mm^3. His examination is within normal limits except for the following findings: tachycardia with a heart rate of 124 beats/min, S$_3$, fine bibasilar rales, and trace pretibial edema.

QUESTIONS

1. What is the most appropriate response?
   a. Order erythropoietin (Epogen/Procrit) 40,000 U/day subcutaneously and transfusion of one single-donor platelet product
   b. Order 2 units of irradiated, filtered, packed red blood cells and one single-donor platelet product
   c. Continue monitoring the CBC every 12 hours
   d. Order furosemide 40 mg intravenously now; transfuse 1 unit of packed red blood cells and one single-donor platelet product

---

ANSWERS

1. Chris has moderately severe cardiomyopathy before the transplant and may have experienced a further decline in his cardiac muscle function as a result of his conditioning regimen. Oxygen delivery is maximized at hematocrits between 30% and 40% (Johnston & Crawford, 1998); however, adequate tissue oxygenation usually can be obtained with an Hgb of 7 to 8 g/dl (Blinder, 1998), and most patients tolerate moderately severe anemia (Hgb of less than 8 g/dl) well (Casciato, 1995). Symptoms such as shortness of breath, chest pain, headache, or dizziness; physical findings such as tachycardia, tachypnea, mental status changes, or severe pallor; and the presence of coexisting disorders such as cardiopulmonary disease must be considered when determining the need for trans-

fusion. Other factors to consider include the degree of physiologic stress and the anticipated recovery time of the hematocrit without transfusion (Johnston & Crawford, 1998). Chris's cardiomyopathy places him at risk for cardiac ischemia and worsening of his CHF as a result of the severe anemia. At day +4 posttransplant, one would not expect erythropoiesis to recover for several more days. Continued monitoring of the CBC would result in unnecessary delay and possible adverse effects. Transfusion with 1 unit of packed red blood cells would likely be inadequate because each unit raises the hemoglobin by 1 g/dl in the average adult (Blinder, 1998). Thus 2 units of packed red blood cells, along with 1 unit of single-donor platelets, should be ordered. Furosemide could be administered between each unit of red blood cells to reduce fluid overload and resulting CHF. The role of Epogen after SCT is still being defined (Hollis & Miller, 1998). Studies suggest that therapy with Epogen may promote erythroid engraftment and decrease overall transfusion requirements (Hollis & Miller, 1998; Johnston & Crawford, 1998). Initiation of Epogen therapy should probably be considered to prevent prolonged anemia and to reduce his overall transfusion requirements (Hollis & Miller, 1998; Johnston & Crawford, 1998). Although the expected time to response is variable, Epogen does not produce an immediate improvement in hematocrit, usually requiring at least 2 weeks of therapy to see an improvement in hemoglobin levels (Johnston & Crawford, 1998). *Answer 1:* **b.**

Case Study continued

Chris is concerned about the possibility of developing human immunodeficiency virus (HIV) from a blood transfusion. Before agreeing to receive the transfusion, he asks to discuss this with you.

QUESTIONS

2. You explain:
   a. The benefits and risks of transfusion therapy in Chris's current situation

b. The options for directed and autologous donations

c. That irradiation of blood products is routinely performed in this unit, which eliminates the risk for blood-borne infections such as hepatitis and CMV

d. That the most common reason for a severe hemolytic transfusion reaction is a failure to identify the unit and recipient properly

---

ANSWERS

2. All blood component therapy has risks, including infection, transfusion reactions, volume overload, and pulmonary edema. Patients' concerns usually focus mainly on transfusion-associated infections such as hepatitis and HIV. Current testing for viral infections includes HIV-1, HIV-2, human T-lymphotropic virus type I (HTLV-1), hepatitis B virus, and hepatitis C virus. The risk of transfusion-associated transmission of HIV-1, HIV-2, and HTLV-1 from screened blood is estimated to be 1 in 500,000 (Blinder, 1998). Estimates of hepatitis B and hepatitis C virus transmission are approximately 1 in 100,000 (Blinder, 1998). Viral infections occur when donors are in the seronegative window period, allowing the infection to escape detection (Blinder, 1998).

Because an autologous transplant recipient will require many transfusions during transplant and is often anemic from previous chemotherapy regimens, autologous blood donation is impractical (Fox, 1998). Although many patients believe blood supplied by family or friends is less likely to transmit blood-borne infections than that from the general blood supply, available data are not consistent with this hypothesis (Menitove, 1994).

The benefits and risks of transfusion therapy must be weighed carefully in each situation. For Chris, the benefits include the need to avoid further injury to his heart muscle through ischemia and to avoid worsening his CHF, as well as to improve his current symptoms of hypoxemia. One alternative to reduce the overall number of packed red blood cell transfusions may be therapy with EpogenProcrit; however, as mentioned, this will not produce the needed improvement in hematocrit in the short term. In each case the indications for transfusion should be recorded in the medical record, and many centers require written informed consent for the transfusion of all blood products.

It has been determined that leukodepletion by either bedside filtration during transfusion or as a result of prestorage leukocyte depletion of the blood product is an effective method of preventing transfusion-associated CMV infection because the virus is transmitted by leukocytes (de Silva,

Contreras, & Warwick, 1998; Fox, 1998). In addition, filtered blood products may also prevent febrile transfusion reactions and delay alloimmunization (Fox, 1998; Johnston & Crawford, 1998; Morgan & Dodds, 1994). However, use of a leukocyte depletion filter does not affect the risk of transmission of hepatitis. Two methods for leukocyte depletion are currently available: bedside filtration using a filter and prestorage leukocyte depletion. Irradiation of blood products does not affect the risk of transmission of CMV or hepatitis. It is true that the most common reason for a severe hemolytic transfusion reaction is a failure to identify the unit and recipient properly. *Answer 2:* **a.**

QUESTIONS

3. During a lecture you are giving on blood product support in the posttransplant patient, you are asked by the staff nurse to explain the rationale for irradiating blood products in patients undergoing transplant. Your response incorporates which of the following concepts?

1. Irradiation inactivates immunologically competent T lymphocytes contained in the blood product.
2. Transfusion-associated GVHD develops when immune-competent allogeneic lymphocytes are transfused into a severely immunocompromised host.
3. Gamma irradiation of the blood product to 2500 cGy is presently the most efficient and effective way to accomplish this.
4. Blood products that have been irradiated cannot be used by other patients because the irradiating process does alter somewhat the efficacy of the blood product.

a. 1, 2, & 3
b. 1 & 3
c. 1, 3, & 4
d. All of these

ANSWERS

3. Transfusion-associated GVHD is a rare but almost uniformly fatal complication of transfusion resulting from the infusion of immunocompetent lymphocytes capable of proliferation, which the recipient is unable to destroy (de Silva, Contreras, & Warwick, 1998; Fox, 1998). The infused lymphocytes recognize host tissues as foreign and mount a reaction. All cellular blood products, except for stem cell grafts and lymphocytes given for graft-versus-tumor effect, must be irradiated to 2500 cGy to prevent transfusion-associated GVHD (Fox, 1998). Blood products that have been irradiated do not alter the efficacy or cellular content of the product and do not harm the recipient in any way. Patients who have undergone allogeneic or autologous HSCT should receive irradiated cellular components, both in the period before SCT and in the posttransplant period (de Silva, Contreras, & Warwick, 1998). *Answer 3:* **a.**

QUESTIONS

4. Which of the following are indications for transfusion in Chris, who has a platelet count of 11,000/mm³?
    1. Fresh minor bleeding of gums, nose, or scattered petechiae
    2. Fever greater than 38° C and active infection
    3. Planned bone marrow aspirate and biopsy
    4. Yesterday's platelet count of 42,000/mm³, independent of transfusion support
    5. Yesterday's platelet count of 10,000/mm³, independent of transfusion support
    6. Concurrent therapy with enoxaparin 60 mg subcutaneously every 12 hours in treatment of venous thrombosis
    7. Outpatient status, therefore will not be returning to the clinic for 3 days
        a. 1, 2, 3, 4, 6, & 7
        b. 1, 2, 3, 5, & 6
        c. All of these except for 5
        d. All of these

ANSWERS

4. The trigger for prophylactic platelet transfusion support is an area of controversy, with some centers maintaining a level more than 10,000/ml for stable patients and others maintaining a level of more than 20,000/ml. Guidelines for platelet transfusion in patients undergoing transplant or aggressive chemotherapy regimens have been proposed by Smith (1995). Most of the literature suggests that patients with a platelet count of less than 5000/ml should be treated with transfusion and that clinical judgment should be used when deciding whether to transfuse patients with platelet counts between 5000 and 15,000/ml (de Silva, Contreras, & Warwick, 1998).

Factors to be considered include the presence of occult or frank bleeding; extensive mucocutaneous ulcerations; abnormalities, such as arteriovenous malformation, or a history of hemorrhage of the central nervous system or GI tract; and the presence of factors such as infection, which increase platelet consumption. The need for hemostasis during procedures such as bone marrow aspirate and biopsy, insertion of central lines, and endoscopy also necessitate transfusion support. Patients in whom the platelet count is declining by more than 50% per day should probably be transfused when they are between 10,000 and 15,000/ml or should have their platelet count rechecked in 12 hours. In fully anticoagulated individuals (e.g., those receiving enoxaparin or heparin), it is advisable to keep the platelet count between 30,000 and 50,000/ml. *Answer 4:* **a.**

QUESTIONS

5. Chris's 15-minute posttransplant platelet increment is 13,000/ml. This finding indicates which of the following?
    a. Platelet refractoriness
    b. Thrombotic thrombocytopenic purpura (TTP)
    c. Hemolytic transfusion reaction
    d. Alloimmunization

6. In response to the development of platelet refractoriness, the appropriate intervention is to:
    a. Send an HLA or lymphocytotoxic antibody screen
    b. Transfuse HLA-matched or HLA-compatible platelets
    c. Transfuse additional units of pooled platelets
    d. Transfuse a unit of apheresis platelets obtained from a family member

ANSWERS

5. Refractoriness to platelet transfusion is a common occurrence in the frequently transfused population. A patient is usually considered refractory if the posttransfusion platelet count increases by less than 5×10^9/L (Johnston & Crawford, 1998). Although a patient showing a platelet increment less than this value is often assumed to be alloimmunized against HLA antigens, it is important to realize that there may be factors inherent in the platelet product or the clinical circumstances that are contributing to the suboptimal transfusion response, including poor quality of platelet concentrates, nonalloimmune mechanisms, and alloimmune mechanisms (de Silva, Contreras, & Warwick, 1998). Platelet refractoriness may develop for multiple reasons, including bleeding, disseminated intravascular coagulation, shortened platelet life span from fever, septicemia, splenomegaly with splenic sequestration, antibiotics, HLA alloimmunization, the development of antiplatelet antibodies or venoocclusive disease (Fox, 1998; Johnston & Crawford, 1998; Smith, 1995). *Answer 5:* **a.**

6. The fastest approach to the problem of platelet refractoriness is to send an HLA or lymphocytotoxic antibody screen to look for anti-HLA antibod-

ies in the patient's serum; if these are present, either HLA-compatible platelets or HLA-matched platelets are then used (de Silva, Contreras, & Warwick, 1998; Fox, 1998). Alloimmunization may occur as a result of red blood cell or platelet transfusions because these components are contaminated by passenger leukocytes (Fox, 1998). After transplant, the hematopoietic stem cell donor or family members may be used as platelet donors because they share many tissue antigens and the recipient is more likely to achieve improved increments with their platelets. Individuals who are candidates for transplantation from an HLA-matched sibling should not receive apheresis products from a family member before transplantation to avoid the risk of allosensitization to donor-specific antigens, which could lead to hematopoietic stem cell graft rejection (Shapiro, Davison, & Rust, 1997).

Methods of preventing or delaying the development of platelet refractoriness and alloimmunization continue to be studied and include the use of high-dose IVIG, the use of leukoreduction filters, and the ultraviolet irradiation of blood products (Johnston & Crawford, 1998). *Answer 6:* **a.**

Case Study continued

Chris is receiving his first transfusion of packed red blood cells. At 45 minutes into the transfusion, Chris reports anxiety, chest tightness, and shortness of breath. His nurse pages you, and when you enter the room, you note that he appears dusky, with mucosal pallor. Examination reveals decreased air entry to the lung bases bilaterally, with scattered wheezing; increased use of the accessory muscles of breathing; tachypnea; tachycardia; and cool, clammy skin. His oxygen saturation on room air is 88%. His temperature is 38.6° C, pulse is 130 beats/min, respiration rate is 34 breaths/min, and blood pressure is 134/82 mm Hg. He denies any areas of body pain; however, he has urticaria on the forearms, neck, and anterior thorax. The nurse has already stopped his transfusion and is infusing normal saline.

QUESTIONS

7. What is the most likely cause of Chris's respiratory distress?
   a. Acute hemolytic transfusion reaction
   b. Febrile, nonhemolytic transfusion reaction
   c. Bacterial contamination
   d. Delayed hemolytic transfusion reaction

ANSWERS

7. Febrile, nonhemolytic transfusion reactions are caused by antibodies in the recipient directed against antigens on the granulocytes or lymphocytes in the donor blood, against immunoglobulin components and other proteins in the plasma of the donor, or as a result of cytokines secreted into the component during storage by leukocytes (Casciato, 1995; Fox, 1998). Clinical symptoms range from low-grade fever to rigors, nausea, vomiting, shortness of breath, urticaria, wheezing, dyspnea, or full-blown anaphylaxis.

An acute hemolytic transfusion reaction results from ABO incompatibility, usually the result of human error during blood preparation or administration. Signs and symptoms include restlessness, fever, chills, tachycardia, tachypnea, chest or low back pain, flushing, and hypotension, which usually develop within the first 30 minutes into the transfusion. Whenever a patient experiences a transfusion reaction, an immediate clerical recheck at the bedside should be performed. A delayed hemolytic transfusion reaction occurs because the patient develops an antibody after transfusion and then hemolyses the transfused cells. A delayed hemolytic transfusion reaction is generally manifested as mild jaundice and elevation in bilirubin and lactate dehydrogenase (LDH) and occurs 5 to 10 days after transfusion (Casciato, 1995). Bacterial contamination of a blood product may cause fevers, rigors, and hypotension, but it would not produce respiratory compromise or urticaria. *Answer 7:* **b.**

QUESTIONS

8. Which of the following actions would you implement first?
   1. O_2 100% by nonrebreather face mask
   2. Benadryl 50 mg intravenous push
   3. Solu-Medrol 125 mg intravenous push
   4. Epinephrine 1:1000 in a dose of 0.1 mg/kg
   5. Infusion of normal saline wide open
      a. 1, 2, 3, & 5
      b. 1, 2, & 5
      c. 1, 2, 3, & 4
      d. 4 only

ANSWERS

8. One would prepare to administer epinephrine and would anticipate intubation and mechanical ventilation. Once epinephrine is administered, Benadryl and Solu-Medrol should follow with remaining supportive measures. Premedication before all future blood products with acetamino-

phen, diphenhydramine, and possibly hydrocortisone is necessary. Maneuvers that remove leukocytes through prestorage leukocyte depletion or washing of red blood cells may be necessary (Fox, 1998). *Answer 8:* **d.**

QUESTIONS

9. Which of the following would *not* be a component of the nutritional assessment for Chris?

- **a.** Height, weight, and ideal weight for height
- **b.** Assessment of the cellular immune system through hypersensitivity testing to common antigens
- **c.** Triceps skinfold measurement
- **d.** Global assessment tools that have undergone psychometric evaluation in the cancer patient population, such as the Subjective Global Assessment of Nutritional Status (SGA)

ANSWERS

9. Assessment of the cellular immune system through hypersensitivity testing to common antigens could be dangerous to the HCT patient who has disorders of immune cell activation and leukocyte function, and response is heavily influenced by the disease itself and the transplant procedure. Percentage of weight loss across time, percentage below or in excess of ideal weight, and calculation of the body mass index (BMI) can all be used in the nutritional assessment process (Apovian, Still, & Blackburn, 1998). Fluid balance and hydration status can affect the accuracy of the weight change determinations, however. Triceps skinfold measurement can help define fat stores in the patient, although the correlation with total body protein stores is unknown (Apovian, Still, & Blackburn, 1998). The SGA is a beneficial tool for nutritional screening in the oncology population (Ottery, 1995). The SGA estimates nutritional status on the basis of medical history (weight and weight history, dietary intake, GI symptoms of more than 2 weeks' duration, functional status, and metabolic demands) and physical examination (five determinations of muscle, fat, and fluid status). On the basis of these features, the patient is categorized as being well nourished, having moderate or suspected malnutrition, or having severe malnutrition. Suggested components of a multidimensional nutritional assessment of the hematopoietic cell transplant patient are outlined in Box 10-3. *Answer 9:* **b.**

QUESTIONS

10. Which of the following is the most reliable indicator of nutritional status during the early posttransplant period?

| BOX **10-3** | **Nutritional Assessment of the Stem Cell Transplant Patient** |

HISTORY AND PHYSICAL ASSESSMENT
Diagnosis
Concurrent medical problems (e.g., diabetes mellitus)
Conditioning regimen used for bone marrow transplant and expected gastrointestinal toxicities
Height, weight, percentage deviation from ideal body weight
Triceps skinfold measurement
Hydration status
Presence of gastrointestinal problems
    Nausea and vomiting
    Diarrhea
    Malabsorption
    Anorexia
    Stomatitis
    Dysphagia/odynophagia
    Dysgeusia
    Early satiety
    Xerostomia
Condition of the oral cavity and teeth
Psychologic responses and cognition
    Anxiety
    Depression
    Pain
Current medications

LABORATORY DATA
Albumin, prealbumin, serum transferrin
Electrolytes, calcium, phosphorus
Liver function tests

DIETARY HISTORY
Food preferences
Ethnic background
Practice of any nonconventional dietary strategies (vegetarian diet)
Availability of a person to assist/provide food preparation
Food allergies
Income

- **a.** Weight
- **b.** Serum albumin
- **c.** LFTs
- **d.** None of these

11. Which of the following laboratory tests will best reveal Chris's term response to nutritional interventions?

- **a.** CBC with differential and quantitative immunoglobulin levels
- **b.** Serum transferrin or prealbumin
- **c.** Triglycerides and LFTs
- **d.** Albumin and total protein

ANSWERS

10-11. Because of their relatively short half-lives (less than 10 days), both prealbumin and serum transferrin are likely measures that will reflect most quickly the interventions to improve nutritional status (Apovian, Still, & Blackburn, 1998; Bergerson, 1998). Visceral protein depletion is reflected with transferrin levels of less than 170 g/dl and prealbumin levels of less than 15 g/dl. It is important to note that in patients who have been heavily transfused and who are iron overloaded, transferrin levels may be an unreliable indicator of nutritional status (Apovian, Still, & Blackburn, 1998). CBC and quantitative immunoglobulin levels may be influenced by the disease statement, previous chemotherapy treatments, and/or the transplant procedure itself. Triglyceride levels are not directly related to the adequacy of an individual's nutritional status. Biochemical measures such as total protein are not reliable indicators of nutritional status because they are affected by a number of factors, including volume status, the severity of illness, and kidney and liver dysfunction (Apovian, Still, & Blackburn, 1998; Chan, 1998; Henry & Souchon, 1998). Body weight is an unreliable indicator of nutritional status during the early posttransplant period because of fluid and electrolyte changes. Weight may increase or remain stable despite loss of lean body tissue, and nitrogen balance is difficult to gauge accurately in the presence of corticosteroid use, diarrhea, impaired renal or hepatic function, and immobility (Henry & Souchon, 1998). Serum albumin, with its relatively long half-life of 21 days, is an insensitive indicator of current nutritional status (Apovian, Still, & Blackburn, 1998). In addition, serum albumin concentration is affected by factors such as hydration, infection, and level of activity. LFTs do not have bearing on nutritional status. *Answer 10:* **d.** *Answer 11:* **b.**

QUESTIONS

12. Which of the following statements about the nutritional management of the SCT patient is *incorrect*?
  a. A multiple-vitamin supplement and folic acid should be taken daily for at least 1 year after the transplant.
  b. Total parenteral nutrition is generally not cost-effective if it is anticipated that such nutrition will be required for less than 1 week.
  c. In the presence of a functional GI tract when oral intake is more than 60% of estimated caloric needs, concurrent total parenteral nutrition may suppress appetite.

  d. A daily iron supplement is needed to provide the necessary building blocks for red blood cell production.

ANSWERS

12. Transplant patients do not require iron supplementation, and in fact, they should avoid such supplementation by taking only multiple vitamins formulated without iron. Transplant patients and others who have received chronic transfusions of packed red blood cells (more than 60 units) have more than adequate iron stores (Menitove, 1994), and additional iron supplementation may contribute to iron overload and resultant oxidant injury of organs. A multiple-vitamin supplement, without iron, and folic acid should be taken daily for at least 1 year after the transplant (Bergerson, 1998). Total parenteral nutrition is generally not cost-effective if it is anticipated that such nutrition will be required for less than 1 week (Bergerson, 1998). *Answer 12:* **d.**

QUESTIONS

13. Which of the following food selections best demonstrates effective patient teaching regarding food choices on the low-microbial diet?
  a. Apple cider, fresh vegetable plate, seafood cocktail
  b. Bottled water, hamburger from a fast food restaurant
  c. Thoroughly microwaved leftovers brought from home by the patient's family
  d. Home cooked food items from a church buffet dinner

14. A staff nurse in your organization asks for consultation with another patient who is returning from the referral center following an allogeneic bone marrow transplant. The patient remains on immunosuppression with FK 506 and Medrol. Your recommendations to the patient and the nurse reflect your knowledge that:
  a. The patient must eat a very restricted diet, limited to only foods that have had sterile food preparation, such as canned items, TV dinners, and foods that are thoroughly cooked.
  b. The patient can eat whatever he or she wants, as long as the food is washed well before it is cooked.
  c. Foods with a high bacillus count (e.g., raw seafood, fresh fruits such as strawberries) are avoided, and bottled water is consumed. Food handling and delivery techniques are modified to reduce the possibility of contamination after preparation.

d. The patient can safely eat whatever he or she wants. Guidelines for a low-microbial diet are no longer followed in most centers.

<hr />

ANSWERS

13-14. Although controversial (Smith & Besser, 2000; Todd, Schmidt, Christain, & Williams, 1999), most transplant programs have guidelines for food selection that are to be followed in the first few weeks following transplantation, until white count recovery is established, and many transplant centers suggest that allogeneic transplant patients continue to follow a prescribed diet while they are receiving immunosuppression. Food is a possible source of pathogenic bacteria, which may colonize and seed the blood through a GI tract damaged by chemotherapy, radiation therapy, GVHD, and neutropenia. A diet with a reduced bacterial content is generally encouraged during periods of neutropenia, for at least 100 days following an allogeneic bone marrow transplant, when full immune reconstitution has not yet been achieved, while receiving immunosuppression, and in the setting of active GVHD (Bergerson, 1998; Henry & Souchon, 1998). The principles of a low-microbial diet, also called a *low-bacteria* or *cooked-food diet,* vary from center to center. The principles of this diet are generally that all foods must be well cleaned and prepared following sanitary practices. Red meat should be cooked until well done to avoid *Escherichia coli,* and raw vegetables and fresh fruits should be avoided. Allogeneic SCT patients must also avoid aged cheeses such as blue cheese, commercially prepared meat and vegetable salads, delicatessen foods, raw or lightly cooked eggs, meat or seafood, and freshly squeezed or unpasteurized juices and ciders (Henry & Souchon, 1998). Dietary guidelines are different among institutions, however, and it is important to learn what restrictions are requested by the transplant center where the patient was treated.

In general, foods that are high in fat, fiber, caffeine, or lactose are eliminated from the diet, as are foods that are highly spiced. The patient receives multiple small feedings every 3 to 4 hours, and once diarrhea has resolved, fat intake is slowly increased. The diet is gradually advanced, adding restricted foods, one per day, to assess tolerance (Gauvreau, Lenssen, Cheney, et al., 1981). *Answer 13:* **c.** *Answer 14:* **c.**

Case Study continued

The attending physician asks you to assess Chris (status post autologous peripheral SCT), now day +14 with a full count recovery to determine his readiness for discharge.

QUESTIONS

15. The priority components of your assessment include all of the following *except:*
   a. Ability to tolerate oral medications, fluid and calorie intake, transfusion support and electrolyte supplementation needs, self-care knowledge and skills
   b. Vital signs, amount of diarrhea and/or vomiting, ability to care for central venous catheter, presence of a caregiver in the home
   c. Current profile of intravenous medications, disease status, hematopoietic engraftment, stage of GVHD
   d. Patient's comfort level with planned discharge, including the presence of anxiety, fear, or concern regarding ability to perform necessary self-care

<hr />

ANSWERS

15. Although the current profile of intravenous medications may be an important factor in planning for ongoing needs, disease status is not a factor that determines readiness for discharge; this is usually assessed 30 to 40 days after transplant. Initial hematopoietic engraftment is assumed because the patient has achieved count recovery. Patients can often have their needs for transfusion support and intravenous electrolyte supplementation met in the outpatient infusion suite. Intravenous electrolyte supplementation can also be achieved in the home through self-administration of electrolytes via an ambulatory infusion pump device. GVHD is not an expected complication of autologous transplantation. Psychologic distress in the form of anxiety, fear, or increased physical complaints can accompany the process of preparing for discharge. Patients and/or their caregivers may be somewhat ambivalent about being discharged because although they want to return home and lead a normal life, they are fearful of being removed from the constant vigilance present in an inpatient setting. Reassurance, frequent clinic visits, the availability of 24-hour telephone advice, and an opportunity to practice all necessary skills before discharge can all help the patient in making the transition from the inpatient to the outpatient setting. See Box 10-4. *Answer 15:* **c.**

Case Study conclusion

Most transplant centers will have unique requirements for continued follow-up care that depends

BOX 10-4 | **Criteria for Hospital Discharge after Stem Cell Transplantation**

Discharge from hospital is usually permitted when the following conditions are true:
- Afebrile for at least 24 hr
- Availability of 24-hr outpatient medical facility
- Availability of family caregiver support
- Independent in basic activities of daily living
- Acute posttransplant complications resolved or controlled
- Evidence of oral intake of at least 1500 ml/day or a plan to meet patient's fluid needs through self-administration of intravenous fluid/fluid administration daily in clinic

- Nausea and vomiting controlled
- Tolerating oral medications
- Availability of appropriate transfusion supporting a clinic environment (i.e., access to irradiated blood products)
- Platelet count supportable with no more frequent than daily platelet product
- White blood cell count greater than 1000/mm^3
- Hematocrit of 25% supportable with no more than daily transfusion of 1 unit of packed red blood cells

TABLE 10-5 | **Early and Late Complications of Autologous and Allogeneic Stem Cell Transplantation**

EARLY (OCCURRING BEFORE DAY +100)	LATE (OCCURRING AFTER DAY +100)
Regimen-related toxicity	Regimen-related toxicity
Cystitis	Cataracts
Pulmonary complications	Neurologic conditions—peripheral and autonomic neuropathies
Renal complications	Gonadal dysfunction
Neurologic complications	Endocrine dysfunction
Nutritional complications	Immunodeficiency
Idiopathic pneumonitis	Infection
Graft failure	Musculoskeletal
Infection	Osteoporosis
Viral	Avascular necrosis
Bacterial	Chronic graft-versus-host disease
Fungal	Relapse of malignancy
Graft-versus-host disease	Secondary malignancy
Relapse	

on protocols. In addition, the frequency of clinic visits will be determined by the kind of complications the patient is experiencing. Some of the complications that may occur within the first few months of transplantation are listed in Box 10-4 and Table 10-5.

CASE 5 STUDY

On day +11 status post related allogeneic SCT, Jeremy Griffin is showing signs of WBC recovery, with his WBC rising to 0.6 and his platelet count stable at 21,000 for 2 days without transfusion support. His nurse reports to you that the patient's face is flushed and that he has a temperature of 38.1° C. His skin feels itchy and hot.

QUESTIONS

1. What posttransplant complication do these symptoms suggest?
   a. Systemic infection
   b. Allergic drug reaction
   c. GVHD of the skin
   d. Varicella-zoster infection

2. What additional components of evaluation would you consider a priority?
   a. Current medications, LFTs, GI symptoms
   b. Transplant conditioning regimen, blood cultures, herpes zoster titer
   c. LFTs, conditioning regimen, herpes zoster titer
   d. Blood cultures, LFTs, herpes zoster titer

3. All of the following organs are common targets of GVHD *except:*
   a. Skin
   b. GI tract
   c. Liver
   d. Heart

1. The usual triad of acute GVHD is rash, hepatic dysfunction, and gastroenteritis with diarrhea and abdominal pain. These symptoms may occur together or alone. *Answer 1:* **c.**

2-3. In general, the first and most common clinical manifestation of acute GVHD is a maculopapular rash, usually occurring near the time of WBC engraftment. In the early stages, the rash may feel pruritic and may be confined to the malar regions of the face, the nape of the neck, ears, shoulders, palms of the hands, or soles of the feet. One of the diagnostic challenges following SCT is to differentiate this rash from drug toxicity as a result of either antibiotics or the conditioning regimen. Skin biopsy may be helpful in determining the diagnosis; however, in the first 3 weeks after SCT, it may be difficult to precisely attribute the histo-

logic changes to GVHD because the conditioning regimen itself can cause similar changes in the skin biopsy.

The second most common organ involved in acute GVHD is the liver. The earliest and most common liver function abnormality is a rise in the conjugated bilirubin and alkaline phosphatase; transaminases may also be elevated.

The third most important organ system affected by acute GVHD is the GI system. High-volume water and sometimes bloody diarrhea can occur, causing fluid and electrolyte losses.

GVHD affects the functioning of the immune system, producing hypogammaglobulinemia and impaired quantities and functioning of T lymphocytes. GVHD-induced immunosuppression increases the risk of infection, independent of the immunosuppressive therapy used to treat it. *Answer 2:* **a.** *Answer 3:* **d.**

CASE 6 STUDY

You are asked to consult regarding a 33-year-old patient who is day +6 status post matched unrelated allogeneic SCT for acute myelogenous leukemia (AML) in second complete remission. She develops abdominal pain, moderate hepatomegaly, bloating, jaundice, pruritus, and a skin rash, and she experiences a 5-kg weight gain. Her laboratory results reflect a WBC count of less than $0.1/mm^3$, Hgb of 10.1 g/dl, Hct of 27.6%, and platelets of $9,000/mm^3$ (with daily transfusion support). LFTs show an alkaline phosphate level of 134, AST U/L of 63 U/L, ALT of 165 U/L, LDH of 1200 U/L, total bilirubin of 3.3 mg/dl, and direct bilirubin 1.8 mg/dl.

QUESTIONS

1. The nurse is concerned that the patient is developing GVHD of the liver. Which of the following features in this case would help distinguish venoocclusive disease from GVHD of the liver?
   a. Evidence of hematopoietic engraftment
   b. Constellation of signs and symptoms
   c. Time frame following transplant
   d. All of these

1. There are several causes of hepatic dysfunction following transplantation, some of which may mimic or coexist with venoocclusive disease. These include drug toxicity, viral hepatitis, and GVHD of

the liver. Viral hepatitis can be excluded with serologic tests and other methods of virus detection. The constellation of signs and symptoms (weight gain, ascites, jaundice, hepatomegaly, and a rising bilirubin) as well as their timing of onset (occurring within the first 20 days after transplant) are relatively specific for venoocclusive disease (Philpott & Kanfer, 1998). In addition, the signs of GVHD (whether of liver, skin, or gut) do not usually occur in the absence of early evidence of engraftment, as manifested by a rising WBC count. The skin rash may represent a petechial rash or may be caused by one or more medications. *Answer 1:* **d.**

QUESTIONS

2. Which of the following would place this patient at a higher risk for the development of acute GVHD?
   a. T-cell depletion
   b. Related, sex-matched donor as source of hematopoietic stem cells
   c. Younger patient/donor
   d. CMV or other viral infections after transplant

2. An unrelated donor or a sex-mismatched donor as the source of hematopoietic stem cells, increasing patient/donor age, and the occurrence of CMV or other viral infections after transplant are all associated with a higher risk for the development of GVHD (Socie & Cahn, 1998). *Answer 2:* **d.**

QUESTIONS

3. Using the clinical grading and staging system for acute GVHD given here, select the correct grade or stage of GVHD for the patients in the following scenarios:

 A. Adam, day +9 status post matched unrelated SCT. He has an erythematous skin rash covering all of his body surfaces, no diarrhea, and a bilirubin of 3.7 mg/dl.
  a. Stage III GVHD of the skin
  b. GVHD clinical grade I
  c. GVHD clinical grade II
  d. Stage IV GVHD of the liver
 B. Anne, day +79 status post related, sibling allogeneic T-cell depleted SCT. She has intermittent malar erythema, diarrhea of 500 to 700 ml/day, and a bilirubin of 2.2 mg/dl.
  a. Stage II GVHD of the skin
  b. Stage I GVHD of the gut
  c. Stage II GVHD of the liver
  d. GVHD clinical grade II

ANSWERS

3. GVHD is graded and staged according to the severity of the symptoms and the organ systems involved. GVHD grading/staging is important in describing patterns of response to therapies and in assessing outcomes of transplantation. The grading system for acute GVHD is given in Table 10-6. Adam demonstrates stage III skin with an erythematous skin rash covering most of his body. With a bilirubin of 3.7 mg/dl, his liver GVHD is stage II. Therefore his overall grade is GVHD clinical grade III.

Anne demonstrates GVHD of the skin stage I, GVHD of the gut stage II, and GVHD of the liver stage I. Therefore her overall grade is GVHD clinical grade II. *Answer 3A:* **a.** *Answer 3B:* **d.**

QUESTIONS

4. Strategies for the prevention or treatment of acute GVHD include all of the following *except:*
 a. Medications such as cyclosporine and tacrolimus that block the activation of donor T cells
 b. Monoclonal antibodies targeted to the interleukin (IL)-2 receptors on T cells
 c. Leucovorin
 d. Corticosteroids

5. All of the following statements about the prevention and treatment of acute GVHD are true *except:*
 a. Immunosuppression is usually discontinued approximately 6 months after HSCT
 b. The increased incidence and severity of GVHD following unrelated donor transplan-

TABLE 10-6 **Staging and Grading System for Acute GVHD**

CLINICAL GRADING OF INDIVIDUAL ORGAN SYSTEMS

ORGAN	GRADE	DESCRIPTION
Skin	+1	Maculopapular eruption over <25% of body area
	+2	Maculopapular eruption over 25%-50% of body area
	+3	Generalized erythroderma
	+4	Generalized erythroderma with bullous formation and often with desquamation
Liver	+1	Bilirubin 2.0-3.0 mg/dl
	+2	Bilirubin 3.1-6.0 mg/dl
	+3	Bilirubin 6.1-15 mg/dl
	+4	Bilirubin >15 mg/dl
Gut	+1	Diarrhea >500 ml/day
	+2	Diarrhea >1000 ml/day
	+3	Diarrhea >1500 ml/day
	+4	Diarrhea >2000 ml/day, or severe abdominal pain, or ileus

OVERALL STAGE

STAGE	SKIN	LIVER		GUT
I	+1 to +2	0		0
II	+1 to +3	+1	and/or	+1
III	+2 to +3	+2 to +3	and/or	+2 to +3
IV	+2 to +4	+2 to +4	and/or	+2 to +4

Note: If no skin disease is present, the overall grade is the higher single organ stage.

tation usually warrant the inclusion of at least three or more strategies for GVHD prevention.

c. Gut rest, hyperalimentation, pain control, and antimicrobial prophylaxis are important aspects of the supportive care of patients with acute GVHD.

d. The emphasis in current research is on methods of completely eliminating GVHD, thereby improving the overall outcomes of transplantation.

6. Patients receiving immunosuppression with Prograf or cyclosporine should be monitored for all of the following adverse effects of these drugs *except:*

    a. Electrolyte abnormalities

    b. Hepatotoxicity

    c. Hypotension

    d. Neurotoxicity

7. Which of the following would be an expected outcome of the teaching provided to patients and families regarding tacrolimus or cyclosporine?

    a. Patient states that headache, tremor, or confusion may occur intermittently on these therapies and do not reflect a serious problem.

    b. Patient states that if a dose of tacrolimus or cyclosporine is missed, 1.5 times the usual dose should be taken at the next regularly scheduled time.

    c. The patient should administer the usual dosage immediately before the clinic visit when drug levels will be drawn.

    d. Because of the many drug-drug and drug-food interactions, the patient takes tacrolimus or cyclosporine exactly as instructed by the health care team and contacts the health care team before starting any new medication and before changing the food/fluid taken with the dose.

8. Steroid doses are tapered orally every morning. The nurse caring for your patient asks why the dose must be administered in the morning. Your answer reflects your understanding that:

    a. This dosing schedule allows the medication to be effective throughout the day.

    b. The psychostimulatory effects of the steroid will have declined by the end of the day so that there is less disruption to the patient's sleep.

    c. Morning steroid administration promotes greater appetite and food intake throughout the day.

    d. The ulcerogenic effect of corticosteroids is blunted by early-morning administration.

9. During the tapering of immunosuppression, all of the following are indications for the patient to be seen in clinic *except:*

    a. New complaints of diarrhea, nausea, or vomiting

    b. Development of fevers

    c. Skin rash

    d. Aching pain in the joints

ANSWERS

4. The pharmacologic therapies commonly used for the prevention or treatment of acute GVHD along with some associated nursing implications are summarized in Table 10-7. Drugs known or suspected to interact with cyclosporine and tacrolimus are listed in Table 10-8.

Strategies for the prevention and treatment of GVHD include the use of medications that block the activation of T cells, monoclonal antibodies that target IL-2 receptors on T cells, and medications such as corticosteroids that inhibit lymphocyte function. Intravenous methotrexate in small doses for the first 2 weeks after the transplant is also a component of some regimens for the prevention and treatment of GVHD. *Answer 4:* **c.**

5. Gut rest, pain control, and antimicrobial prophylaxis coupled with hyperalimentation, if needed, are important aspects of the supportive care of patients with acute GVHD.

While there is a reduced incidence of GVHD associated with T-cell depletion, T-cell depletion has adverse effects on engraftment and results in an increased incidence of infection and leukemic relapse. IVIG has also been reported to significantly decrease the incidence and severity of GVHD, possibly because it reduces the incidence of posttransplant infection. If the patient's symptoms are within acceptable limits or if there is no evidence of GVHD, the immunosuppressive therapy is slowly tapered and eventually discontinued. The plan for tapering is determined by the transplant program, and regular feedback to the transplant team regarding the patient's progress and tolerance of the taper needs to occur. Unrelated HSCT places the patient at significantly increased risks of GVHD, and often, three or more strategies are used to prevent or treat GVHD. In addition, the process of tapering immunosuppres-

TABLE **10-7** Side Effects and Nursing Implications of Selected Immunosuppressants Used in Allogeneic Stem Cell Transplantation

THERAPY	MECHANISM OF ACTION	SIDE EFFECTS	NURSING IMPLICATIONS
Cyclosporine (Sandimmune, Neoral)	Prevents IL-2 gene expression and activation of T lymphocytes	Hypertension, renal toxicity, hirsutism, hypokalemia or hyperkalemia, hypomagnesemia, flushing, paresthesias, tremor, thrombotic thrombocytopenic purpura	Bioavailability differs between oral solution and capsule formulation. Once a regimen is established, patients should be instructed not to change to the formulation. Take with food. Instruct patient on importance of strict adherence to the administration schedule and to notify the health care team immediately if unable to take because of gastrointestinal side effects. Monitor serum creatinine, BUN, potassium. Avoid potassium-sparing diuretics. Coadministration with grapefruit juice may increase cyclosporine levels and should be avoided. Drug-drug interactions can lead to subtherapeutic or toxic cyclosporine levels. Drugs that inhibit or induce cytochrome P450 are most responsible (see Table 10-6). Dosage depends on achieving and sustaining therapeutic blood levels based on laboratory evaluation. Therapeutic monitoring not required once drug is being tapered. Cyclosporine trough levels to be drawn before administration of morning dose. Therefore doses are usually timed for 10 AM and 10 PM to allow trough blood draw at morning clinic visit. Instruct patient to bring dose to clinic and to administer once trough level is drawn. Total daily dose is usually 1.5 mg/kg IV q12h or 3 mg/kg/day as a continuous infusion, with dosage adjusted to achieve therapeutic levels. IV-to-PO conversion is approximately 1:3. Should not be used simultaneously with tacrolimus. Tacrolimus should be discontinued 24 hr before starting cyclosporine. In the presence of increased tacrolimus levels, initiation of cyclosporine should usually be further delayed.
Tacrolimus (Prograf)	Impaired synthesis of IL-2; prevents T-lymphocyte proliferation	Nephrotoxicity, neurotoxicity, hypomagnesemia, hyperkalemia, worsened hyperglycemia, hypertension, hirsutism, hypercholesterolemia, gingival hyperplasia	Take on an empty stomach. Instruct patient on importance of strict adherence to the administration schedule and to notify the health care team immediately if unable to take because of gastrointestinal side effects. Monitor serum creatinine, BUN, potassium, and glucose. Avoid potassium-sparing diuretics. Coadministration with grapefruit juice may increase tacrolimus levels and should be avoided.

Adapted from Bush, W. W. (1999). Overview of transplantation immunology and the pharmacotherapy of adult solid organ transplant recipients: Focus on immunosuppression. *AACN Clin Iss, 10*(2), pp. 253-269; and Solimando, D. (1998). Medications. In Burt, R. K., Deeg, H. J., Lothian, S., & Santos, G. W. (Eds.). *Bone marrow transplantation* (pp. 544-566). Austin: Landes Bioscience.
IL, Interleukin; *BUN*, blood urea nitrogen; *CBC*, complete blood count; *GVHD*, graft-versus-host disease. *Continued*

THERAPY	MECHANISM OF ACTION	SIDE EFFECTS	NURSING IMPLICATIONS
			Drug-drug interactions can lead to subtherapeutic or toxic tacrolimus levels. Drugs that inhibit or induce cytochrome P450 are most responsible (see Table 10-6).
			Dosage depends on achieving and sustaining therapeutic blood levels based on laboratory evaluation. Therapeutic monitoring not required once drug is being tapered.
			Tacrolimus trough levels to be drawn before administration of morning dose. Therefore doses are usually timed for 10 AM and 10 PM to allow trough blood draw at morning clinic visit. Instruct patient to bring dose to clinic and to administer once trough level is drawn.
			Total daily dose is usually 1-2 mg PO q12h or 0.05-0.1 mg/kg/day as a continuous infusion, with dosage adjusted to achieve therapeutic levels.
			IV-to-PO conversion is approximately 1:4.
Steroids	Apoptosis, stabilization of leukocyte lysosomal membrane, inhibition of chemotaxis and cytokine release	Hyperglycemia, hypertension, insomnia, euphoria, depression, gastritis, peptic ulcers, fluid and electrolyte alterations, headache, skin atrophy, blurred vision, cataracts, aseptic necrosis, myopathy, impaired wound healing, cushingoid state, adrenal insufficiency	Usually used in combination with cyclosporine or tacrolimus. Dosage ranges from 0.5-2 mg/kg/day q12h, with tapering scheduled determined based on starting dosage and patient response. Report complaints of visual changes. Consult ophthalmology. Consult physical therapy for proximal muscle-strengthening exercise program. Instruct patient in strategies to prevent or treat hyperglycemia and in diabetic self-management. Administer oral corticosteroids with food or milk to minimize gastrointestinal upset. Administer H_2 blockers as ordered.
Mycophenolate mofetil (MMF; CellCept)	Antimetabolite that selectively inhibits the proliferation of T and B lymphocytes by interfering with purine nucleotide synthesis	Myelosuppression, hypertension, tremor, diarrhea, nausea and vomiting, hypokalemia, hypophosphatemia, hyperkalemia	MMF should be taken on an empty stomach. Dosage ranges from 1-1.5 g q12h depending on institutional guidelines. Monitor CBC at regular intervals and adjust dosage for pancytopenia as ordered. Monitor liver function tests (bilirubin and serum transaminases) at regular intervals and adjust dosage for liver function abnormalities as ordered. Drug interactions with magnesium oxide and aluminum- or magnesium-containing antacids. Cholestyramine may result in decreased MMF absorption with coadministration.
Methotrexate	Irreversible inhibition of dihydrofolate reductase; methotrexate's immunosuppressive activity may be due to inhibition of lymphocyte multiplication	Myelosuppression, mucositis, photosensitivity	Methotrexate prophylaxis for GVHD varies by institution. A common regimen is MTX 5-15 mg/m² on days 1, 3, 6, and 11 posttransplant. Dosages may be adjusted or held for mucositis and renal or liver insufficiency.

Adapted from Bush, W. W. (1999). Overview of transplantation immunology and the pharmacotherapy of adult solid organ transplant recipients: Focus on immunosuppression. *AACN Clin Iss, 10*(2), pp. 253-269; and Solimando, D. (1998). Medications. In Burt, R. K., Deeg, H. J., Lothian, S., & Santos, G. W. (Eds.). *Bone marrow transplantation* (pp. 544-566). Austin: Landes Bioscience.

TABLE 10-8 Drugs Known or Suspected to Interact with Cyclosporine and Tacrolimus		
EFFECTS	**KNOWN INTERACTIONS**	**SUSPECTED INTERACTIONS**
Drugs increasing the serum levels of cyclosporine or tacrolimus	Erythromycin Clarithromycin Itraconazole Fluconazole Ketoconazole Corticosteroids	H_2 antagonists Cephalosporins Thiazide diuretics Furosemide Acyclovir Warfarin Calcium channel blockers (i.e., diltiazem, verapamil, nicardipine) Oral contraceptives Doxycycline Metoclopramide Coadministration with grapefruit juice
Drugs decreasing the serum levels of cyclosporine or tacrolimus Drugs causing additive nephrotoxicity	Phenytoin or phenobarbitone Rifampin or isoniazid Sulfadimidine + trimethoprim (IV) Amphotericin B Aminoglycosides Melphalan Cotrimoxazole-trimethoprim	Sulfinpyrazone Carbamazepine Anticonvulsants Nonsteroidal antiinflammatory agents
Alteration of immuno-suppressive effects		Propanolol Verapamil Etoposide

Adapted from Melocco, T., Kerr, S., & McKenzie, C. (1994). Drug toxicity and interactions posttransplant. In Atkinson, K. (Ed.). *Clinical bone marrow transplantation: A clinical textbook* (pp. 396-409). Cambridge: Cambridge University Press.

sion proceeds over a much longer period. Research has shown that the elimination of GVHD is associated with a higher rate of disease relapse and thus a poorer overall outcome of transplantation. This has been called the *graft-versus-leukemia* (GVL) or *graft-versus-tumor effect.* The GVL effect is an immune response of the donor cells against the recipient's tumor cells. Studies have also shown that it is possible to have the beneficial effects of GVL without clinically apparent GVHD. Current research efforts are oriented toward better understanding the mechanisms of GVHD and of the GVL effect so that strategies can be defined that augment the GVL effect while minimizing or separating it from GVHD (Mavroudis, 1998). *Answer 5:* **d.**

6. Patients receiving immunosuppression with Prograf or cyclosporine should be monitored for electrolyte abnormalities, hepatotoxicity, and neurotoxicity. Hypotension is not associated with Prograf or cyclosporine. *Answer 6:* **c.**

7. Patients taking tacrolimus or cyclosporine should understand that many drug-drug and drug-food interactions can occur. Therefore it is important that the patient take the medication exactly as instructed by the health care team and

contact the team before starting any new medication and before changing the food/fluid taken with the dose. *Answer 7:* **d.**

8. When steroids are tapered, the dosing schedule does not influence therapeutic efficacy. Furthermore, the ulcerogenic and appetite simulation effects of corticosteroids occur irrespective of the schedule or route of administration. However, administering steroids earlier in the day can minimize the sleep disruption that some patients experience when steroids are given in the evening. *Answer 8:* **b.**

9. During steroid tapering, patients often develop bilateral pain in the distal femur and tibia, often occurring at night (Buckley, 1998). This pain responds well to treatment with opioids.

During the process of tapering immunosuppression, it is important that the patient be observed closely for the accelerated development of signs and symptoms of GVHD. This includes the earliest reporting of GI symptoms such as nausea, vomiting, diarrhea, or abdominal pain. The development of a new or worsening skin rash should also be reported immediately. The patient should have LFTs monitored and a clinical examination at least weekly or biweekly. The emergence of symptoms of GVHD while receiving tapering doses of immunosuppression may require a temporary increase in the immunosuppression or a slowing of the rate at which the immunosuppression is tapered. The development of fever may be associated with GVHD, but it may also indicate a bacterial, fungal, or viral infection, especially in a patient who has been receiving long-term immunosuppression. *Answer 9:* **d.**

CASE | STUDY

Charles Jones continued from p. 152. Mr. Jones has been hospitalized for about 45 days since his transplant, and he has developed fairly severe proximal muscle weakness. He will be transferred to a rehabilitation facility to develop better strength and endurance before his transfer home. Mrs. Jones comes to you as the APN for the unit and expresses worry that the staff in the rehabilitation facility may be unfamiliar with the care of patients who have had an allogeneic transplant.

QUESTIONS

1. How do you respond to Mrs. Jones's concerns?
   a. Inform her that you will contact the charge nurse at the rehabilitation facility and offer to send articles on SCT to the staff
   b. Reassure her that you will make regular visits to the rehabilitation facility so that you can monitor the quality of care being provided to Mr. Jones by the rehabilitation staff and assist them in meeting their information needs
   c. Offer to contact the nurse manager, nurse educator, or APN for the rehabilitation unit to discuss the patient's transfer, to discuss his ongoing care needs, and to jointly develop strategies to ensure that the patient's needs continue to be met effectively
   d. Show her an example of the detailed transfer of care summary that accompanies all patients when they are transferred from the transplant unit to another care setting

ANSWERS

1. Transitions in care can expose or intensify feelings of fear, vulnerability, and helplessness. Caregivers in all settings can encourage patients and families to verbalize their feelings and provide reassurance and support as well as encourage realistic planning and problem solving. Although contacting the charge nurse at the rehabilitation facility may be initially helpful, sending articles on transplantation may be of only limited utility in ensuring that Mr. Jones's ongoing needs are met.

Similarly, a detailed transfer of care summary should accompany the patient, but limiting the APN interventions to this approach assumes that simply communicating about patient needs will ensure that those needs are met. Having the APN make regular visits to the rehabilitation facility is probably not practical, evokes liability and territoriality issues, and places unnecessary duress on the APN's time. In addition, this option may reinforce Mrs. Jones's concerns and limit the degree to which she can build trust and confidence in new caregiving personnel. The APN can be helpful by reaching out to the rehabilitation setting to discuss the patient's transfer and ongoing needs; explore their questions, concerns, and issues regarding his care; offer the resources of the transplant center (e.g., literature, ongoing availability for questions); and help them develop strategies to solve problems. Members of the rehabilitation team might also be invited to spend some time observing on the transplant unit so that they can better understand the care needs of patients undergoing transplantation. *Answer 1:* **c.**

Case Study continued

Now 115 days status post allogeneic SCT, Mr. Jones presents at clinic with watery diarrhea of at least 500 ml/day. He indicates that he has been taking a low-residue diet in moderate quantities and consuming at least 1200 ml/day of oral fluids, although most of that oral intake is in the form of cola. He has lost 4 kg since his clinic visit 1 week ago. His immunosuppressive drug level is subtherapeutic, although he states he has been adherent with his usual dose of 1 mg orally every 12 hours.

QUESTIONS

2. What additional laboratory data and physical assessment data are needed to formulate a plan for Mr. Jones?
   a. Abdominal examination, CBC with differential, and orthostatic vital signs

b. Stool cultures, *Clostridium difficile* toxin, abdominal examination, digital rectal examination

c. Stool for *C. difficile* toxin, bacterial and viral stool cultures, LFTs, electrolytes, BUN, creatinine, urine specific gravity

d. Stool for ova and parasites, *C. difficile* toxin, plain films of the abdomen

ANSWERS

2. This presentation is suspicious for either infection (e.g., CMV, adenovirus, rotavirus, enterovirus, *C. difficile*), medication-related toxicity (e.g., antibiotics, promotility GI drugs such as metoclopramide), or GVHD. The tests in answer c will help establish whether there is evidence of GVHD in the liver function tests or on skin examination. Assessment of BUN, creatinine, electrolytes, and urine specific gravity will help gauge the degree of dehydration Mr. Jones is experiencing. Fluid support can then be determined. Plain films of the abdomen might be helpful if Mr. Jones was experiencing severe abdominal pain or had absent bowel sounds and you wanted to evaluate for evidence of obstruction or free air. *Answer 2:* **c.**

Case Study continued

On examination, Mr. Jones's has no skin rashes. He has some mild diffuse abdominal tenderness but no rebound or guarding. Bowel sounds are normoactive and present in four quadrants. There is no organomegaly, and the right upper quadrant is nontender. He has a low-grade temperature of 37.7° C and is tachypneic with respirations of 12 breaths/min, blood pressure of 90/56 mm Hg standing and 130/88 mm Hg lying, and a pulse of 100 beats/min. His LFTs demonstrate a slightly increased alkaline phosphatase, AST, and ALT compared with his previous levels. Total bilirubin and LDH are stable. Hemoglobin and hematocrit are stable; however, there has been a negligible decline in the platelet and total WBC counts.

QUESTIONS

3. What are the most likely differential diagnoses for the diarrhea?
   1. Effects of total body irradiation
   2. *C. difficile* infection
   3. Viral enteritis
   4. GVHD of the GI tract
   5. GI bleeding
   a. 4 & 5
   b. 2, 3, 4, & 5

c. 2, 3, & 4
d. All of these

ANSWERS

3. Diarrhea with crampy abdominal pain is suggestive of infection or GVHD. Microbial entities such as CMV, rotavirus, enterovirus, adenovirus, *C. difficile*, cryptosporidium, *Salmonella*, shigella, or campylobacter are all possibilities. Regimen-related toxicity from total body irradiation and chemotherapy would not be etiologic in symptoms that are occurring more than 100 days after transplantation. GI bleeding is an unlikely cause because his hemoglobin and hematocrit levels are stable; however, this etiology can also be promptly evaluated by sending a stool for guaiac. *Answer 3:* **c.**

QUESTIONS

4. Appropriate interventions include all of the following *except:*
   a. Administering a liter of fluid in the clinic, encouraging Mr. Jones to increase his Gatorade intake, and monitoring his stool output carefully over the next 2 days
   b. Admitting Mr. Jones to the hospital for intravenous immunosuppression, intravenous hydration, and intravenous antimicrobials
   c. Consulting gastroenterology regarding the need for endoscopy
   d. Prescribing Imodium 2 capsules orally after each loose bowel movement; maximum daily dose of 8 capsules

ANSWERS

4. Mr. Jones requires admission for intravenous immunosuppression because in the setting of watery diarrhea of more than 500 ml/day, absorption of his immunosuppressive agent is likely to be erratic. Evidence of his poor drug absorption is provided by his low levels. If this is GVHD of the gut, inadequate immunosuppression will simply worsen the picture. In addition, Mr. Jones requires adequate antimicrobial coverage, and this cannot likely be achieved by the oral route given his diarrhea. Last, his severe orthostatic hypotension clarifies the need for aggressive fluid support. The fact that his hemoglobin and hematocrit levels are normal may reflect his relative hemoconcentration secondary to dehydration; therefore, with rehydration, one would expect to see a decline in his hematocrit, possibly to a level that will require transfusion support. While awaiting the results of stool cultures, Mr. Jones could begin therapy with Imodium or another antidiarrheal agent. Arrangements should be made for consultation with gastroenterology regarding lower endoscopy because a diagnosis of GVHD of the gut would significantly affect the tempo of any further tapering of his immunosuppression, and if infectious, organism-specific antimicrobials can be instituted. *Answer 4:* **a.**

QUESTIONS

5. Which of the following statements is true regarding the diarrhea of GVHD?
1. Chemotherapy-induced diarrhea and GVHD-related diarrhea result from a similar pathophysiology, with the result that both create absorptive and secretory imbalances in the small bowel.
2. Comprehensive assessment of the patient with chemotherapy-related diarrhea requires only documentation of the number of stools per day and stool cultures for bacterial, fungal, and viral pathogens.
3. No data are currently available to support the use of the somatostatin analog octreotide in controlling diarrhea associated with GVHD of the gut; loperamide, diphenoxylate, and codeine are considered the gold standard for the treatment of such diarrhea.
4. The presence of altered mucosal integrity of the gut does not alter the risk of suprainfection by opportunistic pathogens.
   a. 1 & 2
   b. 1, 2, & 3
   c. None of these
   d. All of these

ANSWERS

5. None of the preceding statements is true. Although the histologic damage to the intestinal mucosa in GVHD is similar to damage caused by chemotherapy, resulting in an imbalance of absorptive and secretory functions within the small bowel, the pathophysiology of these two processes is quite different (Kornblau, Benson, Catalano, et al., 2000). Preclinical and clinical studies show that in GVHD of the gut, donor-derived alloreactive cytotoxic T lymphocytes cause apoptosis and necrosis of crypt cells within the intestinal mucosa, whereas chemotherapy induces acute damage to the intestinal mucosa by arresting mitosis of intestinal epithelial cells. The pathophysiologic changes associated with intestinal GVHD as well as mucositis-induced mucosal damage increase the risk of suprainfection by opportunistic pathogens such as *C. difficile, Clostridium perfringens, Bacillus cereus, Giardia lamblia,* cryptospo-

ridium, *Salmonella,* shigella, campylobacter, and rotavirus (Kornblau, Benson, Catalano, et al., 2000). Comprehensive assessment of the patient with diarrhea includes not only the number of stools per day but also the stool volume, the presence of nocturnal stools or episodes of incontinence, the presence of perianal skin breakdown, abdominal pain, cramping, and tenesmus (urgency), as well as the presence of hypoalbuminemia and dehydration. Evaluation should also include a review of medications to identify those that cause diarrhea and a dietary review to identify foods such as dairy products and those with high fat or caffeine content that may stimulate diarrhea. Several small, uncontrolled studies have reported that octreotide is effective in controlling or significantly reducing diarrhea in many patients with GVHD (Ippoliti, Champlin, & Bugazia, 1997). *Answer 5:* **c.**

QUESTIONS

6. Which of the following actions related to nutritional management are most appropriate for Mr. Jones?
   a. Reinitiation of total parenteral nutrition
   b. Initiation of enteral nutrition support with a feeding tube
   c. Trial of an adjusted diet to eliminate foods and drinks containing lactose and caffeine and foods high in fat and fiber
   d. Initiation of nothing-by-mouth (NPO) status for a few days to provide gut rest, followed by the commencement of a diet of clear liquids only

ANSWERS

6. A trial of eliminating lactose, caffeine, fat, and fiber from the diet might be a possible action; however, given that the patient has more than 500 ml/day of watery diarrhea and is dehydrated, gut rest is probably the best initial course of action. GI involvement with GVHD can result in nausea, vomiting, anorexia, abdominal cramping and pain, secretory diarrhea, bloody stools, altered intestinal motility, malabsorption, and ileus. Optimal nutritional support is an important complement to the therapy of acute GI GVHD. Empiric guidelines for the progression of nutrition support in the patient with GVHD have been proposed by Gauvreau, Lenssen, Cheney, et al. (1981). Returning the patient to NPO for a few days, with progression of the diet to clear liquids, is the first stage in the five-stage nutrition plan, and this is clinically indicated in a patient with severe symptoms of intestinal involvement, as manifested by high-volume diarrhea with more than 1000 ml of stool output, accompanied by severe cramping, bloody diarrhea, and nausea or vomiting. In this case Mr. Jones may try adjusting his diet to eliminate lactose, caffeine, and foods high in fat and fiber, coupled with multiple small feedings. His progress with these changes must be monitored. Enteral nutritional support with a feeding tube is contraindicated in bone marrow transplant recipients with diarrhea, nausea, and vomiting secondary to the risks of increasing diarrhea and/or aspiration pneumonia (Bergerson, 1998). Initiation of total parenteral nutrition may be indicated if Mr. Jones's diarrhea persists, a more prolonged period of bowel rest is indicated, or his oral intake decreases to less than 1000 kcal/day or less than 60% of estimated caloric needs for more than 3 to 5 days (Bergerson, 1998). *Answer 6:* **d.**

QUESTIONS

7. You are working with an experienced oncology nursing staff. They have requested assistance with symptom management in patients like Mr. Jones who are experiencing diarrhea. Assuming that you share the staff's assessment that this is an important issue to address on the unit at this time, which of the following strategies would you choose to respond to their request?
   a. Perform a detailed audit of current care delivery practices for patients with diarrhea and conduct a comprehensive staff learning needs assessment
   b. Organize an in-service addressing the problem of diarrhea and presenting current literature addressing assessment, prevention, and management of this symptom complex
   c. Expand your caseload to focus on providing direct care to patients with diarrhea
   d. Work with a small group of interested staff to review the literature and develop an evidence-based protocol for assessment, management, and evaluation of patients with GVHD-associated diarrhea

ANSWERS

7. As the APN in this situation, you have the opportunity to role model evidence-based practice by working with a small group of interested staff to review the literature and develop a protocol, algorithm, or standard of care for the assessment, prevention, and management of diarrhea. Although presenting an in-service may achieve the goal of sharing content, it tends not to involve the adult learner actively. A limited survey of current care delivery practices for patients with diarrhea and a focused staff learning needs assessment could emerge from the small work group; however, a detailed audit or a comprehensive learning needs assessment deflect emphasis from the specific request made by an experienced staff. Expanding your caseload to focus on providing direct care to patients with diarrhea may improve the care provided to those specific patients, but beyond role modeling approaches to problem solving, this solution does little to affect the overall quality of care on the unit and may in fact not be a cost-effective or productive use of the advanced practice expertise. Your direct care and consultation role could be built into the protocol or algorithm, in terms of becoming involved when symptoms do not come under control in the expected time frame or in situations of particular severity. *Answer 7:* **d.**

Case Study continued

Mr. Jones is seen on follow-up day +160 status post related allogeneic transplantation for CML. His early posttransplant course was complicated by CMV reactivation and a skin rash reported as positive for grade II GVHD. Over the past 2 months, Mr. Jones has been doing quite well, although he did experience a flare of gut and liver GVHD that resolved with a modest increase in his steroid dosage. He is currently receiving Medrol 16 mg orally every other day, alternating with 24 mg orally every other day. When seen in clinic, he indicates that he has fatigue, dryness of his mouth and eyes, and mild dysphagia, reporting some difficulty swallowing foods that are dry (e.g., sandwiches). His skin is overall dry, with patches of erythema and flakiness. He is working as an accountant a few hours each day from home. He indicates that his legs are weak and that he has some difficulty climbing stairs or getting up off the toilet. Laboratory data include the following: sodium, 137 mEq/L; potassium, 3.1 mEq/L; chloride, 104 mEq/L; CO_2, 23 mEq/L; glucose, 151 mg/dl; BUN, 36 mg/dl; creatinine, 0.9 mg/dl; magnesium, 1.1 mEq/L; phosphorus, 2.0 mEq/L; and calcium, 8.6 mEq/L.

QUESTIONS

8. All of the following factors place Mr. Jones at greatest risk for the development of chronic GVHD *except:*
   a. His underlying disease
   b. Positive skin or oral biopsy at day +100 posttransplant

c. Use of peripheral blood stem cells instead of bone marrow
d. History of acute GVHD

9. Which of Mr. Jones's symptoms is least likely to be attributed directly to chronic GVHD?
a. Muscle weakness
b. Ocular dryness
c. Skin rash with patches of erythema and flakiness
d. Dysphagia with dry foods

10. All of the following interventions would likely be implemented immediately to address Mr. Jones's leg weakness *except:*
a. Magnesium sulfate 8 g intravenously over 4 hours
b. MagOxide 400 mg orally three times daily, Chloe-Con 20 mEq orally three times daily, and Neutra-Phos 1 packet orally three times daily
c. Electromyographic (EMG) studies and MRI of the pelvis and head of femur bilaterally to rule out avascular necrosis
d. Physical therapy for muscle-strengthening exercises

ANSWERS

8. Traditionally, GVHD that presents beyond day +100 posttransplant is called *chronic GVHD.* It is now thought that symptoms of chronic GVHD, both by clinical and histologic criteria, can occur as early as 50 days after transplant (Chao, 1998).

Risk factors for chronic GVHD are similar to those for acute GVHD and include a positive skin or oral biopsy, a history of acute GVHD, and the use of peripheral blood stem cells. The underlying disease process does not influence the incidence or extent of GVHD. *Answer 8:* **a.**

9. Chronic GVHD may present immediately after the acute process, after an interval in which the patient is free of GVHD, or without any prior evidence of GVHD.

With limited chronic GVHD, there is skin involvement with or without mild hepatic dysfunction. With extensive chronic GVHD, there is more generalized skin involvement, as well as more severe hepatic involvement. There may also be ocular, oral, or other organ involvement (GI tract, lung, genitourinary). Muscle weakness often occurs in patients with GVHD; however, it is generally attributable in large measure to steroid myopathy, rather than being a direct result of GVHD. *Answer 9:* **a.**

10. The cause of Mr. Jones's proximal muscle weakness is most likely steroid myopathy related

to long-term therapy with glucocorticosteroids, coupled with hypomagnesemia and hypokalemia. Mild hypophsophatemia (1.0 to 2.5 mg/dl) is usually asymptomatic. The degree of electrolyte depletion is such that oral therapy alone is likely to be inadequate. Intravenous and oral repletion is indicated. Corticosteroids often produce myopathy, which can be progressive. The weakness typically has an insidious onset but may be sudden. The fluorinated corticosteroids, such as dexamethasone, betamethasone, or triamolone, are more often implicated in the development of steroid myopathy (Teener & Farrar, 1998).

Physical therapy can prevent further decline in the proximal muscle strength, which will inevitably result without immediate implementation of an aggressive program of isometric muscle-strengthening exercises. EMG studies might be indicated if muscle weakness continues to progress despite optimizing the serum electrolytes and engaging in a consistent program of physical therapy.

Table 10-9 summarizes the clinical manifestations, screening/evaluation, and potential interventions for chronic GVHD. *Answer 10:* **c.**

Case Study continued

At day +168 posttransplant, Mr. Jones's CBC demonstrates the following: WBC count, 1.3/mm^3, with 63% neutrophils; Hgb, 8.9 g/dl; Hct, 24.8%; and platelets, 9/mm^3.

Medications
Medrol 30 mg orally twice daily
Prograf 1 mg orally twice daily
Ganciclovir 5 mg/kg twice daily
Itraconazole suspension 200 mg orally twice daily
Zantac 150 mg orally twice daily
Multivites without iron 1 tablet orally daily
Folic acid 1 mg orally daily
Bactrim DS 1 tablet orally on Mondays, Wednesdays, and Fridays
Epogen 40,000 units subcutaneously every week
G-CSF 400 µg subcutaneously every other day
Vitamin B$_{12}$ 1000 µg every month
IVIG 40 g intravenously every 2 weeks

QUESTIONS

11. All of the following etiologies could explain Mr. Jones's pancytopenia *except:*
1. CMV infection
2. GVHD
3. Folate or vitamin B$_{12}$ deficiencies
4. Drug-induced myelosuppression
5. Disease relapse
a. 1, 2, & 4
b. 1, 2, 3, & 4
c. All of these except 3
d. All of these

TABLE **10-9** Chronic Graft-versus-Host Disease: Clinical Manifestations, Screening/Evaluation, and Interventions

ORGAN/SYSTEM	CLINICAL MANIFESTATIONS	SCREENING STUDIES/ EVALUATION	INTERVENTIONS
Dermal	Dyspigmentation, xerosis (dryness), hyperkeratosis, pruritus, scleroderma, lichenification, onychodystrophy (nail ridging/nail loss), alopecia	Clinical examination Skin biopsy—3-mm punch biopsy from forearm	Immunosuppressive therapy Psoralen and ultraviolet irradiation (PUVA) Topical with steroid creams, moisturizers/emollient, antibacterial ointments to prevent suprainfection Avoid sunlight exposure, use sunblock lotion with a large hat that shades the face when outdoors
Oral	Lichen planus, xerostomia, ulceration	Oral biopsy	Steroid mouth rinses, oral PUVA, pilocarpine and anetholetrithione for xerostomia, fluoride gels/rinses Careful attention to oral hygiene; regular dental evaluations
Ocular	Keratitis, sicca syndrome	Schirmer's test, ophthalmic evaluation	Regular ophthalmologic follow-up Preservative-free tears and moisturizing lotions Temporary or permanent lacrimal duct occlusion
Hepatic	Jaundice, abdominal pain	Liver function tests	Actigall 300 mg PO tid
Pulmonary	Shortness of breath, cough, dyspnea, wheezing, fatigue, hypoxia, pleural effusion	Pulmonary function studies, peak flow, arterial blood gas, computed tomography scan of chest	Prevent and treat pulmonary infections Aggressively investigate changes in pulmonary function because these may represent GVHD of lung/bronchiolitis obliterans
Gastrointestinal	Nausea, odynophagia, dysphagia, anorexia, early satiety, malabsorption, diarrhea, weight loss	Esophagogastroduodenoscopy, colonoscopy, nutritional assessment, fecal studies	Referral to gastroenterologist, nutrition support
Nutritional	Protein and calorie deficiency, malabsorption, dehydration, weight loss, muscle wasting	Weight, fat store measurement, prealbumin	Nutritional monitoring, supplementation, symptom-specific interventions
Genitourinary	Vaginal sicca, vaginal atrophy, stenosis or inflammation	Pelvic examination	Efficacy of intravaginal steroid cream currently being evaluated

Based on information from Buchsel, Leum, & Randolph (1996); Chao (1998); Gold, Flowers, & Sullivan (1998); and Seber & Vogelsang (1998).
GVHD, Graft-versus-host disease; *CMV,* cytomegalovirus; *HSV,* herpes simplex virus; *VZV,* varicella-zoster virus; *PCP, Pneumocystis carinii* pneumonia.
Continued

TABLE 10-9 | Chronic Graft-versus-Host Disease: Clinical Manifestations, Screening/Evaluation, and Interventions—cont'd

ORGAN/SYSTEM	CLINICAL MANIFESTATIONS	SCREENING STUDIES/ EVALUATION	INTERVENTIONS
Immunologic	Hypogammaglobulin-emia; autoimmune syndromes; recurrent infections, including CMV, HSV, VZV, fungus, PCP, and encapsulated bacteria	Quantitative immuno-globulin levels, CD4/CD8 lymphocyte subsets	Intravenous immunoglob-ulins and prophylactic antimicrobials (rotating antibiotics, PCP prophylaxis) CMV screening with frequent surveillance cultures and antigen detection
Musculoskeletal	Contractures, debility, muscle cramps	Performance status, formal quality-of-life evaluation, rehabilita-tion needs	Physical therapy

Based on information from Buchsel, Leum, & Randolph (1996); Chao (1998); Gold, Flowers, & Sullivan (1998); and Seber & Vogelsang (1998).

ANSWERS

11. Folate and vitamin B_{12} deficiencies are less likely to cause pancytopenia because the patient is receiving folic acid and vitamin B_{12} supplementa-tion. An important cause of pancytopenia and graft failure following transplantation or high-dose therapy is drug-induced myelosuppression. Agents such as ganciclovir, Bactrim, selected antidepressants, oral hypoglycemic agents, and the benzodiazepines can all cause myelosuppres-sion. *Answer 11:* **c.**

QUESTIONS

12. In determining the cause of his graft failure and developing a plan for its management, all of the following studies would most likely be ordered *except:*

    1. Bone marrow aspirate and biopsy, cytogenetics

    2. CMV antigen and 24-hour urine for creati-nine clearance

    3. CBC with differential

        a. 1 & 2

        b. 2 & 3

        c. 1 & 3

        d. All of these

ANSWERS

12. All of the preceding studies except the CBC with differential would be helpful in suggesting or excluding a cause of the graft failure and/or establishing a plan for its management. A CBC with differential would confirm pancytopenia but would not help clarify the cause. The bone marrow aspirate and biopsy will evaluate marrow function, establish the presence of trilinear hematopoiesis,

and determine cellularity. Cytogenetics are neces-sary to exclude the possibility of leukemic relapse. Chimeric studies (e.g., variable nucleotide tandem repeats [VNTR], restriction fragment length poly-morphisms [RFLP], cytogenetics) will establish the relative percentage of donor and host cells and thus confirm whether the established hematopoie-sis is of host or donor origin. CMV antigen will confirm the outcome of his ganciclovir treatment, and a 24-hour urine for creatinine clearance will help determine whether a dosage adjustment in his ganciclovir is necessary. *Answer 12:* **c.**

Case Study conclusion

Hematopoiesis in the posttransplant patient may be more susceptible to the myelosuppressive influence of various drugs. Ganciclovir is com-monly used for the treatment of CMV infections after SCT and causes dose-dependent myelosup-pression. Its use in patients who have not achieved solid engraftment or its continued use in patients with ganciclovir-induced myelosuppres-sion can result in graft failure. The ganciclovir dosage may also need to be adjusted for renal insufficiency, particularly in the setting of con-comitant use of several nephrotoxic agents (e.g., program, itraconazole). Although H_2-receptor blocking agents are generally safe drugs, both cimetidine and ranitidine have been shown to cause myelosuppression after cytoreductive treat-ment for leukemia and SCT and may need to be avoided. This is also the case with benzodiaz-epines and cotrimoxazole. Risk factors, possible causes for graft failure, and measures to prevent this complication are summarized in Table 10-10.

TABLE 10-10 Graft Failure: Risk Factors, Causes, and Preventive Measures

	RISK FACTORS	CAUSE	PREVENTIVE/SUPPORTIVE MEASURES
Autologous stem cell transplants	Patients with AML, patients extensively pretreated Low cell dose Purged marrow Marrow-suppressive drugs Viral infection	Defective marrow microenvironment, with stromal cell damage Collection of damaged stem cells from extensive previous treatment Drug-induced myelosuppression Viral effects on stroma of bone marrow	Harvest autologous stem cells early, before multiple cycles of potentially stem cell–toxic regimens have been given. Maximize the number of infused cells (the minimum number of autologous peripheral blood stem cells that results in consistent engraftment is at least 1×10^6 CD34+ cells/kg of body weight, below which engraftment may be incomplete or there may be failure of engraftment). Avoid all myelosuppressive drugs after transplantation. Adjust dosages of medications for renal dysfunction. Treat/prevent viral infections. Keep unmanipulated cells as a backup in case of purged or manipulated grafts. Ensure that there is no folate or vitamin B_{12} deficiency. Administer G-CSF and rEPO as needed.
Allogeneic stem cell transplants	Diseases associated with a defective marrow microenvironment, including aplastic anemia and myelofibrosis Stem cell source from HLA-mismatched, unrelated, or cord blood donor Pretransplant transfusions, especially from a related donor T-cell depletion, low cell dose, purging Patients whose clinical condition precludes a sufficiently intensive conditioning regimen Inadequate posttransplant immunosuppression Marrow suppressive drugs Viral infection, including infection with CMV	Defective marrow microenvironment with stromal cell damage Histocompatibility barriers Allosensitization by transfusions Damaged or inadequate number of stem cells infused Persistence of host hematopoiesis Persistence of immunocompetent host lymphocytes GVHD-associated damage to the bone marrow microenvironment Drug-induced myelosuppression Viral effects on stroma of bone marrow	Avoid pretransplant transfusions, especially from relatives. Select histocompatible donors. Ensure that the conditioning regimen is adequately immunosuppressive. Provide sufficient stem cell dose (for peripheral blood stem cells, at least 2×10^6 CD34+ cells/kg of body weight, below which engraftment may be incomplete or there may be failure of engraftment). Use posttransplant immunosuppression with cyclosporine, tacrolimus, and/or methotrexate. Avoid all myelosuppressive drugs after transplantation. Adjust dosages of medications for renal dysfunction. Treat/prevent viral infections. Ensure that there is no folate or vitamin B_{12} deficiency. Administer G-CSF and rEPO as needed. Consider cryopreserving autologous peripheral blood stem cells before allograft for possible use in the event of graft failure or overwhelming clinical problems such as hemorrhage or life-threatening infection.

Adapted from Deeg (1998b); Mehta & Singhal (1998); and Shapiro, Rust, & Davison (1997).
AML, Acute myoblastic leukemia; *G-CSF,* granulocyte colony-stimulating factor; *rEPO,* recombinant Erythropoietin;
CMV, cytomegalovirus; *GVHD,* graft-versus-host disease.

CASE 7 STUDY

Mr. Roger Lofgren is a 63-year-old man with multiple myeloma, day +57 status post autologous peripheral blood SCT, after conditioning chemotherapy with BCNU 300 mg/m^2 and melphalan 140 mg/m^2. He has full hematopoietic engraftment, and his posttransplant course has been complicated by bacterial pneumonia in the first month after transplant, for which he was treated with 5 days of azithromycin. However, Mr. Lofgren has been well ever since. He calls the clinic with profound shortness of breath, dyspnea, a dry cough, and a low-grade temperature. These symptoms have developed over the past 4 days; however, the patient had assumed that they would improve on their own. Physical examination demonstrates tachycardia with heart rate 136 beats/min and regular, tachypnea with a respiratory rate of 44 breaths/min, and diffuse bibasilar inspiratory crackles.

Medications
Axid
Famvir
Daily multiple vitamin

QUESTIONS

1. What are the most likely differential diagnoses in this patient?

    1. Acute pulmonary hemorrhage
    2. Bacterial pneumonia
    3. *Pneumocystis carinii* pneumonia (PCP)
    4. CMV pneumonitis
    5. BCNU pneumonitis
    6. Pulmonary embolism
    7. GVHD of the lung
      a. 1, 2, 3, 4, & 5
      b. 2, 3, 4, & 5
      c. All of these except 7
      d. All of these

ANSWERS

1. Pulmonary complications should be suspected when patients develop acute or insidious onset of shortness of breath, new dyspnea on exertion, cough, diffuse radiographic infiltrates, and/or high spiking fevers. Time to occurrence ranges from the first month after transplant to years after transplant, and overall, 40% to 60% of patients develop pulmonary disease sometime after transplantation. The pulmonary complications of SCT, grouped according to their timeline for develop-

ment, are listed in Table 10-11. Complications arising in the period before day +100 posttransplant occur mainly as a result of conditioning regimen toxicity and the pancytopenia that inevitably follows. During this period, the patient is particularly susceptible to bacterial and fungal infections. The chronic complications occur from 100 days after transplant and beyond. Most

TABLE 10-11 Pulmonary Complications of Stem Cell Transplantation

TIMELINE	COMPLICATION
Acute (before day +30)	Pulmonary edema (secondary to fluid overload, cardiac dysfunction or to allergic reaction to medications/therapy)
	Oropharyngeal mucositis
	Aspiration pneumonia
	Pulmonary hemorrhage/diffuse alveolar hemorrhage (DAH)
	Bacterial or fungal pneumonia
	Atelectasis
	Pleural effusion
	Recall radiation pneumonitis
	Allergic bronchospasm
	Transfusion-associated lung injury (TRALI)
	Adult respiratory distress syndrome (ARDS) and septic shock
Early (before day +100)	Idiopathic interstitial pneumonitis
	Pulmonary embolism
	Viral pneumonia (CMV, HSV, VZV, RSV, adenovirus, parainfluenza, influenza)
	Protozoal pneumonia—PCP
	Fungal pneumonia
	Bacterial pneumonia
	TRALI
	ARDS and septic shock
Late (after day 100)	Idiopathic interstitial pneumonitis
	Bacterial, fungal, or viral pneumonia
	Bronchiolitis obliterans/graft-versus-host disease of the lung

Adapted from Atkinson (1994); Bryant (1994); Crawford (1997); Deeg (1998a); Height & Shields (1995); Long (1998); Philpott & Kanfer (1998); Shapiro, Rust, & Davison (1997).
CMV, Cytomegalovirus; *HSV,* herpes simplex virus; *VZV,* varicella-zoster virus; *RSV,* respiratory syncytial virus; *PCP, Pneumocystis carinii* pneumonia.

chronic complications arise in allogeneic transplant recipients who require long-term immunosuppression and who may also develop GVHD.

In this case, bacterial, protozoal, or viral pneumonias are strong possibilities. GVHD of the lung does not occur in patients who have undergone autologous peripheral blood SCT. The possibility of pulmonary embolism is somewhat less likely given the insidious onset of symptoms. If the patient is not thrombocytopenic, acute pulmonary hemorrhage can be excluded. PCP is an opportunistic organism that usually presents as an interstitial pneumonitis. The peak time for development of PCP after transplant is between 30 and 100 days. Symptoms include dyspnea, a nonproductive cough, and fever. The patient is usually hypoxic. The classical chest x-ray appearance is of bilaterally diffuse perihilar shadowing with an alveolar pattern also described as "ground glass." However, radiologic changes may not be apparent for several days after the development of symptoms and hypoxia.

Idiopathic pneumonitis or idiopathic interstitial pneumonitis occurs most commonly between 30 and 100 days after transplant, although it can also occur beyond day +100 (Atkinson, 1994). Idiopathic interstitial pneumonitis appears to be a direct result of toxicity from the preparative chemotherapy or chemoradiotherapy. Total body irradiation, BCNU, gemcitabine, busulfan, methotrexate, and cyclophosphamide appear to be implicated (Long, 1998). Patient-specific factors that appear to increase the risk of developing idiopathic interstitial pneumonitis include preexisting restrictive lung defects, abnormal diffusing capacity, mantle radiation, and prior exposure to bleomycin. Clinically, it presents with dyspnea, shortness of breath, a nonproductive cough, and fever, and the chest radiograph demonstrates patchy infiltration. Pulmonary function tests predominantly show a restrictive defect. Pathologically, pneumonitis is a tissue reaction. It is characterized by alveolar infiltration and thickening and the formation of hyaline membrane, which later progresses to fibrosis (Height & Shields, 1995). Prompt initiation of corticosteroids (1 to 2 mg/kg/day), followed by a slow taper once improvement is evident, are often able to reverse or limit the pneumonitis (Long, 1998).

At least 50% of patients who undergo SCT experience pulmonary complications, and they are among the most common causes of morbidity and mortality after SCT. For this reason, providers must have a high index of clinical suspicion concerning pulmonary symptoms that occur after transplant and should arrange for their early and appropriate investigation. Moreover, the differential diagnosis and management of pulmonary complications following transplantation can be challenging. When patients develop pulmonary symptoms after they have returned to their home community following transplant, it is strongly recommended that providers in the home community contact staff at the transplant center to discuss management and to determine whether transfer back to the specialty center is indicated to optimize patient management. See Table 10-11. *Answer 1:* **b.**

QUESTIONS

2. All of the following radiologic and laboratory tests are essential in evaluating the patient's respiratory symptoms *except:*
  a. ABGs
  b. Spiral CT of chest
  c. Cultures of blood and sputum
  d. Blood titers for *Mycoplasma, Legionella,* CMV antigen, *Toxoplasma gondii;* polymerase chain reaction (PCR)

ANSWERS

2. All of these are essential except for cultures of blood and sputum. The patient has a dry cough, and although cultures of the blood may identify an organism, they will likely not help tailor specific therapy. Spiral CT of chest will help rule out a pulmonary embolus and will help further characterize the infiltrates noted on chest radiograph. ABGs will evaluate the degree of hypoxemia, establish a baseline, and determine the need for oxygen therapy. Blood titers for *Mycoplasma pneumoniae, Legionella,* and CMV antigen may uncover an infective cause for the symptoms. *Answer 2:* **c.**

Case Study continued

Admission laboratory results reveal the following: WBC count, $12.8/mm^3$; Hgb, 12.6 g/dl; platelets, $208,000/mm^3$; HCO_3, 2 mEq/L; creatinine, 1.2 mg/dl; LDH, 334 U/L; SGOT, 45 U/L; and SGPT, 40 U/L. ABGs on room air reveal the following: pH, 7.48; $Paco_2$, 31 mm Hg; Pao_2, 51 mm Hg; and HCO_3, 27 mEq/L. Reference values for ABGs are as follows: pH, 7.35 to 7.45; $Paco_2$, 35 to 45 mm Hg; Pao_2, 60 to 100 mm Hg; and HCO_3, 22 to 28 mEq/L. Chest radiograph reveals diffuse bilateral infiltrates. CT of the chest demonstrates a ground glass appearance.

QUESTIONS

3. How would you interpret these arterial blood gases?
  a. Respiratory alkalosis with hypoxemia
  b. Respiratory alkalosis with hypocarbia
  c. Respiratory acidosis with hypoxemia
  d. Respiratory acidosis with hypercarbia

ANSWERS

3. It is safe to assume that hypoxemia is the driving force behind the patient's hyperventilatory response. The normal serum bicarbonate level suggests that this is an acute process (Konick-McMahon, 1998). *Answer 3:* **a.**

QUESTIONS

4. The staff nurse learns that the pulmonary team is considering a bronchoscopy with biopsy. She asks why this is required for this patient. What is the best response?
  a. Bronchoscopy with biopsy will likely be necessary to differentiate infectious pneumonia from a treatment-associated or idiopathic pneumonitis.
  b. Bronchoscopy is the only way to obtain data that differentiate the various infectious causes, allowing the physician to tailor the antimicrobial therapy.
  c. It is unlikely that bronchoscopy will ultimately be performed because the risks of bronchoscopy outweigh the diagnostic yield in this patient.
  d. Bronchoscopy will be necessary only if empiric treatment with antibiotics fails to result in clinical improvement.

ANSWERS

4. Bronchoscopy with biopsy is the most effective way of confirming the diagnosis and differentiating idiopathic interstitial pneumonitis from infection (Crawford, 1997). Because of the wide range of possible causes and because appropriate treatment for these etiologies is different, it is important to obtain a tissue diagnosis early in the course of the disease, both to initiate appropriate treatment and to discontinue inappropriate treatments. *Answer 4:* **a.**

Case Study continued

Bronchoscopy with biopsy confirms the diagnosis of idiopathic interstitial pneumonitis, likely secondary to BCNU toxicity, and the patient begins therapy with Medrol 60 mg orally every 12 hours.

QUESTIONS

5. In formulating a plan for supportive therapy, you also recommend all of the following interventions *except:*
  a. Septra DS 1 tablet orally twice daily on Saturday and Sunday and Mycelex troches four times per day
  b. Hormone replacement therapy
  c. H_2-blocker
  d. Counseling regarding the importance of making diet selections that avoid concentrated sugars

ANSWERS

5. High-dose steroids are used in the management of idiopathic interstitial pneumonitis that results from the toxicity of chemotherapy and/or radiation therapy. Steroids are usually started at a dosage of 1 to 2 mg/kg/day and then tapered carefully to prevent clinical deterioration. Generally, they are required over a prolonged period. It is important to be cognizant of the complications of long-term steroid use, including infections with *P. carinii* and fungus, diabetes mellitus, gastritis and ulceration, cataracts, cardiomyopathy, avascular necrosis, and osteoporosis (St. Germain, 1999). Septra DS 1 tablet orally twice a day twice weekly would provide prophylaxis against PCP, and Mycelex troches would prevent the development of oral thrush. Diflucan prophylaxis would also be an alternative. H_2-blocking agents help minimize the chance of gastric ulceration, as does taking the steroids with food or milk. Although there is a risk of osteoporosis with long-term steroid use, before beginning hormone replacement therapy, one would need a more comprehensive analysis of the risks and benefits of such therapy in this patient. Clinical monitoring for the development of hyperglycemia and counseling regarding appropriate diet choices are important components of intervention. *Answer 5:* **b.**

QUESTIONS

6. For the patient who is allergic to sulfa drugs or cannot take Bactrim, all of the following are potential alternative choices to prevent PCP in the patient who has undergone SCT *except:*
  a. Pentamidine
  b. Dapsone
  c. Levofloxacin (Levaquin)
  d. Atovaquone

6. Bactrim (trimethoprim-sulfamethoxazole [TMP-SMX]) DS orally twice daily two to three times a week is the standard prophylaxis of PCP in the patient who has undergone SCT. In patients who are allergic to sulfa drugs or who experience marrow suppression as a result of Bactrim treatment, either pentamidine 300 mg by inhalation every month, atovaquone 1500 mg/day orally, or dapsone 100 mg/day orally is an acceptable substitution. Pentamidine and dapsone have not been shown to have the same efficacy as Bactrim, however, and there is an incidence of breakthrough PCP infection with these therapies (Deeg, 1994). In addition, patients who are hypersensitive to cotrimoxazole will also be hypersensitive to dapsone. Dapsone should not be used in patients with glucose-6-phosphate dehydrogenase (G6PD) deficiency. Patients with asthma may not tolerate inhaled pentamidine (Tebas & Horgan, 1998). Levofloxacin does not have activity against *P. carinii. Answer 6:* **c.**

CASE 8 STUDY

Mrs. Letts is a 43-year-old patient with stage IIIB multiple myeloma with multiple lytic bone lesions of the vertebrae and pelvis. She is now day +66 status post autologous peripheral blood SCT. Her WBC count is $3.6/mm^3$, Hgb is 10.3 g/dl, Hct is 24.6%, and platelets are $39,000/mm^3$; her posttransplant reevaluation indicates remission of her disease, with less than 3% plasma cells in the bone marrow. She comes to transplant clinic reporting a 2-day history of back pain and pruritus of the skin overlying the coccyx. In addition, she is fatigued, has a poor appetite, and has intermittent nausea. She has a low-grade temperature of 37.7° C; remaining vital signs are at her usual baseline.

Medications
Aredia 90 mg intravenously every month
Erythropoietin (EPO) 40,000 units subcutaneously
every week

Mrs. Letts indicates that her family doctor started her on ciprofloxacin 2 days ago, when she telephoned him with complaints of burning and pain with urination. These urinary tract symptoms have not yet resolved, and the rash developed after the first dose of the drug.

QUESTIONS

1. Priority components of your remaining review of systems and physical examination include which of the following?
  a. Musculoskeletal, integumentary, genitourinary, neurologic
  b. Musculoskeletal, integumentary, genitourinary, GI
  c. Abdominal, genitourinary, neurologic
  d. Integumentary, musculoskeletal, neurologic

1. Priority components of your review of systems and physical examination should include the integumentary, neurologic, genitourinary, and musculoskeletal systems. A pulmonary, abdominal, and ophthalmologic examination should also be performed to detect for visceral involvement/dissemination. *Answer 1:* **a.**

Case Study continued

Physical examination reveals painful, raised papules overlying the coccyx, left buttock, left inner thigh, and left labia. Genitourinary examination is otherwise unremarkable. There is tingling dysesthetic pain reported in the left buttock and thigh, but no other focal neurologic deficit such as muscle weakness or sensory loss. There is full range of motion of the left lower extremity without pain or deficit in strength. There is no peripheral edema.

QUESTIONS

2. What is the most likely diagnosis?
  a. GVHD of the skin
  b. Allergic reaction to ciprofloxacin
  c. Herpes zoster reactivation in the left L1-L2 dermatome
  d. Genital herpes

3. Which of the following is accurate with regard to your next steps in the assessment and management of this patient?

a. In the SCT patient, varicella-zoster reactivation always presents with a vesicular rash.

b. It is important in determining the management plan to assess for extradermatomal involvement of the skin and to assess the pulmonary and neurologic systems as well as the abdomen for evidence of visceral dissemination.

c. Accompanying symptoms of herpes zoster reactivation can include high fevers, chills, headache, coagulopathy, and seizures.

d. The presence of pain in the acute phase of infection is a sign of more disseminated involvement.

ANSWERS

2. Varicella-zoster virus reactivation occurs in 20% to 30% of autologous and 20% to 50% of allogeneic patients during the first few months after SCT, with a peak incidence around 4 months after transplant (Burns, 1998). The high incidence of varicella-zoster virus reactivation following SCT, as well as its variable clinical manifestations, require a high index of suspicion for varicella-zoster virus as a potential cause whenever a vesicular rash and/or pain occur in the patient who has undergone SCT (Arvin, 2000). The most likely diagnosis is herpes zoster reactivation in the left L1-L2 dermatome. Following recovery from chickenpox at any time of life, varicella-zoster virus remains latent in the dorsal root ganglia of the spinal cord. Shingles (herpes zoster) is caused by reactivation of virus in the nerves supplying a particular dermatome or small group of adjacent dermatomes. Lesions erupt on the skin in a pattern dictated by its innervation. In otherwise healthy people, there is little spread of the virus, but in SCT patients, local lesion extension, satellite lesions, and visceral dissemination can occur (Westmoreland, 1998). Repeat attacks can occur. Disseminated cutaneous disease is present when there are more than 10 lesions outside the dermatome of primary infection. Cutaneous dissemination occurs in approximately 25% of cases, and visceral dissemination occurs clinically in approximately 10% to 15% of cases. Varicella-zoster reactivation can occasionally present as severe abdominal pain involving the pancreas, intestines, or adrenal glands, without cutaneous involvement (Yagi, Karasuno, Hasegawa, et al., 2000). Visceral dissemination can include the lung, gut, liver, eyes, or central nervous system, and thrombocytopenia or intravascular coagulopathy can occur (Burns, 1998). Chronic GVHD and treatment with immunosuppressive therapy increase the patient's risk of infection. *Answer 2:* **c.**

3. The findings in this patient are typical herpes zoster reactivation in the left L1-L2 dermatome. The painful, erythematous papules grouped in an area of the body, lateralizing to one side of the body and following the dermatomal pattern, and the associated dysesthetic pain, burning, numbing, or tingling sensations are a classical presentation. It may present as burning or tingling of the skin and radicular pain with rash following or as rash and pain simultaneously. Accompanying symptoms of herpes zoster infection may include fever, chills, malaise, headache, or GI disturbances. Seizures or focal neurologic findings indicate possible herpes zoster encephalitis and are ominous occurrences requiring immediate intravenous therapy. Postherpetic neuralgia, with longstanding residual pain from peripheral nerve damage may result.

Immediate antiviral treatment within the first 72 hours of the development of symptoms is indicated. Intravenous antiviral treatment is indicated for disseminated infection in the immunocompromised host, in patients with visceral involvement, and in patients who develop evidence of extradermatomal involvement while taking oral therapy (Woeltje & Ritchie, 1998). Allergic reaction to an antibiotic is unlikely to present with a vesicular rash confined to one side of the body and following a pattern of a dermatome. Genital herpes would not likely produce unilateral symptoms, nor involvement with back pain. The patient underwent autologous transplantation and therefore is not at risk for GVHD. The acute phase of zoster is painful in approximately 75% of patients and does not signal disseminated involvement. *Answer 3:* **b.**

Case Study continued

The patient requires immediate admission for intravenous acyclovir. In discussing room assignment for the patient with the charge nurse, she asks for your recommendation.

QUESTIONS

4. In addition to immediate consultation with the infection control practitioner, your recommendation includes which of the following?

a. Patients infected with varicella-zoster virus should be strictly isolated, including respiratory isolation procedures for patients with visceral dissemination.

b. All staff may care for this patient as long as she has started appropriate antiviral treatment.
c. Because of the anticipated stay of several days, the patient should be assigned to the room that has easiest access to the communal kitchen that patients and families can use to prepare snacks.
d. Respiratory and body substance isolation should be practiced until the patient has completed 48 hours of intravenous antiviral treatment.

acyclovir-resistant strain of zoster. Immediate arrangements for resistance testing will allow the earliest adjustment of therapy.
c. Initial persistence of pain and the development of new lesions indicate the need to increase the dosage of acyclovir to 800 mg/m^2 every 8 hours.
d. Continued emergency of vesicular lesions after instituting intravenous acyclovir indicates the need to administer varicella-zoster immunoglobulin (VZIG).

ANSWERS

4. Staff should wear gloves when direct contact with the patient is anticipated, and a gown should be worn when it is likely that clothing could be soiled by a patient's body fluids. Handwashing between patient visits is essential. Respiratory isolation procedures with a positive-pressure, single room and masks for all staff should be implemented for patients with visceral involvement. Body substance isolation precautions must be continued until visceral involvement has resolved and all cutaneous lesions are crusted (Burns, 1998). Patients who have active varicella-zoster infection should not have contact with other patients, particularly those who are heavily immunocompromised. Patients with zoster infection are infectious to anyone who has never had chickenpox, as well as to others who are immunocompromised, regardless of their prior immune status to varicella-zoster. Staff who do not have protective immunity against varicella-zoster should not care for these patients. *Answer 4:* **a.**

Case Study continued

On the second day of hospitalization, Mrs. Letts continues with intravenous acyclovir at a dosage of 10 mg/kg every 8 hours. However, she continues to have severe dysesthetic pain that radiates from her back down her leg and buttocks. In addition, she notes the development of some new vesicles on her chest and abdomen. She wonders whether her therapy should be changed, because it is not helping.

QUESTIONS

5. Your response incorporates which of the following concepts?
a. It is usual to see the formation of new lesions for 1 to 3 days after beginning acyclovir therapy.
b. Continuing pain and the emergence of new lesions suggest the development of an

ANSWERS

5. It is usual to see the formation of new lesions for 1 to 3 days after beginning antiviral therapy. Studies have showed that time to defervescence and cutaneous healing are not significantly shortened with antiviral treatment; however, the development of varicella pneumonia and mortality from varicella-zoster virus infection are decreased. Resistance testing would be indicated only if the patient developed recurrence of varicella-zoster virus infection while receiving full-dose antiviral therapy, and resistance usually develops only after the treatment of multiple outbreaks. Acyclovir 500 mg/m^2 every 8 hours is the appropriate dosage for a patient with zoster involving more than one dermatome or if visceral disease is suspected/present (Burns, 1998). A dosage increase to 800 mg/m^2 would only prompt renal toxicity. There is no role for VZIG in the treatment of established varicella-zoster virus reactivation. *Answer 5:* **a.**

Case Study continued

After 6 days of hospitalization, the lesions are beginning to crust; however, the patient continues with severe dysesthetic pain as well as pruritus and skin hypersensitivity in the L1-L2 dermatome. The nurse asks you to see the patient and suggest options for pain control.

QUESTIONS

6. In addition to antihistamines, cool compresses, and oatmeal baths for control of pruritus, you might suggest all of the following symptom control options *except:*
a. EMLA cream to areas of skin pain and hypersensitivity, as long as those skin areas are intact and not involved with lesions
b. Gabapentin (Neurontin) 300 mg orally three times daily

c. Nortriptyline (Elavil) 10 mg orally at bedtime

d. Narcotic analgesics

ANSWERS

6. The pain associated with herpes zoster reactivation is called *herpetic neuralgia* or *postherpetic neuralgia.* Herpetic neuralgia or postherpetic neuralgia is more likely to be a neuropathic process than a nociceptive process (Gilden, Kleinschmidt-Demasters, Laguardia, et al., 2000). The role of opioids remains controversial; however, as a single modality, they are somewhat limited because the high dosages required for relief tend to cause sedation, constipation, nausea, and tolerance. Studies have shown that the second-generation anticonvulsant medications such as gabapentin (Neurontin) may be somewhat more effective than the first-generation anticonvulsant agents (e.g., carbamazepine) in the treatment of postherpetic neuralgia (Gilden, Kleinschmidt-Demasters, Laguardia, et al., 2000). Nortriptyline has a role in the treatment of herpetic neuralgia and postherpetic neuralgia; however, the initial dosing of nortriptyline is 25 to 50 mg orally at bedtime. EMLA cream may be helpful in decreasing the hyperesthesia that is also associated with postherpetic neuralgia (Buckley, 1998). *Answer 6:* **c.**

QUESTIONS

7. Your consultation regarding pain control represents which type of consultation?

a. Informal patient-centered consultation

b. Formal patient-centered consultation

c. Program-centered administrative consultation

d. Consultee-centered case consultation

ANSWERS

7. This represents formal patient-centered consultation. The consultation is formal in that the staff nurse has asked for a comprehensive and thorough evaluation of the problem and possible solutions (Barron & White, 1996). Caplan (1970) describes four types of consultation. In client-centered case consultation, the consultant sees the patient directly and completes an assessment of the patient and makes recommendations for the consultee's management of the case. In consultee-centered case consultation, although the goal is also to help the consultee improve patient care, the focus is on the consultee's problem in handling the situation and the goal of the consultation is to assist the consultee in developing the knowledge, skills, confidence, or objectivity to handle the problem. This is not an example of a program-centered administrative consultation because there is no focus on the planning or administration of clinical services for a group of patients. *Answer 7:* **b.**

CASE 9 STUDY

Janet March is a 23-year-old patient who is 2 years status post allogeneic, T-cell depleted, SCT for stage III Hodgkin's disease. Her conditioning regimen consisted of total body irradiation, cyclophosphamide 120 mg/kg, and busulfan 16 mg/kg. Her posttransplant course has been complicated by chronic GVHD of the skin, bronchiolitis obliterans, and repeated viral and bacterial infections of the respiratory tract.

Medications
Medrol
CellCept in treatment of her chronic GVHD

QUESTIONS

1. Which of the following factors contribute to late complications after hematopoietic SCT?

1. Components and dosage intensity of the conditioning regimen
2. Therapies given before the transplant
3. Preexisting medical conditions
4. Side effects of the transplant procedure itself

a. 1, 2, & 4

b. 1, 2, & 3

c. 1 & 4

d. All of these

1. All of these factors influence the development of long-term complications (Harpham, 1998). Long-term complications in both allogeneic and autologous stem cell recipients are multifactorial and result from the interplay of the effects of high-dose chemotherapy, total body irradiation, toxic reactions to therapies, and disease recurrence (Deeg, 1998a). In the setting of allogeneic transplantation, some of the long-term complications are directly related to the transplant itself (e.g., chronic GVHD, immunodeficiency).

The most significant variable is the composition and dose intensity (dose per treatment and total dose) of the transplant conditioning regimen. It is important to consider the effect of the histology, stage, and sites of disease; the composition and dose intensity of previous chemotherapy received; and the use of other treatment modalities such as surgery, radiation, or biologic response modifiers. Preexisting medical conditions (e.g., cardiac disease) or cardiac risk factors (e.g., hypertension, hyperlipidemia, diabetes) should be identified (Harpham, 1998). *Answer 1:* **d.**

QUESTIONS

2. Which of the following studies would most likely be performed in a milestone reevaluation of the allogeneic transplant patient at the 1-year posttransplant evaluation?
1. Pulmonary function tests with DLco, dental evaluation, gynecologic examination with Pap smear
2. DEXA scan, mammogram, ophthalmologic evaluation, testing for hepatitis B and C
3. CD4/CD8 lymphocyte subsets, thyroid-stimulating hormone (TSH), thyroxine (T_4), complete skin examination, CBC with differential
4. CT scans of chest, abdomen, and pelvis; bone marrow aspirate and biopsy with engraftment studies
   a. 1 & 4
   b. 2 & 4
   c. All of these except 2
   d. All of these

2. All of these studies would be a component of the 1-year posttransplant evaluation. Pulmonary function tests permit continued monitoring of lung function. A dental evaluation is indicated secondary to the chronic GVHD as well as the intensity of her previous treatment. Annual gynecologic examinations with Pap smear are part of routine screening for women. The DEXA scan will evaluate for osteoporosis. The risk for breast cancer in a woman treated with previous mantle irradiation and total body irradiation is higher than in the general population (Green, Hyland, Barcos, et al., 2000). Ophthalmic evaluation is indicated because the eyes are targets of acute and chronic GVHD and may show changes related to the conditioning regimen, the treatment of GVHD, and infections. Screening for hepatitis B and C is especially recommended in the long-term follow-up of these patients who have received frequent transfusion support because symptomatic or subclinical hepatitis may be related to transfusion-mediated infections and effective antiviral treatment for hepatitis B and C is available. CD4/CD8 lymphocyte subsets will help gauge the degree of continuing immunocompromise, and the results may shape recommendations regarding immunizations and continuing antimicrobial prophylaxis. Thyroid function tests are indicated because of the risk of hypothyroidism as a result of the total body irradiation. A history of chronic GVHD of skin places a person at risk for basal cell skin cancers. A CBC with differential gauges the quality of the engraftment and screens for the early development of a secondary leukemia or myelodysplastic syndrome. CT scans of chest, abdomen, and pelvis will evaluate the status of solid tumors, and a bone marrow aspirate and biopsy will evaluate the quality of her stem cell engraftment. Individual transplant centers have protocols and practice guidelines that shape the milestone posttransplant evaluation, and the plans for this evaluation should be discussed and coordinated with the transplant center. Routine follow-up examinations should also involve the promotion of healthy lifestyle changes and risk-reduction strategies (e.g., nutrition, exercise, smoking cessation) as appropriate. See Table 10-12 *Answer 2:* **d.**

TABLE 10-12 Evaluation and Screening of Late Effects of Hematopoietic Stem Cell Transplantation

SYSTEM/DIMENSION	POSSIBLE LATE EFFECTS	EVALUATION/SCREENING
Disease status	Relapse/recurrence	Determined based on site of original disease Evaluation for minimal residual disease (if available)
Engraftment	Graft failure/marrow dysfunction with cytopenia	CBC with differential Bone marrow aspirate and biopsy Engraftment studies: to detect differences between DNA of donor and recipient and thus establish engraftment: VNTR (variable nucleotide tandem repeats) or RFLP (restriction fragment length polymorphisms); cytogenetic studies may also be used to establish engraftment if the donor and recipient are of opposite sexes
Immunologic function/recovery	Disorders of B- and T-lymphocyte quantity and function Hypogammaglobulinemia	CD4/CD8 lymphocyte subsets Quantitative immunoglobulin levels Vaccination titers
Cardiopulmonary effects	Interstitial pneumonitis Bronchiolitis obliterans Hypertension, cardiomyopathy, pericardial damage, peripheral vascular disease	Chest radiograph Pulmonary function tests with DL_{CO} Electrocardiogram Echocardiogram History and physical examination
Neurologic effects	Peripheral and autonomic neuropathies Cognitive changes, shortened attention span, difficulty with concentration Leukoencephalopathy Ototoxicity	Health history Neurologic examination Neuropsychologic testing Rehabilitation medicine Audiologic testing
Gastrointestinal effects	Liver dysfunction Malabsorption syndromes	Liver function tests Hepatitis B serologies, hepatitis C-PCR qualitative
Genitourinary effects	Renal dysfunction Radiation nephritis Hematuria, proteinuria Cancer of the bladder	Blood urea nitrogen, creatinine Urinalysis with microscopy 24-hour urine for creatinine clearance, total protein, if indicated

Endocrine
  Thyroid function
  Gonadal function
	Hypothyroidism
	Decreased production of gonadal hormones
		TSH, T_3, T_4, free T_4
		LH, FSH, estradiol (women)
		Pelvic examination
		LH, FSH, testosterone (men)

Hypothalamic-pituitary	Abnormal pituitary gland function	Prolactin levels, FSH, LH, TSH
Ophthalmic	Cataracts	Ophthalmologic examination to include slit-lamp examination and Schirmer's test

Adapted from Buchsel, Leum, & Randolph (1996); Deeg (1998a); Deeg & Socie (1998); Meadows & Fenton (1994); Sanders (1994), Schwartz, Hobbie, & Constine (1994); Constine, Hobbie, & Schwartz (1994); Harpham (1998); Ruccione (1994); and Shalet (1998).
CBC, Complete blood count; *PCR,* polymerase chain reaction; *TSH,* thyroid-stimulating hormone; *LH,* luteinizing hormone; *FSH,* follicle-stimulating hormone; *DXA,* dual-energy x-ray absorptiometry; *MRI,* magnetic resonance imaging; *CT,* computed tomography.

Continued

TABLE 10-12 Evaluation and Screening of Late Effects of Hematopoietic Stem Cell Transplantation—cont'd

SYSTEM/DIMENSION	POSSIBLE LATE EFFECTS	EVALUATION/SCREENING
Dental/oral cavity	Sicca syndrome	
	Caries	
	Periodontal disease	
	Xerostomia	
	Oral malignancy	
Musculoskeletal	Osteoporosis	DXA scan
	Avascular necrosis	MRI if pain in a joint, limited range of motion, or a limp
	Myopathy	MRI, neurologic examination, electromyography
Second malignancy	Nonmelanoma skin cancer	Complete physical examination with biopsy of suspicious lesions; skin photographs may also help monitor status
	Melanoma	
	Breast cancer	Mammogram, self-examination
	Thyroid cancer	History and physical examination, ultrasound, I^{131} scan
	Acute leukemia	CBC with differential
	Myelodysplastic syndrome	Bone marrow aspirate and biopsy (if CBC abnormal)
	Posttransplant lymphoproliferative disorders (PTLD)	CT scans if PTLD suspected
	Cancer of the uterine cervix	Gynecologic examination with Pap smear
	Cancer of the bladder	Urinalysis with microscopic examination to detect microhematuria, urine cytology, follow-up cystoscopy
Integumentary	Increased incidence of benign and malignant nevi	Complete physical examination Skin biopsy of suspicious lesions
Psychologic/rehabilitation; quality of life	Changes in body image, roles, family relationships, lifestyle, occupation, discrimination, overcoming stigma, living with compromises, coping with symptoms	Assessment of individual adjustment, achievement of normal developmental tasks, marital stress, sexual function, body image, rehabilitation needs, symptom distress through systematic and structured evaluation

CASE 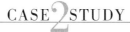 STUDY

Jim Dunstan continued from p. 158. You are discussing the recovery process with Jim, the 19-year-old patient who has undergone autologous transplant for Hodgkin's disease. Although he had a steady girlfriend with him during his initial posttransplant visits, you have noticed that he comes to clinic alone now. He asks, using rather coarse language, about problems he is experiencing in meeting women and achieving an orgasm.

QUESTIONS

1. Your response incorporates which of the following concepts about sexual counseling in the oncology setting?

   a. If patients wish to discuss sexual matters with their health care professionals, they should do so using language that is professional and appropriate. There is no place for slang or coarse expressions on the part of patients.

b. Every patient, regardless of current level of sexual activity, has a perception of himself or herself as a sexual being and is invested in knowing that he or she can function sexually.

c. Appropriate sexual counseling requires the provider to ask specific questions regarding sexual function as a basis upon which to provide information.

d. Jim should be informed that problems with achieving orgasm can be addressed when he has a partner available to participate with him in the counseling process.

ANSWERS

1. A judgmental response does not help create an environment in which the patient feels comfortable to talk about his or her feelings and concerns. Depending on the patient's educational level and background, these may be the only words that they know to express concerns and questions. That stated, it is not necessary for the nurse to use the same language as the patient when responding to the concerns. Simple language and a matter-of-fact approach can help ease the anxieties that both the patient and professional may be feeling in the situation. Ultimately, nurses must assess their own attitudes and beliefs about sexuality. When patients' attitudes and experiences are similar to our own, we tend to judge these as valid, whereas dissimilar attitudes and experiences may be seen as improper or inappropriate (Herson, Hart, Gordon, & Rintala, 1999). If the nurse's attitudes and beliefs run counter to those of the patient and the nurse cannot put aside personal perceptions, the patient may be better served by referral to another clinician who may be more comfortable with the situation. Information and counseling regarding sexuality is usually best received when it addresses the problems with which the patient and his or her partner are currently struggling. It is more important to convey a sense of trust and confidentiality and to legitimize sexual concerns than it is to ask specific questions regarding sexual function. *Answer 1:* **b.**

QUESTIONS

2. All of the following may be barriers to discussing sexual function after cancer treatment *except:*

a. There is too little information available to health professionals regarding sexual health and cancer treatment, and it is often difficult to obtain referral for specialty care of patients with sexual dysfunction.

b. There are too many time constraints.

c. Providers are uncomfortable discussing intimate issues with patients.

d. Patients are often reluctant to directly express sexual concerns to their health care provider.

ANSWERS

2. One of the barriers to addressing sexual counseling in oncology settings is the discomfort that both health care providers and patients may feel in discussing intimate issues. Another restraint may be the time required for sexual counseling. In busy outpatient clinics, the imperative to provide education about the disease, prognosis, and treatment may make it seem like a luxury to include information about the effects of treatment on sexual functioning. In addition, privacy and confidentiality are crucial prerequisites for discussing sexual concerns with patients, and these may be difficult to attain in a busy clinic settings, where several staff members may be present. Although we have a need for more information regarding the effect of cancer and its treatment on sexual health and strategies to promote sexual rehabilitation, there is a growing body of research on sexual health after cancer that can inform and guide our assessment and intervention. *Answer 2:* **a.**

QUESTIONS

3. All of the following statements related to sexual concerns of the post-SCT patient are true *except:*

a. Prolonged hospitalization associated with dose-intensive treatment can significantly alter partner relationships.

b. Libido may be affected by side effects such as nausea and vomiting, pain, fatigue, weakness, and mucositis.

c. Immunosuppression increases the risk of infection or reactivation of genital infections.

d. In hematopoietic SCT, sexual concerns tend to be raised by patients relatively early in the rehabilitative process, with the result that most transplant patients have few sexual concerns at 6 months posttransplant.

ANSWERS

3. Research has shown that sexual concerns and disorders were often presented to the transplant team relatively late in the rehabilitation process. In one longitudinal study of psychosocial adjustment after transplantation, 14% of patients mentioned sexuality as a concern as they were leaving the hospital, with the percentage concerned about this rising to 21% at 6-month follow-up and increasing to 37% at 1-year follow-up (Baker, Zabora, Pollard, & Wingard, 1999). The lengthy hospitalization and an often long posthospitalization convalescence, as well as the effects of the psychologic stress and symptom distress of the cancer experience process, can mean that there are long periods of sexual abstinence. There is a role for staff to encourage other forms of intimacy during this time and to create an environment in the hospital that allows for the privacy that can promote closeness within the partnered relationship. The need for safe sexual practices is key, especially while receiving immunosuppressive medications and while counts are low. *Answer 3:* **d.**

QUESTIONS

4. Your interventions with Jim would probably include all of the following *except:*

  a. A confirmation that these are normal concerns that often involve a gradual recovery, with various kinds of help that may be useful, including reading, counseling, and support groups

  b. Immediate referral for sexual therapy

  c. A discussion of sexual issues that may be arising for him as a result of the treatment, including loss of desire; erectile dysfunction; and the psychologic issues of body image, stigma, isolation, fear of rejection, and lost or impaired fertility

  d. Suggestions regarding additional sources of information and support about these issues, including patient education literature from the American Cancer Society, and the availability of individual and group programs of peer support

ANSWERS

4. Most sexual problems or concerns do not require extensive medical or psychologic treatment. In many patient situations, information about the effect of cancer treatment on sexuality and suggestions for getting one's sex life back to normal are adequate. Many patients will be grateful for simple human understanding and empathic handling of sensitive topics. *Answer 4:* **b.**

QUESTIONS

5. Patients with cancer, especially those who have undergone dose-intensive treatment, may require referral to address one or more of their sexual and reproductive health needs. The critical components of your referral network should include which of the following?

1. A mental health professional who provides sex therapy and sexual counseling

2. A gynecologist or specialist in women's health who can help women make decisions about hormone replacement therapy after cancer

3. Another male patient who has experienced erectile dysfunction and loss in sexual desire

4. A sperm bank that can store semen samples for men about to begin cancer treatment that could potentially damage their infertility

5. A reproductive endocrinologist who can address issues of cancer-related infertility in men and women

  a. 1 & 2

  b. 1, 3, 4, & 5

  c. All of these except 3

  d. All of these

ANSWERS

5. To address the sexual and reproductive health needs of patients following dose-intensive therapies, the APN needs to develop a network of specialists who can provide services for the treatment of sexual problems resulting from cancer therapy, counseling regarding postmenopausal hormone replacement therapy, treatment of female loss of sexual desire and menopausal symptoms, treatment of male loss of sexual desire and erectile dysfunction, provision of sperm banking, and infertility therapy/counseling for survivors who are having trouble conceiving or who have a known impairment in fertility as a result of cancer treatment (Schover, 1999). Sexual desire and erectile dysfunction are usually multifactorial problems that require counseling combined with knowledgeable medical intervention. A urologist or internist specializing in male health is most likely to be knowledgeable about the many medical, surgical, and technologic advances available to treat erectile dysfunction and loss of libido (Costabile, 2000). *Answer 5:* **c.**

QUESTIONS

6. Jim's mother questions you about osteoporosis after reading about it in the waiting room. She is concerned because her mother is disabled by it. Which of the following statements is *incorrect*?

  a. In men, low testosterone as a result of hypogonadism is associated with the development of osteoporosis.

  b. Patients who undergo autologous SCT have less bone loss than those who undergo allogeneic SCT.

c. Therapy-induced damage to bone mass may rapidly become manifest, but it may also remain latent and become apparent only after a number of decades, when the therapy-induced bone loss is augmented by the age-dependent processes of bone loss.

d. Symptoms such as back pain, pain on compression, or pressure over individual sections of the vertebrae suggest the need to begin immediate treatment for osteoporosis.

ANSWERS

6. Symptoms such as sudden violent pain, chronic pain, pronounced loss of height accompanied by characteristic skinfolds and contraction of the back muscles, kyphosis of the spine, pain on pressure, and compression over vertebrae indicate a possible osteoporotic vertebral fracture and must be investigated (Pfeilschifter & Diel, 2000). When these symptoms or signs are present, a radiograph should be taken of the section of the spine in question. In both men and women, the gonadal hormones, estrogen and testosterone, play a fundamental role in maintaining bone mass. Severe bone loss is often observed with both allogeneic and autologous SCT. These patients may start with a lower bone mass because of their underlying illness or earlier chemotherapy. For allogeneic transplant recipients, glucocorticoids and cyclosporine further intensify the degree of bone loss. Accordingly, patients who have undergone autologous SCT seem to have less bone loss than those undergoing allogeneic transplant procedures (Ebeling, Thomas, Erbas, et al., 1999). Osteoporosis is both preventable and treatable. A lack of awareness of the long-term adverse effects of cancer treatment on the skeleton may lead to chronic pain, disability, and a decrease in the quality of life in many patients. The challenge is to make the assessment of the risk of osteoporosis an integral part of the follow-up of patients whose regimens predispose them to skeletal damage so that therapy can be initiated before fractures occur. *Answer 6:* **d.**

QUESTIONS

7. Which of the following would *not* be a key aspect of history taking and examination for Jim related to the problem of osteoporosis?
  a. Family history of osteoporosis, current and previous lifestyle
  b. Current medications, medical history
  c. Vital signs, measures of nutritional status (e.g., weight, prealbumin)

d. Bone pain, point tenderness of the spine, kyphosis, muscle weakness

ANSWERS

7. Key aspects of history taking and examination related to the problem of osteoporosis include family history, level of physical activity, cigarette smoking, calcium intake (past and present), and the presence of comorbid medical conditions (e.g., hyperthyroidism) or the use of medications known to accelerate bone loss (Mahon, 1998; McClung, 1999; Woodhead & Moss, 1998). A family history of osteoporosis or maternal history of fractures suggests genetic factors that may place the patient at increased risk. Examination of the spine for deformity, such as kyphosis, as well as noting the presence of pain or tenderness on palpation over individual sections of the vertebrae (point tenderness) should be performed. Muscle weakness, especially lower extremity muscle weakness, places the patient at increased risk for falls, which is a risk factor for osteoporotic fracture. Although calcium intake and nutritional status may be correlated, weight and prealbumin levels may not reflect current or past calcium intake. Nutritional factors such as milk intolerance, excessive use of alcohol, high caffeine intake, and high consumption of animal protein (e.g., red meat) should be noted. *Answer 7:* **c.**

QUESTIONS

8. Which of the following tests offers the least effective measure of bone mass?
  a. Quantitative ultrasonography
  b. Single energy x-ray absorptiometry
  c. Radiography
  d. Dual-energy x-ray absorptiometry

ANSWERS

8. The definitive technique for measuring bone mass is a bone mineral density test (Woodhead & Moss, 1998). These tests are used to measure bone mass in the spine, hip, wrist, hand, or heel or the entire body and to evaluate its density. Several different types of such tests are currently available; however, they differ in relationship to precision, accuracy, and the type of bone being measured. All of the measures of assessing bone density, except quantitative ultrasound, involve a measurement of the amount of radiation absorbed into the bone being scanned, a technique known as *absorptiometry*. Single-energy absorptiometry has the advantage of being relatively inexpensive; however, it can be used only for measurements at appendicular sites (e.g., the radius). Studies suggest that measurements at the radius are less predictive for spinal and femoral bone mineral densities than direct measurements at these skeletal sites. Dual-energy x-ray absorptiometry is widely used because of its ability to assess bone mass at both axial and appendicular sites and because of the very low dose of radiation associated with its measurement.

Quantitative ultrasound of the heel is also effective in predicting hip fracture; however, because it evaluates the structure and strength of the bone substance rather the bone mass, it is limited to use on the peripheral skeleton. It may therefore be most useful as a screening tool in the general population. Plain radiographs offer the least effective measurement of bone mass. Although they can easily detect bone fractures, they are not sensitive enough to detect osteoporosis until 25% to 40% of bone mass has been lost, by which time, the disease is well advanced. *Answer 8:* **c.**

QUESTIONS

9. Which of the following might be used to prevent the development of osteoporosis in this patient?
  1. Calcium
  2. Fluoride
  3. Bisphosphonates
  4. Androgens
  5. Raloxifene
  6. Hormone replacement therapy
  7. Miacalcin nasal spray
   a. 1, 2, 3, 4, & 6
   b. 1, 3, 5, 6, & 7
   c. All of these except 2
   d. All of these

ANSWERS

9. All of these except for fluoride and androgens might be used to prevent the development of osteoporosis in this patient. Calcium supplementation to 1500 mg with vitamin D supplementation would be recommended because calcium is absorbed from the intestine and used only in the presence of vitamin D. Besides promoting the absorption of calcium, vitamin D regulates serum calcium concentrations (McClung, 1999). Hormone replacement therapy, although controversial in breast cancer survivors, is effective in preventing the development of osteoporosis in patients with therapy-induced menopause.

Raloxifene is classified as a selective estrogen receptor modulator (SERM). It preserves the beneficial effects of estrogens, including protection against cardiovascular diseases and osteoporosis, without stimulating breast and uterine tissues. As with the bisphosphonates, Miacalcin

(calcitonin), administered either by injection or a nasal spray, has an antiresorptive mechanism. It provides an alternative to bisphosphonates, although it is not as potent. *Answer 9:* **b.**

QUESTIONS

10. Which of the following is an adverse effect of hormone replacement therapy?
   a. Decreased risk of breast cancer
   b. Resumption of menstrual bleeding
   c. Decreasing serum concentration of low-density lipoproteins
   d. Decrease in bone pain

ANSWERS

10. Hormone replacement therapy is still very controversial, especially for women with an increased risk of breast cancer (Sands, Boshoff, Jones, et al., 1995; Snyder, Sielsch, & Reveille, 1998). Adverse effects of hormone replacement therapy include breast tenderness, resumption of monthly bleeding, and an increased risk of breast cancer. Bisphosphonates (e.g., pamidronate) and SERMs (e.g., raloxifene) may offer alternatives for patients for whom the risks of hormone replacement therapy outweigh the benefits. Hormone replacement therapy does not directly affect bone pain. Hormone replacement therapy and the SERMs will also decrease the serum concentration of total and low-density lipoproteins, thus producing a favorable effect on cardiovascular health. *Answer 10:* **b.**

QUESTIONS

11. The highest amount of calcium is found in which of the following food items?
   a. 1 cup of whole milk
   b. 1 cup of spinach
   c. 1 cup of yogurt
   d. 1 ounce of cheese

ANSWERS

11. A cup of plain yogurt contains 415 mg of calcium. Spinach contains 278 mg of calcium, a cup of whole milk contains 291 mg, and one ounce of cheese 124 mg. Other foods high in calcium include tofu, collard greens, and soy beans (NIH Consensus Development Panel on Optimal Calcium Intake, 1994). The NIH panel on optimal calcium intake recommends an intake of 1000 mg of calcium daily for women older than 50 who are taking estrogen supplementation and 1500 mg of calcium for postmenopausal women who are not taking estrogen supplementation. A guideline for calcium supplementation in men and women with gonadal dysfunction or those taking antiresorptive agents (e.g., bisphosphonates, SERMs, calcitonin) has not been definitively established. Based on the NIH guidelines, unless there is a clear contraindication (e.g., hypercalcemia), a recommended intake of 1000 to 1500 mg of calcium, along with vitamin D supplementation of 400 IU/day, can be advocated. *Answer 11:* **c.**

QUESTIONS

12. Which of the following statements about preventive measures/risk factors for osteoporosis would not be included in the education you provide to Jim, who is at risk for or experiencing osteoporosis/osteopenia?

- **a.** Regular performance of non–weight-bearing exercise is an essential component of osteoporosis prevention/risk reduction.
- **b.** Nutritional guidelines to reduce osteoporosis risk include a reduction in the intake of alcohol, animal proteins, salt, and caffeine.
- **c.** Medications such as aluminum-containing antacids, glucocorticoids, excessive thyroid replacement therapy, and loop diuretics (e.g., furosemide) are associated with an increased risk of osteoporosis.
- **d.** Osteodensitometry is currently the standard mean of detecting osteoporosis in the early stages and should be performed regularly.

ANSWERS

12. Regular performance of *weight-bearing exercise* (e.g., walking, hiking, stair climbing, dancing, tennis, exercise classes) is an essential component of osteoporosis prevention/risk reduction. The type and amount of exercise required to prevent loss or actually build new bone are unclear. In patients with established osteopenia, the exercise selected should not put any excessive or sudden strain on bones.

A wide variety of medications are associated with an increased risk of osteoporosis or are known to accelerate bone loss (Mahon, 1998; McClung, 1999; Pfeilschifter & Diel, 2000; Woodhead & Moss, 1998). These medications include anticonvulsants, glucocorticoids, anticoagulants, gonadotropin-releasing hormone agonists or antagonists, excessive doses of thyroid hormone, and excessive use of aluminum-containing antacids. Loop diuretics such as furosemide increase urinary calcium excretion. Chemotherapy agents that cause hypogonadism in men and women can also result in osteoporosis. Therapy with antiandrogens for men with prostate cancer can also lead to therapy-induced bone mass deficit. Prolonged bed rest and a sedentary lifestyle are also important risk factors.

Osteodensitometry is currently the standard mean of detecting osteoporosis in the early stages and is indicated in all patients with evidence of vertebral abnormalities or therapy-induced hypogonadism, patients receiving glucocorticosteroid therapy, and patients with tumors that can themselves cause osteopenia (e.g., acute lymphocytic leukemia [ALL], multiple myeloma) (Pfeilschifter & Diel, 2000).

The goals of osteoporosis prevention and treatment are threefold: to prevent further bone loss, to treat the associated pain, and to devise lifestyle modifications to minimize the risk of fractures (Woodhead & Moss, 1998). *Answer 12:* **a.**

CASE 10 STUDY

Jane is a 56-year-old women who underwent autologous peripheral blood SCT for non-Hodgkin's lymphoma almost 2 years ago. Her medical history is significant for splenectomy. She is an elementary school teacher and is hoping to return to full-time work again. She asks for your advice regarding the need for her to be revaccinated.

QUESTIONS

1. Your response incorporates your knowledge that:

- **a.** The most important factor that needs to be taken into account when consider-

ing vaccination after SCT is the individual's immune status.
- **b.** One year after transplant, vaccinations are unlikely to be effective because of poor specific antibody responses in hematopoietic SCT patients.
- **c.** Splenectomized patients or patients who are functionally asplenic (as a consequence of total body irradiation and/or chronic GVHD) are at reduced risk for pneumococcal infection.
- **d.** A single dose of a vaccination is usually sufficient to produce a response in patients who have undergone an SCT.

1. Immune reconstitution after HSCT follows a general pattern developing from immature to mature immune function. Cytotoxic and phagocytic functions recover initially, but the more specialized functions of T and B lymphocytes may remain impaired for a year or even longer (Singhal & Mehta, 1998). The tempo of immunologic reconstitution depends on whether the patient received an allogeneic or autologous stem cell graft, the presence of GVHD, and continuing treatment with immunosuppression (Gold, Flowers, & Sullivan, 1998). All vaccines should be avoided for at least 4 months after transplant because the patient is most likely unable to elicit a response. However, after the first year, patients are likely to respond to booster vaccinations, although multiple doses or courses of vaccination may be required. Two to four weeks after vaccination, the adequacy of the immune response to a vaccine should be measured by the serum level of the specific antibody to establish seroconversion. Splenectomized patients and patients who are functionally asplenic are at increased risk for pneumococcal infection because of their inability to mount an antibody response to the pneumococcal polysaccharide antigen. Patients with Hodgkin's disease and multiple myeloma are also at additional risk to develop pneumococcal infection. *Answer 1:* **a.**

Case Study continued

You recommend vaccination against diptheria and tetanus, *Haemophilus influenzae* type b (HIB), Pneumovax, and the yearly influenza vaccine. In addition, you suggest assessing the adequacy of Jane's antibody titers against measles, mumps, rubella, and varicella.

QUESTIONS

2. Would your recommendations change if Jane was 2 years following matched related sibling allogeneic peripheral blood SCT and receiving low-dose immunosuppression with evidence of mild chronic GVHD of skin only?
   a. Yes, because allogeneic transplant recipients do not require revaccination unless their donor has inadequate antibody titers to poliovirus, tetanus, and diptheria.
   b. Yes, because live vaccines are contraindicated in patients who are immunocompromised.
   c. No, although she may be unable to develop an antibody response to vaccination because of her compromised immune function

   d. No, however, to ensure immunity to measles, mumps, and rubella, vaccination with MMR is also required in patients who have undergone an allogeneic transplant.

2. Singhal and Mehta (1998), Gold, Flowers, and Sullivan (1998), and Ljungman (1999) suggest that patients at 2 years posttransplant, even those with chronic GVHD, may receive vaccination against diptheria, tetanus, HIB, influenza, pneumococcus, inactivated (Salk) polio vaccine, and tetanus. The question of vaccination against meningococcus, hepatitis A, and hepatitis B requires further study in STC recipients (Ljungman, 1999; Singhal & Mehta, 1999). However, after SCT in patients who are otherwise normal, immune responses to vaccination are often compromised. Antibody titers can be tested 2 and 4 weeks after vaccination to evaluate immune responsiveness.

With time, most allogeneic patients and a large proportion of autologous transplant patients lose their immunity to poliovirus, tetanus, diptheria, and measles (Ljungman, Cordonnier, DeBock, et al., 1995; Somani & Larson, 1995). In addition, these patients are at risk of developing infection with *Haemophilus influenzae* and *Streptococcus pneumoniae*, for which effective vaccines are available.

Systematic revaccination after HSCT is a relatively neglected area of study, and even less is known about the return of immune function in patients transplanted using hematopoietic stem cells derived from the peripheral blood. Despite prompt return of normal neutrophil and lymphocyte counts, humoral and cellular immunity may take as long as a year or more to fully recover after SCT (Gold, Flowers, & Sullivan, 1998). It is possible that immune recovery may take longer in recipients of T-cell depleted, HLA-mismatched, or unrelated donor transplants (Singhal & Mehta, 1998). If there is any question about immune competence, serum immunoglobulin levels and CD4+/CD8+ lymphocyte subsets should be determined. When these parameters are low, patients may be considered immunocompromised to some extent.

None of the vaccinations recommended for Jane are live vaccines (Staab, 1998). However, MMR is a live vaccine and generally should not be given to patients receiving immunosuppressive therapy or to those with chronic GVHD, whether requiring therapy or not (Singhal & Mehta, 1998, 1999). Live vaccines such as the MMR carry a risk of inducing uncontrolled infection in the immunocompromised host. *Answer 2:* **c.**

CASE 11 STUDY

John was diagnosed with AML 3 years ago and now is more than 1 year status post allogeneic STC. He and his wife have two children, ages 3½ and 5 years old. John and his wife have not allowed their children to receive any vaccinations because of John's immunocompromised status. During an office visit, John mentions that he anticipates problems once his 5-year-old enrolls in school and must have documented vaccination records.

QUESTIONS

1. What is the appropriate intervention?
   a. Writing a letter to the school explaining that John's children cannot be vaccinated at this time because of his immunocompromised status
   b. Recommending to John that he work with his child's pediatrician to arrange for appropriate childhood vaccinations
   c. Recommending that John discuss this with the transplant center at his next visit with them in 6 months
   d. Vaccinating John's children at this visit with oral polio vaccine, MMR, varicella, and DTaP (acellular pertussis), and setting up a schedule with them for the follow-up vaccinations

ANSWERS

1. John should work with his children's pediatric health care provider to arrange for appropriate childhood vaccinations, discussing with the provider his immunocompromised status. Immunizing contacts and preventing them from acquiring a vaccine-preventable disease may actually be very important to the protection of the immunocompromised individual (McFarland, 1999). Contacts and family members should not receive oral polio vaccine for at least the first year after transplant, and in some patients beyond that, because the patient may be at risk from live virus shedding, which can occur for up to 12 weeks after immunization. Inactivated polio virus vaccine (IPV) may be safely given (McFarland, 1999). Family members can safely receive the MMR vaccine because it does not pass to others (Gold, Flowers, & Sullivan, 1998). The live attenuated varicella vaccine may have to be used with caution or avoided in household contacts of immunocompromised transplant patients, or if contacts/children are vaccinated, the transplant patient should receive acyclovir prophylaxis (Singhal & Mehta, 1999). *Answer 1:* **b.**

REFERENCES

Abdel-Mageed, A., Graham-Pole, J., Del Rosario, M. L. U., et al. (1999). Comparison of two doses of intravenous immunoglobulin after allogeneic bone marrow transplants. *Bone Marrow Transplant, May,* p. 929.

Apovian, C. M., Still, C. D., & Blackburn, G. L. (1998). Nutrition support. In Berger, A. M., Portenoy, R. K., & Weissman, D. E. (Eds.). *Principles and practice of supportive oncology* (pp. 571-588). Philadelphia: Lippincott-Raven.

Atkinson, K. (1994). Interstitial pneumonitis. In Atkinson, K. (Ed.). *Clinical bone marrow transplantation: A clinical textbook* (pp. 360-371). Cambridge: Cambridge University Press.

Arvin, A. M. (2000). Varicella-zoster virus: Pathogenesis, immunity, and clinical management in hematopoietic cell transplant recipients. *Biol Blood Marrow Transplant, 6,* pp. 219-230.

Baker, F., Zabora, J., Pollard, A., & Wingard, J. (1999). Reintegration after bone marrow transplantation. *Cancer Practice, 7*(4), pp. 190-197.

Barron, M. A., & White, P. (1996). Consultation. In Hamric, A., Spross, J. A., & Hanson, C. M. (Eds.). *Advanced nursing practice: An integrative approach* (pp. 165-183). Philadelphia: WB Saunders.

Bearman, S. I. (1995). The syndrome of hepatic veno-occlusive disease after marrow transplantation. *Blood, 85,* p. 3005.

Bergerson, S. (1998). Nutritional support in bone marrow transplant recipients. In Burt, R. K., Deeg, H. J., Lothian, S., & Santos, G. W. (Eds.). *Bone marrow transplantation* (pp. 343-356). Austin: Landes Bioscience.

Blinder, M. A. (1998). Anemia and transfusion therapy. *The Washington manual of medical therapeutics,* 29th ed. (pp. 360-374). Philadelphia: Lippincott Williams & Wilkins.

Bryant, D. (1994). Pulmonary complications. In Atkinson, K. (Ed.). *Clinical bone marrow transplantation: A clinical textbook* (pp. 467-474). Cambridge: Cambridge University Press.

Buchsel, P. C., Leum, E. W., & Randolph, S. R. (1996). Delayed complications of bone marrow transplantation: An update. *Oncol Nurs Forum, 23*(8), pp. 1267-1291.

Buckley, F. P. (1998). Management of pain in the bone marrow transplant patient. In Burt, R. K., Deeg, H. J., Lothian, S., & Santos, G. W. (Eds.). *Bone marrow transplantation* (pp. 357-379). Austin: Landes Bioscience.

Burns, J. M., Tierney, D. K., Long, G. D., et al. (1995). Critical pathway for administering high-dose chemotherapy followed by peripheral blood stem cell rescue in the outpatient setting. *Oncol Nurs Forum, 22*(8), pp. 1219-1224.

Burns, W. H. (1998). Virus infections complications bone marrow transplantation. In Burt, R. K., Deeg, H. J., Lothian, S., & Santos, G. W. (Eds.). *Bone marrow transplantation.* Austin: Landes Bioscience.

Burt, R. K., & Walsh, T. (1998). Infection prophylaxis in bone marrow transplant recipients—Myths, legends and microbes. In Burt, R. K., Deeg, H. J., Lothian, S., & Santos, G. W. (Eds.). *Bone marrow transplantation* (pp. 438-451). Austin: Landes Bioscience.

Bush, W. W. (1999). Overview of transplantation immunology and the pharmacotherapy of adult solid organ transplant recipients: Focus on immunosuppression. *AACN Clin Iss, 10*(2), pp. 253-269.

Caplan, G. (1970). *The theory and practice of mental health consultation.* New York: Basic Books.

Carlson, H. E., & Casciato, D. A. (1995). Metabolic complications. In Casciato, D. A., & Lowitz, B. B. (Eds.). *Manual of clinical oncology*, 3rd ed. (pp. 456-472). Boston: Little, Brown.

Casciato, D. A. (1995). Hematologic complications. In Casciato, D. A., & Lowitz, B. B. (Eds.). *Manual of clinical oncology*, 3rd ed. (pp. 536-555). Boston: Little, Brown.

Chan, B. (2000). The pharmacology of peripheral blood stem cell transplantation. In Buchsel, P. C., & Kapustay, P. M. (Eds.). *Stem cell transplantation: A clinical textbook* (pp. 8.3-8.24). Pittsburgh: Oncology Nursing Press.

Chan, M. F. (1998). Nutritional therapy. In Carey, C., Lee, H., & Woeltje, K. F. (Eds.). *The Washington manual of medical therapeutics*, 29th ed. (pp. 26-38). Philadelphia: Lippincott Williams & Wilkins.

Chao, N. J. (1998). Graft-versus-host disease. In Burt, R. K., Deeg, H. J., Lothian, S., & Santos, G. W. (Eds.). *Bone marrow transplantation* (pp. 478-497). Austin: Landes Bioscience.

Constine, L., Hobbie, L., & Schwartz, C. (1994). Facilitated assessment of chronic treatment by symptom and organ systems. In Schwartz, C. L., Hobbie, W. L., Constine, L. S., & Ruccione, K. S. (1994). *Survivors of childhood cancer: Assessment and management* (pp. 21-79). St. Louis: Mosby.

Cornish, J., Goulden, N., & Potter, N. (1998). Unrelated donor bone marrow transplantation. In Barrett, J., & Treleaven, J. (Eds.). *The clinical practice of stem cell transplantation* (pp. 360-396). Oxford: Iris Medical Media.

Costabile, R. (2000). Cancer and male sexual dysfunction. *Oncology, 14*(2), pp. 195-200.

Coyne, D. W. (1998). Renal diseases. In Carey, C., Lee, H., & Woeltje, K. F. (Eds.). *The Washington manual of medical therapeutics*, 29th ed. (pp. 227-244). Philadelphia: Lippincott Williams & Wilkins.

Crawford, S. (1997). Supportive care in bone marrow transplantation: Pulmonary complications. In Winter, J. (Ed.). *Blood stem cell transplantation* (pp. 231-254). Boston: Kluwer Academic.

de Silva, M., Contreras, M., & Warwick, R. (1998). Blood transfusion support. In Barrett, J., & Treleaven, J. (Eds.). *The clinical practice of stem cell transplantation* (pp. 796-809). Oxford: ISIS Medical Media.

Deeg, H. J. (1994). Delayed complications after bone marrow transplantation. In Forman, S., Blume, K., & Thomas, E. D. (Eds.). *Bone marrow transplantation* (pp. 376-403). Boston: Blackwell Scientific.

Deeg, H. J. (1998a). Delayed complications. In Burt, R. K., Deeg, H. J., Lothian, S., & Santos, G. W. (Eds.). *Bone marrow transplantation* (pp. 515-522). Austin: Landes Bioscience.

Deeg, H. J. (1998b). Graft failure. In Burt, R. K., Deeg, H. J., Lothian, S., & Santos, G. W. (Eds.). *Bone marrow transplantation* (pp. 309-316). Austin: Landes Bioscience.

Deeg, H. J., & Socie, G. (1998). Malignancies after hematopoietic stem cell transplantation: Many questions, some answers. *Blood, 91*(6), pp. 1833-1844.

Ebeling, P. R., Thomas, D. M., Erbas, B., et al. (1999). Mechanisms of bone loss following allogeneic and autologous hemopoietic stem cell transplantation. *J Bone Mineral Res, 14*, pp. 342-350.

Ford, R. N. (1990). Psychosocial and ethical issues in bone marrow transplantation. In Kasprisin, C. A., & Snyder, E. L. (Eds.). *Bone marrow transplantation: A nursing perspective.* Arlington, VA: American Association of Blood Banks.

Fox, M. C. (1998). Transfusions. In Burt, R. K., Deeg, H. J., Lothian, S., & Santos, G. W. (Eds.). *Bone marrow transplantation* (pp. 5-68). Austin: Landes Bioscience.

Fox, M. C. (1998). Transfusions. In Burt, R. K., Deeg, H. J., Lothian, S., & Santos, G. W. (Eds.). *Bone marrow transplantation.* Austin: Landes Bioscience.

Gajewski, J., & Champlin, R. (1998). Bone marrow transplantation from unrelated donors. In Burt, R. K., Deeg, H. J., Lothian, S., & Santos, G. W. (Eds.). *Bone marrow transplantation* (pp. 23-28). Austin: Landes Bioscience.

Gauvreau, J. M., Lenssen, P., Cheney, C. L., et al. (1981). Nutritional management of patients with intestinal graft-versus-host disease. *J Am Acad Dietetics, 79,* pp. 673-675.

Gilden, D. H., Kleinschmidt-Demasters, B. K., Laguardia, J. J., et al. (2000). Neurologic complications of the reactivation of varicella-zoster virus. *N Engl J Med, 342*(9), pp. 635-645.

Gold, P., Flowers, M., & Sullivan, K. (1998). Outpatient management of marrow and blood stem cell transplant patients. In Burt, R. K., Deeg, H. J., Lothian, S., & Santos, G. W. (Eds.). *Bone marrow transplantation* (pp. 524-531). Austin: Landes Bioscience.

Gluckman, E. (1994). Veno-occlusive disease. In Atkinson, K. (Ed.). *Clinical bone marrow transplantation: A clinical textbook* (pp. 356-359). Cambridge: Cambridge University Press.

Graubert, T. A. (1998). Disorders of hemostasis. In Carey, C., Lee, H., & Woeltje, K. F. (Eds.). *The Washington manual of medical therapeutics*, 29th ed. (pp. 343-359). Philadelphia: Lippincott Williams & Wilkins.

Green, D. M., Hyland, A., Barcos, M. P., et al. (2000). Second malignant neoplasms after treatment for Hodgkin's disease in childhood or adolescence. *J Clin Oncol, 18*(7), pp. 1492-1499.

Gupta-Burt, S., & Okunieff, P. (1998). Total body irradiation. In Burt, R. K., Deeg, H. J., Lothian, S., & Santos, G. W. (Eds.). *Bone marrow transplantation* (pp. 109-122). Austin: Landes Bioscience.

Harpham, W. S. (1998). Long-term survivorship: Late effects. In Berger, A., et al (Eds.). *Principles and practice of supportive oncology* (pp. 889-907). Philadelphia: Lippincott-Raven.

Height, S., & Shields, M. (1995). Problems following bone marrow transplantation: Pulmonary complications. In Treleaven, J., & Wiernik, P. (Eds.). *Color atlas and text of bone marrow transplantation* (pp. 169-180). London: Mosby-Wolfe.

Henry, L., & Souchon, V. (1998). Nutritional support. In Barrett, J., & Treleaven, J. (Eds.). *The clinical practice of stem cell transplantation* (pp. 812-825). Oxford: ISIS Medical Media.

Herson, L., Hart, K. A., Gordon, M. J., & Rintala, D. H. (1999). Identifying and overcoming barriers to providing sexuality information in the clinical setting. *Rehabil Nurs, 24*(4), pp. 148-151.

Hollis, L. A. S., & Miller, C. B. (1998). Growth factors. In Burt, R. K., Deeg, H. J., Lothian, S., & Santos, G. W.(Eds.). *Bone marrow transplantation* (pp. 424-435). Austin: Landes Bioscience.

Huey W. Y., & Coyne, D. W. (1998). Dosage adjustments of drugs in renal failure. In Carey, C., Lee, H., & Woeltje, K. F. (Eds.). *The Washington manual of medical therapeutics*, 29th ed. (pp. 549-555). Philadelphia: Lippincott Williams & Wilkins.

Ippoliti, C., Champlin, R., & Bugazia, N. (1997). Use of octreotide in the symptomatic management of diarrhea induced by graft-versus-host disease in patients with hematologic malignancies. *J Clin Oncol, 15*, pp. 3350-3354.

Johnston, E., & Crawford, J. (1998). The hematologic support of the cancer patient. In Berger, A. M., Portenoy, R. K., & Weissman, D. E. (Eds.). *Principles and practice of supportive oncology* (pp. 549-569). Philadelphia: Lippincott-Raven.

Kaplan B., & Mujais, S. (1998). Disorders of renal function and electrolytes. In Burt, R. K., Deeg, H. J., Lothian, S., & Santos, G. W.(Eds.). *Bone marrow transplantation* (pp. 408-422). Austin: Landes Bioscience.

Kapustay, P. M., & Buchsel, P. C. (2000). Process, complications, and management of peripheral stem cell transplantation. In Buchsel, P. C., & Kapustay, P. M. (Eds.). *Stem cell transplantation: A clinical textbook* (pp. 5.3-5.28). Pittsburgh: Oncology Nursing Press.

Kletzel, M., Morgan, E., & Frader, J. (1998). Ethical issues in stem cell transplantation. *J Hematother, 7*, pp. 197-203.

Konick-McMahon, J. (1998). Fluid, electrolyte, and acid-base abnormalities. In Logan, P. (Ed.). *Principles of practice for the acute care nurse practitioner* (pp. 223-235). Stamford, CT: Appleton and Lange.

Kornblau, S., Benson, A. B., Catalano, R., et al. (2000). Management of cancer treatment-related diarrhea: Issues and therapeutic strategies. *J Pain Sympt Manage, 19*(2), pp. 118-129.

Ljungman, P. (1999). Immunization of transplant recipients. *Bone Marrow Transplant, 23*, pp. 635-636.

Ljungma, P., Cordonnier, C., & DeBock, R. (1995). Immunizations after bone marrow transplantation: Results of the European Group for Blood and Marrow Transplantation. *Bone Marrow Transplant, 15*, pp. 455-460.

Long, G. (1998). Regimen related toxicity—First 30 days early toxicity of high-dose therapy. In Burt, R. K., Deeg, H. J., Lothian, S., & Santos, G. W. (Eds.). *Bone marrow transplantation* (pp. 504-514). Austin: Landes Bioscience.

Mahon, S. M. (1998). Osteoporosis: A concern for cancer survivors. *Oncol Nurs Forum, 25*(5), pp. 843-852.

Mavroudis, D. A. (1998). Graft-versus-leukemia effect of allogeneic BMT. In Burt, R. K., Deeg, H. J., Lothian, S., & Santos, G. W. (Eds.). *Bone marrow transplantation* (pp. 499-502). Austin: Landes Bioscience.

McDonald, G. B. (1994). Venoocclusive disease of the liver following marrow transplantation. *Marrow Transplant Rev, 3*(4), pp. 129-134.

McClung, B. L. (1999). Using osteoporosis management to reduce fractures in elderly women. *Nurse Pract, 24*(3), pp. 26-47.

McMahon, K., & Brown, J. K. (2000). Nutritional screening and assessment. *Semin Oncol Nurs, 16*(2), pp. 106-112.

Meadows, A. T., & Fenton, J. G. (1994). Follow-up care of patients at risk for the development of second malignant neoplasms. In Schwartz, C. L., Hobbie, W., Constine, L. S., & Ruccione, K. S. (1994). *Survivors of childhood cancer: Assessment and management* (pp. 319-328). St. Louis: Mosby.

Mehta, J., & Singhal, S. (1998). Graft failure: Diagnosis and management. In Barrett, J., & Treleaven, J. (Eds.). *The clinical practice of stem cell transplantation* (pp. 646-658). Oxford: ISIS Medical Media.

Melocco, T., Kerr, S., & McKenzie, C. (1994). Drug toxicity and interactions posttransplant. In Atkinson, K. (Ed.). *Clinical bone marrow transplantation: A clinical textbook* (pp. 396-409). Cambridge: Cambridge University Press.

Menitove, J. E. (1994). Blood transfusion. In Stein, J. H. (Ed.). *Internal medicine*, 4th ed. (pp. 749-753). St. Louis: Mosby.

Morgan, M., & Dodds, A. (1994). ABO incompatibility and blood product support. In Atkinson, K. (Ed). *Clinical bone marrow transplantation: A clinical textbook* (pp. 291-296). Cambridge: Cambridge University Press.

National Comprehensive Cancer Center Network. (1999). *NCCN practice guidelines for fever and neutropenia.* Rockledge, PA: National Comprehensive Cancer Network.

NIH Consensus Development Panel on Optimal Calcium Intake. (1994). NIH consensus conference on optimal calcium intake. *JAMA, 272*, pp. 1942-1948.

Ottery, F. D. (1995). Supportive nutrition to prevent cachexia and improve quality of life. *Semin Oncol, 22*, pp. 98-111.

Petros, W. P., & Gilbert, C. J. (1998). High-dose alkylating agent pharmacology/toxicity. In Burt, R. K., Deeg, H. J., Lothian, S., & Santos, G. W. (Eds.). *Bone marrow transplantation* (pp. 123-130). Austin: Landes Bioscience.

Pfeilschifter, J., & Diel, I. J. (2000). Osteoporosis due to cancer treatment: Pathogenies and management. *J Clin Oncol, 18*(7), pp. 1570-1593.

Philpott, N. J., & Kanfer, E. J. (1998). Complications in the early post-transplant period. In Barrett, J., & Treleaven, J. (Eds.). *The clinical practice of stem cell transplantation* (pp. 768-785). Oxford: ISIS Medical Media.

Powers, K. M., & Lam, M. (1999). Renal problems. In Logan, P. (Ed.). *Principles of practice for the acute care nurse practitioner* (pp. 1007-1034). Stamford, CT: Appleton and Lange.

Rees, C., Beale, P., & Judson, I. (1998). Theoretical aspects of dose intensity and dose scheduling. In Barrett, J., & Treleaven, J. (Eds.). *The clinical practice of stem cell transplantation* (pp. 17-29). Oxford: Iris Medical Media.

Ruccione, K. S. (1994). Issues in survivorship. In Schwartz, C. L., Hobbie, W., Constine, L. S., & Ruccione, K. S. (Eds.). *Survivors of childhood cancer: Assessment and management* (pp. 329-337). St. Louis: Mosby.

Russell, N. H., & Miflin, G. (1998). Peripheral blood stem cells for autologous and allogeneic transplantation. In Barrett, J., & Treleaven, J. (Eds.). *The clinical practice of stem cell transplantation* (pp. 453-472). Oxford: Iris Medical Media.

St. Germain, D. (1999). Beyond the cure: Late complications of chemotherapy. *Clin Lett Nurse Pract, 3*(4), pp. 1-7.

Sands, R., Boshoff, C., Jones, A., et al (1995). Current opinion: Hormone replacement therapy after a diagnosis of breast cancer. *Menopause, 2*, pp. 73-80.

Sanders, J. (1994). Late effects after bone marrow transplantation. In Schwartz, C. L., Hobbie, W., Constine, L. S., & Ruccione, K. S. (Eds.). *Survivors of childhood cancer: Assessment and management* (pp. 293-318). St. Louis: Mosby.

Schover, L. R. (1999). Counseling cancer patients about changes in sexual function. *Oncology, 13*(11), pp. 1585-1589.

Schwartz, C., Hobbie, W., & Constine, L. (1994). Algorithms of late effects by disease. In Schwartz, C. L., Hobbie, W., Constine, L. S., & Ruccione, K. S. (Eds.). *Survivors of childhood cancer: Assessment and management* (pp. 7-19). St. Louis: Mosby.

Seber, A., & Vogelsang, G. (1998). Chronic graft-versus-host disease. In Barrett, J., & Treleaven, J. (Eds.). *The clinical practice of stem cell transplantation* (pp. 620-634). Oxford: ISIS Medical Media.

Shalet, S. (1998). Endocrine and reproductive dysfunction in adults. In Barrett, J., & Treleaven, J. (Eds.). *The clinical practice of stem cell transplantation* (pp. 850-854). Oxford: ISIS Medical Media.

Shapiro, T. W., Rust, D. M., & Davison, D. B. (1997). Management of stem cell/bone marrow transplantation complications. In Shapiro, T. W., Davison, D. B., & Rust, D. M. (Eds.). *A clinical guide to stem cells and bone marrow transplantation* (pp. 125-253). Boston: Jones and Bartlett.

Singer, G. G. (1998). Fluid and electrolyte management. In Carey, C., Lee, H., & Woeltje, K. F. (Eds.). *The Washington manual of medical therapeutics*, 29th ed. (pp. 39-60). Philadelphia: Lippincott Williams & Wilkins.

Singhal, S., & Mehta, J. (1998). Reimmunization after transplantation. In Barrett, J., & Treleaven, J. (Eds.). *The clinical practice of stem cell transplantation* (pp. 746-756). Oxford: ISIS Medical Media.

Singhal, S., & Mehta, J. (1999). Reimmunization after blood or marrow stem cell transplantation. *Bone Marrow Transplant, 23*, pp. 637-646.

Smith, L. H., & Besser, S. G. (2000). Dietary restrictions for patients with neutropenia: A survey of institutional practices. *Oncol Nurs Forum, 27*(3), pp. 515-520.

Smith, M. R. (1995). Disorders of hemostasis and transfusion therapy. In Skeel, R. T., & Lachant, N. A. (Eds.). *Handbook of cancer chemotherapy*, 4th ed. (pp. 553-572). Boston: Little, Brown.

Snyder, G. M., Sielsch, E. C., & Reveille, B. (1998). The controversy of hormone-replacement therapy in breast cancer survivors. *Oncol Nurs Forum, 25*, pp. 699-706.

Socie, G., & Cahn, J. Y. (1998). Acute graft-versus-host disease. In Barrett, J., & Treleaven, J. (Eds.). *The clinical practice of stem cell transplantation* (pp. 596-618). Oxford: ISIS Medical Media.

Solimando, D. (1998). Medications. In Burt, R. K., Deeg, H. J., Lothian, S., & Santos, G. W. (Eds.). *Bone marrow transplantation* (pp. 544-566). Austin: Landes Bioscience.

Somani, J., & Larson, R. A. (1995). Reimmunization after allogeneic bone marrow transplantation. *Am J Med, 98*, pp. 389-398.

Staab, A. M. (1998). Adult immunization: Recommendations for optimal protection. *Clin Rev, 8*(10), pp. 55-77.

Tebas, P., & Horgan, M. (1998). The immunocompromised host. In Carey, C. F., Lee, H. H., & Woeltje, K. F. (Eds.). *The Washington manual of medical therapeutics*, 28th ed. (pp. 288-301). Philadelphia: Lippincott-Raven.

Teener, J. W., & Farrar, J. T. (1998). Neuromuscular dysfunction and supportive care. In Berger, A. M., Portenoy, R. K., & Weissman, D. E. (Eds.). *Principles and practice of supportive oncology* (p. 475). Philadelphia: Lippincott-Raven.

Todd, J., Schmidt, M., Christain, J., & Williams, R. (1999). The low-bacteria diet for immunocompromised patients: Reasonable prudence or clinical superstition. *Cancer Pract, 7*(4), pp. 205-207.

Wagner, N. D., & Quinones, V. W. (1998). Allogeneic peripheral blood stem cell transplantation: Clinical overview and nursing implications. *Oncol Nurs Forum, 25*(6), pp. 1049-1055.

Walker, F., Roethke, S., & Martin, G. (1994). An overview of the rationale, process, and nursing implications of peripheral blood stem cell transplantation. *Cancer Nurs*, *17*(2), pp. 141-148.

Westmoreland, D. (1998). Other viral infections. In Barrett, J., & Treleaven, J. (Eds.). *The clinical practice of stem cell transplantation* (pp. 710-721). Oxford: ISIS Medical Media.

Williams, L. A., & McCarthy, P. L. (2000). Diseases treated with peripheral stem cell transplantation. In Buchsel, P. C., & Kapustay, P. M. (Eds.). *Stem cell transplantation: A clinical textbook* (pp. 3.3-3.21). Pittsburgh: Oncology Nursing Press.

Woeltje, K F., & Ritchie, D. J. (1998). Antimicrobials. In Carey, C., Lee, H., & Woeltje, K. F. (Eds.). *The Washington manual of medical therapeutics*, 29th ed. (pp. 244-259). Philadelphia: Lippincott Williams & Wilkins.

Woodhead, G., & Moss, M. (1998). Osteoporosis: Diagnosis and prevention. *Nurse Pract*, *23*(11), pp. 18-35.

Yagi, T., Karasuno, T., Hasegawa, T., et al. (2000). Acute abdomen without cutaneous signs of varicella zoster virus infection as a late complication of allogeneic bone marrow transplantation: Importance of empiric therapy with acyclovir. *Bone Marrow Transplant*, *25*(9), p. 1003.

11 Psychosocial Issues

Deborah Boyle

CASE ⎪ STUDY

Mr. Charles Young is a 75-year-old man with inoperable large cell lung cancer who was admitted to the oncology unit 3 nights ago with severe dyspnea. A workup revealed a pleural effusion, and Mr. Young subsequently had a chest tube inserted and then underwent pleurodesis. Diagnosed 3 weeks ago, he had recently started radiation therapy and has seven more treatments to complete his course of palliative radiotherapy.

In addressing Mr. Young's needs during discharge rounds, the staff nurse reports, "He'll probably be discharged tomorrow. The pulmonologist thinks we'll be able to pull the chest tube this afternoon after he sees the film. He can resume the radiation as soon as the tube comes out. His wife will only have to get him to radiation a few more times. That shouldn't be a problem."

You ask about Mr. Young's social support and how he and his wife are coping. The staff nurse replies, "I guess they're doing OK. I really didn't ask. I'm sure the social worker has spoken to them about that." You are concerned about the staff nurse's deferral of the patient and family's psychosocial needs to be the sole domain of the social worker. You decide to speak with the nurse about this outside of the group discharge rounds setting. In the meantime, the unit secretary comes to rounds and says to Mr. Young's nurse via the doorway, "The guy in 64's IV is beeping, and his wife has been up to the desk three times now looking for you. Can you go check on it? She's driving me nuts." You say to the staff nurse, "I'll go with you and see what's up."

As you both leave the nurse's station and begin to walk down the hall, you see an elderly woman pacing outside of Mr. Young's room. "Oh, there you are," she says to the staff nurse. "His IV is beeping, and I'm worried there's an air bubble in there. I need you to check it right away." Without replying, the staff nurse enters the room and begins to assess the IV pump and lines. You introduce yourself to Mr. and Mrs. Young and

mention that you are aware that Mr. Young is getting ready to go home soon. Mrs. Young quickly replies, "Well, I don't know about that. No one has talked to me about any of this, and everyone assumes I can take care of him. I want him to come home, but this is going to be a lot of work." You see Mr. Young look nervously from the IV lines to the staff nurse and to his wife. You decide to attempt to talk with Mrs. Young outside of the patient's room. You ask to Mr. Young, "Is it OK if I borrow your wife for a few minutes and chat in the waiting room while you're getting situated?" Mr. Young says, "That's fine," and you and Mrs. Young leave the room. While walking down the hallway, Mrs. Young begins saying to herself, "I don't know how I'm going to do this. It's just too much for me; I'm not well."

In talking with Mrs. Young, you learn that the couple has been married for 52 years and are childless. Mrs. Young is estranged from her remaining siblings, and Mr. Young has a brother who he is close to. However, he lives 2 hours away. However, Mrs. Young says that they have "church friends" who have been very supportive while Mr. Young has been in the hospital. Mrs. Young tells you that she and her husband are very close. She has never learned to drive, and Mr. Young has been her caretaker up until now. She explains that she has problems with "her nerves" and that Mr. Young has always taken care of everything. Mrs. Young shares, "I'm just a very nervous person, and I don't think I can take care of him. Who's going to take care of me?"

QUESTIONS

1. In addressing your initial concern about the staff nurse's deferral of any psychosocial assessment to be the sole purview of the social worker, you were most likely reacting to:

   a. Staff nurses' frustrations about time constraints

b. Absence of psychosocial content in most basic nursing programs

c. Lack of a holistic orientation in some oncology nurses

d. Territory issues with social workers about psychosocial care

2. Which of the following is a critical example of your assessment of verbal and nonverbal cues that guided your action in Mr. Young's room?

a. Acknowledgment of staff frustration and labeling of the Mrs. Young as "difficult"

b. The anxious greeting of the staff nurse by Mrs. Young and her pacing in the hallway

c. Mr. Young's focusing on IV lines while Mrs. Young verbalized her anxiety

d. Mr. Young's glancing from the nurse to his wife during the verbal exchange

3. In the waiting room, Mrs. Young again states that no one has spoken to her about her husband's discharge. Which of the following is the best response?

a. "Tell me what you do know about it."

b. "Maybe with all that's gone on, you forgot having a conversation about discharge."

c. "Leaving the hospital must be worrisome for you."

d. "I'll be sure someone comes in and goes over everything with you."

4. In assessing the coping needs of Mr. and Mrs. Young, what factor would help you best anticipate how they will cope with the upcoming cancer trajectory?

a. Premorbid coping style

b. Magnitude of imposed role changes

c. Timing of stressors

d. Degree of available social support

5. What should be your first step in considering discharge options with Mrs. Young?

a. Determining whether Mr. Young's brother could come to visit and help

b. Exploring the potential availability of support via their church community

c. Discussing the nature of extended-care facility placement

d. Consulting the social worker about community resources for home care

ANSWERS

1. Since its inception, the specialty of cancer nursing has been articulated, practiced, and lauded for its holistic orientation to care (Welch-McCaffrey, 1986). Oncology nurses have long recognized that patients have biologic, social, and psychologic needs and that the illness of cancer is indeed a family disease. However, the recent predominance of technology, heightened patient acuity, time constraints, role ambiguity, and feelings of inadequacy in psychosocial interventions on the part of nurses often foster the deferral of emotional support to other cancer team members. Yet basic psychosocial support is integral to the core domain of cancer nursing.

Upon hearing the oncology staff nurses' perception of professional responsibility (which conflicted with your opinion), you chose not to discuss this in a group setting but rather to talk with the staff nurse in private. Sizing up the situation quickly also allowed you to seize the moment to role model psychosocial interventions by offering to go to the patient's room with the staff nurse. This provided an opportunity to use a less threatening approach to confronting problem behaviors while concurrently demonstrating more desirable interactions.

Patients and families view the oncology nurse as being a primary support person throughout the cancer continuum. This requires oncology nurses to be proficient in assessing psychosocial needs, providing the basics of emotional support, and recognizing the need to refer to colleagues when appropriate. Box 11-1 outlines key clinical conditions within the realm of basic psychosocial nursing competency.

The advance practice nurse (APN) plays a pivotal role in the provision of information, support, and empathy (Kaplow, 1996). This case study exemplifies how the APN can master a clinical conflict where labeling occurs and insensitive care can prevail. A major portion of the APN's responsibility following this interchange will be to address the staff nurse's perceptions about her responsibilities and to discuss with her how developmental variables affect coping behaviors during the cancer experience. As an element of advocacy, the APN can promote awareness about the unique issues in geriatric oncology, an important subset who represent the majority of patients with cancer, and whose needs have not been systematically addressed to date. By confronting judgmental statements made by staff and role modeling interpersonal competency, the APN can foster a change in attitude and behavior that can be reinforced by subsequent education strategies. *Answer 1:* **a.**

Anxiety
Anger
Affect and mood
   Depressed patient
   Suicidal patient
   Grieving patient
   Hyperactive or manic patient
Confusion
Delusions, hallucinations
   Psychotic patient
Relating to others
   Manipulative patient
   Noncompliant patient
   Demanding, dependent patient
Substance abuse
   Alcohol
   Other substances
Sexual dysfunction
Pain
Nutrition
   Anorexia nervosa or bulimia
   Morbid obesity
Family
   Dysfunction
   Violence

From Gorman, L. M., Sultan, D. F., & Raines, M. L. (Eds.). (1996). *Davis' manual of psychosocial nursing in patient care.* Philadelphia: FA Davis.

2. Anxiety is communicated via the spoken word and by body language. In this case, you assessed the degree of patient and spouse anxiety by responding to both verbal and nonverbal cues. Nervous glances by Mr. Young from his nurse to his wife seemed to be exaggerated by Mrs. Young's anxiety-laden discourse. Your impression was that you needed to defuse this situation by letting the staff nurse resolve the trigger to this crisis by clearing the IV line while attempting to negate Mrs. Young's escalating anxiety by talking to her in private. You also acknowledged Mr. Young's focal point in this episode by involving him in the plan. *Answer 2:* **d.**

3. Similar to assessing the venous access line problem, the staff nurse should have made a basic assessment of discharge planning needs, which included Mr. and Mrs. Young's coping with the transition to home. Once assessing the presence of obstacles to optimal discharge planning (e.g., significant anxiety, emotional distress), the staff nurse could then call in resources such as the social worker to help.

Anxiety is the emotional response that 100% of patients will most surely encounter at some point in their cancer journey. The types of anxiety encountered in cancer care include the following (Massie & Holland, 1992):

- Episodes of acute anxiety related to the stress of cancer and its treatment
- Chronic anxiety disorders that antedate the cancer diagnosis and are exacerbated during therapy
- Anxiety related to medical illness (e.g., metabolic causes, medication side effects, withdrawal states, hormone-producing tumors)

Issues surrounding dependency and burden, from both the patient's and family's perspective, are one of the most prominent worries (D'Errico, Galassi, Schanberg, & Ware, 1999). *Answer 3:* **c.**

4. Of all of the assessment variables key to determining patient and family psychosocial responses to cancer, the most important one is premorbid history, or how the person coped with crisis in the past. Patients and families will often use coping strategies that helped them manage previous conflicts. Past coping behaviors will often predict future responses. Upon identifying coping style, however, we are at risk to pass judgment, particularly if the coping style is distinctly different than our own. Yet mindful of personal bias, it is imperative to determine individual norms. *Answer 4:* **a.**

5. Your initial impression of Mrs. Y was that her norm was one of high anxiety. She confirmed this in your discussion with her, saying this has been her style all of her life. Hence, by knowing this history, you could then expect that anxiety and worry would predominate as Mrs. Young's primary coping strategy in reacting to her husband's grave illness. Also, it would be unrealistic to assume that any intervention would totally relieve Mrs. Young's anxiety. A practical goal would be to minimize, not eliminate, Mrs. Young's anxiety to a level that facilitates teaching and allows her to participate in problem solving. Despite the obvious lack of social support, you could build on what is available (i.e., the church community) to help lessen Mrs. Young's feelings of vulnerability. Once existing social support has been established, determining other community resources that could supplement surrogate family support would be indicated.

Mr. Young had been the primary caretaker for decades. Therefore you can anticipate that his inability to perform in this role will heighten his distress and his fears about his wife's welfare. His emotional response was most likely being validated by Mrs. Young's frantic demeanor in reaction to her husband's life-threatening illness. Certainly, Mr. Young will require supportive intervention in his adaptation to his inoperable cancer, particularly because some degree of respiratory distress will most likely recur.

Regardless of age, significant anxiety can always be expected in cases of new role expectations as well as role reversal. The fact that this couple is elderly and entrenched in patterns of behavior enacted over five decades makes the presumption that new role flexibility is easily accommodated all the more improbable. In addition, whether verbalized or not, this couple is dealing with the finality of their years together.

Anxiety often precludes both the reception and retention of information. Rather than challenge Mrs. Young's perception that no one has spoken to her about discharge, the best response is to acknowledge her worry as both expected and usual in this circumstance. She might then feel that someone is addressing her issues in the context of her husband's cancer. It is no use to ask what Mrs. Young knows because she has already responded that nothing has been communicated. You should ensure that someone comes back and reiterates what has been said, negates her initial statement, and acknowledges her role in decision making. This scenario also validates that patient and family education needs to be reinforced over time. Saying it once does not ensure that the patient and family "got it." It is unrealistic to assume that information will be retained and synthesized easily during the anxiety-laden course of cancer. *Answer 5:* **b.**

QUESTIONS

6. Which drug classification would be most appropriate for management of Mrs. Young's anxiety?
   a. Barbiturates
   b. Benzodiazepines
   c. Adrenergic agonists
   d. Adrenergic antagonists

7. What information will you give Mrs. Young to reassure her that the medication prescription is "not forever"?

8. Which of the following side effects should you teach Mrs. Young to expect from an anxiolytic agent?
   1. Drowsiness
   2. Difficulty concentrating
   3. Dry mouth
   4. Dizziness
      a. 1, 2, & 3
      b. 1, 2, & 4

   c. 2, 3, & 4
   d. All of these

9. Which of the following organ systems are effected by oral lorazepam?
   1. Cardiovascular
   2. Respiratory
   3. Renal
   4. Hepatic
      a. 1 & 3
      b. 2 & 4
      c. All of these
      d. None of these

10. How can you explain increasing the medication being used for Mrs. Young's anxiety at bedtime?
   a. Larger doses are required to manage Mrs. Young's level of anxiety.
   b. Mrs. Young must have used a sleep aid before this stressful time.
   c. Insomnia usually requires larger doses.
   d. Mrs. Young has achieved a level of tolerance.

ANSWERS

6-7. Benzodiazepines are the drugs of choice for anxiety and insomnia management. Mrs. Young's anxiety is situational. With short-term therapy, counseling, and support systems put into place, her anxiety should come into control. It is not a vague, general, longstanding anxiety. *Answer 6:* **b.** *Answer 7:* **See text.**

8. The side effects Mrs. Young should expect are only the selective central nervous system (CNS) effects of oral benzodiazepines, unless mixed with other CNS depressants. However, the intravenous route results in profound hypotension and potential death. *Answer 8:* **b.**

9. Side effects of benzodiazepine are less-general CNS effects. Barbiturates have a high likelihood for causing CNS depression, physical dependence, possible tolerance, and respiratory depression, and they also have the potential for abuse. *Answer 9:* **d.**

10. As benzodiazepine doses are increased, the effects progress from sedation to hypnosis to stupor. Benzodiazepines increase the total sleeping time while shortening the time it takes to fall asleep and facilitating less awakenings during the night. Therefore an increased dose at bedtime is an appropriate intervention for insomnia. *Answer 10:* **c.**

CASE 2 STUDY

On your office message machine, you receive a call from a woman who identifies herself as Mary B. She says she has been referred to you from a nurse in one of the local oncologist's offices and tells you that she needs to talk to someone because she is very concerned about her mother, who is undergoing chemotherapy for pancreatic cancer. Mary states, "She's so depressed, she just lies in bed and won't even get dressed or anything. She keeps talking about my dad who died of colon cancer 2 years ago. I'm really worried about her, and I don't know where to turn. My brother and I are scared she's going to do something to herself. Could you please call me?" You return her phone call, and Mary relates the following story.

Mary's mother was diagnosed with pancreatic cancer 2 months ago at age 61. Initially, she adamantly declined any chemotherapy but, "She was talked into taking something by my brother." Mrs. B. has been receiving weekly 5-fluorouracil (5-FU) with little resolve in her abdominal pain, which is caused by extensive liver metastases. Mary describes her mother's current day as, "Lying on the couch, eating like a bird. We have to force her to take her pain pills, and half the time she doesn't even answer the phone."

You ask Mary what her mother was like before her diagnosis of cancer. Mary replies, "She's never been a dynamo or anything. But when my dad was alive, he always got her going and kept her spirits up." You ask if Mrs. B. has had a problem with depression in the past, and Mary states, "Well, my aunt told me once that when my mom was in her early twenties she had what they called then a 'nervous breakdown.' That's the only mention of Mom having a problem that I know of. I'm pretty sure she's never taken any medication for it over the years, though."

Mary goes on to say, "I've been telling her oncologist how depressed she is, and he keeps saying that's normal for someone in her situation. Last week though, he finally put her on Elavil. My brother has been looking on the Internet for herbal remedies, and now he's trying to convince her to take that St. John's Wort. He keeps saying to my mother, 'Take it Mom, it won't hurt you, it's natural, and I know it will make you feel better.'" Over the phone, Mary begins to cry and says, "I just hate to see her like this. She knows she's dying, but to have her go this way, it's just awful."

QUESTIONS

1. Based on the initial conversation you had with Mary, what risk factor would heighten your suspicion most about a diagnosis of depression in Mrs. B.?
   a. Initial refusal of treatment
   b. Pancreatic primary
   c. Recent loss of spouse
   d. History of a nervous breakdown

2. You acknowledge the need to further assess Mrs. B. for symptoms related to depression. Which of the following signs or symptoms of depression would you be *least* concerned about?
   a. Change in appetite
   b. Social withdrawal
   c. Feelings of worthlessness
   d. Suicide verbalizations

3. In considering amitriptyline (Elavil) for Mrs. B.'s depression, one of your first considerations would be:
   a. Has she received an optimal acute (loading) dose?
   b. Could she be experiencing anticholinergic effects?
   c. What medications has she taken previously?
   d. Is she being compliant?

4. If a selective serotonin reuptake inhibitor (SSRI) were to be used in place of a tricyclic antidepressant, what adverse effect might be most difficult to differentiate in Mrs. B.'s case?
   a. Constipation
   b. Diarrhea
   c. Anxiety
   d. Dry mouth

5. Hearing that Mary's brother is advocating an herbal remedy for his mother and acknowledging that he has been influential is his mother's past decision making, what concerns you most about this future possible scenario?
   a. This form of complementary/alternative medicine has not undergone rigorous clinical trials, and its adverse effects are unknown.
   b. Mrs. B. may not be aware that there are dietary limitations (i.e., no tyramine-containing foods) because of the hypericin

fraction of St. John's Wort, which inhibits monoamine oxidase synthesis.

c. Mrs. B. might begin taking the St. John's Wort while still taking her prescription antidepressant.

d. Mrs. B.'s son is taking control away from his mother when she needs it most.

ANSWERS

1. Using a conservative estimate, 1 of every 4 patients either presents with or develops depression during the course of their cancer experience (Lovejoy, Tabor, & Deloney, 2000). Indicators of depression can be easily attributed to cancer or its therapy, which compromises recognition and treatment of this symptom. Untreated, the anxiety, despair, feelings of helplessness, guilt, and lethargy can become disabling.

Depression in the cancer experience is a challenge to investigate. It can range from normal sadness to a major affective disorder. Although it is the major psychiatric diagnosis used in cancer care, most cases of oncologic depression do not fit the criteria for a major depression (Figure 11-1). Rather, it is a normal response to an unexpected, catastrophic, life-threatening event. Relatedly then, significant mood change may be problematic to evaluate as the cancer patient faces a future threatened by treatment-related uncertainty as well as the prospect of premature mortality.

A number of risk factors have been cited for the development of a major depression during the cancer experience. They include poor functional status, inadequately controlled pain, unrelenting symptom distress, advanced stage of illness, and preexisting mood disorders (Hopwood & Stephens, 2000; Lesko, 1997; Massie & Holland, 1992). A history of depression, panic disorder, or a diagnosis of bipolar disease is the greatest risk factor for the diagnosis of depression during the course of cancer (Fawzy & Greenberg, 1996). It could be assumed that the loss of Mrs. B.'s husband caused intense sadness and that her refusal to accept treatment was her attempt to hasten her death. However, Mrs. B.'s premorbid history of a probable depression would make you most suspect of this risk factor.

Of interest secondarily was the nature of Mrs. B.'s primary tumor. Controversy exists about the nature and prevalence of depression in pancreatic cancer patients. Possible mechanisms of an altered affective state in conjunction with this malignancy include the following (Lesko, 1997):

- Tumor-mediated paraneoplastic syndrome
- Antibody production induced against a protein released by tumor that crosses the blood-brain barrier to bind with serotonin receptors
- Autoantibody production that stimulates antiidiotypic antibodies that act as an alternative receptor for serotonin and reduce its synaptic availability *Answer 1:* **d.**

2. Determination of depression in the cancer patient requires adaptation of the historic ap-

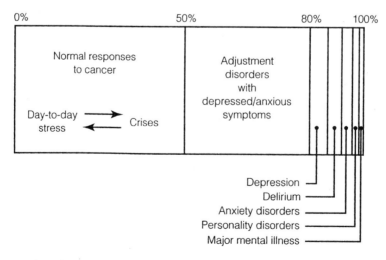

Figure 11-1 Spectrum of psychiatric disorders in cancer. (Derived from PSYCOG prevalence data; Derogatis, L. R., Morrow, G. R., Feting, J., et al. [1983]. The prevalence of psychiatric disorders among cancer patients. *JAMA, 249,* p. 751. From DeVita, V. T., Jr., Hellman, S., & Rosenberg, S. A. [1997]. *Cancer: Principles and practice of oncology,* 5th ed. [p. 2880]. Philadelphia: JB Lippincott.)

proach to symptom recognition (AHCPR, 1993). Classic neurovegetative signs such as anorexia, fatigue, and weight loss are inappropriate indicators of depression in cancer patients because they are uniformly caused by the cancer or its treatment. Hence, diagnosis should be based on psychologic, not somatic, symptoms (Breitbart, Bruera, Chochinov, & Lynch 1995; Fawzy & Greenberg, 1996; Lesko, 1997; Massie & Holland, 1992). Box 11-2 delineates the AHCPR guidelines for diagnosing depression with the Endicott Substitution Criteria for cancer patients (Endicott, 1984). With Mrs. B., a change in appetite would not be a diagnostic criterion for depression. *Answer 2:* **a.**

3. Antidepressant medications, also called *mood elevators,* exert their antidepressant action on the neurotransmitters norepinephrine, serotonin, and dopamine in brain cells. The neurobiology of depression is complex. However, depression is thought to result from deficiencies (either underexpression or overexpression) of neurotransmitter

---

BOX 11-2 | Diagnostic Criteria for Major Depressive Disorder

At least one of the following must be present:
- Depressed mood most of the day nearly every day
- Markedly diminished interest or pleasure in almost all activities most of the day, nearly every day (as indicated either by subjective account or observation by others of apathy most of the time)

At least five of the following symptoms are present during the same time period*:
- Endicott Substitution Criteria (for Physical/Somatic Symptoms)†:
  Tearfulness, depressed appearance
  Social withdrawal, decreased talkativeness
  Brooding, self-pity, pessimism
  Lack of reactivity
- Psychologic/cognitive symptoms:
  Worthlessness/guilt
  Indecisiveness/poor concentration
  Thoughts of death/suicidal ideation

Adapted from AHCPR. (1993). *Depression in primary care: Detection, diagnosis and treatment.* Rockville, MD: US Department of Health and Human Services (Pub. no. 93-0552); Breitbart, W., Bruera, E., Chochinov, H., & Lynch, M. (1995). Neuropsychiatric syndromes and psychological symptoms in patients with advanced cancer. *J Pain Sympt Manage, 10*(2), pp. 131-141; and Endicott, J. (1984). Measurement of depression in patients with cancer. *Cancer, 53*(10, suppl), pp. 2243-2249.
*Symptoms must be present most of the day, nearly daily, for at least 2 weeks.
†Replaces physical/somatic symptoms of change in appetite, weight; sleep disturbance; fatigue, loss of energy; diminished ability to think or concentrate, indecisiveness.

---

receptors responsible for firing impulses through neurotransmitter tracts located in mood-sensitive areas of the brain (Lovejoy, Tabor, & Deloney, 2000). The mechanisms of action differ between the three classifications of antidepressants (i.e., tricyclic antidepressants, second-generation antidepressants, and SSRIs). Hence, their adverse effects differ as well (Gorman, Sultan, & Raines, 1996; Williams, et al., 2000).

In considering psychopharmacologic approaches to depression, the most common error is the prescription of subtherapeutic doses (Abramowitz, 1999). Determining what past medications have been used is also important. However, per her family's report, it is unlikely that Mrs. B. has taken any medications because her initial depression was diagnosed much earlier in her life. One should also consider that there is a lag time of at least 7 to 14 days before improvement is noticed from antidepressant therapy. In the absence of other classic criteria such as improved sleep, increased psychomotor activity, noted efforts at socialization, and mood enhancement, you might be concerned whether the patient was taking her medication (Gorman, Sultan, & Raines, 1996). However, in considering the advanced nature of Mrs. B.'s cancer, her quality of life, and the deleterious effect of symptom distress, the addition of further toxicity in the face of minimal life expectancy would be your primary concern. Amitriptyline (Elavil) is a tricyclic antidepressant associated with a high incidence of sedation and other anticholinergic and cardiovascular symptoms. These anticholinergic corollaries of sedation would be a problem (in lieu of Mrs. B.'s fatigue), as would be dry mouth (she's already anorexic), urinary retention (potential problems of third spacing, dehydration), constipation (taking narcotics, immobile, not eating), and blurred vision (prolonged immobility and weakness). The newer classifications of antidepressants are thought to be more efficacious, have a more benign side effect profile, and are better tolerated (Snow, Lascher, & Mottur-Pilson, 2000). *Answer 3:* **b.**

4. In comparing the toxicities of SSRIs and the tricyclic antidepressants, the tricyclics are more often associated with blurred vision, constipation, dizziness, dry mouth, and tremors. The SSRIs, having weak anticholinergic and antihistamine effects, are more commonly associated with diarrhea, headache, insomnia, and nausea (Lovejoy, Tabor, & Deloney, 2000; Snow, Lascher, & Mottur-Pilson, 2000). For Mrs. B., the potential exacerbation of diarrhea while taking weekly 5-FU is a primary concern and impetus for close monitoring if the SSRIs were to be used. Additional SSRI-related nausea along with increased intraabdominal pressure from her primary and secondary tumors could also be problematic. *Answer 4:* **b.**

5. In the event of a new diagnosis of an advanced cancer for which treatment options are limited and prognosis is poor, patients may turn to complementary or alternative medicines (CAM) (Richardson, 1999). One of the prominent concerns in the use of CAM is patient reluctance to disclose its use to physicians. In Mrs. B.'s case, taking St. John's Wort in conjunction with a prescription antidepressant would be a major concern if she were not to inform her oncologist (Cassileth, 1999; McIntyre, 2000). Other clinical quandaries, such as lack of adverse and efficacy data and dietary limitations related to this CAM therapy, are important but secondary to the disclosure issue. Certainly, the influence of Mrs. B.'s son in decision making is a consideration. However, in the context of a family systems approach to cancer care, acknowledging premorbid norms for the family in question is always paramount in anticipating what might be expected in family behaviors. This mother-son relationship is most likely the result of decades of enculturation. The professional impression and concern about usurping control from Mrs. B. must be evaluated in the context of what is normal behavior for this family. *Answer 5:* **c.**

Case Study continued

You ask Mary what her perception of her mother's willingness to participate in some type of formal emotional support is. Mary responds that she is not sure; however, she remembers that when her father died, her mother spoke several times with the hospice social worker but was not interested in attending a grief group. In fact, Mrs. B. still receives cards from this social worker around the holidays and on the anniversary of her husband's death. Mary states that her mother has been very taken by the social worker remembering her with these gestures of caring. You inquire more about hospice. Mary says her mother had initially refused hospice services but did say, "I might reconsider when I get real bad. I don't want to make this real hard on you and your brother."

You speak to Mary about the possibility of finding out if this social worker is still employed by hospice. You also talk with Mary about communication skills to enhance her comfort in talking with her mother about her concerns. You review some communication strategies that Mary can use with her mom. You reiterate the normalcy of discomfort in talking about such taboo subjects as depression, despondency, dependency, and death. Your objective is to help Mary see that she has choices in taking the next step, that indeed she does have some control in mastering this difficult situation. You help her focus her efforts on what she has control over rather than allowing her to assume responsibility for everyone involved and ending up feeling impotent and overwhelmed. Your goal is to give Mary options, an action plan, in responding to this crisis.

You then ask about her brother. Mary says, "Well, this couldn't have come at a worse time for him. He's recently divorced and has custody of his 7-year-old daughter. He's so angry, sometimes it's hard to even be in the same room with him. You can feel it. I know he's just so mad that we lost Dad and now this with Mom. Plus he was always particularly close with our mom, and his little girl is the light of my mom's life. Since his divorce, Mom has been sort of a surrogate mother to her. But my brother rarely brings her to see Mom now because she looks so bad and he's worried it's going to scare Jocelyn. I think he's really worried Mom's going to do something to herself and that's why he's pushing that herbal medicine on her. I can't really count on my brother for too much except his opinion on everything. He's really going to have a hard time when Mom dies."

QUESTIONS

6. Helping Mary with communication skill mastery implies that you have confidence in your own ability to communicate effectively. Of the statements listed here, which would most indicate your proficiency in helping Mary enhance her communication with her mother?

    a. "Listening with interest and empathy is just as important as talking."

    b. "Validate and confront your mom's feelings. Say to her something like, 'I know your depression is normal in this situation, but I want you to know it's hurting me too.' "

    c. "Your mom may need to reminisce about the good times. Try remembering some of those fun stories when you and your brother were kids. This will also acknowledge the loss of your dad and she might open up."

    d. "Reassure her about Jocelyn. I'm sure she's worried about her. Let your mom know you will always be there for her."

7. In considering Mrs. B.'s potential for suicide, which of the following factors would be of most concern?
 a. Periodic suicidal thoughts since the diagnosis and being middle-aged
 b. Preexisting psychopathology and pain
 c. Family history of suicide in conjunction with refusal of any treatment and support
 d. Pervasive death wish and female sex

8. You acknowledge the possible relationship between anger and anticipatory grief in Mrs. B.'s son. You conclude this based on:
 a. His real and expected losses, which are numerous
 b. His recent divorce and childrearing responsibilities
 c. His attempts to "fix" his mother
 d. His historic close relationship with his mother

9. Knowing that Mrs. B.'s granddaughter Jocelyn is 7 years old, what might be the predominating theme in her perception about death?
 a. Understands that humans are mortal
 b. Views death as sleep
 c. Has feelings of being responsible
 d. Is unable to comprehend

10. What behaviors could be noted in Jocelyn that indicate her processing of her grandmother's grave illness and possible death?
 a. Nightmares
 b. Clinging
 c. Phobias
 d. Aggression

11. Indicators of pathologic or unresolved grief in Mrs. B.'s son following her death might include all of the following *except:*
 a. Repeated verbalizations of guilt
 b. Ongoing tearfulness at the mention of his mother
 c. Neglect of his daughter's needs
 d. Periodic visits to the cemetery

12. The nurses in Mrs. B.'s medical oncologist's office ask your help in developing a formal family bereavement program. Which of the following would be *least* important to consider in the planning?
 a. Education of staff about general aspects of grief reactions
 b. Agreement on a tool to measure dysfunctional grief
 c. Development of a resource list

 d. Involvement of the oncologists in the initiative

ANSWERS

6. Communication is a mandatory skill in cancer nursing. Not taught in most nursing programs other than in psychiatric nursing rotations, interpersonal proficiency enhances nurse-patient-family interactions and facilitates discovery about the nature of psychosocial distress. Less-than-optimal communication not only negates awareness of patient and family emotional concerns but may also promote distancing, isolation, and feelings of abandonment.

Basic to communication skill enhancement is the exploration of the oncology nurse's attitudes and beliefs about psychologic distress. These personal impressions dictate conduct. Some beliefs and their associated behaviors that compromise communication are listed in Box 11-3. Without personal awareness of these beliefs and in the

BOX 11-3 | Beliefs and Behaviors That Compromise Effective Communication

BELIEFS
Talking about sensitive issues takes too much time.
Talking about emotions, particularly those that prompt tearfulness, is detrimental.
Talking about death is taboo.
There is no hope.
Anger is an unwanted emotion that interferes with patient care.

BEHAVIORS
Discounting or devaluing emotional reactions ("I know you're upset, but crying isn't going to help.")
Labeling (stereotyping) ("These older patients never take their meds like they're supposed to.")
Personalizing anger and becoming defensive ("Don't get angry at me. It's the doctor's fault not mine.")
Giving false reassurances ("Don't worry. I'm sure everything will turn out fine.")
Changing the topic ("I know he just gave you some bad news, but I need to know about your pain. Is this new medicine helping?")
Ignoring cues ("He keeps putting on his call light, and when I go in there, he's just fine. All he wants is attention.")

Adapted from Sivesind, D. M., & Rohaly-Davis, J. A. (1998). Coping with cancer: Patient issues. In Burke, C. C. (Ed.). *Psychological dimensions of oncology nursing care.* Pittsburgh: Oncology Nursing Press.

absence of training in effective communication, the psychosocial domain of cancer nursing is imperiled.

Because communication consists of both verbal and nonverbal messages, both the spoken word and body language are key to any interpersonal exchange. Often undervalued, listening is a critical component of effective communication. In helping Mary, you assess that her concerns about her mother's depression have gone unheeded. Listening to Mary then fulfills two objectives. First, it helps you get a history of the crisis at hand. Second, it sends the message to Mary: "Your concerns are credible. I want to hear your story." Listening skills are particularly helpful in supporting families facing cancer. Families often feel they are relegated to an observer status in the cancer drama. When queried, however, families often relate that their world is also in chaos. Yet, not wanting to detract from the resources directed toward the patient's cancer battle, verbalizations about family distress are minimally articulated.

Mastering communication requires skill building in the use of therapeutic verbal responses. Table 11-1 outlines some of these important skills with examples. What is most important is giving the message, "I'm interested, I want to hear more. Tell me what it's like for you." Options b, c, and d limit further exploration of feelings by causing guilt, showing discomfort with depression, imposing unrealistic expectations, and making reassurances with the intent to block further discussion. Personal discomfort with the topic is usually the genesis for limiting conversation (Boyle, 2000). *Answer 6:* **a.**

7. The topic of suicide is laden with anxiety, fear, and guilt. In the cancer experience, suicide is a common concern because of the predominance of loss, grief, and depression. Considered underreported, suicide is often associated with substandard symptom management and impaired quality of life. The mystery surrounding suicide is exacerbated by inconclusive evidence about predictive risk factors. See Box 11-4.

For Mrs. B., risk factors such as previous psychiatric history, presence of advanced illness, pain, and recent loss of her spouse are important risk considerations. Additional determinants include suicide verbalizations and Mrs. B.'s advanced age. While acknowledging overall risk factors, you must also appraise the nature of the suicidal thoughts being articulated. Box 11-5 outlines a framework for synthesizing this information.

The APN in this case study serves as a patient and family advocate in numerous ways. By identifying the need for counseling in this complex situation, the APN intervenes on both the patient's and family's behalf to meet their care needs (McMillan, Heusinkveld, & Spray, 1995). Empowerment was another example of advocacy in outlining Mary's options for intervention (Chafey, Rhea, Shannon, & Spencer, 1998). Reasoning that the patient was at risk for a major depression and possible suicide (particularly in light of her oncologist's minimization of depression), the APN attempted to identify what had worked in the past in an effort to remobilize support options that had been previously accepted by Mrs. B. This serves as a poignant example of the APN actively supporting the

TABLE 11-1	Communication Skills That Enhance Psychosocial Care during the Cancer Experience
SKILL	**EXAMPLE OF APPLICATION**
Listen with interest and empathy	Thoughtful silence with eye contact and attentive body language.
Explore feelings and assist with putting words to feeling	"Tell me what you mean when you said that Susan was quite upset."
Validate emotional reactions	"This must be overwhelming. I can see why you'd be worried."
Inquire about understanding	"Tell me what your understanding is about your dad's cancer."
Clarify misconceptions that may exaggerate anxiety	"What is it about the chemotherapy that worries you the most?"
Use questions and comments that encourage communication	"Really?" "Tell me more about that." "How interesting!"
Respect personal views	"I know you think that pain is God's punishment. But let's talk about how we can manage your discomfort so that you can get to your reunion."
Reassure with realistic hope	"I don't think we can get everything organized for tomorrow, but I do think we can get you home by the weekend."
Summarize results of interaction	"So I need to find out when the hospice nurse can come, and you plan on talking with your wife about the DNR issue, right?"

Adapted from Sivesind, D. M., & Rohaly-Davis, J. A. (1998). Coping with cancer: Patient issues. In Burke, C. C. (Ed.). *Psychological dimensions in oncology nursing care.* Pittsburgh: Oncology Nursing Press.

patient and speaking up for the patient's rights and choices in the context of a moral response (Hamric, 2000). In an effort to increase both awareness and intervention for this undertreated symptom of depression, the APN could subsequently make an appointment to meet with Mrs. B.'s oncologist and office staff to discuss Mrs. B.'s case with them. Because physicians and nurses generally underestimate both the prominence and disabling nature of depression, this patient example could serve to heighten pro-

---

BOX 11-4 | Characteristics of Cancer Patients at High Risk for Suicide

Poor prognosis and advanced illness
Depression and hopelessness
Poorly controlled or uncontrolled pain
Multiple adverse symptoms
Delirium or mild encephalopathy with disinhibition (poor impulse control)
Prior psychiatric history
History of previous suicide attempt or family history of suicide
Professed thoughts of suicide
History of recent death of spouse or friend
History of alcohol abuse
Social isolation or limited available support
Emotional exhaustion
Male gender
Advanced age

Adapted from Lesko (1997); Massie & Holland (1992); Pirl & Roth (1999); Wiener, Breitbart, & Holland (1996).

---

fessional awareness of this important symptom (McDonald, Passik, Dugan, et al., 1999; Passik, Dugan, McDonald, et al., 1998). *Answer 7:* **b.**

8. Some view depression as anger turned inward. For Mrs. B.'s son, he is experiencing multiple sources of frustration and sadness related to numerous losses and added role responsibilities. His real and expected loss of both parents, dissolution of his marriage, and anticipated departure of a stable support figure for both he and his young daughter all result in a coping paradigm of abandonment. It is this duplicity of loss that makes Mrs. B.'s son most at risk for complicated grief. It could be expected then that anger would surface as a predominant coping strategy in someone faced with significant misfortune. *Answer 8:* **a.**

9-10. Feelings of profound loss are not the sole domain of adults. However, in the absence of verbal skills to articulate sadness and grief, children may be perceived to be less affected by loss. The young generally display grief differently than adults using symbolic or nonverbal language to communicate feelings (Gorman, Sultan, & Raines, 1996). School-age children, enmeshed in magical thinking, may feel responsible for the serious illness of a loved one (Table 11-2). Lacking the verbal skills to work though feelings, phobias may result, which emanate from significant anxiety, particularly if the child is isolated from discussion about what is transpiring. In an attempt

---

BOX 11-5 | Assessing Suicidal Thoughts in Terminally Ill Patients

Examine patient's reasons for wanting to end his or her life now:
- Explore the meanings of patient's desires to die.

Assess pain and symptom control:
- Is untreated or undertreated pain contributing to the desire to die?
- Are untreated or undertreated symptoms contributing to the desire to die?
- Is the patient experiencing side effects from medication that can be ameliorated?

Review patient's social supports:
- Has there been a recent loss, conflict, or rejection?
- Are there new fears about abandonment, rejection, or financial burden?
- With whom has the patient spoken about his or her plan?
- How do these persons feel about this plan?

Assess cognitive status:
- Are there cognitive deficits?
- Are there new neurologic signs or symptoms?
- Does the patient understand his or her condition, its implications, and the implications of suicide?
- Is the patient's judgment distorted by hopelessness and other symptoms of depression?

Assess psychologic condition:
- Does the patient have untreated or undertreated anxiety, depression, panic disorder, delirium, or other psychiatric diagnoses?
- How is the patient dealing with issues of loss of control, dependency, uncertainty, and grief?

Explore religious, spiritual, and existential concerns:
- Are there unresolved or distressing questions or concerns in these areas?

From Block, S.D. (2000). Assessing and managing depression in the terminally ill patient. *Ann Intern Med, 132*(3), pp. 209-218.

| TABLE 11-2 | Childhood Meanings of Death | | |
AGE	UNDERSTANDING	IMPACT	BEHAVIORS
<2 yr	Unable to comprehend; no concept, reacts to abandonment	Needs deprivation causes distress	Increased fright response; separation anxiety with parents
3-5 yr	Perceived as sleep	Fear of not being loved; may associate hospital with death	General sadness; clinging; nightmares; regression in toileting; temper tantrums
6-9 yr	Can grasp finality but unable to understand cause and effect	Magical thinking; may feel responsible, associated with punishment, mutilation, violence	Anxiousness when death discussed; avoidance of discussion; fear of punishment; school phobias; preoccupation with health of loved ones
10-12 yr	Understands inevitable nature	Defined in terms of relationships with others	Separation anxiety; afraid to leave home or friends; daydreaming; diminished school performance; aggressive behavior
13-18 yr	Acknowledges own mortality; articulates adult view of death but has limited emotional skill to cope with	Reacts to disruption in lifestyle	Change in relationships with friends; concern about being different than peers; anger; acting out; substance abuse; withdrawal from family; depression

Adapted from Coney, M. (1998). Death, dying and grief in the face of cancer. In Burke, C. C. (Ed.). *Psychological dimensions of oncology nursing care.* Pittsburgh: Oncology Nursing Press; and Gorman, L. M., Sultan, D. F., Raines, M. L. (Eds.). (1996). *Davis' manual of psychosocial nursing in patient care.* Philadelphia: FA Davis.

to protect, parental exclusion of children from the reality of severe illness and death leaves the child feeling abandoned and in need to construct his or her own meaning to what is happening. It appeared that both Mrs. B. and her granddaughter had played influential roles in each other's lives. Imposed separation versus sensitive inclusion could deter resolution of this meaningful relationship and thus foster complicated grief in both Mrs. B. and her young granddaughter. *Answer 9:* **c.** *Answer 10:* **c.**

11. Grief is a normal response to loss. However, distinguishing grief from depression is problematic, particularly in patients anticipating their death. Table 11-3 delineates and contrasts clinical features of each emotional response. It is important to assess the nature and degree of psychologic distress that is potentiating suffering. Then an assessment must be made of whether this emotional distress might be ameliorated by medication or other interventions, similar to the planning used in the management of physical symptom distress.

For family members reacting to the loss of a loved one, numerous factors must be considered in anticipating responses and in determining complicated grief. Variables that influence loss

intensity include the following (Gorman, Sultan, & Raines, 1996):

- Meaning of the loss object to the person (generally the more important the loss is to the person, the more intense the reaction)
- Degree of preparation and past unresolved issues
- Physical health
- Degree of ambivalence in the relationship (generally the more mixed the feelings [i.e., love/hate], the more difficult the grieving process)
- Support system available
- Concurrent stressors

For Mrs. B.'s son, the recent loss of his father, the importance of his mother in his life and her unanticipated illness, the demands of recent single parenthood, and social isolation all contribute to the likelihood of pathologic grief. In addition, feelings of guilt could result in hypervigilance and the imposition of controlling behaviors as a manifestation of confounding anticipatory grief.

Complicated grief is usually determined by its rating on the continuum of expected grief reactions. Complicated grief is often an exaggera-

TABLE 11-3 | Grief Compared with Depression in Terminally Ill Patients

CHARACTERISTIC OF GRIEF	CHARACTERISTIC OF DEPRESSION
Patients express feelings, emotions, and behaviors that result from a particular loss.	Patients experience feelings, emotions, and behaviors that fulfill criteria for a major psychiatric disorder; distress is usually generalized to all facets of life.
Almost all terminally ill patients experience grief, but only a minority develop full-blown affective disorders requiring treatment.	Major depression occurs in 1%-53% of terminally ill patients.
Patients usually cope with distress on their own.	Medical or psychiatric intervention is usually necessary.
Patients experience somatic distress, loss of usual patterns of behavior, agitation, sleep and appetite disturbances, decreased concentration, and social withdrawal.	Patients experience similar symptoms, plus hopelessness, helplessness, worthlessness, guilt, and suicidal ideation.
Grief is associated with disease progression.	Depression has an increased prevalence (up to 77%) in patients with advanced disease; pain is a major risk factor.
Patients retain the capacity for pleasure.	Patients enjoy nothing.
Grief comes in waves.	Depression is constant and unremitting.
Patients express passive wishes for death to come quickly.	Patients express intense and persistent suidical ideation.
Patients are able to look forward to the future.	Patients have no sense of a positive future.

From Block, S. D. (2000). Assessing and managing depression in the terminally ill patient. *Ann Intern Med, 132*(3), pp. 209-218.

tion of normal grief responses. Repeated verbalizations of guilt and self-blame, continued inability to talk about the deceased in the absence of tears, and extreme changes in usual behavior patterns are all indications of problematic grief. In addition, protracted rumination of events leading to the death, obsession and preoccupation with the deceased, self-imposed isolation, and fear of being alone may be indicative of dysfunctional grief. Periodic visits to the cemetery are often a normal gesture of mourning and an attempt to grasp the permanence of death. However, like other grief responses, it is the intensity of behaviors that distinguish between usual and pathologic variations. *Answer 11:* **d.**

12. The well-being of the family and those close to a dying person is part of the cancer team's responsibility (Worden, 1998). In this spirit of holism, the medical oncology staff nurses decided to establish closure with the families who had been in their care by developing a bereavement program. This may have resulted from your discussion with them about depression. In any case, bereavement follow-up is an important supportive intervention following the death of a loved one. Families highly value one final acknowledgment of their loss in the form of a card or call from oncology nurses (Boyle, 2000). Families often view nurses as their strongest ally and their partner in this experience because each has viewed

the patient's struggle firsthand. To create a research-based bereavement program, the following guidelines have been proposed (Hanson & Ashley, 1994):

- Develop written family assessment guidelines, including a list of risk factors for poor bereavement outcomes, to be used as a nursing education tool.
- Conduct in-service education programs to teach nursing staff how to identify families or individuals at risk for poor bereavement outcomes.
- Revise daily clinical nursing assessment charting forms to include documentation of family assessment of coping styles and their use of resources.
- Designate colleagues primarily responsible for the design and implementation of bereavement interventions.
- Develop and distribute to nursing staff a comprehensive resource directory of personnel to whom referrals for assistance with bereavement can be made.
- Develop a packet of resources and make this available to bereaved families following the death of a loved one.
- Provide administrative support for mail and/or telephone bereavement follow-up.

In providing bereavement support, it is not an expectation of office-based oncology staff nurses to formally diagnose family members as having pathologic grief. However, knowledge of risk factors and indices of need should be in the staff nurses' repertoire so that referrals can be encouraged when necessary. In addition to exemplifying the APN's role in mastering psychosocial issues of anger, depression, suicide, and grief, this case study also provides an example of the APN's direct and indirect effect on patient and family knowledge, comfort, coping, anxiety, and satisfaction (Smith & Waltman, 1994). *Answer 12:* **b.**

CASE 3 STUDY

Mr. Sam Kim is a 68-year-old Korean man admitted to the oncology unit for management of intractable pain associated with recurrent multiple myeloma. He is accompanied by his wife and 35-year-old son. Mr. and Mrs. Kim speak limited English, and their son tells you that he will serve as the interpreter for his parents.

In getting Mr. Kim in bed from the wheelchair, you observe that he is grimacing and that any movement seems to exacerbate his pain. Mrs. Kim appears very flustered and anxious. She keeps touching her husband's forehead and straightening his pajama top. Once in bed, Mr. Kim speaks to his wife in Korean, and she then turns to you and makes hand signals referring to drinking from a cup. Their son says that his father is thirsty and would like a drink. Knowing he is not NPO (nothing by mouth) status nor on fluid restriction, you tell Mr. Kim's son that you will show them where the kitchen is and that they can use these facilities as needed. Mr. Kim is told that his son and wife will return shortly. The staff nurse also leaves the room to get the equipment to establish venous access and to check on the pain medication orders.

Upon your return to the room, you ask if you could speak with Mr. Kim's son. He agrees and comes with you to your office. You ask him to tell you his understanding of what is currently evolving related to his father's cancer. Mr. Kim's son says, "The cancer has come back, and the terrible pain is from the myeloma cells getting into his bones. But the doctor says there is other chemotherapy that can be tried to stop it from going anywhere else. As soon as he's better, he's going to take those new drugs." You then ask what his father's understanding is about the status of his myeloma. Mr. Kim's son replies, "Well, he knows he has a tumor, but we don't use the word 'cancer' in front of him because if he knew that, he would just give up. He knows that the medicines he's been taking are for this problem, but he doesn't realize now that they've stopped working." You ask the son if Mr. Kim has an advance directive. He replies, "No," and says that it is not necessary because he will make any decisions about his father's care. In fact, he clarifies, he, not his father, is to be consulted first on any matter relating to his father's health. He then politely excuses himself and says he has to check on his parents.

After initiating Mr. Kim's patient-controlled analgesia, the staff nurse says to you, "I think he understands more than he can speak. We did OK getting him settled while his son was with you. He's really a sweet man. I definitely think he's the type who minimizes his pain, though, and won't complain. He's sleeping now. Dr. Thompson was just on the floor, and he said Mr. Kim's bone scan is a disaster. He's lit up like a Christmas tree with bone mets down his spine and in both hips, plus he has a hairline fracture in his left femur, and his rib cage looks like Swiss cheese. He's a mess. I can't believe he went this long at home on just Percocet." The staff nurse then asks you about your conversation with Mr. Kim's son. Upon hearing that Mr. Kim does not have an advance directive and learning the specifics of his son's instructions about information disclosure, the staff nurse becomes angry. She responds, "Well, that's crazy. This man needs to know how bad off he is. Can you imagine what would happen if we had to code him and do chest compressions? I wouldn't do that to my dog."

QUESTIONS

1. Your best response to the staff nurse at this time would be:

   a. "I agree with you, but it's probably an accepted part of Korean culture. We have to honor his wishes."

b. "Aren't you being judgmental basing what's right on your own personal values?"
c. "I hear your concern, but we have to assess this situation further."
d. "This might be an appropriate call to the Ethics Consultation Team."

2. In contemplating the dynamics of decision making, what is the most important factor to consider?
   a. Developmental stage of the ill person
   b. Degree of emotional dependence
   c. Functional role of the ill person
   d. Ethnicity and religion

3. In anticipation of the need for translation, the use of family members in this capacity needs to be considered in light of all the following *except:*
   a. Modification of information to protect the patient
   b. Degree of proficiency in English
   c. Knowledge of medical terminology
   d. Matching of age and gender with the patient

4. In comparing the concept of a "good" or "appropriate" death, the Asian version would most likely be characterized by which of the following?
   a. Patient is informed that "death is near" to prepare for final journey.
   b. Patient is surrounded by family in a specialized hospice unit.
   c. Family may openly cry, chant, or pray.
   d. Invasive tubes are removed to purify the soul at the time of death.

5. Two characteristics of end-of-life care that all patients and families desire regardless of culture are:
   a. Absence of spiritual distress and sense of contributing to others
   b. Sense of completion and saying good-bye
   c. Being pain free and coherent
   d. Family presence and self-determination

ANSWERS

1. A basic premise of cultural competency is that examination of one's own culture is necessary before gaining familiarity with others. In the absence of such introspection, personal bias may lead to dismissal of others' cultural beliefs as primitive or irrational (Leonard & Plotnikoff, 2000). Because the culture of the dominant race is rarely disputed, negative labeling of minority cultures usually prevails. This practice must be actively challenged as we evolve into the twenty-first century, when diversity will increase and the global imperative becomes realized.

Individual cultures are learned in childhood and create a blueprint for living and problem solving that structures the behavior of its group members (Iwamoto, 1995). This enhances the group's sense of norm that is challenged when members are confronted with cultural standards distinctly different than their own. Because nurses bring their personal cultural heritage to work with them, appreciation of "mine versus yours" values is imperative to actualize true cultural sensitivity.

Even in the context of optimal cultural awareness, caution should be used about viewing cultural groups as uniform and homogeneous. As in any group, individual variation must be expected. Some factors that influence ethnic individuality are listed in Box 11-6. *Answer 1:* **c.**

2. Although geographically diverse and politically unique, immigrants from countries on the Asian continent are unified by several predominant cultural norms. In Asian relationship-centered cultures, the concept of familial-self supersedes the Anglo individualized-self orientation to life. An intense emotional connectedness and interdependence results in a closely knit extended Asian family system in which decision making is not the sole domain of the ill person (Nilchaikovit, Hill, & Holland, 1993). Rather, in the face of illness, a patriarchal model is used whereby the male spouse, father, or eldest son becomes the principal decision-maker and family spokesperson determining the better good for the family as a whole.

Closely related is the dominant principle of filial piety. Love, loyalty, honor, and respect are extended to elder parents in Asian cultures by the provision of care in old age and the assumption of responsibility to make decisions on their behalf. Mr. Kim's son has assumed the role of culturally

BOX **11-6** | **Prevailing Characteristics of Cultural Distinction**

Generation
Length of time in host country
Language spoken
Social network
Education background
Economic status
City versus rural residence in native country
Motivation for acculturation

From Boyle, D. A. (2000). Pathos in practice: Exploring the affective domain of cancer nursing. *Oncol Nurs Forum,* 27(6), pp. 915-919.

prescribed dutiful protector. Because cancer is routinely viewed as a terminal illness and death is a subject not to be discussed, shielding his father from the devastation of bad news could be expected. In addition, there may also be the culturally dictated fear that to talk about death invites its presence (Hallenbeck, Goldstein, & Mebane, 1996). *Answer 2:* **d.**

3. The aforementioned beliefs are germane to translation issues. In an effort to offset anxiety and fear, the family translator may edit the message without the health professional's knowledge. Other considerations include how proficient the translator is in English as well as in his or her native tongue. Does the translator understand medical terminology and is he or she able to make these translations correctly? Finally, of least importance, is the matching of gender and age with that of the patient. A well-respected family member can generally be used as a translator. However, the exception to this practice is the case of a genitourinary topic of discussion where embarrassment may prevail with a translator of the opposite sex. Last, children should never be used as translators. Their emotional frailty and intellectual naiveté puts them in a vulnerable position, particularly during the context of life-and-death discussions. The Office of Civil Rights has published a strong statement to negate this practice in health care settings (Office of Civil Rights, DHHS, 1964). *Answer 3:* **d.**

4. In the case of Mr. Kim, his son was enacting the role expected of him. Response a makes assumptions about what has transpired without having knowledge of cultural norms. Response b will most likely solicit defensiveness on the part of the staff nurse, which would block further exploration and the potential for education. Response d implies that a problem has occurred and help is needed, but whose problem is it? Response c fosters more in-depth consideration of the nature of this scenario rather than taking a reactionary stance with the ultimate potential to elicit conflict between family and staff. Because ethnicity and religion provide a template for living, beliefs associated with culture and spirituality all underscore decision making. Other variables, such as patient age, emotional maturity, and the ill person's role in the family constellation, are important but remain secondary to cultural identity.

Despite the recent American prioritization of what constitutes a "good death," confusion prevails (Steinhauser, Clipp, McNeilly, et al., 2000). This is perhaps related to the diversity of people experiencing dying firsthand. "Appropriate" death is dictated by culture. Discussing the nearness of death with the person experiencing it is not always welcome. Care of family members in institutions associated with dying may be avoided in an attempt to negate the likelihood of death. The status of the body at the time of death is often specified by religious beliefs. However, the most common Asian religious denominations (i.e., Christianity, Buddhism, Confucianism, and Shamanism) embrace the rituals of tears and litany around the time of dying. *Answer 4:* **c.**

5. Acknowledging that communication style and emotional expression are heavily influenced by culture, you would not anticipate that the ability to say good-bye is important in all cultures. Experiencing some pain may be indicative of righteous suffering as a prelude to God's acceptance (Lipson, Dibble, & Minarik, 1996). It has already been stated that self versus family determination is not a universal goal. Regardless of participation in formal religious practices, all people have a spiritual dimension integrating beliefs that permeate all aspects of one's life (Gorman, Sultan, & Raines, 1996). Experiencing a sense of peace with one's life in the absence of spiritual turmoil is a highly valued state. This, coupled with a validated sense of self-worth in terms of service to others, is a construct at the end-of-life revered by most ethnic and religious denominations. *Answer 5:* **a.**

Case Study continued

The morning after Mr. Kim's admission, you find the staff nurse caring for him and inquire about his night and current status. The staff nurse tells you, "He had a terrible night, didn't sleep at all, and his output is minimal. We're worried he's going into renal failure. He's short of breath and his O_2 sats are dropping. He's at his nadir, and he may be septic. His son has been here with him all night. I think he's crashing."

You decide to visit Mr. Kim and assess his status. Just outside his room, you hear multiple female voices speaking Korean in the form of a chant. Upon reaching his bed, you see a group of women with Bibles in hand praying around Mr. Kim. During this chanting, Mrs. Kim is attempting to feed her husband. You also notice the presence of numerous religious pictures on the wall above Mr. Kim's head and statues on his bedside stand. Mr. Kim's son appears in the doorway and tells you that these women are from his parents church and have come to pray for his father's recovery. Minutes later, the medical resident following Mr. Kim approaches with a medical student. He interrupts the women praying and says he needs to speak with Mr. Kim in private. He asks that everyone leave the room. You say to the resident, "The family needs a few more minutes together. Can we talk outside?" The resident impatiently agrees and leaves the room with you.

In the hallway, the resident immediately says, "I need to have a serious talk with Mr. Kim, and I have this medical student with me who speaks Korean. He should be a DNR, and I want to talk to him about this before he codes. It'll save us all a lot of trouble. I can't let his son make irrational decisions. The man is competent even though he doesn't speak English, and he has a right to decide his own destiny. This conspiracy of silence has got to stop." Soon after the resident makes this statement, Mr. Kim's son comes out of his father's room. He says to the resident, "You are to talk to me about decisions regarding my father's care." The resident states, "I know you want what's best for your father, but he needs to know how sick he is. If we were to administer emergency treatment on him if he stopped breathing, we might only add to your father's pain. I want to make him a DNR, and I need to talk with him about this. He has a right to make his own decisions about what he wants done and to die with some dignity."

QUESTIONS

6. Not being bilingual in Korean and English, you feel unable to participate in the prayer intervention for Mr. Kim. However, you could best demonstrate spiritual sensitivity by:
   a. Standing silently while the group prays
   b. Calling the chaplain and soliciting their presence
   c. Leaving the group to their private religious gathering
   d. Acknowledging the importance of this ritual to Mr. Kim's son

7. In observing Mrs. Kim's behavior, you accurately postulate that:
   a. Mrs. Kim feels powerless, and feeding her husband makes her feel like she is contributing to his recovery.
   b. Elder women are primarily responsible for caregiving and nurturance.
   c. Families must take care of all the patient's needs during illness.
   d. Nutritional sustenance ensures long life.

8. The ethical principle implied in the discourse with the resident is most representative of which of the following?
   a. Justice
   b. Beneficence
   c. Respect
   d. Futility

ANSWERS

6. Individuals are a complex sum of biologic, psychologic, sociocultural, and spiritual dimensions. For many, cancer generates an existential crisis that prompts life review and questioning of one's meaning and purpose in life. Death, a common yet mysterious and enigmatic milestone, may elicit anguish and varying levels of fear. In the face of uncertainty, many will rely on a higher power for guidance and sustenance.

Spirituality and religion are two distinct but complementary entities. Spirituality is characterized by the capacity to seek purpose and meaning, to have faith, to love and forgive, to worship, to see beyond the present, and to rise above suffering (Rousseau, 2000). Religion embraces structured belief systems based on principles that dictate codes of conduct and ethical behavior. At the core of religions are rituals, ceremonies, and a participative community that exemplify religious doctrine, particularly as it relates to life after death. Hence, within the scope of these definitions, nurses have the capacity to meet spiritual needs, regardless of one's own religious orientation.

You sensed the importance of religion by your observations. Seeing the women praying and noticing the religious objects in his room, you became aware of the potential strength religion was offering Mr. Kim and his family. As a measure of respect, your best action would be to stand quietly with the group, honoring their time of prayer. This body language demonstrates a comfort, an acceptance of this effort to help Mr. Kim during this time of crisis. Other actions, such as calling in the chaplain or leaving, give a message of discomfort. Although it would be a good idea to share your thoughts with Mr. Kim's son, it is your actions in the presence of Mr. Kim that are most likely to send the message of support. This example of body language is particularly critical in Mr. Kim's situation, acknowledging the communication barrier that interferes with verbal exchange (Worden, 1998). *Answer 6:* **a.**

7. In many Asian societies, and in the Korean culture in particular, the woman's role is to nurture and care for the sick. This responsibility is not age related. Women in general are expected to provide bedside care, which at times can be labeled as excessive by Western standards (Lipson, Dibble, & Minarik, 1996). Total care is offered, including feeding and bathing the patient, sleeping in a cot in the patient's room, and assisting with all functional needs. Ambulation or movement may be discouraged in an effort to minimize discomfort and save energy for recovery. Women are action-oriented, and the patient becomes the passive recipient of family care. Although Mrs. Kim may indeed feel powerless and there is the general view that eating improves one's capacity to heal, it is her culturally derived caregiving responsibility that underscores your observations of Mrs. Kim. Your awareness of this norm in the Korean culture was also the impetus for showing Mrs. Kim and her son where the kitchen was upon admission because you anticipated that bringing in food from home for Mr. Kim would be done. *Answer 7:* **c.**

8. The response of the medical resident was not uncommon. Conflict around end-of-life decision making abounds when cultural beliefs clash. Usually, these conflicts generate from strong feelings about quality of life (Iwamoto, 1995). Although the resident's concern about Mr. Kim's comfort was well-intended, he was making judgments without appreciating the role of culture during this time of crisis. To promote optimal participation in decision making, all patients should be asked about the extent to which they wish their family to be involved. When indicated, it is important to ask who the designated decision-maker will be at the outset (Davison & Degner, 1998). With the help of an interpreter, most likely the resident would have discovered that Mr. Kim did indeed both designate and expect his son to make decisions on his behalf, regardless of his state of competency.

Rousseau (2000) stated that physicians must respect the diverse beliefs of patients, be willing to listen and engage in discussion, and provide for the rituals and ceremonies that bring meaning to their patients' lives. As a corollary to the Asian view of filial piety, the oldest son is responsible for his parents, and he is charged to preserve their lives at all cost. To agree to a "No Code" or to stopping life support is to invoke dishonor on the family in the Korean community (Boyle, 1998). In general, most laypersons have little understanding of or misconceptions about DNR orders (Jezewski & Finnell, 1998). Also, we must remember that the existing literature on advance directives is dominated by the North American view of patient self-determination as an ideal (Voltz, Akabayashi,

Reese, & Sass, 1998). Like all other indications for individualized assessment, life-and-death decision making must be founded on the patient's, not the health professional's, norm.

The resident's role was not to "change the son's mind" but rather to fully inform him as the designated decision-maker about the outcomes of a resuscitation effort specific to Mr. Kim's case. There was an opportunity to talk about the nature of this, which could have then facilitated an informed decision, regardless of what the resident thought was "right." In addition, the resident had not established a relationship with the family; hence trust had not been built. In knowing the patient, the resident would have had information about this family's decision-making norm. In this case the absence of a relationship and trust interfered with communication during this time of turmoil and stress (Blatt, 1999; Stagno, Zhukovsky, & Walsh, 2000).

The resident voiced his opinion emanating from several ethical principles. Beneficence, or the avoidance of unnecessary suffering, injury, or harm, was strongly stated, as was the principle of respect (Smith & Bodurtha, 1995). The futility of treatment was also mentioned, centered around Mr. Kim's progressive myeloma. What was implied but not stated related to the concept of justice, the equitable distribution of resources among individuals. With his statement referring to the prospect of, "Saving us all a lot of trouble," the resident indicated that extra work could be in store for the health professionals involved in Mr. Kim's care if the wrong decision was made about future treatment efforts.

Physician attitudes in this case were a major deterrent to optimal patient-centered decision making. This was particularly troublesome in light of the context of Mr. Kim's limited life expectancy. The on-the-spot problem solving demonstrated by the APN is an example of immediate conflict resolution that requires further individual follow-up with the resident. In addition, formal education on the ethical implications of working with a culturally diverse patient population would be in order as a component to housestaff education.

Ethical issues are central to the clinical practice of oncology nursing (Ersek, Scanlon, Glass, et al., 1995). Undertreatment of pain, truth telling, treatment refusal, informed consent, and DNR orders are all priority concerns present in this case study. The APN again proved to be a patient and family advocate. Being culturally astute and recognizing a conflict in the making, the APN chose to intervene with the intent to provide a forum for education and discussion rather than assertion and confrontation. *Answer 8:* **a.**

REFERENCES

Abramowicz, M. (Ed.). (1999). Drugs for depression and anxiety. *Med Lett, 41*(1050), pp. 33-38.

AHCPR. (1993). *Depression in primary care: Detection, diagnosis and treatment.* Rockville, MD: US Department of Health and Human Services (Pub. no. 93-0552).

Blatt, L. (1999). Working with families in reaching end-of-life decisions. *Clin Nurse Specialist, 13*(5), pp. 219-223.

Block, S. D. (2000). Assessing and managing depression in the terminally ill patient. *Ann Intern Med, 132*(3), pp. 209-218.

Boyle, D. A. (2000). Pathos in practice: Exploring the affective domain of cancer nursing. *Oncol Nurs Forum, 27*(6), pp. 915-919.

Boyle D. M. (1998). The cultural context of dying from cancer. *Int J Palliative Nurs, 4*(2), pp. 70-83.

Breitbart, W., Bruera, E., Chochinov, H., & Lynch, M. (1995). Neuropsychiatric syndromes and psychological symptoms in patients with advanced cancer. *J Pain Sympt Manage, 10*(2), pp. 131-141.

Cassileth, B. R. (1999). Evaluating complementary and alternative therapies for cancer patients. *CA Cancer J Clin, 49*(6), pp. 362-375.

Chafey, K., Rhea, M., Shannon, A., & Spencer, S. (1998). Characteristics of advocacy for practicing nurses. *J Prof Nurs, 14*(1), pp. 43-52.

Davison, B. J., Degner, L. F. (1998). Promoting patient decision making in life and death situations. *Semin Oncol Nurs, 14*(2), pp. 129-136.

D'Errico, G. M., Galassi, J. P., Schanberg, R., & Ware, W. B. (1999). Development and validation of the cancer worries inventory: A measure of illness-related cognitions. *J Psychosocial Oncol, 17*(3/4), pp. 119-137.

Endicott, J. (1984). Measurement of depression in patients with cancer. *Cancer, 53*(10, suppl), pp. 2243-2249.

Ersek, M., Scanlon, C., Glass, E., et al. (1995). Priority ethical issues in oncology nursing: Current approaches and future directions. *Oncol Nurs Forum, 22*(5), pp. 803-807.

Fawzy, F. I., & Greenberg, D. B. (1996). Oncology. In Rondell, J., & Wise, M. (Eds) *Textbook of consultation liaison psychiatry* (pp. 673-694). Washington, DC: American Psychiatric Press.

Gorman, L. M., Sultan, D. F., & Raines, M. L. (Eds.). (1996). *Davis' manual of psychosocial nursing in patient care.* Philadelphia: FA Davis.

Hallenbeck, J., Goldstein, M. K., & Mebane, E. W. (1996). Cultural considerations of death and dying in the United States. *Clin Geriatr Med, 12*(2), pp. 393-406.

Hamric, A. B. (2000). What is happening to advocacy? *Nurs Outlook, 48*(3), pp. 103-104.

Hanson, J. L., & Ashley, B. (1994). Advanced practice nurses' application of the Stetler Model for research utilization: Improving bereavement care. *Oncol Nurs Forum, 21*(4), pp. 720-724.

Hopwood, P., & Stephens, R. J. (2000). Depression in patients with lung cancer: Prevalence and risk factors derived from quality of life data. *J Clin Oncol, 18*(4), pp. 893-903.

Iwamoto, R. (1995). Cultural influences on quality of life. *Qual Life Nurs Chall, 3,* pp. 68-73.

Jezewski, M. A., & Finnell, D. S. (1998). The meaning of DNR status: Oncology nurses' experiences with patients and families. *Cancer Nurs, 21*(3), pp. 212-221.

Kaplow, R. (1996). The role of the advanced practice nurse in the care of patients critically ill with cancer. *AACN Clin Iss, 7*(1), pp. 120-130.

Leonard, B. J., & Plotnikoff, G. A. (2000). Awareness: The heart of cultural competence. *AACN Clin Iss, 11*(1), pp. 51-59.

Lesko, L. M. (1997). Psychologic issue. In DeVita, V. T., Hellman, S., & Rosenberg, S. A. (Eds.). *Cancer: Principles and practice,* 5th ed. (pp. 2879-2891). Philadelphia: Lippincott-Raven.

Lipson, J. G., Dibble, S. L., & Minarik, P. A. (Eds.). (1996). *Culture and nursing care: A pocket guide.* San Francisco: UCSF Press.

Loney, M. (1998). Death, dying and grief in the face of cancer. In Burke, C. C. (Ed.). *Psychosocial dimensions of oncology nursing care* (pp. 152-179). Pittsburgh: Oncology Nursing Press.

Lovejoy, N. C., Tabor, D., & Deloney, P. (2000). Cancer-related depression: Part II–Neurologic alterations and evolving application to psychopharmacology. *Oncol Nurs Forum, 27*(5), pp. 795-808.

Massie, M. J., & Holland, J. C. (1992). The cancer patient with pain: Psychiatric complications and their management. *J Pain Sympt Manage, 7*(2), pp. 99-109.

McDonald, M. V., Passik, S. D., Dugan, W., et al. (1999). Nurses' recognition of depression in their patients with cancer. *Oncol Nurs Forum, 26*(3), pp. 593-599.

McIntyre, M. (2000). A review of the benefits, adverse events, drug interactions and safety of St. John's Wort: The implications with regards to the regulation of herbal medicines. *J Alternative Complement Med, 6*(2), pp. 115-124.

McMillan, S. C., Heusinkveld, K. B., & Spray, J. (1995). Advanced practice in oncology nursing: A role delineation study. *Oncol Nurs Forum, 22*(1), pp. 41-50.

Nilchaikovit, T., Hill, J. M., & Holland, J. C. (1993). The effects of culture on illness behavior and medical care: Asian and American differences. *Gen Hosp Psychiatry, 15*(1), pp. 41-50.

Office of Civil Rights, Department of Health and Human Services, Title VI of the Civil Rights Act of 1964.

Passik, S. D., Dugan, W., McDonald, M. V., et al. (1998). Oncologists recognition of depression in their patients with cancer. *J Clin Oncol, 16*(4), pp. 1594-1600.

Pirl, W. F., & Roth, A. J. (1999). Diagnosis and treatment of depression in cancer patients. *Oncology, 13*(9), pp. 1293-1302.

Richardson, M. A. (1999). Research in complementary/alternative medicine therapies in oncology: Promising but challenging. *J Clin Oncol, 17*(11S), pp. 38-43.

Rousseau, P. (2000). Spirituality and the dying patient. *J Clin Oncol, 18*(9), pp. 2000-2002.

Sivesind, D. M., & Rohaly-Davis, J. A. (1998). Coping with cancer: Patient issues. In Burke, C. C. (Ed.). *Psychological dimensions of oncology nursing care* (pp. 4-26). Pittsburgh: Oncology Nursing Press.

Smith, J. E., & Waltman, N. L. (1994). Oncology clinical nurse specialists perceptions of their influence on patient outcomes. *Oncol Nurs Forum, 21*(5), pp. 887-893.

Smith, T. J., & Bodurtha, J. N. (1995). Ethical considerations in oncology: Balancing the interests of patients, oncologists and society. *J Clin Oncol, 13*(9), pp. 2464-2470.

Snow, V., Lascher, S., & Mottur-Pilson, C. (2000). Pharmacologic therapy of acute major depression and dysthymia. *Ann Intern Med, 132*(9), pp. 738-742.

Stagno, S. J., Zhukovsky, D. S., & Walsh, D. (2000). Bioethics: Communication and decision-making in advanced disease. *Semin Oncol, 27*(1), pp. 94-100.

Steinhauser, K. E., Clipp, E. C., McNeilly, M., et al. (2000). In search of a good death: Observations of patients, families and providers. *Ann Intern Med, 132*(10), pp. 825-832.

Voltz, R., Akabayask, A., Reese, C., & Sass, H. M. (1998). End-of-life decisions and advance directives in palliative care: A cross-cultural survey of patients and health care professionals. *J Pain Sympt Manage, 16*(3), pp. 153-162.

Welch-McCaffrey, D. (1986). Role performance issues for oncology clinical nurse specialists. *Cancer Nurs, 9*(6), pp. 287-294.

Wiener, I., Breitbart, W., & Holland, J. (1996). Psychological issues in the care of dying patients. In Rundell, J., & Wise, M. (Eds.). *Textbook of consultation liaison psychiatry* (pp. 804-831). Washington, DC: American Psychiatric Press.

Williams, J. W., Mulrow, C. D., Chiquette, E., et al. (2000). A systematic review of newer pharmacotherapies for depression in adults. *Ann Intern Med, 132*(9), pp. 743-756.

Worden, J. W. (1998). Bereavement care. In Berger, A. M., Portenoy, R. K., & Weissman, D. E. (Eds.). *Principles and practice of supportive oncology* (pp. 767-772). Philadelphia: Lippincott-Raven.

12 Pain

Rita Wickham

CASE | STUDY

You have been following Shirley Jackson in the clinic. She is a 56-year-old African American woman who was diagnosed with Duke's stage B_2 colon cancer several years ago. She was initially treated with surgical resection and postoperative adjuvant chemotherapy consisting of 5-flououracil (5-FU) and leucovorin. She did well until about 1 year ago, when she had symptoms of cramping, fullness, and "constipation." She was diagnosed to have recurrent colon cancer, with regional and hepatic metastases. She was restarted on chemotherapy (irinotecan), but this was discontinued 3 months ago because of further tumor progression.

About 5 months ago, Mrs. Jackson started to have pain that was not relieved by occasional acetaminophen or ibuprofen. Her oncologist started her on hydrocodone 5 mg plus acetaminophen 500 mg (Vicodin). The instructions on her bottle of medication say "one or two tablets every 4 hours as needed." She tells you that she almost always takes only one tablet and tries to stretch out the time by taking the pill about every 6 hours. Initially, this dose was somewhat effective, but she says it didn't help at all after about a month and a half. She wonders if she can take Motrin (ibuprofen) instead her of Vicodin.

QUESTIONS

1. What are the most likely reasons that Mrs. Jackson would take only one Vicodin?
   1. She did not want to take too much pain medicine.
   2. Her pain was controlled.
   3. Her pain assessment did not include an exploration of common patient concerns.
   4. Her physician told her she should save the pain medicine for when the pain got "really bad."
      a. 1 & 2
      b. 2 & 4
      c. 1 & 3
      d. All of these

2. What alternative intervention would you most appropriately have taught Mrs. Jackson at this point?
   a. Telling her to increase the Vicodin to two tablets every 4 hours
   b. Telling her to increase the Vicodin to two tablets every 6 hours
   c. Starting her on sustained-release oxycodone (Oxycontin) 40 mg every 12 hours
   d. Starting her on sustained-release morphine (MS Contin) 15 mg every 12 hours

3. If Mrs. Jackson had increased the number of Vicodin tablets she was taking and now told you that she was taking two tablets every 4 hours, you would know this to be:
   a. An optimal dose of both acetaminophen and hydrocodone
   b. Too much acetaminophen
   c. Too much hydrocodone
   d. Both too much acetaminophen and Vicodin

4. If Mrs. Jackson had started taking over-the-counter (OTC) ibuprofen, a nonsteroidal antiinflammatory drug (NSAID) three 600-mg tablets four times a day in addition to an optimal dose of Vicodin, you would say the relative safety of this option is:
   a. Safe because acetaminophen and NSAIDs inhibit prostaglandin synthesis in different sites
   b. Safe because both acetaminophen and ibuprofen are nonopioids
   c. Unsafe because the dose of ibuprofen is too large
   d. Unsafe because using both may increase the risk for renal toxicity

1. Poorly alleviated pain is an unfortunate problem that is more prevalent than would be expected, given the wide spectrum of currently available analgesics, which could alleviate at least 70% to 90% of all cancer-related and other pain (Portenoy, 1995). Patient/family barriers may be one impediment to optimal pain control, and the advanced practice nurse (APN) should address patient worries about taking pain medication so that these concerns can be discussed and allayed. Mrs. Jackson may be concerned about taking strong pain medicines, or she might be having side effects she does not like. It is not unusual for patients (or their family members) to be concerned about taking morphine in particular, or other strong opioid analgesic, and they often believe they can become addicted or "hooked" if they take too much. Side effects and costs may also be an impediment to the patient (Ersek, Kraybill, & Du Pen, 1999). Other patients worry that they may become tolerant to the analgesic and hold back on taking opioids for severe pain now so that there will be something left if the pain worsens later (Von Gunten & Von Roenn, 1994). Patients' concerns about taking opioids are often not addressed when these medications are ordered.

In addition, the prescribing physician or APN may not have addressed side effects of opioids that often are initially bothersome, especially mental dullness; feeling "spacey," light-headed, or sleepy; or having nausea or constipation (Ersek, Kraybill, & Du Pen, 1999). The APN should provide details about new analgesics, including how and when to take them and any potential side effects. The APN should supplement these details with written materials to help reduce or alleviate patient concerns and plan management strategies. You can also stress to Mrs. Jackson that it is not unusual for some patients to be reluctant to report pain to their physician or nurse (because of concerns about distracting their physician from treating their underlying cancer, fears that increasing pain means worsening cancer, and wanting to be seen as a good patient) (Von Gunten & Von Roenn, 1994). Patients who are older, have lower incomes, or are less educated may be more likely to have concerns about taking opioid analgesics (Ward, Goldberg, Miller-McCauley, et al., 1993). *Answer 1:* **c.**

2. Three important dosing principles you would consider with Mrs. Jackson are (1) recognizing potential maximum doses of analgesics you prescribe or recommend, (2) maximizing dosages of prescribed analgesics before deciding whether they are helpful or not, and (3) using the analgesic ladder approach to make an educated guess about which analgesics *might* be helpful. Knowledge of optimal and maximum dosages is particularly important with nonopioid medications, which have a ceiling effect. That is, increasing a daily dose to a higher-than-recommended dose usually

does not increase analgesia, but it may increase toxicity or side effects. *Answer 2:* **b.**

3. Side effects are a particularly important consideration for acetaminophen because it is included in many prescription-strength combination analgesics used for moderate pain, and it is also available in many OTC products. The prescriber may have forgotten that if Mrs. Jackson were to take Vicodin as ordered (two tablets every 4 hours), her 24-hour dose of acetaminophen would be 6000 mg. The maximum dose of acetaminophen should not exceed 4000 mg (some clinicians recommend no more than 3500 mg/day with chronic use), and a single dose should not exceed 1000 mg. Lower dosages may be prudent for cachectic patients, those with a history of chronic alcohol use (three or more drinks per day), or those with altered hepatic function. Individuals who take larger-than-recommended doses over a sustained time could experience inadvertent overdoses of acetaminophen. This can potentially lead to acute liver failure (which may cause elevated aminotransferase, bilirubin, and prothrombin levels), hepatic coma, or death, as well as renal failure (evidenced by increased serum creatinine) (Schiødt, Rochling, Casey, & Lee, 1997). Toxicity caused by longer-term use is not reversed by acetylcysteine, which is the antidote for acute acetaminophen overdose. Furthermore, the maximum daily doses of acetaminophen or NSAIDs should probably be adjusted for weight and decreased for persons who weigh 50 kg or less (AHCPR, 1994).

The exact mechanism of action for acetaminophen is not known, but it probably increases the pain threshold by blocking prostaglandin synthesis via both the cyclooxygenase-1 (COX-1) and the cyclooxygenase-2 (COX-2) pathways in the central nervous system (CNS) (Gold Star Multimedia, 2000). Acetaminophen has no effect on cyclooxygenase inhibition in peripheral tissues and thus no antiinflammatory property. *Answer 3:* **b.**

4. NSAIDs, on the other hand, exert analgesic properties largely in the periphery. Their antiinflammatory action is thought to result from inhibition of prostaglandin synthesis by interfering with COX-2 at sites of injury in peripheral tissues. Although it is true that acetaminophen and NSAIDs have different mechanisms of action and might be safely administered concomitantly, both agents pose some risk for renal toxicity (papillary necrosis with secondary interstitial nephritis) (De Broe & Elseviers, 1998; Duarte, 1997). The risk increases with long-term use, but the APN would need to carefully weigh whether underlying disease states or other factors outweigh the risks for adverse effects if considering this recommendation.

With the exception of two new selective COX-2 inhibitors, celecoxib (Celebrex) and rofecoxib (Vioxx), available NSAIDs inhibit both COX-1 and COX-2. COX-1 is a "housekeeping" enzyme that is always present in most tissues, including the gastrointestinal (GI) tract, kidneys, and platelets, whereas COX-2 is induced during an inflammatory response. It has been proposed that nonselective NSAIDs block both COX-2, which causes analgesia, and COX-1, which leads to adverse effects. Celebrex and Vioxx were therefore developed to be active only at COX-2 receptors. These drugs are no more effective as analgesics than older NSAIDs, but patients are statistically significantly less likely to experience dyspepsia (indigestion) (i.e., incidence 23.5% with Vioxx and 25.5% with other NSAIDs), as well as perforation, ulcer, or bleeding (1.3% versus 1.8%, respectively) (Langman, Jensen, Watson, et al., 1999). To date, COX-2 inhibitors have not been associated with any interference of platelet aggregation. The clinical significance of these modest differences should be considered when choosing an NSAID, and the APN should remember that selective COX-2 inhibitors do not eliminate the risk of renal toxicity. Thus these expensive agents are justified for patients at greatest risk for clinically significant GI ulcers and hemorrhage, that is, those who are older than 75 years of age or who have developed a complicated ulcer while taking a nonselective NSAID (Peterson & Cryer, 1999). COX-2 inhibitors for these patients would be less costly than concomitant use of a nonselective NSAID and omeprazole (Prilosec), a proton pump inhibitor, or misoprostol (Cytotec), a prostaglandin E_1 analog.

Many OTC and prescription nonselective NSAIDs are available, and none is clearly more efficacious than another. One meta-analysis found ibuprofen to be less likely to cause serious upper GI complications, but comparative studies had small sample sizes (Gøtzsch, 2000). However, based on such data, as well as low cost and availability in many dosage strengths, ibuprofen may be the most suitable "standard" NSAID for patients who are not at high risk for adverse GI effects. Summary data regarding several NSAIDs are included in Table 12-1 (not a totally inclusive list) (Gold Star Multimedia, 2000). The risks for particular adverse effects vary, but the greatest risk for all NSAIDs is GI tract effects, followed by effects on platelet aggregation and renal function. Furthermore, if one NSAID causes adverse effects, it is controversial as to whether switching to another

will be more efficacious. The APN should consider the following several important points when recommending or prescribing *any* NSAID.

Adverse GI effects may be minor or serious, and minor effects do not always herald serious effects. Minor adverse effects include dyspepsia, which is experienced by 10% to 20% of patients taking NSAIDs (Wolfe, Lichtenstein, & Singh, 1999), as well as nausea and vomiting, abdominal pain, heartburn, diarrhea, constipation, and flatulence. H_2-receptor blockers, such as ranitidine (Zantac), may reduce the symptoms of indigestion but do not protect against serious complications and are thus not recommended. Omeprazole 20 or 40 mg/day not only is more effective than misoprostol 800 µg/day in alleviating dyspepsia, preventing ulcers, and healing established ulcers, but also has fewer side effects. The risk for serious adverse effects (i.e., ulcers of the stomach and small bowel, and rarely, obstruction) is approximately 7% in patients with osteoarthritis, and 1% to 3% of such patients may experience life-threatening GI bleeding or perforation. Although chronic users such as patients with rheumatoid and osteoarthritis are at greatest risk, more than 100,000 people in the United States are hospitalized each year because of such complications. Risk factors that definitely increase the risk for GI ulcers are advanced age (linear association), history of ulcer, concomitant use of corticosteroids, higher dosages of NSAIDs or using more than one NSAID simultaneously, and serious systemic disorder. GI infection with *Helicobacter pylori,* cigarette smoking, and alcohol consumption may increase risk.

Nonselective NSAIDs can interfere with platelet aggregation, thereby affecting clotting. This effect is related to the pharmacokinetics of the drug administered, and platelet inhibition reverses shortly after the drug is stopped. Aspirin is the exception; the effect on platelet aggregation is irreversible, so clotting is impaired for 7 to 10 days after aspirin is stopped.

Renal effects may also occur with NSAID use. These effects include acute tubular necrosis and renal papillary necrosis. Acute reversible renal failure has also been documented in chronically ill patients who were taking a COX-2 inhibitor (Perazella & Eras, 2000). Age is a risk factor, and elderly patients are at greatest risk.

Less common adverse effects of NSAIDs include central nervous system (CNS) effects, cardiovascular (CV) effects, and hypersensitivity reactions. The spectrum of CNS adverse effects is wide and includes tinnitus (especially with salicylates), dizziness, sedation, headache, and insomnia. NSAIDs may cause confusion in elderly patients, and this

TABLE 12-1 Nonopioid Analgesics for Adults

DRUG	DOSING	REPORTED ADVERSE EFFECTS	COMMENTS	COST
Acetaminophen (Tylenol)	325-650 mg PO/PR q4-6h 1000 mg PO/PR tid-qid Maximum dose: 4 g/day	Hepatotoxicity Nausea and vomiting, anorexia Acute renal tubular necrosis Hemoglobinemia with acute overdose	Use longer than several months has been associated with hepatotoxicity and nephrotoxicity Use cautiously in patients with impaired hepatic function; use for <5 days in patients with stable liver disease; contraindicated in alcoholic patients Chronic use discouraged in patients with renal disease	650 mg qid, $3.00-$7.20/mo (generic)
Aspirin (ASA, Ecotrin, Bayer, Empirin, etc.)	325-650 mg PO/PR q4h prn 1000 mg PO/PR q6h Maximum dose: 4 g/day	GI: minor and serious Thrombocytopenia with irreversible inhibition of platelet aggregation Renal: papillary necrosis CNS: tinnitus, hearing loss, dizziness Other/rare: Stevens-Johnson syndrome, hypersensitivity	Prophylactic MI/CVA dosages (80-325 mg/day) do not preclude using another NSAID Use cautiously in patients with coagulopathy or thrombocytopenia Monitor LFTs in patients taking large doses	650 mg PO qid, <$5.00/mo (generic)
Ibuprofen (Motrin, Advil, Nuprin, Excedrin IB, etc.)	400-800 mg 3-4 times a day Maximum dose: 3200 mg/day	GI: minor and serious Platelet effect, reversible in 24-48 hr after stopping ibuprofen Renal: acute renal failure, azotemia, cystitis, hematuria Other: ocular—blurred vision or visual impairment (reversible); pancreatitis—<1%	Misoprostol does not lower risk for GI ulcers No dosage adjustments needed for renal impairment Lower dosages for fever (200-400 mg q4-6h) or headache (100-400 mg q4-6h)	600 mg qid, <$10.00/mo (generic OTC)
Choline magnesium trisalicylate (Trilisate)	2-3 g/day PO in 2-3 divided doses	GI: minor CNS (1%-2%): dizziness, drowsiness, headache, tinnitus (<20%)	Use cautiously in patients with history of peptic ulcer GI irritation, antiplatelet effect less than with aspirin Dosages should be decreased in patients with renal impairment (no definitive recommendations)	1500 mg bid $30.00-$40.00/mo (generic)
Naproxen (Aleve, Anaprox, Naprosyn, etc.)	250-500 mg PO bid Maximum dose: 1000 mg/day	GI: minor (3%-9%) Reversible thrombocytopenia Renal (<1%): nephritic syndrome CNS (3%-9%) CV: peripheral edema: (3%-9%), dyspnea, CHF (<1%)	Rare effect on white blood cells Drug accumulates in patients with renal impairment, increased risk for toxicity Preexisting hepatic disease increases risk for hepatic complications, increases LFTs Use cautiously in patients with CHF or condition predisposing to fluid retention	375 mg PO q8h, $70.00-$80.00/mo

AUC, Area under the curve; *CHF,* congestive heart failure; *CNS,* central nervous system; *CV,* cardiovascular; *CVA,* cerebrovascular accident; *GI,* gastrointestinal; *Hct,* hematocrit; *Hgb,* hemoglobin; *LFTs,* liver function tests; *MI,* myocardial infarction; *NSAID,* nonsteroidal antiinflammatory drug; *OTC,* over the counter; *PT,* prothrombin time; *PTT,* partial thromboplastin time.

TABLE **12-1** Nonopioid Analgesics for Adults—cont'd

DRUG	DOSING	REPORTED ADVERSE EFFECTS	COMMENTS	COST
Ketoprofen (Orudis, etc.)	25-50 mg PO q6-8h Maximum dose: 300 mg/day	GI: minor (3%-12%); serious (<1%) Reversible platelet dysfunction CNS (1%-3%) CV (2%): peripheral edema worsening CHF	Decrease dosage 33%-55% if creatinine clearance <10 ml/min No documented renal effects, but possible Use cautiously in patients with CHF or condition predisposing to fluid retention	50 mg PO tid, $70.00-$80.00/mo
Toradol (Ketorolac)	<65 yr: 30 mg IM/IV q6h; ≥65 and/or with de-creased renal func-tion: 15 mg IM/IV q6h Maximum dose: 120 mg/day if renal function normal, 60 mg/day if renal func-tion de-creased	GI: minor (1%-12%); serious (<1%) Hematologic: purpura, thrombocytopenia, anemia, transient decrease in Hgb/Hct Renal (<1%) CNS: headache (17%), dizziness or drowsi-ness (3%-14%), sei-zures (<1%) CV: peripheral edema (3%-9%)	Short-term use only (≤5 days) in patients unable to take oral NSAID; oral therapy is included in this time frame Higher risk (5.4%) of serious GI toxicity increases in elderly with long-term oral administration Coagulopathy can result in postoperative and post-dental procedure bleeding Risk for renal toxicity increases with long-term use (2%-3%)	30 mg IM q6h, $20.00-$30.00/day 10 mg PO q6h, $4.00-$5.00/day
Diflunisal (Dolobid)	250-500 mg PO bid; may in-crease or decrease according to re-sponse and tolerance Maximum dose: 1.5 g/day	GI: minor (3%-9%); severe (1%-3%) Renal impairment/ hematuria (<1%) CNS (1%-9%): dizzi-ness, somnolence, insomnia, tinnitus Hepatotoxicity (<1%)	Derivative of salicylic acid: contraindicated for patients with NSAID hypersensitivity Renal impairment results in drug accumulation and increases risk of toxicity	500 mg PO bid, $40.00-$50.00/mo
Celecoxib (Celebrex)	200 mg/day PO as single or divided dose Hepatic impairment: decrease dosage by 50%	GI: mild (2%-9%); serious (<0.1%) Hematologic: anemia (0.6%); no effect on platelets, PT, PTT Anaphylactoid reactions: <2%	Impaired renal or hepatic function, advanced age (effect greater in women than in men), and Afri-can race significantly al-ter the pharmacokinetics Dyspepsia and abdominal pain most common adverse effects leading to withdrawal from clinical trials	100 mg PO once a day, $40.00-$50.00/mo
Rofecoxib (Vioxx)	Start at 12.5 mg once a day Maximum dose: 25 mg/day	GI: minor and serious (serious GI bleeding and 1 GI obstruction have been reported) Slight increase in LFTs; rare severe hepatic effects Anemia; no effects on platelets, PT, PTT	Impaired hepatic function, advanced age may alter pharmacokinetics Contraindicated for pa-tients who have had an allergic-type reaction after taking aspirin or other NSAID Reduces renal clearance of methotrexate, increases AUC by 23	12.5 mg tablet once a day, $70.00-$80.00

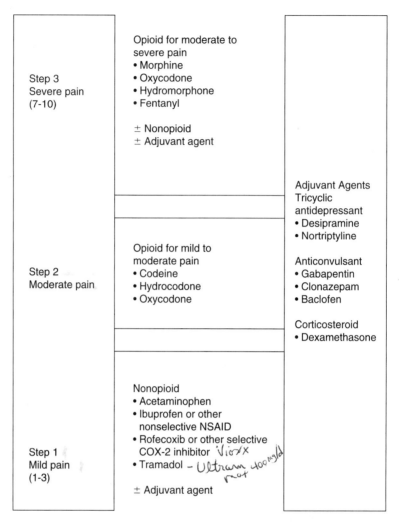

Figure 12-1 Pain ladder. *NSAID,* Nonsteroidal antiinflammatory drug. (Courtesy WHO, 1999.)

risk is greatest with indomethacin (Tannenbaum, Davis, Russell, et al., 1996). CV effects are exacerbation of congestive heart failure (CHF) or peripheral edema. Hypersensitivity reactions are rare, are most commonly documented with salicylates, and can lead to urticaria, angioedema, bronchospasm, and shock. Patients at greatest risk are those who have chronic urticaria or asthma. NSAIDs, including COX-2 inhibitors, should be used with extreme caution in any patient who has experienced a hypersensitivity reaction.

A rare, but potentially fatal, adverse effect that is particularly important to cancer patients can occur with coadministration of an NSAID and methotrexate (Tannenbaum, et al., 1996). Patients who have received more than 15 mg of methotrexate per week for treatment of arthritis experienced decreased creatinine clearance and decreased renal clearance of methotrexate. Vioxx administered in a similar fashion reduced metho-

trexate clearance, which resulted in a 23% increase in area under the cure (AUC). Therefore NSAIDs can cause fatal methotrexate toxicity, especially in patients receiving high-dose therapy, so the APN should monitor renal function and methotrexate levels carefully when an NSAID is administered (Gold Star Media, 2000).

Nonopioids: NSAIDs and acetaminophen (step 1): At this point, you know that Mrs. Jackson's pain seems to be continuous and uncontrolled. You use the ladder approach (World Health Organization, 1990) (Figure 12-1), which is useful to manage cancer-related and other types of pain. NSAIDs and acetaminophen are useful as single agents for mild pain and should probably be used more often with analgesics indicated for more severe pain with an inflammatory component (e.g., bone metastases, fungating lesions, arthritis). Oral formulations are most commonly used, but parenteral and rectal forms are available for some drugs (Table 12-2). In

TABLE 12-2 | Oral Laxatives

CLASS	EXAMPLES/ COMMON DOSES	MECHANISM OF ACTION	COMMENTS
Bulk forming	Raw bran: 1-3 tablespoons Psyllium (Metamucil): 3-6 g qd-tid Methylcellulose (Citrucel): 2.4-4.8 g qd-tid	↑ Stool bulk and softness by taking water into the bowel lumen ↑ Rate of transit and bacterial metabolism	Onset of action 12-72 hr Contraindicated for patients with poor oral intake of water, fecal impaction; may lead to obstruction Requires intake of 1.5-2 L PO fluids/day May ↓ appetite; do not take before meals or with milk
Stool softeners	Docusate sodium (Colace): 100-200 mg qd-tid Docusate calcium (Surfak): 240 mg/day	Softens stool, nonabsorbed Some gut secretory, motility effects	Onset of action may be as long as 3 days when used alone Not laxatives; not habit forming May be hepatotoxic or potentiate the hepatotoxicity of other drugs
Lubricating laxatives	Mineral oil: 5-45 ml qhs	Lubricates stool for easier passage Decreases water absorption	Onset 6-8 hr Not recommended for elderly or immobile patients Do not use on a regular basis: impairs absorption of fat-soluble vitamins May cause aspiration pneumonia if inhaled
Saline laxatives	Milk of magnesia: 15-30 ml qhs Citrate of magnesia (Magnesium citrate): 200-240 ml prn	Osmotic action: draws water into the bowel from the bowel wall	Onset 6-10 hr Need good fluid intake to prevent dehydration and maximize laxative action Contraindicated in impacted patient Magnesium citrate is the most reliable and has the fastest onset of action (5-6 hr) Can cause cramping and bloating Magnesium toxicity in patients with renal insufficiency
Stimulant (irritant) laxatives	Cascara: 5 ml prn (up to 2-3 times per wk) Senna (Senokot): 1-2 tabs qd-bid Bisacodyl (Dulcolax): 10-15 mg qd Castor oil: 15-60 ml qd prn	Acts primarily on the colon Increases gut mucosa secretion Increases gut motility May require gut bacteria for activation	Onset 6-10 hr Cramping, dehydration, fluid and electrolyte imbalance may occur Risk of hepatotoxicity (danthron) when combined with docusate Castor oil may cause cramping
Hyperosmotic laxatives	Lactulose: 5-60 ml qd-bid Sorbitol: 15-60 ml qd-bid Polyethylene glycol-saline (GoLYTELY): 200-1000 ml prn	Nonabsorbable salts or sugars Stimulates peristalsis Increases intraluminal pressure	Lactulose may take 24 hr or longer to work Lactulose may cause flatulence, cramps, diarrhea, and electrolyte imbalance Sorbitol is less expensive than lactulose and may be more tolerable
Combination stool softener + laxative	Docusate sodium + casanthrol (Peri-Colace) Docusate sodium + senna (Senokot S)	Softens stool Stimulates peristalsis	Onset 8-12 hr Peri-Colace available as syrup or capsule Indicated for patients taking opioid analgesics; dosage is titrated to desired frequency of bowel movements

Adapted from Alessi, C. A., & Henderson, C. T. (1988). Constipation and fecal impaction in the long-term care patient. *Clin Geriatr Med, 4,* pp. 583-584; and Portenoy, R. K. (1987). Constipation in the cancer patient: Causes and management. *Med Clin North Am, 71,* pp. 303-311.

teaching patients and staff, an important reminder is that all nonopioid drugs have a ceiling effect, so increasing the dosage over what is maximally recommended does not enhance analgesia but does increase the risk for adverse effects.

The ladder (see Figure 12-1) highlights the three types of analgesics—nonopioids, opioids, and adjuvant agents—that may be useful to control different types of pain. Cancer patients often experience pain from more than one cause. Approximately 42% of patients have pain caused by bone or joint lesions, 28% have visceral pain, 28% have soft tissue infiltration, and 28% have peripheral nerve injuries (Caraceni, Portenoy, working group of the IASP Task Force on Cancer Pain, 1999). The patient's pain intensity directs which step of the ladder is a reasonable starting point. Thus a patient who has moderate or severe pain would not be started on step 1. You realize that Mrs. Jackson may require an opioid indicated for moderate to severe pain. If step 2 analgesics were prescribed, the dosage would be maximized and the patient assessed frequently. If pain was not controlled, the patient might be rapidly escalated to step 3 analgesics. Because Mrs. Jackson has not been taking her Vicodin regularly, it would be reasonable to instruct her to first try increasing her Vicodin to two tablets every 6 hours around the clock (assuming she was not experiencing any other unmanageable side effects). You will follow up with her tomorrow if the Vicodin is effective to control her pain. *Answer 4:* **d.**

Case Study continued

Mrs. Jackson begins taking Vicodin at a dosage of two tablets every 6 hours. For a few weeks, this decreases her pain from 8 to 3 on a 0 to 10 scale (0 being no pain and 10 being worst possible pain), but her pain then worsens to 7. You collaborate with the oncologist to start her on sustained-release oxycodone (Oxycontin) 10 mg every 12 hours, plus oxycodone 5 mg as needed. Within several days, you instruct Mrs. Jackson to increase the dosage of Oxycontin to 20 mg every 12 hours and to take one 5-mg capsule of oxycodone every 3 to 4 hours (she takes two or three doses a day). This regimen initially helps her pain somewhat, but you ultimately increase her Oxycontin to 80 mg every 12 hours plus oxycodone 15 mg every 3 to 4 hours as needed. At this point, Mrs. Jackson tells you that her pain is usually a 2 or 3, which is satisfactory to her.

However, Mrs. Jackson now telephones to tell you that the pain is "awful" and that she is having problems with constipation. You tell her to come to the office. When she arrives, you can see that she has lost some weight and muscle mass over the last few months. You start by reviewing Mrs. Jackson's pain history with her. Her abdominal pain has increased to the point that she "cannot stand it." She rates her pain as "12." Her pain is a vaguely diffuse "hurt" throughout her abdomen, and when it worsens, it is accompanied by cramping that makes her "roll up in a ball." Her pain sometimes awakens her at night and interferes with social and other activities during the day. Her physical examination is unremarkable except for her abdomen, which is slightly distended. She has bowel sounds in all four quadrants; however, she cannot tolerate palpation or even light percussion, and she asks that you not do either because they increase her abdominal cramping a great deal. Gentle examination reveals a left lower quadrant (LLQ) mass that is approximately 10 by 10 cm. It is not possible to determine whether her liver is enlarged because of her abdominal pain. She states that she occasionally passes flatus but that she has not had a bowel movement in 5 days. She has not had any nausea, vomiting, or diarrhea.

QUESTIONS

5. If you asked Mrs. Jackson to describe her pain and she said it was "a dull ache," this would indicate which of the following types of pain?
   1. Nociceptive
   2. Neuropathic
   3. Visceral
   4. Not severe
      a. 2 & 3
      b. 1, 2, & 3
      c. 1 & 2
      d. All of these

6. What elements should you include in your focused assessment of Mrs. Jackson?
   1. Inspection, palpation, percussion, and auscultation of her abdomen
   2. Assessment of her liver span
   3. Inspection, auscultation, palpation, and percussion of her abdomen
   4. Detailed pain assessment
   5. Bowel elimination history
   6. Peripheral neurologic examination
      a. 1, 2, & 4
      b. 1, 4, & 5
      c. 2, 3, 4, & 5
      d. 2, 3, 4, & 6

7. The frequency of normal bowel movements has been defined as:
   a. Once or twice a day
   b. Twice a week
   c. From two per day to four per week
   d. From three per day to three per week

8. Which finding in Mrs. Jackson's abdominal assessment would aid you in determining whether the LLQ mass is tumor or stool?
   a. The consistency of the mass
   b. The presence of hyperactive bowel sounds
   c. Percussion of tympany over the LLQ mass
   d. Accompanying hepatomegaly

9. If Mrs. Jackson were experiencing constipation secondary to her Vicodin, what would you recommend that she do to manage this?
   a. Nothing because it will resolve on its own
   b. Take prune juice or have a hot cup of tea with lemon every morning and then sit on the toilet
   c. Take lactulose 30 ml every 4 hours until achieving a bowel movement
   d. Take senna plus docusate or plus docusate twice a day

ANSWERS

5. Your focused assessment considers the natural history of Mrs. Jackson's disease, investigates her chief complaints (pain and constipation), and includes a thorough physical examination of her abdomen. Early colon cancer is asymptomatic, but mass effects may eventually cause symptoms such as constipation alternating with diarrhea, fatigue, and palpitations (secondary to decreased hemoglobin from occult bleeding). The liver is the most common site of metastases from colon and rectal cancers because of venous blood drains directly from the GI tract to the liver. Hepatomegaly may occur in stage IV disease, but the liver, lungs, intestine, and other abdominal organs do not have nociceptors and thus become painful. Inflammation, distension, or stretching, such as of the enervated liver capsule, may cause severe pain. An enlarged liver may lead to painful compressive symptoms in the stomach and intestines ("squashed stomach syndrome") that results in anorexia and nausea. Both nociceptive and neuropathic pain may be described as an "ache." *Answer 5:* **c.**

6. If you have not previously done so, you will do a complete baseline pain assessment now, which gives you a picture of your patient's pain. This allows you to estimate pain severity and possible underlying pathogenic causes, which will influence your decisions about analgesics choices and will allow you to be more focused in subsequent assessments. Your pain assessment will include a pain history, with questions that address the physical aspects of pain; a focused history of potential related problems (e.g., constipation); and a focused physical examination. Your findings may lead you to order or recommend laboratory or visualization procedures.

APNs are familiar with the critical assessment elements for a major symptom, which include location; intensity; quality; onset and pattern over time; aggravating and alleviating factors; effects of pain on important life activities, sleep, and mood; a thorough analgesic history; any concerns the patient has about taking pain medications; and the patient's goals for pain relief.

Remember that the patient may have pain in more than one site, and these may have different causes. Therefore each pain site should be assessed separately. Pain may be localized, diffuse, radicular, or referred. Patients who have localized pain can easily point out on a drawing of a body figure or their own body where their pain is felt. An example is pain that results from metastasis to bone, a somatic pain, in which the pain message is transmitted to the CNS via nociceptors. Somatic pains are usually responsive to opioid and nonopioid analgesics.

A patient who has obstruction of a hollow abdominal structure may experience visceral pain, which is typically described as diffuse or difficult to localize (the patient may say it is "all over" his or her abdomen). Visceral organs are insensitive to cutting or burning, as occurs during surgical procedures, but distension, ischemia, and inflammation that affect normal motility and secretion are stimuli for visceral pain (Cervero & Laird, 1999; Regan & Peng, 2000). Visceral pain may be referred to other nonvisceral structures, such as shoulder or back pain with pancreatic cancer or cholangiocarcinoma. In addition, the patient may have accompanying autonomic symptoms, such as nausea and vomiting or diaphoresis. Visceral pain may be relieved with a combination of analgesics (i.e., nonopioid, opioid, plus adjuvant) or may respond to a local anesthesia procedure. Pain from nonvisceral causes may also be referred in some cases. For instance, the patient who complains of pain in a thigh or knee without obvious pathology in that site may be experiencing pain referred from the third lumber vertebral body (L3) or from the ipsilateral hip (Cleary, 2000). Interventions will depend on whether the underlying pain seems to be visceral or neuropathic.

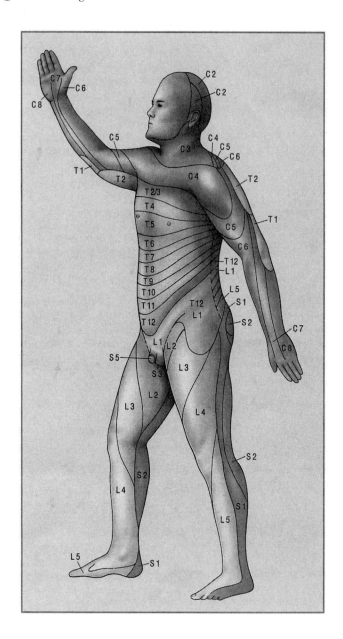

Figure 12-2 Dermatome areas. Vertebral body metastases or spinal cord compression related to infiltration of cancer into foramen or between vertebral bodies may cause radicular pain that radiates from the corresponding area of the neck or back to some of or the total area innervated. For instance, a patient who describes pain in the hip and groin may have disease at L1. (From Habif, T. P. [1995]. *The diagnostic manual of herpesvirus infections* [p. 57]. Research Triangle Park, NC: Burroughs Wellcome.)

In addition, some patients experience nerve root compression or impending spinal cord compression secondary to bone metastases (lytic or blastic), tumor infiltration between vertebral bodies or into vertebral foramen, or paraspinal disease. Their pain may initially be localized, but eventually they develop radicular pain that radiates from the back toward the periphery along one or more dermatomes. These patients may say that their pain goes up and down their back or may not always tell you about back pain first because they perceive a more peripheral site to be more painful. A dermatome map is useful in figuring out that a patient who tells you he or she has pain in the groin might have a vertebral metastasis at about L1 (Figure 12-2). The words the

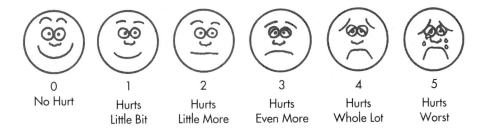

0	1	2	3	4	5
No Hurt	Hurts Little Bit	Hurts Little More	Hurts Even More	Hurts Whole Lot	Hurts Worst

Original instructions:
Explain to the person that each face is for a person who feels happy because he has no pain (hurt) or sad because he has some or a lot of pain. **Face 0** is very happy because he doesn't hurt at all. **Face 1** hurts just a little bit. **Face 2** hurts a little more. **Face 3** hurts even more. **Face 4** hurts a whole lot. **Face 5** hurts as much as you can imagine, although you don't have to be crying to feel this bad. Ask the person to choose the face that best describes how he is feeling.
   Rating scale is recommended for persons age 3 years and older.

Figure 12-3 Faces pain rating scale. (From Wong, D. L., Hockenberry-Eaton, M., Wilson, D., et al. [Eds.]. [2001]. *Wong's essentials of nursing*, 6th ed. St. Louis: Mosby.)

patient uses to describe the quality of pain tend to reflect neuropathic pain, which results from infiltration, compression, inflammation, or other damage to nervous system structures (Regan & Peng, 2000). Neuropathic pain may require other or additional adjuvant medications in addition to opioid and nonopioid analgesics for adequate control.

There are several reliable and clinically practical measures of pain intensity. These include numerical rating scales, such as the 0 to 10 scale in which 0 is no pain and 10 the worst pain (some practitioners/institutions use 0 to 5 or 0 to 7); a verbal descriptor scale that uses words understandable to the patient (i.e., none, mild, moderate, severe), or a pediatric faces scale (cartoon or photograph), which are useful for children and adults who cannot rate their pain on a numerical scale, who have expressive aphasia, or who do not speak English (Figure 12-3). You might also find it useful to use pain scales that have been translated into several languages (McCaffery & Pasero, 1999). A pain intensity card that includes at least two of these measures would be convenient for ongoing assessments and also help you use the same tool consistently with a given patient. When assessing pain intensity/severity, you should ask the patient to rate his or her pain now, the worst pain, and the least pain in the last 24 hours.

To ascertain the quality of your patient's pain, you ask, "What does your pain feel like?" Tearnan and Cleeland (1990) found that 11 words accounted for 67% of all words cancer patients use, which were (in order of prevalence) ache, dull-ache, sharp, stabbing, burning, throbbing, dull, continual, hurting, pressure, and shooting. These words most often describe the sensory aspects of pain. Patients offered evaluative words only occasionally but were more likely to do so if they had high pain ratings. Examples of evaluative words include severe, horrendous, unbearable, terrible, hell, excruciating, and bad.

Which words patients used did not vary between patients with different malignancies. Quality words may also provide clues as to whether pain is predominantly nociceptive or neuropathic (many pain syndromes have both components), which may direct your choices of analgesics. It is useful to remember that *ache* was the most common word used by patients, who by other descriptive words had either nociceptive or neuropathic pain (or both), so aching or dull pain can represent very severe pain. If you suspect neuropathic pain, you can ask the patient if his or her pain is electric, shocklike, stabbing or grabbing, spasmlike, or accompanied by numbness and tingling (if the patient does not offer these words).

Ask the patient when the pain started and what is has been like over time. For instance, it may have been mild pain at the onset a few weeks or months ago but now is more severe, or it may have started a few days or weeks ago and been severe all along. If pain is severe, it may represent a pain emergency.

When asked about what makes the patient's pain worse, all too often the answer is movement or activity. In terms of what makes the pain better, ideally the response *should* be the pain medicine, rest, change in position, pressure, massage, or other measures.

During your comprehensive pain assessment, you gather important general survey information from your observations of and communication with a patient. For example, you note your patient's general appearance and demeanor, mental status (e.g., alert, somnolent, confused), whether he or she seems rested or fatigued, how he or she holds body position (straight and comfortable versus other), and his or her facial appearance (e.g., relaxed, worried, angry, depressed, in pain). It is also important to ask patients how they usually express their pain, such as if they let people know they are in pain or if they are the "strong, silent type." You would also ask them specific questions regarding the effects pain has had on activities important to them, sleep, and mood. Questions might include the following: Does your pain affect your job? housework? relationships with others? time with friends and family? other leisure-time activities? Does pain keep you from going to sleep or does it wake you up? Does pain interfere with your ability to think and concentrate? Does your pain make you feel depressed or anxious? It may be useful to explore if the pain has any meaning to the patient, such as the concern that increasing pain means worsening cancer or some other problem.

The APN must take a thorough analgesic history and keep this information up to date. Medications to ask about include all analgesics the patient has taken over time, including both OTC and prescription drugs. As mentioned earlier, you should pay close attention to the amount of acetaminophen the patient is taking. If analgesics have been changed, you should estimate whether the patient was taking optimal doses of previously ordered analgesics and whether particular drugs were discontinued because of inadequate pain relief or because of adverse effects. When gathering information from a hospitalized patient, particularly one admitted for pain control, you need to not only confirm which analgesics he or she was taking but also calculate as closely as possible how much medication (opioids, nonopioids, and adjuvant medications) the patient was taking over 24 hours. This is important because if you find out only what was ordered, the initial doses of analgesics administered in the hospital may be *less* than what the patient was *actually taking* at home.

As mentioned earlier, patient concerns about taking pain medications may be a formidable barrier to adequate pain management. Thus you will explore common barriers to reporting pain and taking pain medications to address them. This is also the time to address the patient's goal for pain treatment, which may change over time.

In addition, your pain assessment will include a focused physical examination. In Mrs. Jackson's

case, her pain is most likely visceral, and she denies increased weakness. Therefore your examination will focus on her site of pain. As you palpate painful sites, you should note if this increases pain or causes any unusual pain sensations such as allodynia (see discussion of neuropathic pain on previous page). If she had vertebral body disease or other neurologic indications or if she clearly had a neuropathic component to her pain, a detailed neurologic examination is in order. If indicated, you should palpate muscles to ascertain bulk and tone during passive movements; test strength against resistance and gravity; and assess for abnormal movements (fasciculations or myoclonus), sensory changes, vibration, proprioception, gait, and reflexes (deep tendon and Babinski) (Portenoy, 1997).

Physical assessment of the abdomen is necessary to try to identify the basis for Mrs. Jackson's symptoms (e.g., bowel obstruction with visceral pain, pain from an enlarged liver, other abdominal tumor mass). Assessment may be difficult because of her increased pain intensity. The usual sequence of abdominal assessment is inspection of the contours, auscultation for bowel sounds, palpation, and percussion. This order of techniques is necessary because manipulation of the bowel by palpation or percussion for tympany and masses can erroneously change the frequency or intensity of bowel sounds for several minutes. Thus a patient who has no or few bowel sounds may actually be perceived to have bowel sounds present. You should assess her liver borders because you know that she has liver metastases, which may be accompanied by an enlarging liver. During palpation for abdominal masses, you should note the consistency of any masses found. In an easily palpable colon, stool is indentable and mobile and the site typically is not tender. Conversely, if a colonic mass were tumor, the palpable mass would be hard, not indentable, and fixed, and palpation would likely induce tenderness. In addition, obstruction by tumor might be accompanied by high tinkling bowel sounds or no bowel sounds (Fallon & O'Neill, 1997). A digital rectal examination is also needed to check for hard stool or tumor masses in the rectum, although most bowel obstructions occur in the small bowel.

There are multiple causes of constipation in cancer patients (Box 12-1) (Levy, 1991; Prather & Ortiz-Camacho, 1998; Romero, Evans, Fleming, & Phillips, 1996). A bowel history is important in Mrs. Jackson's case because her report of constipation could reflect local obstructive effects of tumor (intermittent or incomplete bowel obstruction, which can progress to complete obstruction) and because constipation is the most common side

BOX 12-1 **Factors That May Increase Constipation in Cancer Patients**

DRUGS

Opioids
Antacids (aluminum and calcium containing)
Anticholinergic agents (i.e., belladonna, antihistamines)
Antidiarrheal agents
Antihistamines
Barium
Bismuth
Calcium channel blockers
Calcium supplements
Diuretics
Iron
NSAIDs
Ondansetron
Phenothiazines
Sucralfate
Tricyclic antidepressants

NEUROTOXIC CHEMOTHERAPY AGENTS

Vincristine
Vinblastine
Navelbine
Cisplatin

MECHANICAL PROBLEMS

Local progression of colon cancer
Intraabdominal or pelvic disease
External compression by tumor or lymphadenopathy

Strictures
Anal fissure
Hemorrhoids
Malignant ascites

METABOLIC CONDITIONS

Diabetes mellitus
Hypothyroidism
Hypercalcemia
Hypokalemia
Uremia

OTHER CONDITIONS

Spinal cord compression
Cauda equina syndrome
Sacral plexus involvement
Depression
Degenerative joint disease
Immobility
Cognitive impairment
Cardiac disease

OTHER SYMPTOMS OF CANCER

Anorexia/poor oral intake
Weakness
Debility
Inactivity/bed rest
Poor fluid intake
Inability to reach toilet

NSAIDs, Nonsteroidal antiinflammatory drugs.

effect of chronic opioid use (Mrs. Jackson has been taking Vicodin and then oxycodone for quite some time). Opiate receptors in the small bowel become bound with exogenously administered opioids, which results in slowed bowel transit time and greater water extraction from feces, which results in dry, hard, and difficult-to-pass stool. *Answer 6:* **c.**

7. Normal bowel movements are arbitrarily defined as regular, easy, and complete passage of formed stool at least three times per week and no more than three per day (McShane & McLane, 1985). Conversely, constipation is defined as bowel movements that are infrequent (compared with what is normal for the patient), dry, and hard stools that result in straining during bowel movements, a sense of incomplete evacuation, or some combination of these (Levy, 1992; Prather & Ortiz-Camacho, 1998). *Answer 7:* **d.**

8. Not only does constipation cause accompanying abdominal discomfort, but it also can lead to impaction (the inability to pass a collection of hard

stool) with overflow diarrhea, or obstipation (the absolute inability to pass stool). Impaction and obstipation require manual removal of stool from the rectum by disimpaction, followed by an enema (tap water or oil retention) or suppositories (docusate or glycerin) before implementing laxatives and stool softeners. Therefore a thorough baseline bowel history should always be taken in at-risk patients who have abdominal complaints or who take potentially constipating drugs (Box 12-2). *Answer 8:* **a.**

9. Prophylactic management to prevent constipation secondary to opioids is imperative and should include recommending a stool softener and a laxative, such as senna and docusate (combination product or single agents). When possible, the patient should use products that are available as store brands or generic agents because these are considerably less expensive than brand name products. Stool softeners and laxatives often have to be titrated upward as opioid dosages are increased, but there is no direct relationship between the dosages of each. Other agents, such

When was your last bowel movement?

What is the *usual* pattern of your bowel movements (frequency, amount, consistency)? Normal bowel movements are easily passed and not accompanied by cramping or straining.

What has your recent pattern (over the last few weeks, or since you started taking your pain medicine) of bowel movements been like?

Do you have any cramping or discomfort in your abdomen/stomach or nausea?

Do you usually use bran, laxatives, stool softeners, suppositories or enemas, or anything else to keep your bowels regular? Did you start having to take laxatives, etc., before you started taking strong pain medicine?

Do you ever have to manually remove stool from your rectum?

Do you *feel* constipated (use words the patient understands)?

Do you have any of these other problems: a full feeling in your abdomen, cramping, nausea, poor appetite, or intermittent diarrhea?

as sorbitol or mineral oil, may subsequently be added, with care, to a laxative regimen. Typical recommendations for functional constipation, such as adding bulk (bran, psyllium, or methylcellulose) to the diet, increasing fluid intake, and increasing exercise will not alleviate opioid-related constipation and may increase bloating and abdominal discomfort. Similarly, lactulose is not a first-line product because it has a relatively long lag time to onset, which may actually lead to diarrhea, and is more expensive than other laxatives. If you decide that a nonabsorbable sugar might help the patient, sorbitol is a better choice. *Answer 9:* **d.**

Case Study continued

You consult with the oncologist because Mrs. Jackson's pain is now an emergency and because of the possible risk of bowel obstruction. Although her dosage of oxycodone could be increased at home, you decide to admit her for pain control and workup of possible bowel obstruction. She is admitted to the oncology unit on Friday afternoon. The housestaff physician starts Mrs. Jackson on a continuous intravenous (CIV) morphine (MSO_4) drip of 1 mg/hr. Concerned that Mrs. Jackson may have a gastric ulcer, the physician orders Prilosec 20 mg orally, once an obstruction is ruled out. An abdominal flat plate rules out frank obstruction.

Admission Medication Orders
MSO_4 1 mg/hr intravenously
MSO_4 1 to 2 mg intravenous push (IVP) as needed
Prilosec 20 mg
Senokot 1 tablet every morning as needed

After being away for a long weekend, you visit Mrs. Jackson in the hospital. When you enter her room, you note that Mrs. Jackson is in bed. She is awake and alert, her grooming is neat and clean, but she is not wearing any makeup, nor is her hair styled. She is still on the MSO_4 drip, which has been increased to 3 mg/hr, and her medication record shows that she requires occasional boluses of 1 mg (two doses in the last 24 hours). Now, 4 days after being admitted to the hospital, she rates her pain as 8. The worst pain in the last 24 hours was "higher than 10!" and least pain was 6 to 7. She would like her pain to be less but "doesn't want to take too much of that morphine." MSO_4 has helped her pain somewhat, but taking Prilosec intensifies the cramping pain. Mrs. Jackson is distressed because the resident insists she *has* to take the Prilosec and she does not want to be a bad patient. Although the pain makes her feel a little down, she tries not to think about it and prays quite a lot.

QUESTIONS

10. What factor or factors might preclude Mrs. Jackson from receiving increased doses of morphine?
   a. Mrs. Jackson's reluctance to take morphine
   b. The registered nurse's (RN) lack of time to reassess Mrs. Jackson's pain
   c. The housestaff physician's perception that cancer pain is inevitable
   d. All of these

11. The patient who takes an opioid for pain experiences signs of physical withdrawal when he or she suddenly stops taking the medication indicates that the patient is:
   a. Addicted to the opioid
   b. Physically dependent on the opioid
   c. Tolerant to the opioid
   d. Psychologically dependent on the opioid

12. If the staff RNs caring for Mrs. Jackson upon admission wanted to confirm that the dose of intravenous MSO_4 1 mg/hr was appropriate, you would help them calculate the equianalgesic dose. Her approximately equivalent dose of intravenous MSO_4 to oxycodone (Oxycontin 80 mg every 12 hours, plus oxycodone 15 mg three times a day) is:

    a. 2 mg/hr
    b. 4 mg/hr
    c. 6 mg/hr
    d. 8 mg/hr

13. Which of the following assessment factors are critical to optimal pain management?
    a. Pain intensity, pain relief, amount of opioid taken, family's concerns
    b. Pain intensity, pain relief, side effects of opioids, amount of opioid taken
    c. Pain intensity, pain behaviors, side effects of opioids, satisfaction
    d. Pain intensity, pain relief, side effects of opioids, satisfaction

---

ANSWERS

10. Health care provider barriers to pain control have, unfortunately, not changed in many instances. Nurses, physicians, and pharmacists often have insufficient education regarding pain assessment and management concepts; still do not assess pain in a systematic and consistent fashion; and have concerns about prescribing, administering, or dispensing controlled substances, while fearing addiction, tolerance, and side effect occurrence in patients (AHCPR, 1994; Pargeon & Hailey, 1999). One survey found that more than half of the physicians had misconceptions regarding tolerance. Twenty percent believed that addiction was a potential problem when using morphine for cancer pain, that pain from cancer was inevitable, and that pain was not likely to be totally relieved (Elliot & Elliot, 1992). Even oncologists, who often care for patients with increasing pain from progressive cancer or cancer therapy, may have knowledge deficits. For example, 86% of almost 900 medical oncologists in one study agreed that pain is undertreated in most cancer patients, and they believed that only 51% of the patients in *their* practice had good or very good pain control (Von Roenn, Cleeland, Gonin, et al., 1993). Nurses may compound the problem of inadequate pain management. Twenty percent of the nurses surveyed believed that patients could attain and maintain complete pain control, and only one third agreed that they would call the physician if their patient was experiencing continuing pain (Howell, Butler, Vincent, et al., 2000). These barriers may seem insurmountable, particularly in settings where health care professionals have few clinical models to help them incorporate knowledge and practice pain management skills. *Answer 10:* **d.**

11. One major issue is that health care professionals may have misconceptions regarding the risks for addiction from opioids prescribed for pain. Some clinicians use three terms, *addiction* (more appropriately termed *psychologic dependence*), *physical dependence,* and *tolerance,* interchangeably. *Psychologic dependence* is "a pattern of compulsive drug use characterized by a continuous craving for an opioid and the need to use the opioid for effects other than pain relief" (AHCPR, 1994, p. 185). A second definition is that it is "a compulsive use of a substance resulting in physical, psychological, or social harm to the user, and continued use despite that harm" (Rinaldi, Steindler, Wilford, et al., 1988). Drug abusers or addicts would thereby jeopardize family and social relationships, job, and health by getting and using medically approved drugs for unapproved uses. The risk of addiction occurring in any patient with cancer is extremely low. One classic paper estimates the risk for iatrogenic addiction to be less than 1% (Porter & Jick, 1980). When a patient's pain is controlled, the opposite is more likely to occur and the patient will be more able to partake in family and social activities. Furthermore, the most recent reports regarding drug abuse substantiates that from 1990 to 1996, the medical prescription of opioid analgesics increased by 6.6%, whereas the reported abuse of these agents decreased from 5.1% to 3.8% (Joranson, Ryan, Gilson, & Dahl, 2000). Conversely, nonopioid analgesics, alcohol in combination with other drugs, illicit drugs, and other prescribed drugs (e.g., amphetamines, antidepressants, antipsychotics, benzodiazepines, sedatives) are much more likely to be abused.

Physical dependence, on the other hand, is a predictable physical consequence that results from continuous binding of exogenous opioids to opioid receptors. The significance of physical dependence is that if opioids are suddenly withdrawn, physical withdrawal syndrome will occur. Symptoms such as restlessness, tremor, and rhinorrhea will be mild and perhaps unnoticeable in a patient who has been taking regular doses of morphine for 1 or 2 weeks and stops taking the opioid. However, patients who have been taking larger doses and for a longer period can have more severe symptoms of withdrawal if they stop taking the opioid analgesic. Furthermore, patients will have more pronounced and dramatic physical withdrawal syndrome if naloxone (Narcan) is administered, even after one dose of morphine (Payne, 1998).

Tolerance is also a physiologic process by which a given dose of opioid that once relieved pain no longer produces the same degree and duration of analgesia. The mechanisms of tolerance in humans are not well understood, and there is no predictable pattern for its occurrence. Some individuals with malignant and chronic benign pain remain on the same dosage of opioid for an extended time. It is more likely that patients with cancer who require higher dosages of opioid analgesics are experiencing progressive cancer that is causing increasing pain rather than tolerance to analgesic effects of their opioid. One positive note is that tolerance also occurs to most side effects of opioids, except for constipation and delirium.

Other issues that might be pertinent to Mrs. Jackson are ethnicity and gender. There is evidence that physicians underestimate pain severity, as well as the effects of pain on activities and sleep, in African American and Hispanic patients (Todd, Deaton, D'Adamo, et al., 2000). Furthermore, they are more likely to underestimate pain in women than in men.

Systems barriers have also been major obstacles to pain control. Pain management has a low priority, and health care providers have not had to be accountable for pain assessment, documentation, and control. Although triplicate prescriptions for class II opioids (morphine, hydromorphone, oxycodone, fentanyl, methadone, and meperidine) are no longer required, the pall of their dampening effect on the prescription of opioids for severe pain remains. Furthermore, pharmacists who hold misconceptions regarding opioid analgesics may impede the availability of these drugs in hospital or community pharmacy. Systems barriers are the major focus the new Joint Commission on Accreditation of Health Care Organization's (JCAHO) pain standards (1999), which are rapidly being implemented in hospitals and other health care settings. The new standards represent a major initiative to address the inadequacy of pain management and recognize the right of all patients for pain control. A summary of the standards is included in Box 12-3 (Phillips, 2000; www.jcaho.org). Specific details for particular care sites can be found at the JCAHO website. The power of these new standards is that health care providers and institutions will have to demonstrate compliance. APNs will likely be called on to provide education (formal and informal via consultation) for students, nurses, physicians, and patients to address health care provider and systems barriers and to impart leadership to implement the JCAHO pain standards. APNs often are responsible for the development of pain management algorithms in quality assurance efforts to improve pain control (Ersek, Kraybill, & Du Pen, 1999). *Answer 11:* **b.**

BOX **12-3** | **New JCAHO Pain Standards**

Rights and ethics: Organizations must recognize the right of patients to appropriate assessment and management of pain. The organization must make an organizational commitment to pain management that may be reflected in their mission statement, their patient bill of rights, or detailed service standards.

Assessment of individuals with pain: The existence of, nature of, and intensity of pain must be assessed in all patients or clients. To comply, the organization must develop policies and procedures for pain assessment and ensure that staff members are competent to manage pain (e.g., through new staff orientation and continuing education/pain competencies).

Documentation: All assessments should be recorded in a manner that facilitates reassessment and follow-up.

Care of individuals with pain: The organization must have policies and procedures that support appropriate prescribing/ordering of effective pain medications, such as policies for intraspinal or continuous intravenous infusions of opioids.

Education of patients or clients with pain: The organization is responsible for educating individuals with pain regarding the importance of pain management as a goal of treatment, dispel misconceptions, etc.

Continuum of care: Care providers must address the patient's need for symptom management, including pain, in discharge planning, which may include postdischarge follow-up.

Improvement in organizational performance: Quality improvement activities must incorporate pain management performance issues, that is, collect data to monitor its performance in appropriate and effective pain management.

---

12. Calculation for Mrs. Jackson, who has been receiving Oxycontin 80 mg every 12 hours, plus oxycodone 15 mg, one tablet three times a day, is as follows:

- Her 24-hour total dose of oxycodone is $(80 \text{ mg} \times 2) + (15 \text{ mg} \times 3) = 205 \text{ mg}$.
- Because there is no parenteral formulation of oxycodone, you next convert the oral oxycodone to oral morphine: $205 \text{ mg}/20 \text{ mg} = x/30 \text{ mg}$
  $(30 \times 205 \text{ mg}) \div 20 \text{ mg} = x \text{ mg}$
  $307 \text{ mg oral morphine} = x$

- Then calculate the parenteral dose of morphine (divide by 3): $307 \div 3 = 102$ mg parenteral morphine/24 hr.
- Divide by 24 hours to calculate the hourly rate: 102 mg $\div$ 24 hours = 4.25 mg/hr. Thus the closest equianalgesic dose is 4 mg/hr.

Because Mrs. Jackson's pain was severe when she was admitted to the hospital, her dose of parenteral morphine should have been at least the calculated equianalgesic dosage. You should encourage her nurses to assess her pain intensity and control frequently and to document these and the degree of her satisfaction with her pain control. This will empower the staff to convince the reluctant resident physician to improve the order guidelines for intravenous morphine to "titrate to pain." *Answer 12:* **b.**

13. Ongoing assessment is less time-consuming, unless a major change in pain occurs. As the APN, you are likely to play an ongoing role in teaching staff nurses, residents, attending physicians, and pharmacists about basic concepts of pain management, including assessment, pharmacologic and nonpharmacologic management, the importance of accurate and thorough documentation, and the establishment of the *patient's* goal of pain relief. Empowering the patient to believe that his or her goals are more important than being seen as a good patient is often an initial and vital step. Patients have a right to refuse therapies without being made to feel guilty. Medicating patients against their will (in Mrs. Jackson's case, it was Prilosec) is unethical and illegal and may constitute battery. You can help health care professionals develop consistent methods to document pain and relief in prominent places on the inpatient or outpatient clinical record and to make pain highly visible by recording pain as the "fifth vital sign" on the graphic sheet (*JAMA*, 1995).

Because pain is a subjective experience, the patient's own rating of his or her pain severity/intensity is the gold standard of assessment. Believing what patients report is difficult for some physicians and nurses who want to rely on objective measures of pain. When patients' pain ratings are compared with those of their physicians and nurses, professionals often think that patients have less pain than they report and exaggerate their pain severity; thus pain assessments of patients and care provides often do not correlate (Drayer, Henderson, & Reidenberg, 1999).

Documentation of baseline and consistent, regularly scheduled reassessment are the keys to optimal pain control. The measures of effectiveness for pharmacologic and nonpharmacologic interventions include the amount and duration of pain relief from an intervention. In addition, patients must be specifically asked if they are having any side effects that they do not like from the intervention, and the bottom line is the degree of satisfaction patients have with their pain control. One strategy to find out how effective analgesics are is to ask patients how their pain compares with that of yesterday and offer them the alternatives of "the same," "worse," or "better." If they rate it as better, you should see if you can help them quantify the improvement (i.e., 10%, half). Similarly, you should ask them if their pain is controlled well enough, or if they would like it to be better. Offering options decreases the chance that you will ask leading questions and bias patients' responses.

All opioid agonists act primarily by binding to mu (for morphine or morphinelike) opioid receptors in the CNS. They may have some effects at other receptors, such as kappa and delta receptors, which may also play a role in analgesia and in adverse effects. Opioids may have peripheral effects in sites of inflammation that are just beginning to be understood (American Pain Society, 1999). Opioids are classified as those indicated for mild to moderate pain and those indicated for moderate to severe pain.

Opioids for mild to moderate pain (step 2): Opioids for mild to moderate pain are formulated as low-dose preparations and are usually combined with acetaminophen, occasionally with another nonopioid, or as a single product (e.g., oxycodone, codeine) (Table 12-3). Examples include codeine 30 to 60 mg (combined with acetaminophen), oxycodone with acetaminophen (Percocet) or aspirin (Percodan), hydrocodone with acetaminophen (Vicodin, Lortabs) or ibuprofen (Vicoprofen), and propoxyphene with acetaminophen (Darvocet). All combination products are limited by the dosage and side effects of the adjuvant nonopioid drug. Patients must be reminded to report all pain relievers they take, including OTC medications, so that they do not exceed the maximally recommended dose of acetaminophen. The use of propoxyphene (in Darvon and Darvocet) is discouraged because propoxyphene is only one half to one third as potent as codeine; is expensive; and has a metabolite, norpropoxyphene, that has a long half-life for neurotoxic side effects (Perin & Pasero, 2000). One newer product is tramadol (Ultram), which is indicated for mild to moderate pain. Ultram has a similar mechanism of action to codeine. A potential benefit is that it does not contain acetaminophen or aspirin but has a low dose of a tricyclic antidepressant (TCA).

TABLE 12-3 | Oral Opioids Indicated for Moderate Pain (WHO Steps I/II)

MEDICATION	USUAL STARTING DOSAGE	COMMENTS
Codeine (with acetaminophen 325 mg or aspirin 325 mg) Tylenol no. 2 (15 mg codeine) Tylenol no. 3 (30 mg codeine) Tylenol no. 4 (60 mg codeine)	60 mg q3-4h	Schedule III agent Total dose should not exceed maximum dose of aspirin or acetaminophen (i.e., 12 tabs/day)
Hydrocodone (with acetaminophen 500 mg) Lortab (5 mg hydrocodone) Vicodin (5 mg hydrocodone) Lortab ES (7.5 mg hydrocodone + acetaminophen 750 mg) Vicodin ES (7.5 mg hydrocodone + acetaminophen 750 mg)	10 mg hydrocodone q3-4h	Same as codeine Total dose should not exceed maximum dose of acetaminophen (i.e., 5 of ES products and 8 of regular) Often ordered q4-6h, which exceeds duration of action
Oxycodone Roxicodone (only oxycodone) Percocet (oxycodone 5 mg plus acetaminophen 500 mg) Tylox (oxycodone 5 mg plus acetaminophen 500 mg) Percodan (oxycodone 5 mg plus aspirin 500 mg)	10 mg q3-4h	Same as codeine Oxycodone alone increases the usefulness of this drug, but 5-mg tablets limit higher dosages
Tramadol (Ultram)	50 mg qid	Acts as a mu receptor agonist but not classified as an opioid Acts as serotonin reuptake inhibitor Seizures may occur at dosages of >400 mg/day

Adapted from Payne, R. (1998). Pharmacologic management in pain. In Berger, A., Portenoy, R. K., & Weissman D. E. (Eds.). *Principles and practice of supportive oncology* (pp. 61-107). Philadelphia: JB Lippincott.

Opioids for moderate to severe pain (step 3): Morphine is the natural strong opioid derived from the opium poppy, and it has long been held as the prototypical strong opioid. Advantages of morphine include a short duration of action; a short half-life of immediate-release oral and parenteral products; the wide availability of formulations, including sustained-release formulations (MS Contin, Oramorph, Kadian); and the low cost of generic oral immediate-release morphine (MS IR). Morphine has two active metabolites: morphine-3-glucoronide (M3G) and morphine-6-glucoronide (M6G). M6G is thought to result in analgesia, whereas M3G may be responsible for myoclonus and increased pain, especially when large doses are given long term (Payne, 1998).

Hydromorphone (Dilaudid) and oxycodone are also strong opioids that have a short duration of action and a short half-life. Their use may be limited in that Dilaudid is available only as an immediate-release drug (sustained-release products will be commercially available soon) and because small dose preparations are typically stocked. That is, a hospital may have only 1- and 2-mg tablets of Dilaudid on formulary, whereas 4- and 8-mg tablets are also available. Meperidine

(Demerol) is a short-acting opioid, but it has a half-life of 15 to 30 hours. Its use is discouraged because its metabolite, normeperidine, accumulates with sustained use (greater than a few days) and the risk for CNS excitatory effects (myoclonus and grand mal seizures) increases. Furthermore, the parenteral or oral potency is poor, and it can interact with monoamine oxidase (MAO) inhibitors to cause severe respiratory depression or CNS excitation (Payne, 1998).

Fentanyl is estimated to be 50 to 100 times more potent that morphine. It is highly lipophilic and thus can be administered transdermally (Duragesic) and transmucosally (Actiq). When administered intravenously, fentanyl has a very short half-life, but transdermal administration effectively changes it to a long-acting drug with a relatively long time period until a steady state is achieved. This is because fentanyl must transverse the skin to reach the bloodstream and CNS, and the skin and fat stores act as drug stores, so drug levels fall slowly after patches are removed. Therefore, when suggesting Duragesic, colleagues and patients should be reminded that it takes at least 12 to 14 hours and as long as 24 hours for fentanyl to reach steady state after application. Fifty percent of the drug concentration will fall in a similar time period after removal (Payne, 1998). On the other hand, transmucosal fentanyl is indicated for breakthrough cancer-related pain and is occasionally used as a single analgesic by patients who have significant side effects with other opioids. You should carefully instruct the patient how to use Actiq: The unit is swabbed or painted over the buccal mucosa and not sucked on. The entire dose should be applied within 15 minutes. Part of the dose absorbs through the mucosal, where it rapidly reaches the bloodstream and then the spinal cord (lipophilic drugs cross the dura more rapidly than hydrophilic drugs). The remainder is swallowed and undergoes first-pass metabolism, similarly to other oral drugs. The potency of transmucosal fentanyl to IV morphine has been estimated to be approximately 8:1 to 14:1 in postoperative patients (Lichtor, Sevarino, Hoshi, et al., 1999); 800 µg of Actiq produces similar analgesia (amount and duration) to morphine 10 mg intravenously.

Levorphanol (Levo-Dromoran) and methadone (Dolophine) are longer-acting agents that have long half-lives. Thus they are more difficult to use because they must be titrated upward more slowly than shorter-acting drugs. Either agent may be a useful alternative for patients who have dose-limiting side effects with other opioids, and methadone has the advantage of having a very low cost.

Equianalgesia is a useful concept applicable to opioids for moderate to severe pain (Table 12-4) (AHCPR, 1994; APS, 1999; Ferrell & McCaffery, 1997). Equianalgesia provides an approximate estimate of equivalent doses and therefore is useful when converting from one drug to another (i.e., oxycodone to morphine) and from one dosage form to another (i.e., oral to intravenous). Because equianalgesic conversions are not exact, the patient may achieve better pain relief with another drug. When converting from one drug to another, it also may be prudent to reduce the calculated equianalgesic dose by 25% (if the patient's pain was well controlled with the first analgesic). To determine equianalgesia, you calculate the 24-hour dose of the first analgesic, convert to the 24-hour dose of the desired analgesic, and then divide by the appropriate interval (i.e., divide by 2 if a sustained-release product is to be administered every 12 hours or by 24 if an intravenous drug is to be administered as a continuous infusion). *Answer 13:* **c.**

Case Study continued

Mrs. Jackson's condition seems to be worsening. Her abdominal tenderness is not lessening, and the Prilosec makes the cramping unbearable. She refuses a computed tomography (CT) scan with contrast because this test increased her pain and cramping the last time it was performed. In addition, her left thigh is larger than her right thigh. A deep venous thrombosis (DVT) in her left leg is confirmed, and you suspect this is related to the left low abdominal mass occluding venous and lymphatic return. You broach the topic of hospice care to Mrs. Jackson.

QUESTIONS

14. Because of the nature of her disease, you anticipate that which of the following will be the best analgesic for Mrs. Jackson?
1. CIV hydromorphone
2. Sublingual morphine
3. Oral oxycodone (Oxycontin)
4. Transdermal fentanyl
   a. 1 & 2
   b. 1 & 4
   c. 2 & 3
   d. Any of these

15. As Mrs. Jackson's condition worsened, she was unable to take oral medications. If her family wanted to help her stay at home, the best analgesic options for a patient who does not have a central venous catheter include which of the following?
1. Rectal or vaginal administration of Oxycontin
2. Continuous subcutaneous infusion of morphine
3. Sublingual morphine
4. Intraspinal morphine
   a. 1 & 2
   b. 1, 2, & 3
   c. 2 & 3
   d. All of these

16. In selecting nondrug interventions for a patient such as Mrs. Jackson, you know that all of the following are true *except:*
   a. Nondrug treatments should always be used in addition to analgesics.
   b. The nurse must always assess the patient's level of fatigue, cognitive status, and ability to concentrate before selecting nondrug measures.
   c. Family/friends should always be involved in implementing nondrug measures, such as massage, to the patient.
   d. The nurse should always assess the patient's past use of nondrug measures.

TABLE **12-4** Equianalgesia: Commonly Used Opioids for Moderate to Severe Pain

OPIOID	PARENTERAL	ORAL	DURATION OF ACTION	COMMENTS
Morphine sulfate (IR, MS Contin, Oramorph, Roxanol)	10 mg	30 mg	3-4 hr	Standard of comparison; available as immediate-release and controlled-release tablets, rectal suppositories Has two main metabolites: morphine-3-glucuronide (M3G) and morphine-6-glucuronide (M6H); only M6G is active at opioid receptor and causes analgesia and side effects
Fentanyl (transdermal— Duragesic; transmucosal— Actiq)	100 μg	—	48-72 hr	Duragesic patches available in 25, 50, 75, 100 μg/hr Equianalgesic conversion is controversial (manufacturer-recommended conversion is often too low); using oral:parenteral ratio for MSO$_4$, Duragesic 1 μg/hr ≈ PO MSO$_4$ 2 mg/24 hr Toxic metabolite (norfentanyl) may accumulate Actiq indicated for breakthrough pain when other analgesics lead to excessive side effects; start with 200 μg
Oxycodone (Roxicodone, Oxycontin)	—	20 mg	3-4 hr	Equivalence to morphine ranges from 1:1 to 1:2 (average 1:1.5) Often compounded with acetaminophen or aspirin, which limit use to mild to moderate pain
Hydromorphone (Dilaudid)	1.5 mg	7.5 mg	3-4 hr	Also available as rectal suppository; 3 mg rectally ≈ 650 mg of aspirin Sustained-release product will probably receive U.S. Food and Drug Administration approval soon
Levorphanol (Levo-Dromoran)	2 mg	4 mg	4-6 hr	Long half-life; accumulates on days 2-3
Methadone (Dolophine)	10 mg	15-20 mg	3-4 hr	Long half-life; accumulates on days 2-5
Meperidine* (Demerol)	75 mg*	300 mg	2-3 hr	Toxic metabolite (normeperidine) accumulates with repetitive doses, causing central nervous system excitation; avoid high and frequent doses, chronic use (>7 days), and in patients with impaired renal function

*Not recommended.

ANSWERS

14. You apply a basic pain management principle to administer oral analgesics whenever possible and to consider cost, invasiveness, and burden to the patient and family when oral drugs are not possible. Another route of administration other than orally should be anticipated in Mrs. Jackson's case. Although oxycodone is an excellent analgesic, it is not available as a parenteral drug, so selecting another analgesic with a wider variety of formulations is probably wise. Although some nurses and physicians advocate sublingual morphine, in reality, all of the drug will be swallowed

because morphine is hydrophilic and thus poorly absorbed through the oral mucosa (Payne, 1998). Intravenous morphine might be an alternative, but this may require the patient to have some type of central venous catheter inserted at great cost, and the costs of intravenous morphine, the pump, and other supplies for intravenous infusion are substantial. Starting transdermal fentanyl (Duragesic) at this point is probably the most reasonable alternative when there is time to find the dose that relieves Mrs. Jackson's pain. This can be done by starting an intravenous infusion of fentanyl at 25 μg/hr (with 12.5-μg bolus doses) and titrating the dose by 10% to 20% to pain relief, and then converting to the same dose in patch form (Mercadante, Caligara, Sapio, et al., 1997; Miser, Narang, Dothage, et al., 1989). Alternatively, a conservative equianalgesic dose to Mrs. Jackson's present analgesic can be started, and she can be supplemented with oxycodone as the dose of Duragesic is increased (generally every 2 to 3 days). Cancer patients who have severe pain and have taken only codeine or who are opioid naive can use Duragesic (Vielvoye-Kerkmeer, Mattern, & Uitendaal, 2000). Such patients are started at 25 μg and the dosage titrated every 2 to 3 days as needed. Duragesic is often more acceptable to older patients than taking sustained-release tablets because it seems less burdensome and there is less constipation with Duragesic than with morphine (Payne, Mathias, Pasta, et al., 1998; Radbruch, Sabatowski, Loick, et al., 2000). *Answer 14:* **b.**

15. Analgesic tablets and capsules (including morphine sustained release, oxycodone, methadone, naproxen, and ibuprofen) that have been administered orally can be administered rectally with comparable pain relief (amount and duration) (De Conno, Ripamonti, Saita, et al., 1995; Maloney, Kesner, Klein, & Bockenstette, 1989; Warren, 1996). Because of the venous anatomy of the rectum, drugs administered via this route avoid first-pass hepatic metabolism. Oral formulations may be more practical to administer because a wider variety is available and larger doses of drugs can be given, and probably at a lower cost. In addition, if more than one tablet is administered or if rectal irritation seems to be a problem (which may be less common with sustained-release tablets than with rectal suppositories), the pills can be placed in a gel capsule before administration. In women, the vagina provides another mucosal surface for administration. The rectal or vaginal route may be objectionable to some patients, but it is worth exploring as an alternative.

Another feasible alternative for the patient who does not have a central venous catheter is continuous subcutaneous infusion of opioid (Bruera, Brenneis, Michaud, et al., 1988; Miller, McCarthy, O'Boyle, & Kearney, 1999; Storey, Hill, St. Louis, & Tarver, 1990). As with intravenous continuous infusions, drugs that have a short duration of action and a short half-life are the drugs of choice for continuous subcutaneous infusion. Based on cost, morphine is used most often, and hydromorphone is an alternative for patients who have intolerable side effects with morphine or who require the smallest possible

volumes because of limited subcutaneous tissues. Both drugs are relatively nonirritating and can be combined with haloperidol (Haldol) or metoclopramide (Reglan) for the patient who is also experiencing nausea. A home infusion pump that has the capability of delivering a continuous infusion plus bolus doses is desirable, but no other special equipment is needed. An area on the chest, upper arm, upper thigh, or abdomen is prepped as for an intravenous insertion, and a small-gauge (e.g., 27-gauge) winged infusion needle is inserted subcutaneously. A Band-Aid over the wings stabilizes the needle, and a transparent dressing promotes observatory insertion of the site. The needle is changed according to policy and procedure, which may be every 72 hours in the hospital or at a longer interval in the patient's home. Continuous subcutaneous infusion is contraindicated in a few patients who develop induration at the insertion site with drug leakage from the skin. Intraspinal opioid infusions are indicated in a relatively small number of patients who cannot achieve adequate pain control or who have unmanageable severe side effects when opioids are administered orally or parenterally. *Answer 15:* **a.**

16. Analgesics are the foundation of cancer pain control. Although nonpharmacologic drug measures do not replace analgesics, they may decrease the emotional suffering from pain, enhance coping, promote a sense of control, contribute to comfort and pain relief, decrease fatigue, and enhance sleep (McCaffery & Pasero, 1999). There are many nondrug interventions that might be acceptable to and helpful for selected patients, including cutaneous stimulation (i.e., application of heat or cold, massage, vibration), distraction (useful for brief periods), and relaxation techniques. One potential way the nonpharmacologic measures might be effective is because of the interaction that occurs between the nurse and the patient when teaching a technique or performing a procedure, such as a massage. Patients should be informed that nonpharmacologic measures are not used instead of pharmacologic measures, but rather in a synergistic attempt with analgesics. It is useful to explore with the patient what experiences he or she has had with nonpharmacologic methods, if these were successful, if there were any problems with what was tried, and how he or she feels about trying other measures. If the patient is in severe pain, very fatigued, or unable to think or concentrate, he or she will not be able to learn and use techniques such as relaxation, but massage or application of heat or cold might be helpful. When teaching a nonpharmacologic method, you should see if the family or other caregivers want to be involved. Some might be glad to be able to do something for the patient, whereas others may feel overwhelmed and already overly burdened. *Answer 16:* **c.**

CASE 2 STUDY

You are consulted to see Jonathan Moore, a 35-year-old white man who was completely well until 4 months ago, when he began to experience low back pain that radiated toward his right hip. The pain was bothersome enough that he saw his family physician, who initially ordered a plain film radiograph. No abnormality was seen, and the physician suggested an OTC NSAID for "back strain." Mr. Moore took ibuprofen for almost 3 weeks, during which time the pain steadily worsened. The pain now extends to his right hip. A CT scan of his abdomen and pelvis demonstrated a small mass in the right kidney and multiple small defects in his right acetabulum. Several needle biopsies of the bone lesions were performed, which finally confirmed metastatic renal cell carcinoma. The time from initial onset of symptoms and confirmation of diagnosis was approximately 6 weeks.

Present Analgesics
Sustained-release morphine (MS Contin) 240 mg every 12 hours
Morphine immediate release (MS IR) 30 to 60 mg orally every 3 to 4 hours as needed
Gabapentin (Neurontin) 300 mg three times a day
Clonazepam (Klonopin) 2 mg three times a day

Mr. Moore appears healthy and has not lost any weight. His current laboratory values are within normal limits, except for his serum calcium, which is 11.0 mg/dl (normal is 8.5 to 10.5 mg/dl). When you enter his room, you note that he appears sleepy and is having sudden and intense myoclonic jerks of his arms and legs every few minutes. He is able to participate in his pain history, but his thinking seems to be slow and disjointed. A few of his comments do not make sense, and you are not sure whether he is confused. He says his pain is in his left sacrum and hip, and it does not radiate to the groin or thigh. Despite regularly administered opioid and adjuvant analgesics, his pain at rest is 7 to 8 (on a 0 to 10 scale). He gets up only to use the bedside commode, and this activity, as well as the myoclonic jerks, brings on immediate episodes of greatly increased pain (rating of 10). He describes his pain as sharp and constant, and he denies shooting pain, numbness, tingling, or burning. The orthopedic surgeon consulted for potential stabilization of Mr. Moore's acetabulum states this cannot be done because there is virtually no bone to repair and because Mr. Moore's life expectancy is short. Radiation therapy is begun, but moving Mr. Moore from bed to cart causes him excruciating pain. He is given MS IR 60 mg before he goes to radiation therapy, but it is not possible to know exactly when he will leave, and the dose is often given a few minutes before he is to transfer to the cart.

QUESTIONS

1. If Mr. Moore has confusion related to his analgesics, what is the most appropriate management strategy?
   a. Decreasing the dose of morphine and adding a second opioid analgesic, such as hydrocodone plus acetaminophen (Vicodin, Lortabs)
   b. Maintaining the present dose and route of morphine because the confusion is likely to abate
   c. Changing the morphine to a continuous infusion because this route is associated with fewer side effects
   d. Discontinuing the morphine and starting another opioid indicated for moderate to severe pain

2. Gabapentin (Neurontin) is usually suggested for:
   a. Neuropathic pain with a burning quality
   b. Neuropathic pain with a paroxysmal, lancinating/stabbing quality
   c. Nociceptive pain with an aching quality
   d. Nociceptive pain with a throbbing quality

3. Which side effect of an opioid is most likely to be dose limiting?
   a. Sedation
   b. Constipation

c. Delirium
d. Myoclonic jerks

4. In light of the data you have collected regarding Mr. Moore, which intervention might be a useful adjunct to his analgesics?
   a. Hydroxyzine (Vistaril)
   b. Lorazepam (Ativan)
   c. Pamidronate (Aredia)
   d. A neurolytic procedure/block

5. Which of the following patients is most likely to be experiencing respiratory depression from an opioid?
   a. A 65-year-old patient who is opioid naive, was started on oxycodone 10 mg every 4 hours around the clock yesterday, has a respiratory rate of 10 breaths/min, and is very sedated
   b. A 65-year-old patient who has been taking Oxycontin 40 mg every 12 hours for 2 months, received lorazepam 3 mg intravenously yesterday afternoon for a procedure, has a respiratory rate of 10 breaths/min, and is sedated
   c. A 75-year-old patient who has been taking MS Contin for 2 months and has a respiratory rate of 11 breaths/min during nights
   d. A 75-year-old patient who has been taking codeine 60 mg every 4 hours, has now changed to MS Contin 30 mg every 12 hours, has moderately elevated liver function tests (LFTs), has a respiratory rate of 10 breaths/min, and is easily arousable

ANSWERS

1. As discussed previously, pain assessment is critical in determining the nature of pain (nociceptive versus neuropathic versus visceral), and the pain ladder helps match analgesic choice to the pain intensity and underlying cause or causes. In Mr. Moore's case, his pain ranged from 7 or higher, so an opioid for severe pain is appropriate. Because he has bone involvement, an NSAID might also help. *Answer 1:* **d.**

2. Neuropathic pain is common in cancer patients and may be caused by spinal cord or nerve root compression, plexopathies (cervical, brachial, and lumbosacral), postsurgical, chemotherapy, radiation syndromes, phantom limb pain, acute herpes zoster, or postherpetic neuralgia (Martin & Hagen, 1997). Because Mr. Moore has extensive bony spread, you should assess him for neuropathic pain by asking him about the quality of his pain (What does it feel like?). He never offered any of these words, and when asked specifically, he denied burning, stabbing, grabbing, electric, unusual or different pain; numbness; tingling; and so on—words that are usually indicative of neuropathic pain. Patients may also experience allodynia, which is pain that results from normally innocuous stimuli, such as light pressure from clothing or bedding. Physical examination of the painful area may or may not reveal vasomotor changes, such as cool skin, dystrophic changes, and absence of sweating (these signs can also occur with ischemic pain, which is thought to be a variant of neuropathic pain). Neuropathic pain arises from injury to the peripheral nervous system (or occasionally the CNS), which causes abnormal nerve healing, altered connections, and the generation of ectopic/aberrant pain messages. Some clinicians think that opioids are not effective for neuropathic pain, but in reality, opioids may be somewhat helpful.

There is no clear, evidence-based recommendation for which agents to use for neuropathic pain, but TCAs and anticonvulsants are the mainstay agents (Cameron, 1992; Watson, 1994). TCAs modulate pain transmission in afferent pathways by decreasing the action potentiation and progression of pain to the spinothalamic pathway and in the efferent (descending) pathways by altering serotonin and/or norepinephrine release and reuptake, whereas the mechanism of action of anticonvulsants is not known (Hansen, 1999). If Mr. Moore did have a neuropathic component to his pain (burning, numbness, or tingling), the first recommendation would be a nonsedating TCA (e.g., desipramine, imipramine); if he described stabbing or grabbing pain, an anticonvulsant would be chosen (e.g., Neurontin) (Cameron, 1992; Egbunike & Chaffee, 1990; Martin & Hagen, 1997). Therefore, if Mr. Moore said that he had shooting, stabbing, or grabbing pain going down from his back or hip to his groin or leg, you would probably recommend Neurontin. Because of his young age, relative health, and severe pain, you would probably be aggressive and suggest starting at 300 mg three times a day and escalating every 1 to 2 days if he did not have dose-limiting side effects. When Neurontin is efficacious, the results are often quite dramatic, and the number of paroxysms of pain falls off rapidly. *Answer 2:* **b.**

3. Health care providers, patients, and their families are concerned about the adverse effects of opioids. Unfortunately, they overestimate the risk for respiratory depression, which is very rare, and underestimate or do not recognize the risk for more common adverse effects. In some instances adverse effects increase with higher dosages of opioid, to the point of becoming dose limiting. Adverse effects occur more often in the short time after an opioid is started and resolve as tolerance to the effect occurs. A useful approach is to know the relative likelihood of adverse effects, anticipate when they are likely to occur, and manage in a prompt fashion. In addition, when a patient experiences an adverse effect, the question of whether this is a manageable side effect and/or whether the patient will develop tolerance to this effect should be considered. The more common adverse effects (constipation, sedation or mental clouding, nausea) are manageable or resolve in a short time in most instances. Sedation after the onset of opioid analgesics may be an effect of the analgesic or may mean that a patient who has been experiencing severe pain is finally able to sleep. Therefore the addition of a stimulant is not indicated unless it is several days after the medication has been started and the patient is still very sleepy. Similarly, mental clouding or fuzziness usually improves, but the patient often perceives these as intolerable when they do not resolve. More serious psychomimetic reactions (dysphoria, vivid daydreams or nightmares, depersonalization, hallucinations, and panic) are usually dose limiting and require conversion to another opioid (Lehmann, 1997). Fortunately, a replacement drug is likely to be just as effective or be associated with fewer side effects because opioids are not structurally identical and not completely cross-tolerant (Galer, Coyle, Pasternak, & Portenoy, 1992).

Therefore the patient should be asked if he or she feels confused or mixed up, or if he or she is having vivid dreams or hallucinations. Most patients do not volunteer this information because they think they are "going crazy." Sometimes confusion is mild, and a nurse unfamiliar with the patient might miss it, but as the dosage of the opioid is escalated, confusion usually worsens and is more easily identified. Some clinicians advocate using haloperidol for opioid-induced confusion, yet its use for this purpose has not been proven helpful. Mild to moderate nausea can be managed with a regularly scheduled antiemetic (prochlorperazine 10 mg intravenously or orally, or metoclopramide 10 mg intravenously or orally four times a day) for about a week. Few patients develop severe nausea accompanied by vomiting, but unfortunately, this side effect is often dose limiting. Tolerance to less common adverse effects, such as urinary retention (a smooth muscle effect), myoclonic jerks, and urticaria, usually develops. Respiratory depression, the least common adverse effect, can also resolve with tolerance. In

Mr. Moore's case, Klonopin was helpful in alleviating his myoclonic jerks. *Answer 3:* **c.**

4. Other adjuvant drugs may be useful for particular situations, such as a small dose of stimulant (e.g., methylphenidate [Ritalin]) for nonresolving sedation or a corticosteroid for impending spinal cord compression (Table 12-5) (Bruera & Watanabe, 1994). It has been suggested that a new psychostimulant, modafinil (Provigil), may also be useful to alleviate sedation from opioids. Modafinil is a schedule C-IV drug, but there is no literature reporting doses used. A bisphosphonate or a radiopharmaceutical may be useful to alleviate pain and lessen opioid requirements for some patients who have bone metastases. Both pamidronate (Aredia) and strontium-89 are selectively taken up by and "stabilize" bone and have been shown to be reduce pain by approximately 30% to 60%, respectively (Pereira, Mancini, & Walker, 1998; Pons, Herranz, Garcia, et al., 1997). Strontium-89 is very expensive and affects other blood cells, whereas pamidronate is much less costly and does not affect bone marrow progenitor cells. Some patients who have severe and relatively localized pain may benefit from a neurolytic procedure. Collaborating with the anesthesiologist in your practice setting who specializes in these procedures may prevent your patient from experiencing unnecessary pain or adverse effects of analgesics. Unfortunately, a neurolytic procedure will not benefit Mr. Moore, who has more generalized pain.

The myth about potentiators is still operating with hydroxyzine (Vistaril), often given in combination with an opioid (usually Demerol). The evidence strongly supports that the commonly used dose (Vistaril 25 mg) does not enhance analgesia. Although doses of at least 75 to 100 mg would provide added analgesia, these doses could depress respirations (Glazier, 1990). Although some clinicians advocate the use of benzodiazepines, such as lorazepam (Ativan) and diazepam (Valium), there is no compelling evidence that they have analgesic properties (Reddy & Patt, 1994). Benzodiazepines are thus best reserved for limited use for acute muscle spasm and for anxiety that accompanies pain. An exception is clonazepam (Klonopin), which is the drug of choice for myoclonic jerks (Cameron, 1992) (see Table 12-5). *Answer 4:* **c.**

5. Pain is usually the antidote for the rarely occurring opioid-induced respiratory depression. There are virtually no helpful guidelines for nurses and physicians to anticipate at-risk patients, the

TABLE 12-5 **Adjuvant Analgesics**

AGENT	DOSAGE RECOMMENDATIONS	COMMENTS
TRICYCLIC ANTIDEPRESSANTS		
Desipramine (Norpramin)	Start at 25-75 mg q$_{AM}$, ↑ dose by 25 mg q2-4days to a maximum of 300 mg	Sedation greatest with amitriptyline Anticholinergic effects greatest with amitriptyline, less with nortriptyline and imipramine, least with desipramine
Nortriptyline (Pamelor)	Start at 25-50 mg q$_{AM}$, ↑ as above to 300 mg	Orthostasis greatest with imipramine, less with amitriptyline and desipramine, least with nortriptyline Onset of analgesic effect in 1-2 wk, maximum at 4-6 wk
Imipramine (Trofanil)	Start at 10-25 mg q$_{AM}$ or q$_{PM}$, ↑ as above to 300 mg	Common error: doses are not rapidly? Increased after initial dose to relief or side effects If side effects occur, change to another agent in the class
Amitriptyline (Elavil)	Start at 10-25 mg qhs, ↑ as above to 150-300 mg	
ANTICONVULSANTS		
Gabapentin (Neurontin)	Start at 100 mg tid, ↑ each dose by 100 mg every 1-2 days to 1600-2400 mg	Most common adverse effects: sedation (13%), dizziness/light-headedness (8%), nausea (8%), confusion (2.4%)
Carbamazepine (Tegretol)	Start at 100 mg tid, ↑ every 2-4 days by 100 mg to 200-400 mg tid	Risk for aplastic anemia, 0.4% with long-term use; monitor complete blood count q2wk for 4-6 wk
Phenytoin (Dilantin)	Start at 100 mg tid, ↑ as above by 25-50 mg/dose to 350-500 mg/day	Can induce central nervous system excitation
Baclofen (Lioresal)	Start at 5-10 mg tid, ↑ as above by 10 mg/day to 80 mg/day in divided doses	Indicated for trigeminal neuralgia, post-herpetic neuralgia, painful legs syndrome, etc.
Valproic acid (Valproate)	Start at 125 mg tid, ↑ as above to 500-1000 mg tid	Side effects: sedation, dizziness, nausea, rare confusion
Clonazepam (Klonopin)	Start at 0.5 mg bid, ↑ each dose by 0.5 mg as above to 8 mg/day	Drug of choice for myoclonic jerks
CORTICOSTEROIDS		
Dexamethasone (Decadron, Prednisone)	16-24 mg/day 40-100 mg/day	Emergency management for increased intracranial pressure and spinal cord compression Effects: antiinflammatory, antiemetic, appetite stimulant, mood elevation Side effects (e.g., hyperglycemia, dysphoria, myopathy) may occur with long-term use
STIMULANTS		
Methylphenidate (Ritalin, Dextroamphetamine)	5 mg at 8 AM, add second dose at 1 PM, ↑ to 10 mg prn 2.5 mg as above, ↑ to 7.5 mg each dose	Decrease sedation and improve mentation Dextroamphetamine may decrease appetite
OTHER		
Cyclobenzaprine Flexeril Benzodiazepines (lorazepam, diazepam)		May be useful for particular patients who have muscle spasms Not first line for cancer patients Useful if anxiety is another component of cancer or pain experience

sequence of events associated with respiratory depression, and how to confirm it as an adverse effect. Patients who are opioid naive are at greatest risk, whereas opioid-tolerant patients undergoing rapid titration of their dose are at smaller risk. Elderly patients may be a greater risk because they *may* have decreased hepatic or renal function. Impaired renal function is probably more important, particularly with drugs that have toxic metabolites (e.g., morphine, fentanyl, meperidine) that are renally excreted. If the patient is opioid tolerant and new-onset sedation occurs, opioid-induced respiratory depression will be at the bottom of the differential diagnosis list. This is a concept the APN may frequently have to remind housestaff physicians and staff nurses about. Thus other causes of sedation should be ruled out before administering naloxone to a cancer patient who has pain.

Respiratory depression or profound sedation (level 4) precedes (Pasero, Portenoy, & McCaffery, 1999) and results in a falling respiratory rate (Box 12-4). A patient whose respirations are 8 per minute or less is considered to have respiratory depression, but he or she should be assessed in light of what is normal for him or her. For instance, a patient who is breathing deeply and comfortable and has a respiratory rate of less than 10 breaths/min may not be respiratory depressed. Therefore the patient whose sedation score is 3 or more should not be given naloxone (Narcan). Because pulse oximetry may be useful in assessing whether oxygenation is declining, starting an opioid-naive patient on an opioid is a reasonable recommendation. In addition, staff should be reminded that large doses of benzodiazepine premedications before procedures can induce profound and lasting sedation in some patients and will not be reversed by naloxone. *Answer 5:* **a.**

Case Study continued

You advise the housestaff physician to discontinue morphine because Mr. Moore still has severe pain despite relatively large doses, as well as dose-limiting adverse effects, including confusion, depression, and distressing myoclonic jerks. In addition, he is receiving Neurontin and large doses of clonazepam, which may also be causing sedation. Although Klonopin would be appropriate for myoclonic jerks, a much greater dose than is usually recommended (see Table 12-5) was started, and even this dose was not effective. Neurontin is not a first-line choice because Mr. Moore's pain does not clearly indicate a neuropathic component. You have discussed potential options with Mr. Moore, including oral Oxycontin with oxycodone as needed for pain at rest and incident pain or a continuous intravenous infusion of Dilaudid. He opts for Oxycontin first, because he hopes to leave the hospital soon and this would be easier to take. You thus suggest Oxycontin and oxycodone to the resident.

Unfortunately, although the dose of Oxycontin is escalated, Mr. Moore has only "some" pain control if he stays in bed and does not move. Attempts to sit up or move are still accompanied by severe pain. He is given oxycodone before activities. Because the onset of action is too slow and usually increases his sedation, he is converted to intravenous Dilaudid. You ask Mr. Moore if you can contact his wife, still at home and visiting infrequently. You recommend that his family be closer to him. He appreciatively says yes, and you consult with the social worker to find out what types of living accommodations are available. After talking with Mr. Moore's mother, it is decided that the wife and son will stay with her. This increases the psychosocial support for all.

Mr. Moore does not respond to therapy, and his condition declines rapidly. He is now terminally ill, and he and his family agree to the care goal of comfort. His dose of intravenous Dilaudid is now 115 mg/hr, and bolus doses of 30 mg every 10 minutes as needed are ordered, which is controlling his pain without sedation or other side effects. A nurse from another floor floats to the oncology unit and is assigned to take care of Mr. Moore. She is shocked at the size of the dose, which she thinks will kill the patient. When she sees you, she asks you if his dose should be decreased and says it is "against my ethics to give a big dose that will make him die."

BOX 12-4	Sedation Scale

S = Sleep, easy to arouse
1 = Awake and alert
2 = Slightly drowsy, easily aroused
3 = Frequently drowsy, arousable, drifts off to sleep during conversation
4 = Somnolent, minimal or no response to physical stimulation

From McCaffery, M., & Pasero, C. (1999). *Pain. Clinical manual*, 2nd ed. (p. 267). St. Louis: Mosby.

QUESTIONS

6. Reasons to avoid polypharmacy when starting analgesics include all of the following *except:*

   a. Drugs from different classes may have interactions with each other.

   b. Adverse effects may be related to other chronic diseases.

   c. Analgesics from different classes can have overlapping adverse effects.

   d. Ability to assess amount of analgesia from particular agents becomes more confusing.

7. Calculate equianalgesic dose of Oxycontin for Mr. Moore based on his current dose of morphine (MS Contin 240 mg every 12 hours, MS IR 30 mg every 3 hours).

8. The nurse who appealed to ethics in Mr. Moore's case would probably justify her position using the bioethical concept of:

   a. Autonomy

   b. Beneficence

   c. Nonmaleficence

   d. Justice

ANSWERS

6. Although analgesics from different classes may be needed to control a patient's pain, initial polypharmacy should be avoided. Mr. Moore provides ample evidence of why this is so: His pain is not controlled, and he is having intolerable, and perhaps unmanageable, side effects from one or more of his analgesics or adjuvant agents (morphine, Neurontin, or Klonopin). You are thus left with the difficult decision about how to proceed. All three drugs can cause sedation. Because gabapentin does not seem to be indicated, it could be rapidly titrated down and discontinued. The dose of Klonopin is much higher than would usually be ordered to quell myoclonic jerks and should be escalated down. The bottom line is that his pain is not being controlled, and a different opioid is the best option. The best plan is to start with and titrate the best agent for the severity of pain (opioid for severe pain), assess effectiveness and adverse effects, and then sequentially add other drugs. There are no known interactions between agents in different classes. *Answer 6:* **a.**

7. You can demonstrate to the medical and nursing staff how to use an equianalgesia table (see Table 12-4) to convert Mr. Moore's morphine to oxycodone. His 24-hour total dose of morphine is (240 mg × 2) + (30 mg × 8) = 480 mg + 240 mg = 720 mg. Oral morphine 30 mg is equivalent to 20 mg of oral oxycodone, so you multiply the 24-hour

dose of morphine by ⅔. Thus 720 mg × ⅔ = 480 mg of oxycodone in 24 hours. The every-12-hour dose is therefore calculated as 240 mg of Oxycontin, but you would probably suggest a lower dosage (160 mg every 12 hours) and oxycodone 30 mg every 3 hours as needed. Encouraging the staff nurses to assess Mr. Moore's pain frequently and to offer the as-needed doses every 3 to 4 hours is consistent with your consultative role. The next day you would increase the every-12-hour dose of Oxycontin by considering the amount of the as-needed doses administered (e.g., 180 mg/24 hr; thus new Oxycontin dosage is 250 mg every 12 hours). *Answer 7:* **480 mg in 24 hours or 120 mg every 12 hours.**

8. The nurse appeals to ethics (her own) to ask whether the dosage should be decreased. In fact, this is a clinical issue rather than an ethical one, and it relates to the nurse's lack of knowledge regarding opioids for severe pain and her own personal discomfort. The APN is confronted by such issues with many nurses and patients and in many settings (e.g., hospital, clinic, home care). Helping nurses and families clarify the issues and deal with ethical conflicts is an important role for the APN.

   The reasons behind resistance to large opioid doses usually surround not wanting to harm the patient (nonmaleficence). Nonmaleficence is one of four broad bioethical principles: autonomy, beneficence, nonmaleficence, and justice (Beauchamp & Childress, 1994). The APN assists the staff in recognizing Mr. Moore's autonomy (the opposite of paternalism) by informing him and assisting him to make decisions regarding his pain management options. Beneficence means that we as health care providers have a responsibility or duty to benefit patients. Beneficence is reflected in the JCAHO pain standards: Because all patients have a right to pain control, health care providers have a corresponding duty to do their best to control pain.

   Nonmaleficence means that health care providers should avoid causing harm to patients. In practical terms, this might relate to not managing adverse effects of opioids or to prescribing technologies that a patient or family could not afford or manage at home (e.g., intraspinal opioids delivered by pump in a patient who could be managed with oral or parenteral analgesics) (Whedon & Ferrell, 1991). However, nurses and physicians sometimes incorrectly equate increasing dosages of opioid analgesics with "dangerous" side effects or euthanasia (Angell, 1982; Hammes & Cain, 1994; Mount, 1996). Colleagues should be reminded that the intent is palliation of pain (or other symptoms, such as dyspnea), not at the cost of increased sedation, and that this goal can be accomplished for most patients. The concern that morphine (or another strong opioid) could shorten life is addressed in the principle of double effect, which recognizes that although an opioid could hasten death, the primary intent is to relieve pain and suffering. Therefore administering morphine is ethically justified. Double effect may be a moot point because there is evidence that morphine use does *not* depress respirations or shorten life in patients with advanced disease (Thorns, 2000; Walsh, 1984). Furthermore, it seems as likely that a patient whose pain is relieved may be more relaxed and might actually live for a slightly longer time.

The principle of justice means that scarce resources will be distributed fairly (Whedon & Ferrell, 1991). Thus a patient should be able to get the medications he or she needs to control pain. This is not always the case because analgesics are very expensive and not all individuals have coverage. Therefore, when assessing patients' needs, you should always ask about this so that you can assist patients in finding coverage for needed analgesics, such as through pharmaceutical company drug assistance programs. *Answer 8:* **c.**

CASE 3 STUDY

Mrs. Dorothy Bennett, a 73-year-old white woman, was diagnosed with a low-grade retroperitoneal lymphoma 4 years ago. She had a complete response to chemotherapy and did well until 2 years ago, when she received radiation therapy to a single metastasis in her abdomen. She again did well until 3 months ago, when she had the onset of mild pain in her left upper arm. Her physical examination is within normal limits. She was started on conservative treatment with an OTC NSAID followed by Vicodin.

Mrs. Bennett is married and lives with her 82-year-old husband. Both have chronic health problems but appear younger than their stated ages. Mr. and Mrs. Bennett have four adult children who live nearby, and they describe their family as very close. Mrs. Bennett seems to look to her husband and children for guidance, which is a change for her because she used to be so independent and active before she became ill. Mrs. Bennett is in relatively good nutritional and physical health, but she is somewhat deconditioned because of decreased physical activity.

Mrs. Bennett now takes Oxycontin 40 mg in the morning and 20 mg in the evening, plus an occasional 5-mg tablet of oxycodone. Despite this, her pain is worsening. Her daughter calls and tells you that Mrs. Bennett had been spending most of the day lying on the sofa. She thinks this is because of her mother's unrelieved pain, but other family members think the oxycodone is making their mother too sleepy. The daughter is also concerned because Mrs. Bennett has low back pain that is somewhat relieved with massage.

You consult with the oncologist and schedule Mrs. Bennett for a plain radiograph, chest CT, and bone scan. A large destructive mass of the left humerus, consistent with metastatic disease, is noted. No other metastases are found, and Mrs. Bennett undergoes surgical resection of the tumor-involved bone with a graft from the left ileum. After surgery, Mrs. Bennett is hospitalized on the gerontology rehabilitation unit. She received morphine 15 mg orally every 4 hours as needed and Vicodin (hydrocodone 5 mg plus acetaminophen 500 mg) one tablet every 4 hours as needed. Two weeks later, she is transferred to the oncology unit because she still has severe pain in her left hip that is interfering with ambulation and she is extremely constipated. She is started on a morphine drip of 1 mg/hr, and over 4 days, the dosage is increased to 10 mg/hr.

QUESTIONS

1. If Mrs. Bennett still rated her pain as 7 and she was not having dose-limiting side effects, you would suggest that her dosage be increased to:
   a. 11 mg/hr
   b. 12 mg/hr
   c. 14 mg/hr
   d. 16 mg/hr

2. The 24-hour dose of oral morphine equianalgesic to Mrs. Bennett's intravenous dose is:
   a. 120 to 240 mg
   b. 240 to 360 mg
   c. 360 to 480 mg
   d. 480 to 720 mg

3. If the housestaff physician asked about how to convert Mrs. Bennett from intravenous morphine 10 mg/hr to oral morphine, your initial advice would be:

   a. Convert half of the dose to oral morphine IR (45 mg every 6 hours) and continue CIV at 5 mg/hr
   b. Convert half of the dose to sustained-release oral morphine (120 mg every 12 hours) and continue CIV at 5 mg/hr
   c. Convert the entire dose to oral morphine IR (MS Contin 120 mg every 6 hours)
   d. Convert the entire dose to sustained-release oral morphine (240 mg every 12 hours)

ANSWERS

1. When a patient's pain is not satisfactorily controlled, the opioid dosage should be titrated upward. There are no clear guidelines as to appropriate dosage increases. Doses equal to 10% to 25% of the 24-hour total dose of analgesic are recommended for rescue doses (Payne, 1998). A similar rule of thumb usually works as well when titrating opioid analgesics upward (or downward to avoid physical withdrawal and emergent pain): For moderate to severe pain, the dose is increased by 15% to 25%. Some clinicians advocate larger increases for severe pain, but if this is done, the patient may become somewhat sedated and the nurses and physicians may be reluctant to increase doses further. The 15% to 25% rule is practical for opioids administered by any route. In Mrs. Bennett's case, 15% of 10 mg/hr is 1.5 mg and 25% is 2.5%, so you would recommend that Mrs. Bennett receive a bolus dose of 2 mg intravenously (to rapidly increase her serum level) immediately before increasing the hourly intravenous (or continuous subcutaneous infusion if she were receiving morphine by that route) rate of morphine to 12 mg/hr. *Answer 1:* **b.**

2. Although the equianalgesic dose of oral morphine to parenteral morphine is calculated as 3:1, patients sometimes require a smaller dose of oral morphine to maintain pain control. This is more likely to be true when the patient is receiving larger doses of morphine (more than 10 mg/hr). Therefore you would use the estimates of 2:1 and 3:1 and show the intern that the dose of oral morphine might range from 480 to 720 mg/24 hr. Elderly age would be one consideration in leaning toward the more conservative estimate. *Answer 2:* **d.**

3. In addition, it is practical to convert part of a dose of parenteral morphine to oral morphine for the same reason. You should suggest using the conservative estimate to convert 50% of the intravenous dose (i.e., 5 mg/hr) to oral morphine (5 mg × 2 = 10 mg/hr orally, × 24 hours = 240 mg ÷ 2). Starting Mrs. Bennett on MS Contin 120 mg every 12 hours and continuing the intravenous infusion at 5 mg/hr will allow the staff to assess her response (pain control and side effects) and increase the intravenous dose if needed. If this strategy is effective, the remaining intravenous morphine can be converted to oral morphine the following day. If not, the doses can be adjusted accordingly. *Answer 3:* **b.**

Case Study continued

You are again called to see Mrs. Bennett because yesterday her morphine drip was discontinued and she was converted to MS Contin 180 mg every 8 hours, plus 30 mg of morphine IR every 4 to 6 hours for breakthrough pain. Within 8 hours of the first oral dose, she became quite sedated and the evening dose was held. The resident wanted to give Mrs. Bennett naloxone (Narcan) and wrote an order for "Narcan 0.4 mg IVP, if no response may repeat." The oncology nurses consult with you because they realize this is an incorrect order. No Narcan is given, and the MS Contin dosage is changed to 90 mg every 12 hours.

The next morning, you talk to the staff RN caring for Mrs. Bennett, who says she thinks that perhaps Mrs. Bennett's pain is "not quite as bad as she says it is." When you ask the RN if Mrs. Bennett is having any adverse effects of morphine (other than sedation), particularly confusion, the nurse states, "Oh, no. She is as sharp as a tack!" When you go in to see Mrs. Bennett, she is in a wheelchair and waiting for assistance to return to bed. Her entire left arm is immobilized in a soft cast and plastic orthotic device. You help her back to bed and find that she is steady on her feet. She tells you that her left arm does not hurt at all anymore but that her left hip (the site where bone was taken for the graft) hurts. She says the pain is dull, nonradiating, and rated as 2 to 3 when she is not moving, but rated as 10 when walking. When you ask her if she has any side effects from the morphine that she does not like, she mentions bowel movements. You specifically ask her if morphine makes her feel mixed up or confused, she says, "Well, when I was on the IV, I thought there was a dog on my face." She did not tell anyone this because she thought they would think she was crazy.

QUESTIONS

4. Which of the following are true regarding naloxone (Narcan)?
   1. Narcan can be given via IVP.
   2. Narcan can induce pain.
   3. Narcan can induce cardiac arrhythmias, hypertension, and sudden death.
   4. Narcan can be titrated to reversal of respiratory depression without return of pain.
      a. 1, 2, & 3
      b. 1, 3, & 4
      c. 2, 3, & 4
      d. All of these

5. Which of the following statements about breakthrough/incident pain are true?
   1. It is a transitory pain that increases to moderate or severe pain.
   2. One type is end-of-dose failure.
   3. It may be spontaneous or precipitated by a recognizable event.
   4. It may be nociceptive or neuropathic.
      a. 1, 2, & 3
      b. 2, 3, & 4
      c. 1, 3, & 4
      d. All of these

6. Assume that the physician had agreed with the nurse that Mrs. Bennett's pain seemed out of proportion to her disease and ordered an intravenous placebo. If Mrs. Bennett said her pain was relieved after administration, what would this mean?
      a. It does not tell you anything.
      b. Mrs. Bennett's pain is not severe.
      c. Mrs. Bennett has drug-seeking behaviors.
      d. Mrs. Bennett is exhibiting pseudoaddiction.

ANSWERS

4. As discussed earlier, nurses and physicians must be relatively certain that a patient is experiencing respiratory depression, in which case naloxone (Narcan) is lifesaving. Mrs. Bennett is somewhat sleepy but easily arousable, so she does not need Narcan. In other instances patients who enter the terminal phase of their disease and experience deep sedation or coma related to brain metastases, hepatic failure, hypercalcemia, sepsis, or some other problem are incorrectly assumed to be experiencing respiratory depression, despite being on stable doses of opioids for longer than 1 week. As a consultant, educator, or primary caregiver, the APN can help the staff decide when they should and should not give Narcan and how to give this drug safely.

Narcan can induce not only immediate pain but also physical abstinence syndrome. This syndrome includes the signs and symptoms of anxiety and irritability: chills, diaphoresis, goose flesh, nausea and vomiting, runny nose and tearing, abdominal cramping, and diarrhea. Furthermore, rapid administration is dangerous and can cause sudden death from cardiac or respiratory arrest, hypertension, ventricular tachycardia and fibrillation, and pulmonary edema (Andree, 1980; Burke & Dunwoody, 1990; Flacke, Flacke, & Williams, 1977; Schwartz & Koenigsberg, 1987). Narcan should be administered slowly to any patient, even when opioid overdose is confirmed. The 0.4-mg ampule should be reconstituted with 9 ml of sterile normal saline (NS) in a 10-ml syringe (total volume of 10 ml), and 1 ml should be administered every 2 to 3 minutes. *Answer 4:* **c.**

5. One definition of breakthrough pain is a transitory increase from pain that is at least fairly well controlled (moderate or less) to more severe pain (Portenoy, Payne, & Jacobsen, 1999). Any type of pain the patient is experiencing (somatic, visceral, or neuropathic) can have breakthrough pain and can occur under several circumstances (Patt & Ellison, 1998). In-depth assessment is the rule; one pain type, incident pain, is predictable and occurs with movement or other activity. Some patients actually experience end-of-dose failure, whereby their dose of analgesic should be increased or the interval decreased. In fewer instances patients' flares of pain occur spontaneously and are not related to analgesic dosing. Some patients benefit from an interventional procedure (surgery, radiation therapy, anesthetic block, radiopharmaceutical, or bisphosphonate).

Guidelines for managing breakthrough pain are the same as those for chronic pain, and oral routes are recommended when feasible because they promote patient independence, do not require special technology or nursing care, and are the least costly (Patt & Ellison, 1998). This strategy may be effective for end-of-dose failure, for neuropathic pain, and for patients who have predictable pain (e.g., prescribing extra doses of short-acting opioid for pain that occurs with activity). However, using oral opioids for unpredictable flares of somatic or visceral pain may be problematic because of the delay in onset of action of oral drugs, which may lead to increasing sedation or other side effects. Intravenous or subcutaneous boluses might be a solution, but they are more difficult and costly for a patient who is relatively stable and at home.

One new option for managing breakthrough pain is transmucosal fentanyl (Actiq). As mentioned previously, fentanyl is absorbed through the mucosa, resulting in higher serum levels than oral drug (peak plasma level in 23 minutes versus 101 minutes, respectively) (Simmonds, 1999). Actiq is available in several dosage strengths, from 200 to 1600 µg, and patients are usually started on the smallest dose (200 µg). The manufacturer of Actiq can provide the patient six free doses to assess whether this will be a helpful option. If you can observe the patient, you can make sure he or she is using the Actiq unit correctly and give the patient another if he or she is not experiencing satisfactory relief 15 minutes after completing the first Actiq dose (Rhiner & Kedziera, 1999). In addition to teaching patients how to use the product, you should instruct them not to smoke or drink hot beverages; otherwise, the oral pH will be altered. Alcohol is avoided because it can potentiate the opioid effect. Actiq is intentionally made to look unattractive to children. *Answer 5:* **d.**

6. The use of placebos without the patient's knowledge and consent presents ethical and legal issues, as well as being clinically uninformative. Administering placebos involves being deceitful to the patient, not believing the patient, and violating the nurse's obligation to be truthful and respectful of the patient's right to informed consent. Placebo administration also violates the patient's autonomy (McCaffery, Ferrell, & Turner, 1996; Rushton, 1995). Some clinicians incorrectly believe that patients who respond to placebos do not have "real" or severe pain or are drug seekers. In truth, the placebo effect is very powerful—15% to 58% of patients respond to drug and surgical placebos. The placebo response is somewhat related to expectations of relief (Turner, Deyo, Loesser, et al., 1994). Nurses often induce placebo effects in their patients when they tell them they are going to do a procedure or give a medication that will "really help." APNs can help nurses recognize these problems and develop a policy regarding the nurses' response to an order for a placebo based on the Oncology Nursing Society position statement on the use of placebos (McCaffery, Ferrell, & Turner, 1996). *Pseudoaddiction* refers to the health care provider's perception that a patient is addicted because he or she asks for analgesics more often than ordered when in fact the requests are due to inadequate dosing. *Answer 6:* **a.**

Case Study conclusion

Mrs. Bennett is started on Actiq 200 µg before ambulation, which relieves her incident pain without disagreeable sedation. Further diagnostic tests after hospital discharge confirm sacral disease, which is treated with external beam radiation therapy. Her pain is almost totally gone, and she continues on chemotherapy.

REFERENCES

Agency for Health Care Policy and Research (AHCPR). (1994). *Clinical practice guideline. Management of cancer pain.* Rockville, MD: US Department of Health and Human Services, Agency for Health Care Policy and Research (AHCPR Publication No. 94-0592).

Alessi, C. A., & Henderson, C. T. (1988). Constipation and fecal impaction in the long-term care patient. *Clin Geriat Med, 4,* pp. 571-588.

Andree, R. A. (1980). Sudden death following naloxone administration. *Anesth Analges, 59,* pp. 782-784.

Angell, M. (1982). The quality of mercy. *N Engl J Med, 306,* pp. 98-99.

Anonymous. (1995). Quality improvement guidelines for the treatment of acute pain and cancer pain. American Pain Society Quality of Care Committee. *JAMA, 274,* pp. 1874-1880.

Beauchamp, T. L., & Childress, J. R. (1994). *Principles of biomedical ethics,* 4th ed. (pp. 120-394). New York: Oxford University Press.

Bruera, E., Brenneis, C., Michaud, M., et al. (1988). Use of the subcutaneous route for the administration of narcotics in patients with cancer pain. *Cancer, 62* pp. 407-411.

Bruera, E., & Watanabe, S. (1994). Psychostimulants as adjuvant analgesics. *J Pain Sympt Manage, 9,* pp. 412-415.

Burke, D. F., & Dunwoody, C. J. (1990). Naloxone: A word of caution. *Orthop Nurs, 9*(4), pp. 44-46.

Cameron, L. B. (1992). Neuropsychotropic drugs as adjuncts in the treatment of cancer pain. *Oncology, 6*(10), pp. 65-72.

Caraceni, A., Portenoy, R. K, working group of the IASP Task Force on Cancer Pain. (1999). An international survey of cancer pain characteristics and syndromes. *Pain, 82,* pp. 263-274.

Cervero, F., & Laird, J. M. A. (1999). Visceral pain. *Lancet, 353,* pp. 2145-2148.

Cleary, J. F. (2000). Cancer pain management. *Cancer Control JMCC, 7*(2), pp. 120-131 (accessed at oncology.medscape.com on 5/12/00).

De Broe, M. E., & Elseviers, M. M. (1998). Analgesic nephropathy. *N Engl J Med, 338,* pp. 446-452.

De Conno, F., Ripamonti, C., Saita, L., et al. (1995). Role of rectal route in treating cancer pain: A randomized crossover clinical trial of oral versus rectal morphine administration in opioid-naïve cancer patients with pain. *J Clin Oncol, 13,* pp. 1004-1008.

Drayer, R. A., Henderson, J., & Reidenberg, M. (1999). Barriers to better pain control in hospitalized patients. *J Pain Sympt Manage, 17*, pp. 434-440.

Duarte, R. A. (1997). Nonsteroidal anti-inflammatory drugs. In Kanner, R. (Ed.). *Pain management secrets* (pp. 167-171). Philadelphia: Hanley & Belfus.

Egbunike, I. G., & Chaffee, B. J. (1990). Antidepressants in the management of chronic pain syndromes. *Pharmacotherapy, 10*, pp. 262-270.

Elliot, T. E., & Elliot, B. A. (1992). Physician attitudes and beliefs about use of morphine for cancer pain. *J Pain Sympt Manage, 7*, pp. 141-148.

Ersek, M., Kraybill, B. M., & Du Pen, A. (1999). Factors hindering patients' use of medications for cancer pain. *Cancer Pract, 7*, pp. 226-232.

Fallon, M., & O'Neill, B. (1997). ABC of palliative care: Constipation. *BMJ, 315*, pp. 1293-1296.

Ferrell, B. R., & McCaffery, M. (1997). Nurses' knowledge about equianalgesia and opioid dosing. *Cancer Nurs, 20*, pp. 201-212.

Flacke, J. W., Flacke, W. E., & Williams, G. D. (1977). Acute pulmonary edema following naloxone reversal of high-dose morphine anesthesia. *Anesthesiology, 47*, pp. 376-378.

Galer, B. S., Coyle, N., Pasternak, G. W., & Portenoy, R. K. (1992). Individual variability in the response to different opioids: Report of five cases. *Pain, 49*, pp. 87-91.

Glazier, H. S. (1990). Potentiation of pain relief with hydroxyzine: A therapeutic myth? *DICP Ann Pharmacother, 24*, pp. 484-488.

Gold Star Media. *Clinical pharmacology.* Accessed at www.gsm.com on 6/1/00.

Gøtzsch, P. C. (2000). Clinical review. Non-steroidal anti-inflammatory drugs. *BMJ, 320*, pp. 1058-1061.

Hammes, B. J., & Cain, J. M. (1994). The ethics of pain management for cancer patients: Case studies and analysis. *J Pain Sympt Manage, 9*, pp. 166-170.

Hansen, H. C. (1999). Treatment of chronic pain with antiepileptic drugs: A new era. *South Med J, 92*, pp. 642-649.

Howell, D., Butler, L., Vincent, L., et al. (2000). Influencing nurses' knowledge, attitudes, and practice in cancer pain management. *Cancer Nurs, 23*, pp. 55-63.

Joranson, D. E., Ryan, K. M., Gilson, A. M., & Dahl, J. L. (2000). Trends in medical use and abuse of opioids. *JAMA, 283*, pp. 1710-1714.

Langman, M. J, Jensen, D. M., Watson, D. J, et al. (1999). Adverse upper gastrointestinal effects of rofecoxib compared with NSAIDs. *JAMA, 282*, pp. 1929-1933.

Lehmann, K. A. (1997). Opioids: Overview on action, interaction and toxicity. *Support Care Cancer, 5*, pp. 439-444.

Levy, M. H. (1991). Constipation and diarrhea in cancer patients. *Cancer Bull, 43*, pp. 412-422.

Lichtor, J. L., Sevarino, F. B., Hoshi, G. P., et al. (1999). The relative potency of oral transmucosal fentanyl citrate compared with intravenous morphine in the treatment of moderate to severe postoperative pain. *Anesthes Analges, 89*, pp. 732-738.

Maloney, C. M., Kesner, R. K., Klein, G., & Bockenstette, J. (1989). *Am J Hospice Care, July/Aug*, pp. 34-35.

Martin, L. A., & Hagen, N. A. (1997). Neuropathic pain in cancer patients: Mechanisms, syndromes, and clinical controversies. *J Pain Sympt Management, 14*, pp. 99-117.

McCaffery, M., Ferrell, B. R., & Turner, M. (1996). Ethical issues in the use of placebos in cancer pain management. *Oncol Nurs Forum, 23*, pp. 1587-1593.

McCaffery, M., & Pasero, C. (1999). Pain—Clinical manual, 2nd ed. St. Louis: Mosby.

McShane, R. E., & McLane, A. M. (1985). Constipation. Consensual and empirical validation. *Nurs Clin North Am, 20*, pp. 801-807.

Mercadante, S, Caligara, M., Sapio, M., et al. (1997). Palliative care rounds. Subcutaneous fentanyl infusion in a patient with bowel obstruction and renal failure. *J Pain Sympt Manage, 13*, pp. 241-244.

Miller, M. G., McCarthy, N., O'Boyle, C. A., & Kearney, M. (1999). Continuous subcutaneous infusion of morphine vs. hydromorphone: A controlled trial. *J Pain Sympt Manage, 18*, pp. 9-16.

Miser, A. W., Narang, P. K., Dothage, J. A., et al. (1989). Transdermal fentanyl for pain control in patients with cancer. *Pain, 37*, pp. 15-21.

Mount, B. (1996). Morphine drips, terminal sedation and slow euthanasia: Definitions and facts, not anecdotes. *J Palliat Care, 12*(4), pp. 31-37.

Pargeon, K. L., & Hailey, B. J. (1999). Barriers to effective cancer pain management: A review of the literature. *J Pain Sympt Manage, 18*, pp. 358-368.

Pasero, C., Portenoy, R. K., & McCaffery, M. (1999). Opioid analgesics. In McCaffery, M., & Pasero, C. (Eds.). *Pain: Clinical manual*, 2nd ed. (pp. 161-299). St. Louis: Mosby.

Patt, R. B., & Ellison, N. M. (1998). Breakthrough pain in cancer patients: Characteristics, prevalence, and treatment. *Oncology, 12*, pp. 1035-1046.

Payne, R. (1998). Pharmacologic management of pain. In Berger, A., Portenoy, R. K., & Weissman, D. E. (Eds.). *Principles and practice of supportive oncology* (pp. 61-107). Philadelphia: Lippincott-Raven.

Payne, R., Mathias, S. D., Pasta, D. J., et al. (1998). Quality of life and cancer pain: Satisfaction and side effects with transdermal fentanyl versus oral morphine. *J Clin Oncol, 16*, pp. 1588-1593.

Perazella, M. A., & Eras, J. (2000). Are selective COX-2 inhibitors nephrotoxic? *Am J Kidney Dis, 35*, pp. 937-940, 976-977.

Pereira, J., Mancini, I., & Walker, P. (1998). The role of bisphosphonates in malignant bone pain: A review. *J Palliat Care, 14*(2), pp. 25-36.

Perin, M. L., & Pasero, C. (2000). Problems with propoxyphene. *Am J Nurs, 100*(6), p. 22.

Peterson, W. L., & Cryer, B. (1999). COX-1-sparing NSAIDs—Is the enthusiasm justified? (editorial). *JAMA, 292*, pp. 1961-1963.

Phillips, D. M. (2000). JCAHO pain management standards are unveiled. *JAMA, 284*, pp. 428-429.

Pons, F., Herranz, T., Garcia, A., et al. (1997). Strontium-89 for palliation of pain from bone metastases in patients with prostate and breast cancer. *Eur J Nucl Med, 24*, pp. 1210-1214.

Portenoy, R. K. (1987). Constipation in the cancer patient: Causes and management. *Med Clin North Am, 71*, pp. 303-311.

Portenoy, R. K. (1995). Pharmacologic management of cancer pain. *Semin Oncol, 22*(suppl 3), pp. 112-120.

Portenoy, R. K. (1997). The physical examination in cancer pain assessment. *Semin Oncol Nurs, 13*, pp. 25-29.

Portenoy, R. K., Payne, D., & Jacobsen, P. (1999). Breakthrough pain: Characteristics and impact in patients with cancer pain. *Pain, 81*, pp. 129-134.

Porter, J., & Jick, H. (1980). Addiction rare in patients treated with narcotics. *N Engl J Med, 302*, p. 123.

Prather, C. M., & Ortiz-Camacho, C. P. (1998). Evaluation and treatment of constipation and fecal impaction in adults. *Mayo Clin Proc, 73*, pp. 881-887.

Principles of analgesic use in the treatment of acute pain and cancer pain. (1999). Glenview, IL: American Pain Society.

Radbruch, L., Sabatowski, R., Loick, G., et al. (2000). Constipation and the use of laxatives: A comparison between transdermal fentanyl and oral morphine. *Palliative Med, 14*, pp. 111-119.

Reddy, S., & Patt, R. B. (1994). The benzodiazepines as adjuvant analgesics. *J Pain Sympt Manage, 9*, pp. 510-514.

Regan, J. M., & Peng, P. (2000). Neurophysiology of cancer pain. *Cancer Control JMCC, 7*(2), pp. 111-119 (accessed at http://oncology.medscape.com/moffit/CancerControl/2000 5/21/00).

Rhiner, M., & Kedziera, P. (1999). Managing breakthrough cancer pain: A new approach. *AJN, 99* (3, suppl), pp. 3-12.

Rinaldi, R. C., Steindler, E. M., Wilford, B. B., et al. (1988). Clarification and standardization of substance abuse terminology. *JAMA, 259*, pp. 555-557.

Romero, Y., Evans, J. M., Fleming, K. C., & Phillips, S. F. (1996). Constipation and fecal incontinence in the elderly population. *Mayo Clin Proc, 71*, pp. 81-92.

Rushton, C. H. (1995). Placebo pain medication: Ethical and legal issues. *Pediatr Nurs, 21*, pp. 166-168.

Schiødt, F. V., Rochling, F. A., Casey, D. L., & Lee, W. M. (1997). Acetaminophen toxicity in an urban county hospital. *N Engl J Med, 337*, pp. 1112-1117.

Schwartz, J. A., & Koenigsberg, M. D. (1987). Naloxone-induced pulmonary edema. *Ann Emerg Med, 16*, pp. 1294-1296.

Simmonds, M. A. (1999). Management of breakthrough pain due to cancer. *Oncology, 13*, pp. 1103-1108.

Storey, P., Hill, H. H., St. Louis, R. H., & Tarver, E. E. (1990). Subcutaneous infusions for control of cancer symptoms. *J Pain Sympt Manage, 5*, pp. 33-41.

Tannenbaum, H., Davis, P., Russell, A. S., et al. (1996). An evidence-based approach to prescribing NSAIDs in musculoskeletal disease: A Canadian consensus. *Can Med Assoc J, 155*, pp. 77-88.

Tearnan, B. H., & Cleeland, C. S. (1990). Unaided use of pain descriptors by patients with cancer pain. *J Pain Sympt Manage, 5*, pp. 228-232.

Thorns, A. (2000). Opioid use in last week of life and implications for end-of-life decision-making. *Lancet, 356*, pp. 398-399.

Todd, K. H., Deaton, C., D'Adamo, A. P., & Goe, L. (2000). Ethnicity and analgesic practice. *Ann Emerg Med, 35*, pp. 11-16.

Turner, J., Deyo, R. A., Loesser, J., et al. (1994). The importance of placebo effects in pain treatment and research. *JAMA, 271*, pp. 1609-1614.

Vielvoye-Kerkmeer, A. P., Mattern, C., & Uitendaal, M. P. (2000). Transdermal fentanyl in opioid-naive cancer pain patients. An open trial using transdermal for the treatment of chronic pain in opioid-naive patients and a group using codeine. *J Pain Sympt Manage, 19*, pp. 185-192.

Von Gunten, C. F., & Von Roenn, J. H. (1994). Barriers to pain control: Ethics & knowledge. *J Palliat Care, 10*(3), pp. 52-54.

Von Roenn, J. H., Cleeland, C. S., Gonin, R., et al. (1993). Physician attitudes and practice in cancer pain management: A survey from the Eastern Cooperative Oncology Group. *Ann Intern Med, 119*, pp. 121-126.

Walsh, T. D. (1984). Opiates and respiratory function in advanced cancer. *Rec Results Cancer Res, 89*, pp. 115-117.

Ward, S. E., Goldberg, N., Miller-McCauley, V., et al. (1993). Patient-related barriers to management of cancer pain. *Pain, 52*, pp. 319-324.

Warren, D. E. (1996). Practical use of rectal medications in palliative care. *J Pain Sympt Manage, 11*, pp. 378-387.

Watson, C. P. N. (1994). Antidepressant drugs as adjuvant analgesics. *J Pain Sympt Manage, 9*, pp. 392-405.

Whedon, M., & Ferrell, B. R. (1991). Professional and ethical consideration in the use of high-tech pain management. *Oncol Nurs Forum, 18*, pp. 1135-1143.

Wolfe, M. M., Lichtenstein, D. R., & Singh, G. (1999). Gastrointestinal toxicity of nonsteroidal antiinflammatory drugs. *N Engl J Med 340*, pp. 1888-1899.

Wong, D. L., Hockenberry-Eaton, M., Wilson, D., et al. (Eds.). (2001). *Wong's essentials of nursing*, 6th ed. St. Louis: Mosby.

World Health Organization. (1990). Cancer pain relief and palliative care: report of a WHO expert committee. *WHO Technical Report Series, 804*, pp. 1-73.

13 Genetics

Rita Wickham
Sarah McCaffery

CASE 1 STUDY

You are scheduled to see Sally McGowan, a 44-year-old white woman, in the interdisciplinary breast cancer clinic today. Sally is concerned because there is "so much cancer" in her family, and she wonders if she should have "that breast cancer gene test." She also thinks her 15-year-old daughter should get the test but is not worried about her 18-year-old son, because "he can't get breast cancer." She tells you that her mother, sister, and an aunt on her father's side were diagnosed with breast cancer; her brother has cancer; and her grandfather died of cancer. You explore Sally's family history with her to help her identify her breast cancer risk factors (see Chapter 1) and to determine whether you should recommend a consultation with the cancer genetic counselor (who might be an oncology advanced practice nurse [APN] with subspecialist education in cancer genetics).

QUESTIONS

1. Sally's reports of cancer in which of the following family members would lead you to believe that she may have inherited a mutated cancer susceptibility gene?

1. Her mother was diagnosed with breast cancer when she was 66 and is now 72.
2. Her 48-year-old brother was recently diagnosed with lung cancer.
3. Her sister was diagnosed with breast cancer at age 50.
4. She thinks one paternal aunt died of breast cancer in her 80s.
   - **a.** 1, 3, & 4
   - **b.** 3 only
   - **c.** None of these
   - **d.** All of these

2. If Sally's mother had been diagnosed with breast cancer at an earlier age (e.g., 35 years), and both the mother and Sally's sister had been confirmed to have the same disease-associated

mutation in BRCA1, Sally's risk of having the same mutation in BRCA1 would be:
   - **a.** 10%
   - **b.** 25%
   - **c.** 50%
   - **d.** 100%

3. The "red flags" that raise your suspicion that a patient may have an increased risk for cancer because of inheritance of a susceptibility gene mutation include:

1. Cancer in two or more first- or second-degree relatives
2. Cancers usually occurring in patients older than 60 years of age, being diagnosed at a younger age
3. Diagnoses of multiple primary cancers or bilateral tumors in paired organs
4. Evidence of autosomal recessive transmission
   - **a.** 1 & 2
   - **b.** 1, 2, & 3
   - **c.** 1, 3, & 4
   - **d.** All of these

4. You know the response to Sally's request for the BRCA gene test for her daughter would be based on:
   - **a.** Medical indication: A gene test is indicated because the daughter has a high risk of carrying the same gene mutation and would thus probably develop breast cancer.
   - **b.** Legal rights: The parents can make gene testing decisions for their minor children.
   - **c.** Psychosocial benefit: Such information will aid the child and family.
   - **d.** Ethical considerations: The child's autonomy regarding decision making may be influenced by the parent's wishes.

5. When completing a family history to assess for inherited cancer susceptibility risk, you ideally need information regarding how many generations?

    a. One
    b. Two
    c. Three
    d. Four

6. Based on the information Sally initially gave you, construct her family pedigree. What other information do you need to help you determine whether there is a familial pattern?

ANSWERS

1. Cancer is a genetic disease and occurs because of mutations in genes and chromosomes. Initial mutations in solid tumors usually involve changes in cancer susceptibility genes (suppressor genes, proto-oncogenes, or DNA damage repair genes) that have critical roles in normal cells. Suppressor genes inhibit uncontrolled cell division and promote cellular differentiation. Proto-oncogenes regulate normal cell division, and DNA damage repair genes correct errors that occur during DNA replication. These genes are very large (thousands of base pairs long), and a mutation in a single base pair (point mutation) may be sufficient to alter or inactivate the function of a protein that gene codes for. Point mutations are common initiating events, but frank cancer results from the accumulation of multiple mutations. Proto-oncogenes may be converted to oncogenes by several mechanisms, including point mutations, chromosomal translocations, gene amplification, and retroviral insertion (MacDonald & Lessick, 2000).

Deleterious genetic mutations, the hallmark of malignant diseases, are acquired during life to cause sporadic cancers, whereas the first mutation is inherited in hereditary malignancies. Most malignancies are sporadic, so mutations are present only in tumor tissues. On the other hand, up to 5% to 10% of malignancies are hereditary. Because the individual inherits one mutated allele of a cancer susceptibility gene from an affected parent, this germline mutation is present in all body cells. An inherited mutation can thus be detected by a gene test, if one is available.

Inheritance of cancer susceptibility genes usually follows a Mendelian autosomal-dominant transmission pattern (although there are a few autosomal recessive syndromes). Thus each child, male and female, has a 50% chance of inheriting the mutated allele from the affected parent. The child inherits a second, normal allele from their other (unaffected) parent. When a tumor suppressor gene is involved, the normal copy initially allows cells to function normally. Cancer arises sometime during adulthood, when the normal allele acquires a somatic, cancer-inducing mutation. *Answer 1:* **d.**

2. Every individual who inherits a mutated cancer susceptibility gene mutation does not necessarily develop cancer because these genes have reduced or incomplete penetrance (Loescher, 1999). Different genes, dietary and environmental factors, and lifestyle may modify gene expression and cancer occurrence in mutation carriers (Fearon, 1997). In addition, when cancers occur predominantly in one gender (e.g., breast cancer), the pedigree may seem to show that cancer skips generations. Therefore, if Sally carries a mutated allele, each of her children has the same risk of having the mutated allele (50%). Although Sally's daughter has a much greater risk of having breast cancer, her carrier son can pass it on to his sons and daughters. In a few instances, tumors related to an inherited mutation, such as familial retinoblastoma, Wilms' tumor, and medullary thyroid cancer in multiple endocrine neoplasia type 2, arise in very young children. Most often, hereditary cancers demonstrate age-related penetrance; that is, they arise earlier during adulthood than expected, incidence increases with age, and frequency is greater than with sporadic tumors (Table 13-1) (Calzone, 1997; Fearon, 1997; Offit, 1998). *Answer 2:* **c.**

3. According to the American Society of Clinical Oncology (ASCO, 1996), physicians who consider offering an actual gene test to a patient should know what the potential benefits, limitations, and risks of particular gene tests are; know what the appropriate treatments for that cancer are; and be able to adequately communicate this information to the patient in the form of informed consent. ASCO (1996) proposed three categories for considering cancer predisposition testing. The considerations include (1) whether there is a strong family history of cancer, (2) whether a test can be adequately interpreted, and (3) whether knowing the results would influence medical management (Table 13-2). It is likely that advances in knowledge regarding the genetics of cancer will continue on a rapid pace, and oncology APNs are increasingly likely to take a greater part in such patient education, counseling, and informed decision making in the future. The Oncology Nursing Society has recognized this in two position statements: The Role of the Oncology Nurse in Cancer Genetic Counseling (1997) and Cancer Genetic Testing and Risk Assessment Counseling (1997). These statements recognize that generalist

TABLE 13-1 Selected Hereditary Cancers

SYNDROME/CONDITION	PRIMARY MALIGNANCY	OTHER CANCERS OR CLINICAL MANIFESTATIONS	GENE [CHROMOSOME]	MODE OF INHERITANCE/ TYPE OF GENE
Familial breast cancer 1	Breast	Ovarian cancer, prostate cancer, colon cancer	BRCA1 [17q21]	Autosomal dominant/ tumor suppressor
Familial breast cancer 2	Breast	Male breast cancer, ovarian cancer, pancreatic cancer	BRCA2 [13q12-13]	Autosomal dominant/ tumor suppressor
Familial adenomatous polyposis	Colorectal	Colorectal adenomas, duodenal and gastric tumors, desmoid tumors, osteomas, thyroid cancer	APC [5q21-22]	Autosomal dominant/ tumor suppressor
Hereditary nonpolyposis colorectal cancer	Colorectal	Endometrial, ovarian, gastrointestinal, urinary tract cancers	MSH2 [2p16], MLH1 [3p21-22], PMS1 [2q32], PMS2 [7p22]	Autosomal dominant/ DNA damage repair
Familial retinoblastoma	Retinoblastoma	Osteosarcoma	RB1 [13q14.3]	Autosomal dominant/ tumor suppressor
Li-Fraumeni syndrome	Sarcomas, breast cancer	Brain tumors, leukemia, adrenocortical carcinoma	p53 [17p13.1]	Autosomal dominant/ tumor suppressor
Hereditary prostate cancer	Prostate	Unknown	PCA1 [10q25], ? HPC1 [p24-q25]	Autosomal dominant/ unknown
Neurofibromatosis	Neurofibromas (type 1), acoustic neuromas and meningiomas (type 2)	Neurofibrosarcoma, AML, brain tumors (type 1); gliomas, ependymomas (type 2A)	NF1 [17q11.2], NF2 [22q12.2]	Autosomal dominant/ tumor suppressor
Multiple endocrine neoplasia type 1 (MEN 1)	Pancreatic islet cell	Parathyroid hyperplasia, pituitary adenoma	MEN 1 [11q13]	Autosomal dominant/ oncogene
Multiple endocrine neoplasia type 2 (MEN 2)	Medullary thyroid	Familial medullary thyroid only Type 2A: pheochromocytoma, parathyroid hyperplasia Type 2B: pheochromocytoma	RET [10q11.2]	Autosomal dominant/ oncogene
Wilms' tumor	Wilms' tumor	WAGR (Wilms', aniridia, genitourinary abnormalities, mental retardation)	WT1 [11p13] WT2 [11p15.5]	Autosomal dominant/ tumor suppressor
Ataxia telangiectasia	Lymphoma	Cerebellar ataxia, immunodeficiency, breast cancer	ATM [11q22.3]	Autosomal recessive/ DNA damage repair
Xeroderma pigmentosum	Skin cancer, melanoma	Pigmentation abnormalities, hypogonadism	XPB, XPD, XPA/multiple complementation groups	Autosomal recessive/ DNA damage repair
Fanconi's anemia	AML	Esophageal, skeletal abnormalities	FACC [9q22.3], FACA [16q24.2]	Autosomal recessive/ unknown
Von Hippel-Lindau syndrome	Renal	Pheochromocytomas, retinal angiomas, hemangioblastoma	VHL [3p25-26]	Autosomal dominant/ tumor suppressor

AML, Acute myoblastic leukemia.

TABLE 13-2 Categories for Considering Cancer Gene Predisposition Testing

GROUP 1 TESTS

For families with well-defined hereditary syndromes
For which either a positive or a negative result will change medical care
And for which genetic testing is considered part of standard management of affected families

SYNDROME	GENE TESTED	CHARACTERISTICS/COMMENTS*
Familial adenomatous polyposis (FAP)	APC	Hundreds to thousands of colonic polyps Diagnosed in late teens or early twenties; at-risk individuals require colonoscopy/sigmoidoscopy starting at age 10-12 yr and repeated every 1-2 yr ≥100 polyps to make diagnosis Virtually all patients will die of metastatic colon cancer by age 50 if not treated with prophylactic colectomy
Multiple endocrine neoplasia (MEN) 2A, 2B	RET	Hallmark tumor of all syndromes is medullary thyroid carcinoma (MTC) Syndromes characterized by earlier onset and variable aggressiveness (MEN 2B > MEN 2A > MTC) RET testing is gold standard (age <5 yr) Treatment: prophylactic thyroidectomy Surveillance for other associated tumors
Retinoblastoma	RB1	Most common pediatric eye tumor in children Diagnosis based on strabismus and/or leukocoria ("white eye") Median age at diagnosis, 18 mo, most tumors diagnosed in children <4 yr Treatment varies from cryotherapy or photocoagulation to enucleation plus radiation therapy Genetic counseling and continuing surveillance for associated tumors is important
von Hippel-Lindau (VHL) syndrome	VHL	VHL syndrome is very rare; linked with cancer predisposition and tendency to form cysts High penetrance: 90% affected by age 45 and 99% by age 65 Multifocal or bilateral renal cell carcinoma in 25% of cases Surveillance for pheochromocytoma and other associated tumors

GROUP 2 TESTS

Hereditary syndromes with a high probability of linkage to known cancer susceptibility genes and
For which the medical benefit of the identification of a heterozygote ("carrier") is presumed but not established
Potential clinical value and reliability of the test is based on research studies

SYNDROME	GENE TESTED	CHARACTERISTICS
Hereditary nonpolyposis colon cancer (HNPCC)	MSH2, MLH1, PMS1, PMS2	Rare, but more common than FAP Diagnosis relies of pedigree appraisal MLH1 and MSH2 account for >90% of mutations Patients may have synchronous or metachronous tumors of the colon (multiple sites) and other sites (uterus, stomach, ovary, small intestine, ureter, kidney) More commonly right-sided tumors
Hereditary breast ovarian syndrome (HBOS)	BRCA1, BRCA2	Relative risk for breast cancer related to mutated BRCA1 or BRCA2 >50% (general population risk 2%) Male breast cancer risk is 6% by age 70 in presence of BRCA2 mutation Founder effect: particular mutations are seen with greater frequency in some populations (e.g., Ashkenazi Jewish, African Americans, Swedish)
Li-Fraumeni syndrome	p53 (TP53)	Families characterized by multiple cases of soft tissue sarcomas, breast cancer, and other tumors (leukemia, brain, adrenocortical, lung, pancreas, and skin) Sarcoma, brain tumor, leukemia usually occur in childhood, breast cancer between 15 and 44 yr No proven way to screen for associated tumors

Adapted from American Society of Clinical Oncology. (1996). Statement of the American Society of Clinical Oncology: Genetic testing for cancer susceptibility. *J Clin Oncol 14*, pp. 1730-1736.
*From Offit, K. (1998). *Clinical cancer genetics* (pp. 39-65). New York: Wiley-Liss; and Lindor, N., Greene, M., & The Mayo Familial Cancer Program. (1998). The concise handbook of family cancer syndromes. *J Natl Cancer Instit 90*, pp. 1039-1071.

Continued

TABLE **13-2** Categories for Considering Cancer Gene Predisposition Testing—cont'd

GROUP 3 TESTS

Tests for individuals without a family history of cancer in which significance of detecting a germline mutation is not clear

Or tests for hereditary syndromes for which germline mutations have been identified in only a small number of families

Or for which the medical benefit of identifying a heterozygote is not established

SYNDROME	GENE TESTED	CHARACTERISTICS
Melanoma and melanoma-associated syndromes	P16, CDK4	10%-15% of patients diagnosed with melanoma have a family history Median age of onset midforties Multiple primary lesions more common than with sporadic cases Early and regular surveillance is critical for family members with family history or multiple dysplastic nevi
Ataxia telangiectasia-associated suscepti-bilities (AT)	ATM	Extremely rare: 1 in 30,000 to 1 in 100,000 Progressive cerebellar ataxia diagnosed about time a child learns to walk leading to wheelchair use by age 10 yr Telangiectasia usually begin in sun-exposed areas and conjunctiva, onset >7 yr of age; may have other cutaneous manifestations Endocrine and immune abnormalities may occur Usually fatal by age 30 yr

Adapted from American Society of Clinical Oncology. (1996). Statement of the American Society of Clinical Oncology: Genetic testing for cancer susceptibility. *J Clin Oncol 14*, pp. 1730-1736.

and advanced practice oncology nurses must increase their knowledge of genetics and that only APNs in oncology who have specialized education in genetics should provide cancer genetic counseling. However, all oncology APNs must recognize that medical, psychosocial, and ethical issues must be recognized and addressed before and after genetic testing. *Answer 3:* **c.**

4. By and large, gene testing in children, even adolescents, should be deferred until adulthood because children cannot legally provide consent and must rely on surrogate decision makers (their parent or parents). Therefore children may be uniquely vulnerable to the psychosocial risks of testing, including subtle coercion by the parent, and may surrender their future autonomy by knowing results they themselves might not choose to know (Elger & Harding, 2000; Wilfond, Rothenberg, Thomson, & Lerman, 1997). The central issue in decision making for testing should be, "Does benefit outweigh risk?" There are a few early childhood tumors in which knowing gene status affects medical treatment. Because there are several characteristics of inherited cancer risk syndromes differentiating them from sporadic cancers, these red flags would make one consider genetic testing in children. A hereditary predisposition might be suspected if any of the following are true (Lindor, Greene, & The Mayo Familial

Cancer Program, 1998; Tinley & Lynch, 1999; Weitzel, 1996):

- Cancer is diagnosed at an unusually young age, often 15 to 20 years earlier than expected.
- There is a high rate of the same cancer in a family, especially if this is a rare tumor.
- One family member has multifocal cancer in one organ, or bilateral cancers in paired organs.
- One family member has multiple primary cancers.

Up to this point, Sally's family history does not provide sufficient evidence of a hereditary cancer syndrome. Her mother was postmenopausal (age 66) when she was diagnosed with breast cancer, and her sister was at least perimenopausal. *Answer 4:* **b.**

5. By taking a comprehensive family history, expanding on the history as indicated, and constructing a family pedigree, a visual picture of the family relationships and health history develops (Dimond, Calzone, Davis, & Jenkins, 1998; Johnson & Christianson, 1999; Offit, 1998) (Figure 13-1). When possible, at least three generations should be considered, including information about relatives affected and unaffected with cancer and age at diagnosis (and death if applicable). Ex-

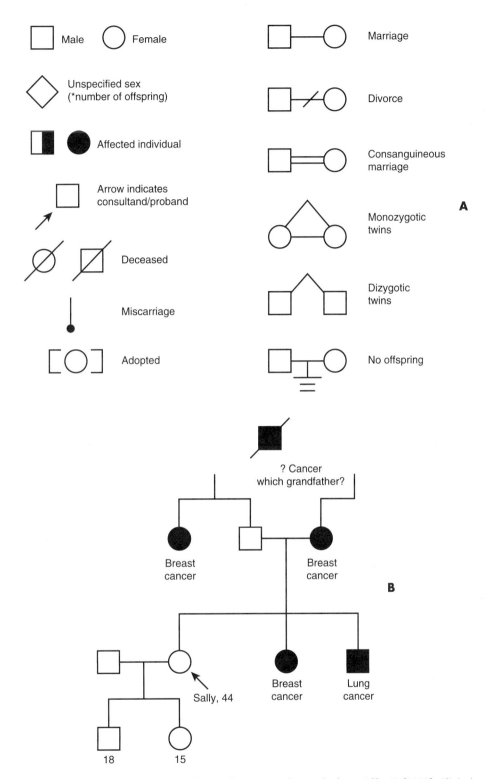

Male   Female   Marriage

Unspecified sex
(*number of offspring)   Divorce

Affected individual   Consanguineous
marriage

Arrow indicates
consultand/proband   Monozygotic
twins   **A**

Deceased   Dizygotic
twins

Miscarriage

Adopted   No offspring

? Cancer
which grandfather?

Breast
cancer   Breast
cancer   **B**

Breast
cancer   Lung
cancer

Sally, 44

18   15

Figure 13-1 A, Common pedigree symbols. **B,** Sally's preliminary pedigree. (**A** from Offit, K. [1998]. *Clinical cancer genetics* [p. 11]. New York: Wiley-Liss.)

Suggested Family History Questions

PATIENT'S PERSONAL HISTORY

1. Have you ever had cancer? If so, list the following:
   Type/site of cancer
   Age at diagnosis
   Type(s) of treatment
   Date(s) of treatment
2. Have you ever had more than one cancer? If so, list same information as in (1) for each cancer
3. Have you ever been told that you have "precancerous" lesions: for example, colon polyps, atypical moles, cervical dysplasia, breast biopsies showing lobular carcinoma in situ, or atypical hyperplasia?
4. What is your ethnic/religious background; for example, Jewish or Mormon?

FAMILY HISTORY (BLOOD RELATIVES ONLY)

1. Have any of your first-degree relatives (father, mother, brothers, sisters, or children) ever had cancer?
   For each family member with cancer, list the following:
   Type/site of cancer
   Age at diagnosis
   More than one cancer
2. Have any of your second-degree relatives (grandparents, aunts, uncles, nieces, or nephews) ever had cancer?
   For each family member with cancer, list the following:
   Type/site of cancer
   Age at diagnosis
   More than one cancer
3. Has anyone else in your family ever had cancer? If so, list the following:
   Relationship to patient
   Type(s) of cancer
   Age at diagnosis

From Loescher, L. J. (1999). The family history component of cancer genetic risk counseling. *Cancer Nurs, 22,* pp. 96-102.

amples of useful questions are included in Box 13-1 (Loescher, 1999). *Answer 5:* **c.** *Answer 6:* **See Figure 13-1.**

Case Study continued

You get more information from Sally about cancer in her family history. Starting with her siblings, she tells you she has two sisters, Marge and Mary. Marge is 50 years old, is in good health, and has two daughters (ages 28 and 26) who are alive and well. Mary is 52 years old and has three children (two sons, ages 19 and 14, and a 16-year-old daughter) who are healthy. Mary was diagnosed with breast cancer when she was 50. According to Sally, Mary had a mastectomy and then received radiation therapy and chemotherapy, and she is "OK." Sally says that she and Mary do not talk about Mary's breast cancer yet because Mary "doesn't take things too well." Sally's 48-year-old brother was diagnosed with lung cancer 2 months ago, but she knows he smoked a lot—she estimates one or two packs a day since he was a young teenager. Her father died from a heart attack when he was 65. Sally thinks her father's sister died of breast cancer when she was in her eighties, but his two brothers are in their early eighties and relatively well. She does not know about anyone else who had cancer on her father's side of the family (her paternal grandparents died from unknown causes when they were approximately 70 years old). Sally's mother is 72 and was diagnosed with breast cancer when she was 66. She took tamoxifen for 5 years after her mastectomy and is doing well. Sally's mother has one brother who is alive and well. Sally recalls that her maternal grandmother died from "some kind of cancer" when she was in her sixties, and she thinks her maternal grandfather died from liver cancer.

QUESTIONS

7. Construct Sally's revised pedigree (Figure 13-2).

8. Sally reveals that she would be interested in learning more about a possible hereditary link to breast cancer in her family. She hesitates though because she says that she does not want the actual test right now. You inform Sally that genetic counseling can include:
   1. Careful analysis of her pedigree by a team of specialists
   2. Confirmation of a suspicious hereditary link to cancers in family
   3. Discussion of surveillance/medical treatment options
   4. Discussion of risk and benefits of gene testing
   5. Genetic testing
   6. Genetic counseling and psychologic support for Sally and other receptive family members
   a. 1, 2, & 3
   b. 1, 2, 3, & 5
   c. 1, 3, 5, & 6
   d. All of these

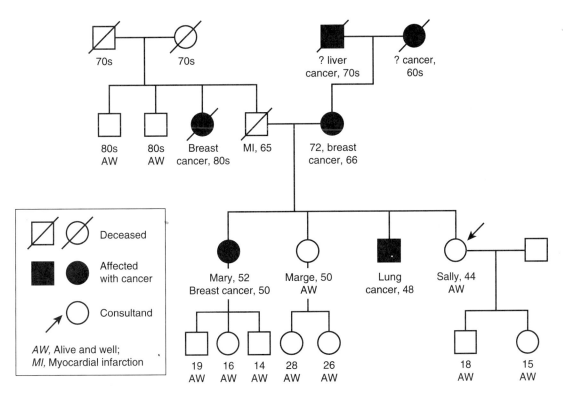

Figure 13-2 Sally's revised pedigree.

9. If Sally had been diagnosed with breast cancer when she was 40 years old, the altered gene that would most likely be responsible for the prevalence of cancer in her family is:
  a. BRCA1/BRCA2
  b. TP53
  c. APC
  d. MLH1/MSH2/MSSH6/PMS1/PMSS2

10. If Sally wants to increase her knowledge regarding her risk for breast cancer, this may be accomplished by:
  a. Performing a gene test
  b. Applying risk information from the general population
  c. Calculating her risk based on two or more models (e.g., Gail, Claus, Couch/Weber)
  d. a or c

ANSWERS

7. Although several members of her family appear to have had cancer, Sally's revised pedigree does not show a pattern of autosomal-dominant transmission of a germline mutation associated with a known hereditary cancer syndrome. Most family members were diagnosed in their fifties to eighties, or when we expect cancer incidence to increase because of age. In addition, it is possible that her grandfather did not have cancer at all, but some other problem with his liver unrelated to cancer. The family history provided by patients is often inaccurate and must be substantiated. Inaccuracy may be related to lack of medical knowledge, how family members communicate with one another, and the closeness of the relationship (i.e., reports of cancer are more likely to be accurate in first- and second-degree relatives and less so in more distant relatives) (Douglas, O'Dair, Robinson, et al., 1999). In addition, her brother was a heavy smoker, and lung cancer is not associated with a hereditary link. *Answer 7:* **See Figure 13-2.**

8. You would refer Sally to a high-risk cancer genetic risk clinic to help her investigate her concerns, particularly if you had recognized a clearly suspicious history pointing to a hereditary cancer link. This is critical because of the necessity of confirming the family history (by obtaining and reviewing actual medical histories, pathology, and autopsy reports of family members) before progressing toward genetic screening. In addition, you can point out that the high-risk clinic is staffed by several team members, each who contributes expertise in risk evaluation and nondirective genetic counseling, as well as explaining informed consent, providing psychologic support, and making recommendations for surveillance and follow-up (MacDonald, 1997). Oncology APNs are increasingly becoming educated to take on roles in such settings, and they often help patients address issues surrounding decision making, including personal and family values and dynamics, perception of risk, cultural influences, and emotional response. Family issues are particularly important when the person seeking genetic counseling (the consultant) does not have cancer. Ideally, a gene test is performed on a family member who already has been diagnosed with cancer to identify the specific disease-causing mutation in that family before screening other family members for that mutation. Therefore the consultant may need to address this with the affected family member or members, who may or may not desire testing. In addition, oncology APNs are uniquely prepared to address education and advocacy issues. You know that genetic counseling does not necessarily include a gene test, but gene testing should always be preceded by and followed up with extensive education, counseling, and psychosocial support. *Answer 8:* **d.**

9. Although several gene mutations have been associated with hereditary breast cancer, you know that mutations in the BRCA (breast cancer) genes are most commonly implicated in inherited breast cancer risk. The lifetime risk for breast cancer associated with a BRCA1/BRCA2 mutation is estimated to be 50% to 85%, and lifetime ovarian cancer risk with a BRCA1 mutation is 20% to 60% and 10% to 20% with a BRCA2 mutation (Penson, Seiden, Shannon, et al., 2000). Commercial tests are available for BRCA1 and BRCA2, as well as for several other cancer susceptibility genes. As mentioned, these tests are offered when appropriate and in the context of genetic counseling. Many individuals may attend an initial educational session regarding genetic testing but not all choose to have the test performed. Reasons include concerns about insurance, finding out that a test may not be informative, and the potential of emotional upheaval (Penson, et al., 2000). There are three possible outcomes of gene tests: positive, indeterminate, and

negative. Recommendations for BRCA mutation-positive patients center around earlier clinical surveillance (beginning at age 25) and more frequent surveillance (annual or semiannual clinical breast examination and annual mammography) (Burke, Daly, Garber, et al., 1997). At this time, there is limited evidence to support therapeutic options, such as chemoprevention or prophylactic bilateral mastectomy and oophorectomy. Indeterminate mutations are a source of consternation because their clinical significance is not known. That is, it is not possible to inform the patient if an identified mutation is a harmless polymorphism (an alternative, normal form of a gene) or a disease-causing mutation. Finally, even patients who do not have a mutation have the same risk for developing a particular cancer as the general population. *Answer 9:* **a.**

10. If Sally were to refuse gene testing, the high-risk team would use two or more of the models developed to calculate breast cancer risk (Claus, Risch, & Thompson, 1994; Couch, DeShano, Blackwood, et al., 1997; Frank, Manley, Olopade, et al, 1998; Gail, Brinton, Byar, et al., 1989; Shattuck-Eidens, 1995) (Table 13-3). The Gail Model and the Claus Tables are used the most frequently because they vary in how risk is determined and each has limitations. The Couch/Weber model can be used to estimate the risk for having a BRCA1/BRCA2 mutation. *Answer 10:* **d.**

Case Study continued

Whether Sally does or does not opt for a gene test, as her primary oncology APN, you will continue to follow Sally with recommended screening and surveillance. If she had a test and it was negative, you will continue to stress to her that a gene test predicts the risk for and not the actual occurrence of cancer. Thus a patient whose predicted risk to develop cancer is 50% to 80% may never actually develop cancer, whereas another individual's lifetime risk (e.g., 11% risk to develop breast cancer at age 85) may never develop cancer. Therefore you continue to educate all of your patients, and other nurses, about the importance of self-care behaviors and cancer screening at recommended intervals. You continue to increase your knowledge regarding cancer genetics. Internet sites for health care professionals, as noted in Table 13-4, can serve as a starting point for resources.

TABLE 13-3 Breast Cancer Risk Calculation Models

MODEL	RISK DETERMINATES	PROS	CONS
Gail	Age Number of first-degree relatives with breast cancer Menstruation age Age of first live birth Race Number of breast biopsies History of atypical hyperplasia	Calculates 5-yr and lifetime (90 yr) risk of breast cancer of consultant (person seeking genetic counseling) compared with another woman of same age without same risk factors	Does not consider known predictors of hereditary risks for breast and ovarian cancer Does not consider second-degree or more distant relatives No age at onset of cancer factored into risk calculations No ovarian cancer factored into risk calculations Cannot use model if woman has cancer
Claus	Age of onset of breast cancer for woman having one, two, or more first- or second-degree relatives with breast cancer	Considers both maternal and paternal breast cancers Calculates 10-yr and lifetime (80 yr) risk of breast cancer	Does not consider total number of breast and ovarian cancers Does not factor in ovarian cancer May underestimate risk for breast cancer in BRCA1 or BRCA2 mutation carriers and may overestimate risk in nonmutation carriers

Couch/Weber	Average age of onset of breast and/or ovarian cancer	Can calculate risk in which family history is any of the following:
		Breast cancer only
		  A relative with breast and ovarian cancer
		  Different family members have breast or ovarian cancer
		Considers non-Jewish and Ashkenazi Jewish families risks for BRCA1 mutations
			Does not consider relationship of affected family member to consultant
			Does not calculate risk of detecting BRCA2 mutation

Frank	Breast cancer diagnosed before age 50 yr Have at least one first- or second-degree relative with breast cancer younger than 50 yr or with ovarian cancer at any age	Calculates mutation detection risk based on various ages of onset of breast cancer Risks calculated for both BRCA1 and BRCA1 mutations	Cannot use table if relatives diagnosed after age 50, if proband does not have breast/ovarian cancer, or if only one first-degree relative has breast/ovarian cancer
Shattuck-Eidens	Single affected family member, sister pairs, and families with breast and/or ovarian cancer in three or more relatives younger than age 50	Calculates risk of BRCA1 mutations	Does not consider clear dominant pedigrees with vertical transmission No risk calculated for mother and daughter diagnosed No BRCA2 risk calculated

TABLE 13-4 | Internet Resources on Genetics

SITE	WEB ADDRESS AND SITE DESCRIPTION
GenBank: National Center for Biotechnology Information	www.ncbi.nlm.nih.gov/Web/Genbank/GenbankOverview.html DNA sequences available to public
Genentech	www.gene.com Commercial site: biotechnology company developing pharmaceuticals based on genetic knowledge
Genetics Professional Societies: FASEB	www.faseb.org/genetics/ Contains links to various genetic societies
Genome Database: Hospital for Sick Children, Toronto, Canada	http://gdbwww.gdb.org/gdb Human genome regions, maps, genome variations
Human Genome Mutation Database	www.uwcm.ad.uk/uwcm/mg/hgmd0.html Gene mutation databases from the University of Wales College of Medicine
Myriad Laboratories	www.myriad.com Commercial site, genetic tests and therapeutics
National Center for Genome Resources	www.ncgr.org Information regarding the National Center for Genome Resources, software and current research
OMIM: Online Mendelian Inheritance In Man	www.ncbi.nlm.nih.gov/Omim/ Catalog for human genes and genetic disorders
Yahoo Human Genetics	www.yahoo.com/Science/Biology/Genetics//Human_Genetics/ Links to various sites related to gene therapy, genetic disorders, gene testing services, Human Genome projects, human cloning, journals, Web dictionaries, etc.
International Society of Nurses in Genetics (ISONG)	http://nursing.creighton.edu/isong/ Clinical practice, educational resources; links to other genetic sites
CancerNet (National Cancer Institute)	http://cancernet.nci.nih.gov/clinpdq/cancer_genetics/ Links to cancer genetics overview, elements of cancer genetics risk assessment and counseling, glossary, and patient education
Robert Lurie Cancer Center	www.cancergenetics.org Excellent site for physicians/advanced practice nurses; includes case studies
Oncolink	http://oncolink.upenn.edu Excellent site for cancer-related information, links to PDQ
Children's Hospital Medical Center, Cincinnati	www.cincinnatichildrens.org/traininged/training/gpnf Information regarding summer program in genetics for nursing faculty

REFERENCES

American Society of Clinical Oncology. (1996). Statement of the American Society of Clinical Oncology: Genetic testing for cancer susceptibility. *J Clin Oncol, 14*, pp. 1730-1736.

Burke, W., Daly, M., Garber, J., et al. (1997). Recommendations for follow-up care of individuals with an inherited predisposition to cancer. II. BRCA1 and BRCA2. Cancer Genetics Studies Consortium. *JAMA, 277*, pp. 997-1003.

Calzone, K. A. (1997). Genetic predisposition testing: clinical implications for oncology nurses. *Oncol Nurs Forum, 24*, pp. 712-718.

Claus, E., Risch, N., & Thompson, W. D. (1994). Autosomal dominant inheritance of early-onset breast cancer. *Cancer, 73*, pp. 643-651.

Couch, F., DeShano, M., Blackwood, K., et al. (1997). BRCA1 mutations in women attending clinics that evaluate the risk of breast cancer. *N Engl J Med, 336*, pp. 1409-1515.

Dimond, E., Calzone, K., Davis, J., & Jenkins, J. (1998). The role of the nurse in cancer genetics. *Cancer Nurs, 21*, pp. 57-75.

Douglas, F. S., O'Dair, L. C., Robinson, M., et al. (1999). The accuracy of diagnoses as reported in families with cancer: a retrospective study. *J Med Genet, 36*, pp. 309-312.

Elger, B. S., & Harding, T. W. (2000). Testing adolescents for a hereditary breast cancer gene (BRCA1): Respecting their autonomy is in their best interest. *Arch Pediatr Adolesc Med, 154*, pp. 113-119.

Fearon, E. R. (1997). Human cancer syndromes: clues to the origin and nature of cancer. *Science, 278*, pp. 1043-1050.

Frank, T. S., Manley, S. A., Olopade, O. I., et al. (1998). Sequence analysis of BRCA1 and BRCA2: Correlation of mutations with family history and ovarian cancer risk. *J Clin Oncol, 16*, pp. 2417-2425.

Gail, M., Brinton, L., Byar, D., et al. (1989). Projecting individualized probabilities of developing breast cancer for white females who are being examined annually. *J Natl Cancer Instit, 81*, pp. 1879-1886.

Johnson, V. P., & Christianson, C. (1999). Taking a family history. In *Clinical genetics: A self study for health care providers.* Accessed at www.vh.org/Providers/Textbooks/ClinicalGenetics/Contents.html on 10/14/00.

Lindor, N., Greene, M., & The Mayo Familial Cancer Program. (1998). The concise handbook of family cancer syndromes. *J Natl Cancer Instit, 90*, pp. 1039-1071.

Loescher, L. (1999). The family history component of cancer genetic risk counseling. *Cancer Nurs, 22*, pp. 96-102.

MacDonald, D. J. (1997). The oncology nurse's role in cancer risk assessment and counseling. *Semin Oncol Nurs, 13*, pp. 123-128.

MacDonald, D. J., & Lessick, M. (2000). Hereditary cancers in children and ethical and psychosocial implications. *J Pediatr Nurs, 15*, pp. 217-225.

Offit, K. (1998). *Clinical cancer genetics.* New York: Wiley-Liss.

Oncology Nursing Society. *ONS position on cancer genetics testing and risk assessment counseling* (1997, revised 8/2000). Available at www.ons.org/xp6/ONS/Information.xml/Journals_and_P. . ./Cancer_Genetic_Testing.xm.

Oncology Nursing Society. *ONS position statement. The role of the oncology nurse in cancer genetic counseling* (1997, revised 8/2000). Available at www.ons.org/xp6/ONS/Information.xml/Journals_. . ./Role_of_the Oncology_Nurse.xm.

Penson, R. T., Seiden, M. V., Shannon, K. M., et al. (2000). Communicating genetic risk: pros, cons, and counsel. *The Oncologist, 5*, pp. 152-161.

Shattuck-Eidens, D., McClure, M., Simard, J., et al. (1995). A collaborative survey of 80 mutations in the BRCA1 breast and ovarian cancer susceptibility gene: Implications for presymptomatic testing and screening. *JAMA, 273*, pp. 534-541.

Tinley, S. T., & Lynch, H. T. (1999). Integration of family history and medical management of patients with hereditary cancer. *Cancer, 86*, pp. 2525-2532.

Weitzel, J. N. (1996). Genetic counseling for familial cancer risk. *Hosp Pract, 31*, pp. 57-69.

Wilfond, B. S., Rothenberg, K. H., Thomson, E. J., & Lerman, C. (1997). Cancer genetic susceptibility testing: ethical and policy implications for future research and clinical practice. *J Law Med Ethics, 25*, pp. 243-251.

14 Laboratory Value Assessment

Esther Muscari Lin

CASE ▎ STUDY

Jackie Powell, a 49-year-old African American woman, following her fifth cycle of high-dose cisplatin and paclitaxel (Taxol) for recurrent ovarian cancer, finds herself battling protracted nausea and vomiting. Believing that she just has the same flu that has affected her family, she attempts to "ride it out" without calling her health care practitioner. On the third day, when she is not feeling much better, she calls a friend to bring her to her care providers' offices. Upon presentation to the advanced practice nurse (APN) she reports her "intake and outputs" as follows: (1) She has not kept anything down for 3 days but really has not wanted to eat anything anyhow, (2) she is so thirsty but vomits everything, and (3) the only good thing is the drainage from her rectovaginal fistula seems to have decreased despite continued abdominal cramping.

QUESTIONS

1. What will provide the most additional information about Jackie's volume status at this moment?

- **a.** Orthostatic blood pressure (BP) readings and pulses
- **b.** Orthostatic BP readings
- **c.** Serum sodium, potassium, blood urea nitrogen (BUN), and creatinine
- **d.** Serum sodium and potassium

Case Study continued

Jackie's supine BP is 100/68 mm Hg with a weak pulse rate of 64. She does not have a fever and her respirations appear weak and shallow. Jackie's coloring is pale and washed out as she walks in on the arm of her good friend Mary. As Jackie tries to answer your questions, Mary often contributes to the answers with clarifications or corrections.

QUESTIONS

2. Based on the information presented, what fluid and electrolyte imbalances is Jackie at risk for?
- **1.** Hypokalemia
- **2.** Hypovolemia
- **3.** Metabolic alkalosis
- **4.** Hypomagnesemia
    - **a.** 1, 2, & 3
    - **b.** 2, 3, & 4
    - **c.** 1, 2, & 4
    - **d.** All of these

3. What are the signs in this case of hypokalemia?
- **1.** Confusion
- **2.** Bradycardia
- **3.** Anuria
- **4.** Weakness
    - **a.** 1, 2, & 3
    - **b.** 1, 2, & 4
    - **c.** 1, 3, & 4
    - **d.** All of these

4. Which of the following is *not* a major contributor to hypokalemia?
- **a.** Magnesium deficiency
- **b.** Hypoaldosteronism
- **c.** Extracellular volume contraction
- **d.** Gastrointestinal losses

5. What is the minimum laboratory work that is necessary?

ANSWERS

1. Because of Jackie's hypovolemic state, the easiest and quickest pieces of information for that moment arise from the orthostatic vital signs. Of particular note and concern is that both the BP and pulse are low. If the BP is low, the heart rate should have been tachycardic in attempt to compensate for the decreased pressure. Bradycardia can be associated with severe hypokalemia and needs further follow-up.

Hearing Jackie's 3-day history of gastrointestinal (GI) losses tells the APN immediately that fluid has been lost and not retained. Renal function will only confirm what you are finding on examination.

An easy and quick means of assessing anyone's volume status regardless of cause for losses is pulse and BP in the lying, sitting, and standing positions. For a young person, tachycardia in light of hypotension (mild or moderate) would be expected as a sign of compensatory functioning. Although the pulse may not increase as much in the older individual with hypotension, orthostatic changes can still be identified as the BP drops more than 10 mm Hg from a recumbent to standing position. *Answer 1:* **a.**

2-4. Because the majority of the total body potassium (K) is intracellular, it is difficult to ascertain how much is lost during significant deficits. In the event of metabolic alkalosis or elevated glucose, K moves into the cell, lowering the serum K. Because K has a role in a number of important physiologic processes at the cellular level, deficiencies are reflected in nonspecific symptoms. The clinical manifestations of hypokalemia are usually a result of altered membrane potential that affect the function of excitable tissue. Symptoms can include muscle weakness, malaise, myalgias, tetany, constipation, or ileus. The cardiac alterations usually require a potassium less than 3.0 mEq/L to occur. Causes of hypokalemia and signs and symptoms commonly seen with a low potassium can be found in Box 14–1.

Metabolic alkalosis (high serum HCO_3) can commonly occur when there is extracellular volume depletion/contraction and hypokalemia. The volume depletion triggers antidiuretic hormone (ADH) release and resultant sodium (Na) and water retention. This worsens the hypokalemia because Na is reabsorbed in exchange for urinary excretion of K.

Increased aldosterone production contributes to hypokalemia because of the action on the distal tubules secreting potassium. In the oncology population, increased aldosterone production is usually the result of a hormone-secreting tumor.

Loop or thiazide diuretics, amphotericin B, the aminoglycosides, ganciclovir, or penicillin derivatives, all of which are used in the oncology population, contribute to renal losses of K. *Answer 2:* **d.** *Answer 3:* **b.** *Answer 4:* **b.**

| BOX 14-1 | Hypokalemia |

CAUSES

Redistribution as a result of catecholamines, insulin, or alkalemia
Decreased dietary intake
Increased renal losses as a result of drugs
Magnesium deficiency
Increased renal losses as a result of mineral and glucocorticoid excess
Excessive gastrointestinal losses
Metabolic alkalosis

SIGNS AND SYMPTOMS

Muscle weakness
Hyporeflexia
Fatigue
Muscle cramps
T-wave flattening
ST-segment depression
Prominent U wave
Prolonged PR interval
Increased P-wave amplitude
Polydipsia

From Chernecky, C. C., & Berger, B. J. (Eds.). *Advanced and critical care oncology nursing. Managing primary complications.* Philadelphia: WB Saunders; Okuda, T., Kurokawa, K. & Papadakis, M. A. (1998). In Tierney, L. M., McPhee, S. J., & Papadakis, M. A. (Eds.). *Current medical diagnosis & treatment,* 37th ed. (pp. 824-849). Stamford, CT: Appleton and Lange.

5. The fluid and electrolyte losses via the GI tract (emesis and fistula) immediately bring to mind hypokalemia, hypovolemia, metabolic alkalosis, hypomagnesemia, and hypoglycemia as potential consequences. The minimum amount of blood work necessary to confirm suspicions and identify potential underlying causes, as well as any damage to renal function, include a chemistry panel consisting of Na, K, magnesium (Mg), glucose, BUN, creatinine, urinalysis with specific gravity, and urine electrolytes. The adrenal glands and renal system control normal serum potassium levels. Hypokalemia (less than 3.5 mEq/L), a common occurrence in the oncology population, results because of GI losses, renin-secreting tumors, interference with K reabsorption in the renal tubules from medications, or ectopic adrenocorticotropic hormone–secreting tumors. *Answer 5:* **See text.**

QUESTIONS

6. Which of the following could be a significant contributor to confusion in Jackie?
   a. Cisplatin
   b. Taxol
   c. Hypernatremia
   d. Intracellular volume contraction

7. What other problems need to be ruled out immediately before further intervention?
  1. Sepsis
  2. Disseminated intravascular coagulation (DIC)
  3. Small bowel obstruction
  4. Adrenal tumor
     a. 1 & 2
     b. 2 & 4
     c. 3 & 4
     d. 1 & 3

8. What are the probable causes in this case for hypomagnesemia?
  1. Fistula
  2. Emesis
  3. Hypokalemia
  4. Taxol
     a. 1, 2, & 3
     b. 2, 3, & 4
     c. 1, 3, & 4
     d. All of these

ANSWERS

6. Increased Na levels because of dehydration, syndrome of inappropriate antidiuretic hormone secretion (SIADH), diabetes insipidus, or hyperadrenocortical secretion are characterized by altered mental states. Jackie has other possible reasons for being slightly confused, including fatigue from being so ill for 3 days straight, brain metastasis, or sepsis. As the electrolyte panels are analyzed, the reasons for the confusion being electrolyte related will surface and other potential causes are ruled out. *Answer 6:* **c.**

7. The presentation of nausea and vomiting in a person with a history of abdominal surgery always makes small bowel obstruction a possibility. The combination of vomiting and decreased stool output raises a flag of suspicion. Although a fever is not reported, the lowered BP and GI upset pose infection and sepsis as a distant possibility requiring evaluation. DIC always occurs as a result of some other underlying event, such as trauma, infection, or malignancy. It is not of concern at this point, especially when there are no indicators of thrombosis or bleeding. An adrenal tumor could be a cause of the hypokalemia but would be considered only if other causes are not identified for the low potassium. It also does not require immediate evaluation because there are other more life-threatening events that could occur. *Answer 7:* **d.**

8. Renal loss of magnesium occurs with cisplatin therapy and poses an additional insult to Jackie's potassium level. Magnesium deficiency is usually associated with malabsorptive syndromes. For GI losses to incur hypomagnesemia, a large amount of diarrhea needs to occur. This is a possibility with any type of rectal fistula. An excessive loss of fluids through emesis would also have to occur, but the possibility of losses through the two routes could be sufficient enough to result in hypomagnesemia. In addition, hypokalemia is commonly seen in association with hypomagnesemia (Okuda, Kurokawa, & Papadakis, 1998). *Answer 8:* **a.**

QUESTIONS

9. Appropriate intervention for Jackie's dehydration and her potassium of 2.5 mEq/L is reflected in which of the following orders?
  a. 1 L of normal saline with 110 mEq/L of potassium at 200 ml/hr
  b. 1 L of D_5W with 110 mEq/L of potassium at 200 ml/hr
  c. 1 L of D_5W with 200 mEq/L of potassium at 100 ml/hr
  d. 1 L of normal saline with 200 mEq/L of potassium at 100 ml/hr

10. Which of the following orders is an appropriate intervention for Jackie's magnesium level of 1.2 mEq/L?
  a. Magnesium oxide 1g orally every day
  b. Magnesium sulfate 2 g/200 ml intravenously to infuse over 1 hour
  c. Hold on magnesium doses until potassium level is within normal range
  d. Magnesium oxide 500 mg twice a day

11. If unfamiliar with appropriate dosages for electrolyte repletion, what approaches could you take to meet the patient's needs?

12. What are the implications of choosing rapid infusion of potassium and/or magnesium?

ANSWERS

9. Because of the severity of Mg and K deficiencies combined with Jackie's GI upset and dehydration, the speediest method of replenishing her is through the intravenous (IV) route. Oral K can contribute to nausea and vomiting in some people. IV K repletion should not exceed 20 mEq/hr, and then only in a unit where very close monitoring exists. Depending on institutional protocol, K level, cardiac status, and rate of repletion, a cardiac monitor during infusion may be indicated, especially when rates exceed 10 mEq/L (Pearson, 2000; Singer,

1998). If the repletion rate exceeds 20 mEq/hr, many institutions require electrocardiographic (EKG) monitoring. Parenteral K needs adequate dilution, and because of its potential vein damage and discomfort, doses exceeding 10 mEq/L should be administered through a central line. Hydration should consist of normal saline and not dextrose because of the tendency for K to move from the extracellular space intracellularly in the presence of glucose. *Answer 9:* **d.**

10. Oral magnesium can result in diarrhea if taken in large doses or not spaced out during the day, lowering the K and Mg levels even further. Mg can be infused relatively quickly, and normal levels can be achieved without cardiac monitoring. It is important to correct Mg in the face of hypokalemia; otherwise, the potassium will not correct itself despite K infusions. Magnesium sulfate 1 to 2 g can be administered over 15 minutes, then repeated if necessary based on the follow-up laboratory work (Pearson, 2000). *Answer 10:* **b.**

11. Using the pharmacist, reference books, policies, critical pathways, or institutional computer programs to learn dosing, potential side effects, and what precautions to monitor for is a means to safe drug administration. It is impossible to expect safe drug administration from memory, especially during the initial experiences of electrolyte repletion. *Answer 11:* **See text.**

12. Of major importance is the recognition of how quickly values can change, pushing the laboratory value to the other extreme with IV administration. Therefore instituting standardized orders and systems checks contributes to safe fluid and electrolyte repletion. *Answer 12:* **See text.**

QUESTIONS

13. Practical methods of evaluating and monitoring the fluid and electrolyte interventions for Jackie include which of the following?
1. Measurement of all secretions and excretions while hospitalized
2. Serum electrolytes and renal panel at least weekly until stable
3. Orthostatic vital signs
4. Urine specific gravity
5. Cardiac rate, rhythm, and form
   a. 1, 3, & 5
   b. 1, 3 & 4
   c. 2, 3, & 4
   d. 1, 2, 4, & 5

ANSWERS

13. Because of the rapid rate at which electrolytes change with IV repletion, frequent serum levels need to be drawn during the initial periods when the patient is receiving hourly K and Mg. Once the levels rise to safer levels and the repletion rates decrease, the time between blood draws can increase. If the level is unstable, with the patient in the hospital receiving IV electrolytes, the serum level should be checked at least twice a day until the patient's losses and repletion requirements are stabilized. For the outpatient receiving oral repletion, the frequency of laboratory work will depend on the contributing causes. If there are recurrent episodes of GI losses or changes in the drug dose, more frequent laboratory checks are needed. It is the patient's condition, drug dose, and stability that should determine blood draw frequency. *Answer 13:* **b.**

CASE 2 STUDY

Susan Chambers is a 51-year-old white female 4 years status post a right mastectomy and reconstructive surgery. Susan was a stage 2 at diagnosis and underwent 6 months of Cytoxan, adriamycin, 5-fluouracil (5-FU) (CAF) therapy. She is estrogen receptor/progesterone receptor (ER/PR) positive and has been taking tamoxifen 10 mg orally ever since the completion of chemotherapy. Susan was initially prescribed 20 mg/day but experienced significant nausea that threatened drug compliance. She presents at her annual appointment with complaints of malaise and not feeling quite right. With further inquiry, she tells you that on some days she is sleeping almost all day. Although unfamiliar with Susan, you evaluate her because you have agreed to cover for your colleague while he is on vacation.

QUESTIONS

1. As you begin your assessment, which of the following aspects will contribute the most information in attempt to identify a possible cause?

a. Medication list
b. Weight
c. History of postpartum depression
d. Date of menarche cessation

c. The more rest a person gets, the better the chances are of feeling better.
d. The episodes and intensity of accompanying symptoms are less.

ANSWERS

1. There are so many possible reasons for Susan's reported symptoms. As the APN completes the review of systems, findings assist in narrowing down possible causes. Anemia-related fatigue will be reflected in cardiopulmonary findings of shortness of breath, tachycardia, dizziness, difficulty concentrating, forgetfulness, confusion, withdrawal from usual activities, and possibly depression. Identifying the daily pattern of fatigue and viewing it within the context of lifestyle changes, disease status, medications, stresses, and changes to these areas can identify contributors to fatigue. Fatigue, being multidimensional and a result of many causes, requires learning about every aspect of a person's life and disease course. Learning not only when the fatigue began but how it has changed and compares with previous episodes of fatigue can identify causes as well. *Answer 1:* **a.**

Case Study continued

During the family history, Susan repeatedly reminds you that her mother died of breast cancer at the age of 52, as did her mother's sister. Susan's younger sister was diagnosed with stage 1 infiltrating ductal breast cancer 1 year ago at the age of 49.

QUESTIONS

2. As you learn how long Susan has been feeling this way, what is the rationale for identifying all health care providers involved in Susan's care?
  1. Duration of the problem is identified.
  2. Unhelpful treatment options can be identified.
  3. Potential problems can be ruled out.
  4. Obtaining past records can contribute to your assessment.
    a. 2 only
    b. 1 & 2
    c. 3 & 4
    d. All of these

3. Within your assessment of Susan's presenting problems, which characteristic of fatigue is consistent with fatigue in the patient with a cancer diagnosis?
  a. Fatigue is often unrelieved by rest.
  b. Distraction is a successful intervention.

ANSWERS

2. Reviewing Susan's medical records provides concrete facts unaffected by memory and detail the attempted interventions and the success of those efforts. Reviewing the providers in her care also contributes to understanding the disease experience Susan has had and the possible problems that have occurred and that may be reoccurring. It also provides a means for the APN to consider the differential diagnoses she is presented with. The APN could easily contact one of Susan's providers and discuss assessment and thoughts, intercorporating the providers' previous findings and interventions, if directed at the same problems. Continuity of care occurs when Susan's story of cancer is put together in a chronologic fashion with information from all care providers. *Answer 2:* **d.**

3. The frequent need for rest periods that usually do not relieve the fatigue is characteristic of cancer-related fatigue (CRF) because it is a different experience than the fatigue a healthy person experiences. The fact that this present bout of fatigue is a new onset and is not in association with any oncologic occurrences or treatments warrants further evaluation. CRF does not respond or improve with rest or sleep, which contributes to feelings of hopelessness, frustration, and even depression. When a person experiences fatigue, accompanying symptoms may be more intense and the combination can contribute to a decreased quality of life (Nail, 2000). Fatigue assessment should include some type of rating scale for comparisons over time but should also include an evaluation of the person's sleep patterns and habits. Because CRF is so common and multifactorial, the quality of a person's sleep can be overlooked, yet may be a major cause of being tired. *Answer 3:* **a.**

Case Study continued

Susan describes her daily routine as arising at 7 AM, showering, eating breakfast, and then resting on the couch until 10:30 AM. Then she does some work at the computer, which seems to be taking her longer and longer to complete, and at noon, she takes a nap until 2 PM, when she gets something to eat before returning to the computer. Her husband comes home at 5:30 PM, at which time he cooks dinner now while she rests on the couch. He complains to her that she is short-tempered with him and has no right to take out her frustrations on him.

QUESTIONS

4. If the fatigue Susan is feeling is anemia related, name two pulmonary symptoms that you would expect Susan to report.

    1. _____

    2. _____

5. Because fatigue is the most common symptom experienced by patients with cancer, why would you aggressively evaluate Susan's reports of fatigue?

    a. Susan is frustrated with feeling tired.

    b. This fatigue does not match Susan's usual pattern.

    c. Susan's fatigue is accompanied by malaise.

    d. Susan's fatigue is abnormal as evidenced by the interference with activities of daily living.

ANSWERS

4. Cardiopulmonary symptoms of dyspnea, orthopnea, palpitations, and chest pains can occur with anemia as a result of decreased oxygen availability (Worrall, Tompkins, & Rust, 1999). Signs and symptoms will vary depending on the cause of the anemia and the rate of onset (Blinder, 1998). Because Susan has not had recent myelosuppressive therapy, an anemia associated with decreased red blood cell (RBC) production is not expected. *Answer 4:* **See text.**

5. Patients commonly report frustration with ongoing fatigue, and even depression, which warrants a thorough assessment and evaluation of possible contributing factors. Because fatigue is usually multifactorial, differentiating the causes can result in at least interventions for some if not all causes. In Susan's case, her presentation of fatigue is strikingly severe and disruptive to her life. However, the key point in this assessment is that this experience is different from her previous experiences and has been the impetus for her visit to the health care team. *Answer 5:* **b.**

Case Study continued

During the physical examination, you note slight tenderness along Susan's lumbar sacral spine, which Susan says has contributed to her not sleeping well the last few weeks. Examination is otherwise unremarkable. In addition to the routine mammogram and chest radiograph, laboratory work consisting of a complete blood count

(CBC) with differential and routine chemistries are drawn.

Results
Normal mammogram and chest radiograph
White blood cell (WBC) count: 5000/mm^3 (5000 to 10,000/mm^3)
Hemoglobin (Hgb) and hematocrit (Hct): 13 g/dl and 38%, respectively (12 to 18g/dl and 35% to 45%, respectively)
Platelets: 150,000/mm^3 (150,000 to 300,000/mm^3)
Na: 142 mEq/L (135 to 145 mEq/L)
K: 4.0 mEq/L (3.5 to 5.0 mEq/L)
BUN: 15 (10 to 15 mg/dl)
Creatinine: 1.2 (0.5 to 1.5 mg/dl)
Alkaline phosphatase: 480 U/L (30 to 120 U/L)

QUESTIONS

6. From your assessment at this point, what knowledge causes you to order an ionized calcium, albumin, and a liver panel (liver enzymes and bilirubin)?

Case Study continued

Test Results
Ionized Ca: 5.0 mg/dl (4.4 to 5.0 mg/dl)
Albumin: 3.5 g/dl (3.5 to 5.0 g/dl)
alanine aminotransferase (ALT/SGPT): 300 U/ml (5 to 35 U/ml)
alkaline phosphatise (AST/SGOT): 250 U/ml (8 to 20 U/ml)
GGT: 100 IU/L (5 to 25 IU/L)
Total bilirubin: 1.4 mg/dl (0.1 to 1.2 mg/dl)
Direct bilirubin: 1.0 mg/dl (0.1 to 0.3 mg/dl)
Indirect bilirubin: 0.4 mg/dl (0.1 to 1.0 mg/dl)

QUESTIONS

7. As you collaborate with the physician about how to proceed with Susan's care, what is of utmost concern in your list of possible causes?

    a. Lytic lesions

    b. Hepatocellular disease

    c. Renal disease

    d. Unconjugated bilirubinemia

8. Seeing Susan's blood work results, what is the most likely thing you would question yourself about regarding her physical examination?

    a. Was there thoracic spine tenderness?

    b. Was there high-pitched tinkling on abdominal auscultation?

    c. Was the liver palpable on examination?

    d. Was she leaning on her friend because of femur tenderness/discomfort?

ANSWERS

6-7. Because breast cancer metastasizes to bone, liver, and lung, disorders of those systems are always under suspect for recurrence. Because recurrence does not necessarily become obvious on routine follow-up, abnormal symptoms reported by patients require scrutiny. Knowing that Susan was a stage 2 at diagnosis places her at an increased risk of recurrence, and the potential metastatic sites become the focus of additional assessment. Considering these sites, one considers what the signs and symptoms of metastasis would be. Bony disease results in lytic lesions; elevated lactate dehydrogenase (LDH), alkaline phosphatase, and calcium because of osteoblastic action; and pain (often in the weight-bearing bones). With metastatic bone disease and the osteoclastic action of tumor cells, calcium levels can be elevated. Hypoalbuminemia can alter serum calcium levels because calcium is complexed primarily to albumin (which is synthesized in the liver). Ionized or free calcium is unaffected by albumin levels and should be measured in patients with nutritional disorders, liver dysfunction, and fluid overload. Liver metastasis does not result in significant liver impairment until a large majority of the liver is consumed with disease. However, elevated transaminases, LDH, and alkaline phosphatase are early indicators of hepatocyte destruction. As liver cell death progresses, hepatocellular uptake of bilirubin is impaired as evidenced by a rising bilirubin level. Jaundice does not usually become apparent until the direct bilirubin reaches 2.0 mg/dl (Lin, 1998). The combination of elevated transaminases and abnormal conjugated and total bilirubin focuses the immediate concern on hepatocellular disease. Even if there is metastatic disease to the bone, Susan could be on the verge of hepatic failure, which makes finding the causes of liver dysfunction the first priority. *Answer 6:* **See text.** *Answer 7:* **b.**

8. The APN's review of the patient's chief complaint, physical examination, and laboratory work is done within the framework of the APN's oncology knowledge. To see such highly elevated transaminases can lead a practitioner to stop and reconsider his or her physical examination because the laboratory work is so significant for liver disease. One is drawn to the abdominal and, in particular, the liver examination. Because the alkaline phosphatase is also elevated, bone involvement from tumor and destruction is a very real possibility. Susan's report of pain was limited to her lower back, and although the APN might have accepted Susan's explanation and not have delved into this area for further assessment, it is something that can be asked about over the telephone or in subsequent clinic visits. *Answer 8:* **c.**

Case Study continued

After speaking with Susan at length, you and your collaborating physician decide to recheck the liver panel in 1 week. You counsel Susan to avoid alcohol and over-the-counter pharmacologic agents and to hold all prescribed medications, including the tamoxifen. Depending on the repeat liver panel results, an abdominal computed tomography (CT) scan will be recommended. You note your recommendations in your clinic visit note.

At 1 week, when Susan returns to the clinic for her blood draw, she is notably jaundiced. On examination, she has right upper quadrant tenderness and the liver is palpated at 2 cm below the right costal margin.

Laboratory Results
ALT: 350 U/ml (5 to 35 U/ml)
AST: 260 U/ml (8 to 20 U/ml)
GGT: 200 IU/L (5 to 25 IU/L)
Total bilirubin: 2.4 mg/dl (0.2 to 1.2 mg/dl)
Direct bilirubin: 2.2 mg/dl (0.1 to 0.3 mg/dl)
Indirect bilirubin: 0.2 mg/dl (0.1 to 1.0 mg/dl)

QUESTIONS

9. What other signs reflective of hyperbilirubinemia would the APN most likely find on Susan's physical examination?

10. What critical risk factors from Susan's history do you need to ask her about?
  1. Transfusions
  2. Mononucleosis exposure
  3. Neutropenia history
  4. Pharmacologic use
     a. 1 & 2
     b. 2 & 3
     c. 3 & 4
     d. 1 & 4

11. Because the abdominal CT scan is negative, a liver biopsy is planned. In the interim, what further information could you collect that might contribute to identification of a cause or contributing factors?
  a. Bone marrow biopsy
  b. Abdominal ultrasound
  c. Urobilinogen
  d. Viral serologies

12. How would you interpret –HBsAg and +anti-HBs on blood work?
  a. Previous exposure to hepatitis B with recovery and immunity achieved

b. Previous exposure to hepatitis A with recovery and immunity achieved

c. Active infection with hepatitis B and active immunity occurring

d. Active infection with hepatitis A and active immunity occurring

---

ANSWERS

9. Signs of hyperbilirubinemia include a yellowish hue to the sclera, mucous membranes, and skin; dry, flaky, itchy skin; darkened urine; and lightening of the stool color (Lin, 1998). As the liver becomes engorged and increased in size, the capsule stretches, resulting in right upper quadrant pain that can extend to the back. *Answer 9:* **See text.**

10-11. The etiology behind hepatocellular death in the person with a cancer history includes recurrent or metastatic disease in the liver; venoocclusive disease; graft-versus-host disease; viral hepatitis, with the most significant risk from hepatitis B virus, which accounts for approximately 15% to 20% of hepatic failure cases across all patient populations; and drug (legal and illegal) use. Acetaminophen is a common drug, as are the nonsteroidal antiinflammatory drugs (NSAIDs). Tamoxifen, a nonsteroidal antiestrogen, is metabolized extensively in the liver into several metabolites (Pearson, 2000). Illegal drugs such as cocaine and alcohol abuse are the other major agents with potentially major hepatocellular insult. *Answer 10:* **d.** *Answer 11:* **d.**

12. The specific viruses causing viral hepatitis are hepatitis A virus (HAV), B virus (HBV), C virus (HCV), D virus, and E virus. Epstein-Barr virus, herpes virus, and cytomegalovirus are also possible hepatocellular insults. The prodromal symptoms of a viral hepatitis can be vague and very similar to side effects from chemotherapy. They include anorexia, nausea, vomiting, malaise, or flulike symptoms. During active infection, the antigens of the virus are present and symptoms occur within 2 to 3 months of exposure. As the virus resolves, antibodies to the virus begin to be detected in the blood within 2 months of the symptoms or 4 to 6 months after viral exposure (Friedman, 1998). *Answer 12:* **a.**

Case Study continued

The liver biopsy results are consistent with intrahepatic cholestasis from a cause other than malignant disease. At this point, the APN decides to review the history with Susan to make sure all risk factors were covered. On repeat questioning, Susan admits to doubling up on the tamoxifen dose at times, thinking a larger dose would decrease her risk of recurrence. She also acknowledges that she did not stop the tamoxifen at the first indication of elevated liver enzymes, but since she became jaundiced, she did hold the medication.

QUESTIONS

13. Blood work is scheduled to be repeated in 1 week. What further laboratory values require monitoring?

a. Prothrombin time (PT)

b. Albumin

c. White cell differential

d. Creatinine

ANSWERS

13. Because of hepatic responsibility for production of clotting factors, PT and activated partial thromboplastin time (aPTT) can be prolonged and might require factor repletion and vitamin K administration. Increased risk of bleeding would also require in-depth education and monitoring for occult bleeding. *Answer 13:* **a.**

CASE 3 STUDY

Hermann Ritchey is a 65-year-old white man with a history of a squamous cell carcinoma of the tongue, treated with a radical neck dissection and a chemotherapy regimen of 5-FU and cisplatin 12 months ago. At the time of diagnosis, he was unaccompanied and reported that he lived alone in the back room of a bar owned by an ex-brother-in-law because he had difficulty "making ends meet." He has a history of missing follow-up appointments, and when trying to reach him, his telephone is often disconnected.

Upon presentation, he appears somewhat disheveled, is very thin and gaunt, and requires a good deal of coaxing to answer any questions. He is referred to the nutrition support clinic run by the general surgeon with whom you share a collaborative practice. You evaluate him for a folic acid deficiency.

QUESTIONS

1. Which of the following values do you expect to be present on Hermann's CBC?

TABLE 14-1 Laboratory Values for Common Anemias

ANEMIA CLASSIFICATION	DIFFERENTIAL DIAGNOSIS	SUPPORTING LABORATORY RESULTS
Microcytic	Iron deficiency	Below-normal iron, below-normal transferrin, below-normal hemoglobin, below-normal ferritin, and above-normal total iron-binding capacity (TIBC)
	Thalassemia	Normal/above-normal iron, normal/above-normal ferritin, normal TIBC, and normal transferrin
	Sideroblastic	Normal/above-normal iron, above-normal ferritin, above-normal transferrin, above-normal sideroblasts, and normal/above-normal TIBC
Macrocytic	Folate deficiency	Below-normal folate, above-normal iron, above-normal ferritin, and normal TIBC
	B_{12} deficiency	Below-normal B_{12}, below-normal ferritin, below-normal/normal iron, and above-normal TIBC
Normocytic	Anemia of chronic disease	Below-normal iron, normal/above-normal ferritin, below-normal transferrin, below-normal TIBC, and normal/above-normal reticulocyte count
	Hemolytic	Above-normal reticulocyte count, above-normal lactate dehydrogenase, below-normal haptoglobin, and positive Coombs' (autoimmune)

From Worrall, L. M., Tompkins, C. A., Rust, D. M. (1999). Recognizing and managing anemia. *Clin J Oncol Nurs, 3*(4), pp. 153-160.

a. Elevated mean corpuscular volume (MCV)
b. Low RBC distribution width
c. Decreased MCV
d. Elevated hemoglobin

2. What other values would be consistent with a folic acid deficiency?
a. Normal B_{12} vitamin levels
b. Decreased B_{12} vitamin levels
c. Prolonged PT
d. Elevated mean corpuscular hemoglobin concentration

3. What type of anemia is caused by a folic acid deficiency?
a. Microcytic
b. Macrocytic
c. Aplastic
d. Normocytic

ANSWERS

1. Anemias can be classified according to their red blood size (MCV) and diagnosed with serum iron and ferritin levels. See Table 14-1.
   Folic acid deficiency is identified by an increased MCV and decreased hematocrit. If serum LDH or indirect bilirubin is elevated, the cause is more likely RBC destruction or ineffective erythropoiesis (Blinder, 1998). *Answer 1:* **a.**

2. Accompanying the increased MCV are below-normal serum folic acid and RBC folate levels. *Answer 2:* **a.**

3. Folic acid and B_{12} deficiencies result in megaloblastic anemias because the deficiency causes abnormalities in DNA synthesis, which leads to altered hematopoietic cell morphology and decreased RBC production (Worrall, Tompkins, & Rust, 1999). Although B_{12} deficiencies require years to develop, folic acid deficiency may develop within a few months because of decreased intake, malabsorption, or increased utilization in the case of a hemolytic anemia or pregnancy. *Answer 3:* **b.**

QUESTIONS

4. What risk factors need to be assessed in Hermann?
   1. Dietary intake of fruits and vegetables
   2. Dietary intake of red meat
   3. Regular alcohol intake
   4. Medication list
   a. 1, 2, & 3
   b. 2, 3, & 4
   c. 1, 3, & 4
   d. All of these

5. What symptoms did Hermann most likely describe when he presented with his anemia?
   1. Anorexia
   2. Headache
   3. Dizziness
   4. "Racing" heartbeat
   a. 1, 2, & 3
   b. 1, 2, & 4
   c. 2, 3, & 4
   d. All of these

6. What additional laboratory work, at the minimum, *must* be considered for anemia evaluation after Hermann's Hgb and Hct were determined to be low?

a. Stool hemoccult, reticulocyte count, and MCV

b. Reticulocyte count, MCV, and total iron-binding capacity (TIBC)

c. MCV review, serum ferritin, and TIBC

d. TIBC, MCV, and prealbumin

7. The dietitian creates a diet plan to help restore Hermann's folic acid levels. What contributions can you offer to the dietitian's plan of care knowing that Hermann lives alone, often eating precooked foods, and is still consuming alcohol on a frequent basis?

1. Fax the missing and necessary food items to the Meals on Wheels coordinator

2. Consult with the rehabilitation counselor within the cancer center regarding past attempts and possible new options for Hermann

3. Recommend a drug change from the phenytoin he takes for a history of seizures

4. Schedule Hermann to see the dietitian annually during his follow-up visit to the cancer center

a. 1, 2, & 3

b. 1, 2, & 4

c. 2, 3, & 4

d. All of these

8. How will you plan to monitor Hermann once the plan of care is initiated?

BOX 14-2 | **Folic Acid/Folate Deficiency: Oncology Patients at Risk**

DIETARY ISSUES

Prolonged inadequate intake

Neutropenic patient who has been counseled to avoid fresh fruits and vegetables

Consistently overcooked food

Alcohol abuse

ABSORPTION ISSUES

Liver disease

Drugs that interfere with folic acid absorption

Diabetes mellitus

Steatorrhea

Gastrectomy

Jejunal bypass/resection

Leukemia/lymphoma

INCREASED REQUIREMENTS

Hyperthyroidism

Skin diseases

Rapid cell turnover

Malignancy

Adapted from Worrall, L. M., Tompkins, C. A., & Rust, D. (1999). Recognizing and managing anemia. *Clin J Oncol Nurs, 3*(4), pp. 153-160.

the red cell produces changes in mucosal cells, glossitis, anorexia, and diarrhea disturbances. In B_{12} deficiency, there are profound neurologic impairments, beginning with paresthesias and progressing to decreased vibration and position sense (Linker, 1998). See Table 14-2 and Box 14-3. Anemias are characterized by decreased hemoglobin and hematocrit. *Answer 5:* **a.**

6. Anemia evaluation begins with a CBC and reticulocyte count. The reticulocyte count indicates the status of marrow function, which would be low in the case of marrow failure, aplastic anemia, iron or folate anemia, and the anemia of chronic disease. The reticulocyte count is elevated with RBC destruction and blood loss. The red cell morphology guides further laboratory work depending on microcytic or macrocytic cell size. Stool testing for occult bleeding should occur during the physical assessment when reports of fatigue, dizziness, or stool color change are reported and/or when anemia is suspected. Most anemia cases are iron deficiency anemias resulting from blood loss or, in the case of the oncology patient, an anemia of chronic disease caused by altered hemopoiesis. Other necessary laboratory work includes a ferritin, TIBC, and in some cases, an erythropoietin level. However, an early assessment

---

ANSWERS

4. The risk factors related to the anemias depend on the classification type. Microcytic or iron deficiency anemias most commonly result from acute or chronic blood loss, whereas the macrocytic anemias are caused by a B_{12} or folate deficiency (Abramson & Abramson, 1999; Erickson, 1996; Little, 1999) (Box 14-2).

Folic acid is found in citrus fruits and green leafy vegetables with daily requirements of 50 to 100 µg/day, and body stores consist of enough folate (approximately 5000 µg), which is enough to last 2 to 3 months (Linker, 1998). Within the oncology population, a number of factors place a patient at risk for a megaloblastic anemia. *Answer 4:* **c. See Box 14-2.**

5. The signs and symptoms of folate deficiency anemia are not as obvious as those associated with a microcytic anemia. The megaloblastic state of

TABLE **14-2** History and Physical Examination	
HISTORY	**PHYSICAL EXAMINATION**
GENERAL	
Recent blood loss, surgery, trauma, chronic infection, family history of anemia, malaise, weight loss, age, exposure to radiation or chemical toxins, and occupation	Lethargy, apathy, and fever
GASTROINTESTINAL	
Nausea, vomiting, diarrhea, dysphagia, dyspepsia, pica, night sweats, cold intolerance, diet, constipation, tarry stools, abdominal pain, painful tongue, and history of gastrointestinal disease	Cheilitis (inflammation of the lip), atrophic glossitis, beefy red or shiny tongue, stomatitis, abdominal distension, hepatosphenomegaly ascites, and occult blood loss
GENITOURINARY	
Hematuria and history of renal disease	—
MUSCULOSKELETAL	
Muscle weakness, decreased strength, and bone pain	—
CARDIOPULMONARY	
Dyspnea, orthopnea, hemoptysis, palpitations, and chest pain	Tachycardia, systolic murmur, bruits, intermittent claudication, ankle edema, arrhythmias, postural hypotension, and tachypnea
NEUROLOGIC	
Headaches, paresthesias of feet and hands, changes in vision, changes in taste, changes in hearing, vertigo, tinnitus	Confusion, impaired judgment, irritability, ataxia, weakness, retinal hemorrhage, loss of sensation or proprioception (position sense in toes), and spasticity
SEXUAL/REPRODUCTIVE	
Pregnancy history, menorrhagia, and metrorrhagia	—
HEMATOLOGIC	
History of inflammatory disorders and transfusion	Generalized lymphadenopathy
INTEGUMENT	
Early graying of hair	Pale skin and mucous membranes, blue or pale white sclera, poor skin turgor, brittle spoon-shaped fingernails, jaundice, petechiae, ecchymosis, nasal or gingival bleeding, poor healing, dry brittle thinning hair, and skin ulcerations
MEDICATIONS	
Use of vitamin/iron supplements, aspirin, anticoagulants, birth control pills, anticonvulsants, antimicrobials, nonsteroidal anti-inflammatory drugs, oral hypoglycemics, and methyldopa	—

From Worrall, L. M., Tompkins, C. A., Rust, D. M. (1999). Recognizing and managing anemia. *Clin J Oncol Nurs, 3*(4), pp. 153-160.

BOX 14-3 Symptoms and Signs of Anemia in Cancer Patients

CARDIORESPIRATORY SYSTEM
Exertional dyspnea
Tachycardia, palpitations
Cardiac enlargement, eccentric hypertrophy
Increased pulse pressure, systolic ejection
    murmur
Risk of life-threatening cardiac failure

CENTRAL NERVOUS SYSTEM
Fatigue
Dizziness, vertigo
Depressive moods
Impaired cognitive function

GASTROINTESTINAL SYSTEM
Anorexia
Nausea

GENITAL TRACT
Menstrual problems
Loss of libido

VASCULAR SYSTEM
Low skin temperature
Pale skin, mucous membranes, and conjunctivae

IMMUNE SYSTEM
Impaired T-cell and macrophage function

From Ludwig, H., & Fritz, E. (1998). Anemia in cancer patients. *Semin Oncol, 25*(3), pp. 2-6.

step is to determine whether occult bleeding is occurring (Figure 14-1, p. 290). *Answer 6:* **a.**

7. Faxing the necessary information to other health care providers is an example of ensuring good transition and continuity of care. The plan of care can be successful only when all care providers involved are knowledgeable about the action plan. The therapeutic effects of phenytoin (Dilantin) may be decreased by folic acid; therefore Hermann's seizure threshold may decrease as folic acid replenishment occurs (Pearson, 2000). A drug change would most likely be performed in consultation with the prescribing health care provider. Alcohol rehabilitation should be offered to Hermann. Programs offered by rehabilitation centers meet specialized needs for many people, and the APN's input and knowledge of what Hermann has experienced because of his cancer can enhance the treatment plan. Creativity in finding programs that will accept the resources Hermann has is often challenging but within the role of the APN. Networking with numerous community groups can many times lead to resources for people with limited resources and support systems. The APN is often the key to knowing many of the resources available and matching patients with appropriate groups. Close and frequent follow-up, especially in the beginning of Hermann's treatment plan, will be necessary. Follow-up provides support and encouragement while also troubleshooting early in the treatment plan with feedback that can alter the plan as the patient's needs and challenges arise. *Answer 7:* **d.**

8. Folic acid repletion in the oral form is continued until the deficiency is corrected. Total correction can occur within 2 months and rapid improvement can be seen within a week, as evidenced by reticulocytosis and an improved sense of well-being (Linker, 1998; Little, 1999). *Answer 8:* **See text.**

CASE 4 STUDY

Mrs. Jean Stuart is the 72-year-old mother of a patient you have been caring for over the last 2 years. She always accompanies her 50-year-old son David to his clinic appointments and has been a very assertive advocate for David. He has been transfusion dependent following an autologous bone marrow transplant for non-Hodgkin's lymphoma. This week David arrives unaccompanied and mentions that his mom has not been feeling too well. He is concerned that caring for him is wearing her out. Within a few days of David's appointment, he calls and asks you for a favor. He tells you that he thinks his mother's eyes are yellow and would appreciate it if "you could check her out."

QUESTIONS

1. Upon arrival, Mrs. Stuart is indeed icteric. What body areas are usually affected by a yellowish hue when someone is jaundiced?
   a. Sclera, mucous membranes, skin
   b. Sclera, skin
   c. Sclera, skin, nares
   d. Sclera, skin, nailbeds

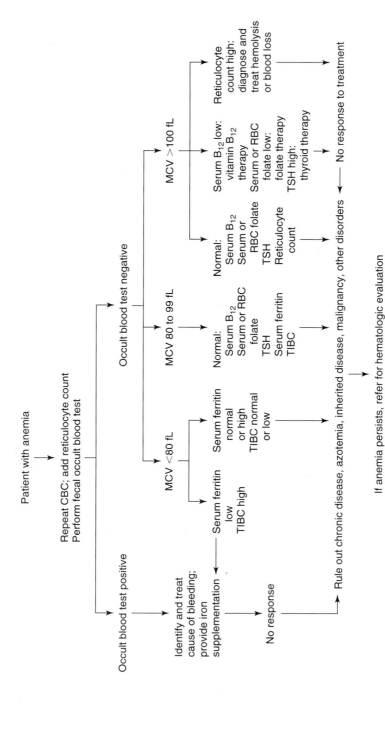

Figure 14-1 Protocol for the initial investigation of a patient with anemia. *CBC,* Complete blood count; *MCV,* mean corpuscular volume; *RBC,* red blood cell; *TIBC,* total iron-binding capacity; *TSH,* thyroid-stimulating hormone. (From Abramson, S. D., & Abramson, N. [1999]. "Common" uncommon anemias. *Am Fam Physician, 59*(4), pp. 851-858.)

2. What is the lowest possible level that the bilirubin generally needs to be for jaundice to be apparent?
- **a.** 1.5 mg/dl
- **b.** 2.0 mg/dl
- **c.** 4.0 mg/dl
- **d.** 3.0 mg/dl

3. Within your health history of Mrs. Stuart, what signs and symptoms could you correlate with the jaundice?
1. Epigastric pain
2. Chills and a fever
3. Rash
4. Oily skin
  - **a.** 1, 2, & 3
  - **b.** 2 & 4
  - **c.** 2 & 3
  - **d.** All of these

4. To identify the cause of the jaundice, differential diagnoses that need to be ruled out include all of the following *except:*
- **a.** Prehepatic dysfunction
- **b.** Intrahepatic dysfunction
- **c.** Extrahepatic dysfunction
- **d.** Posthepatic dysfunction

5. On physical examination, which of the following signs are consistent with advanced hepatocellular disease?
1. Ascites
2. Splenomegaly
3. Palmar erythema
4. Skin excoriations
  - **a.** 1, 2, & 3
  - **b.** 1, 3, & 4
  - **c.** 2, 3, & 4
  - **d.** All of these

ANSWERS

1. Jaundice, the yellowish discoloration of the skin, sclera, and mucous membranes, results from bile pigment deposition. *Answer 1:* **a.**

2. Jaundice becomes clinically evident when the bilirubin reaches and exceeds 2 mg/dl. If someone is not observed in daylight, it is possible for an individual to present with an elevated bilirubin as high as 4 mg/dl (Lin, 1998). An elevated bilirubin can occur for a number of reasons. See Box 14-4. *Answer 2:* **b.**

3. In addition to the yellowish hue associated with jaundice, lightening of the stool and darkening of the urine occurs because conjugated

---

| BOX **14-4** | **Hyperbilirubinemia: Reasons for Elevation** |

I. Elevated unconjugated/normal conjugated levels
  A. Excess production
    1. Red cell destruction/hemolysis, exceeding liver capacity
    2. Hemolytic transfusion reaction
    3. Gilbert's syndrome (hereditary disorder of bilirubin uptake failure)
II. Elevated conjugated/normal unconjugated
  A. Extrahepatic biliary tree obstruction of main or common hepatic duct or common bile duct
    1. Gallbladder disease
    2. Common bile duct stones
    3. Primary or metastatic carcinoma
    4. Carcinoma of ampulla of Vater or common bile duct
    5. Pancreatic carcinoma
    6. Pancreatitis or pancreatic pseudocyst
  B. Intrahepatic obstruction/intrahepatic cholestasis
    1. Alcoholic cirrhosis
    2. Primary biliary cirrhosis
    3. Steroids
    4. Venoocclusive disease
    5. Hodgkin's disease
    6. Graft-versus-host disease
    7. Hepatocellular carcinoma
    8. Metastatic consumption of liver spaces
    9. Sepsis
III. Elevated conjugated and unconjugated
  A. Parenchymal damage associated with decreased hepatocellular bilirubin uptake, intracellular protein binding failure, or impaired bilirubin secretion
    1. Cirrhosis
    2. Metabolic disorders
    3. Viral hepatitis (acute or chronic)
    4. Space-occupying tumors that have metastasized to the liver
    5. Graft-versus-host disease
    6. Acute and chronic inflammatory diseases

Adapted from Lin, E. M. (1998). Jaundice. In Preston, F. A., & Cunningham, R. S. (Eds.). *Clinical guidelines for symptom management in oncology. A handbook for advanced practice nurses.* (pp. 51-57). New York: Clinical Insights Press.

bilirubin is soluble and is excreted in the urine. See Box 14-5 for other signs and symptoms of jaundice. *Answer 3:* **a.**

4. Ascites and edema occur because of decreased plasma oncotic pressure, sodium retention, and portal venous hypertension (Ghalib, 1998). Skin excoriation can occur because of pruritus that accompanies jaundice, as well as upper quadrant

BOX **14-5** | Jaundice: Signs and Symptoms

Yellow tint of sclera, mucous membranes, and skin
Lightened stool color/darkened urine
Pruritus/skin excoriation
Xanthomas
Left or right upper quadrant/epigastric pain radiating to back
Colicky abdominal pain
Fever/shaking chills
Rash and arthralgias
Chills, fever, and abdominal pain

ADVANCED DISEASE
Abdominal venous distension and ascites
Peripheral edema
Testicular atrophy
Gynecomastia
Bleeding
Encephalopathy

pain, colicky abdominal pain, fever, shaking chills, rash, arthralgias, chills, and fever.

Chronic hepatocellular disease and portal hypertension can also accompany testicular atrophy, splenomegaly, a prominent abdominal venous pattern, palmar erythema, and gynecomastia (Lin, 1998). *Answer 4:* **a.**

5. With advanced hepatocellular disease, encephalopathy, prolonged PT, GI bleeding, sepsis, hypoglycemia, renal failure, electrolyte abnormalities, and coagulopathies can occur (Berger, Wrigley, & Ladaika, 1998). *Answer 5:* **d.**

Case Study continued

Liver enzyme levels are high and alkaline phosphatase is greater than 300 U/L. The bilirubin is 3.0 mg/dl, with the conjugated level at 1.8 mg/dl.

QUESTIONS

6. Knowing this, what cause of the jaundice is immediately ruled out?
   a. Alcoholic cirrhosis
   b. Hemolysis
   c. Infection
   d. Carcinoma of the ampulla of Vater

ANSWERS

6. Diagnosis of the cause of jaundice is made by ruling out or excluding other possibilities. The first step in analyzing bilirubin levels is to look at the conjugated (direct) and unconjugated (indirect)

results. The reason for an elevated unconjugated or indirect bilirubin is excess bilirubin production because of severe hemolysis, a hemolytic transfusion reaction, or a hereditary disorder. Intrahepatic or extrahepatic obstruction results in elevated conjugated or direct bilirubin levels. In some cases parenchymal damage leading to jaundice can cause elevations in both, with the conjugated level eventually being higher. The inability for bilirubin to reach the liver causes it to be unable to be conjugated with glucuronide, so it becomes soluble in bile and can be excreted into bile canaliculi. Therefore the urine will be negative for bilirubin. Mrs. Stuart's blood work results reveal an elevated conjugated bilirubin; therefore a prehepatic abnormality of severe hemolysis, hemolytic transfusion reaction, or a hereditary disorder of bilirubin uptake failure is ruled out early in the assessment process. An intrahepatic obstruction is within intralobular biliary canaliculi, resulting in intrahepatic cholestasis. This is associated with alcoholic cirrhosis, drugs or toxins, viral hepatitis, steroids, venoocclusive disease, graft-versus-host disease, hepatocellular carcinoma, and sepsis (Lin, 1998). An extrahepatic abnormality would involve some type of biliary tree obstruction involving the hepatic ducts or common bile duct and is seen in association with gallbladder disease, common bile duct stones, primary or metastatic disease, pancreatic cancer, pancreatitis, or a pancreatic pseudocyst. *Answer 6:* **b.**

Case Study continued

Mrs. Stuart is scheduled for a right upper quadrant ultrasound. In discussing the plan for determining the cause or causes of her jaundice, David encourages his mother to not worry by telling her that because she has not had any pain, she "will be fine." He states out loud how he knows that chronic pain is often a sign that accompanies cancer.

QUESTIONS

7. Should the APN quickly correct David and tell him that carcinoma is high in the list of possible causes? What is the value or "rationale" behind your decision?

8. What is the ultrasound finding that results in Mrs. Stuart being scheduled for an endoscopic retrograde cholangiopancreatography (ERCP)?
   a. Dilated ducts
   b. No duct dilation or constriction
   c. Presence of gallstones
   d. A large cyst

9. Which laboratory values on Mrs. Stuart's blood work would contribute to evaluating hepato-cellular function?
   a. WBC count with differential
   b. BUN and creatinine
   c. Albumin and PT
   d. Albumin, calcium, and PT

10. Mrs. Stuart questions why she needs to provide a urine sample. What is your rationale?
   a. To check for white cells indicative of a viral infection
   b. To check for urine bilirubin indicative of a nonhemolytic cause
   c. To check for urine electrolytes indicative of advanced liver disease
   d. To check for drug accumulation because of poor liver metabolism abilities

ANSWERS

7. It is at the APN's discretion as to whether she corrects David's statement. The APN needs to weigh the value of telling David in front of his mother just as she is about to undergo a test that painless jaundice is a common finding in individuals with pancreatic cancer. Because she has seen them regularly over the past few years, the APN knows their knowledge level, ability to handle new information, coping mechanisms, and support systems. To correct David at this point might result in an emotional discussion that deserves the appropriate time and private setting. These are all factors that the APN is well positioned to answer. *Answer 7:* **See text.**

8. An ultrasound visualizes the bile ducts and shows whether they are dilated, suggesting a distal obstruction but not necessarily identifying the obstruction. A CT scan identifies an obstructive lesion and any anatomic changes. An ERCP or percutaneous transhepatic cholangiography (PTC) is used to locate an obstruction and biopsy the tissue. A PTC can help differentiate between large bile duct obstruction and parenchymal causes. *Answer 8:* **a.**

9. A low albumin and prolonged PT can be suggestive of hepatocellular injury and suppressed synthesis capability. *Answer 9:* **c.**

10. A urine bilirubin in combination with the direct and indirect serum values help rule out hemolysis as the cause. *Answer 10:* **b.**

Case Study continued

Diagnosed with pancreatic cancer, Mrs. Stuart is unable to be treated surgically because of the

extent of the disease. She refuses participation in any clinical trial and vocalizes her hopes that she can finally "give her life in exchange for her son's." Some other members on the periphery of David's health care team are quite concerned at Mrs. Stuart's approach and belief that she can change his disease course with her "sacrifice." They ask you to step in and revisit their discussion about a clinical trial treatment option because you are caring for David and know his family well.

QUESTIONS

11. You refuse for all of the following reasons *except:*
   a. This may be a value Mrs. Stuart places on her illness and impending death.
   b. This is Mrs. Stuart's articulation of accepting the severity of her illness with some meaning or hope attached.
   c. It is none of your business because David is in your care and not his mother.
   d. Your history with David and his mother has provided you with the opportunity to appreciate the depth of the mother's understanding and philosophy of cancer and death.

ANSWERS

11. Caring for David includes caring for his family as well. Therefore Mrs. Stuart is in your goals of care as you care for David. It is within patients' rights to refuse treatment and choose palliative and supportive care. As they make their decisions, the meaning of their illness, their life, and their relationships enter into the process. Understanding Mrs. Stuart provides the APN with a wonderful opportunity to support Mrs. Stuart in her decision making and advocate on her behalf as opposed to setting out to "change her mind." Learning the meaning of her illness to her and listening to her are all examples of people's rationales for choosing their treatment options. It is an option to not receive treatment and the ultimate decision lies with each person. *Answer 11:* **c.**

Case Study continued

Mrs. Stuart requests you to oversee her hospice care with the goal to remain at home "at all costs."

QUESTIONS

12. As Mrs. Stuart's disease progresses, she experiences significant back pain. In working with the hospice nurses, you recommend removing meperidine from Mrs. Stuart's as-needed drug list for which major reason?

a. There is no role for meperidine in the person with cancer.
b. It can constrict the sphincter of Oddi.
c. The principle mode of actions is not at the opiate receptors.
d. It can contribute to hypertensive effects and subsequent headaches.

13. In Mrs. Stuart's last days, the hydration is stopped and a continuous narcotic drip maintained. Mr. Stuart questions about how his wife can be comfortable as she becomes dehydrated. Your best explanation includes all of the following *except:*
a. As Mrs. Stuart's body shuts down, the fluid would contribute to body edema.
b. Fluid in the lungs can result in the "gurgle sound" often associated with death.
c. Frequent oral care and lip moisturizer can ease the oral discomfort.
d. The fluid would hasten her death.

ANSWERS

12. Palliative care principles of comfort and dignity in the last stage of life guide the care Mrs. Stuart receives. In addition to the value of administering other narcotics for pain relief, meperidine should be avoided in the patient with hepatic failure. Meperidine constricts the sphincter of Oddi, contributing further to bilirubin buildup. *Answer 12:* **b.**

13. Fluid other than what the person is able to take in on his or her own can contribute to fluid overload for the dying person's body. Dehydration diminishes the fluid in the oral cavity that the person needs to manage and can assist in drying up secretions that would otherwise cause gurgling or choking sounds. As Mrs. Stuart dies, her body functions decrease accordingly with slow multisystem organ failure. The less fluid that is administered, the less the kidneys need to process. The additional fluid would serve to prolong Mrs. Stuart's life without contributing to any type of quality existence. *Answer 13:* **d.**

QUESTIONS

---

14. In a discussion with David 3 months after the loss of his mother, you inquire into how he is doing without his "health care companion." Which of the following responses suggest potentially unhealthy coping?
a. "My mother had been telling me ever since I was diagnosed 10 years ago that she would do anything if she could

take my place with this cancer. Well, she got her wish."
b. "I feel stronger since her death, as if she is taking care of me from a distance."
c. "Have you noticed how my counts are improving and my transfusion requirements are less? You see there really was something to her hopes for exchanging her life for mine."
d. "I really didn't need my mother to accompany me all those years. It is much easier parking and walking up here. I don't need to worry about her getting tired waiting for me, and so forth."

ANSWERS

14. The bereavement process takes time that is marked by certain milestone dates. It was clear even to you while caring for David that his mother was often focused on what she could do for her son. She had almost feelings of guilt that cancer should happen to her son and there was nothing she could do for him. Contributing something tangible to him was so important to her as she often voiced her inability to control what was occurring to him. Answers a, b, and c reflect a means for David to adjust to his mother's death. These are examples of David incorporating her death into some type of meaning and goodness in his present life. Answer d could suggest that David is denying the value his mother had in his life and the role she played in his own illness and recovery. Further discussion is warranted to explore these feelings of denial and to allow him the opportunity to vent in a safe and supportive environment. *Answer 14:* **d.**

REFERENCES

Abramson, S. D., & Abramson, N. (1999). "Common" uncommon anemias. *Am Fam Physician*, 59(4), pp. 851-858.
Berger, B. J., Wrigley, M., & Ladaika, J. C. (1998). Hepatic encephalopathy. In Chernecky, C. C., & Berger, B. J. (Eds.). *Advanced and critical care oncology nursing. Managing primary complications* (pp. 220-243). Philadelphia: WB Saunders.
Blinder, M. A. (1998). Anemia and transfusion therapy. In Carey, C. F., Lee, H. H., & Woeltje, K. F. (Eds.). *The Washington manual of medical therapeutics* (pp. 360-371). Philadelphia: Lippincott Williams & Wilkins.
Erickson, J. M. (1996). Anemia. *Semin Oncol Nurs, 12,* pp. 2-14.
Friedman, L. S. (1998). Liver, biliary tract, and pancreas. In Tierney, L. M., McPhee, S. J., & Papadakis, M. A. (Eds.). Stamford, CT: Appleton and Lange. pp. 628-665.

Ghalib R. (1998). Hepatic diseases. In Carey, C. F., Lee, H. H., & Woeltje, K. F. (Eds.). *The Washington manual of medical therapeutics* (pp. 329-342). Philadelphia: Lippincott Williams & Wilkins.

Lin, E. M. (1998). Jaundice. In Preston, F. A., & Cunningham, R. S. (Eds.). *Clinical guidelines for symptom management: A handbook for advanced practice nurses* (pp. 51-57). Baltimore: Clinical Insights Press.

Linker, C. A. (1998). Blood. In Tierney, L. M., McPhee, S. J., & Papadakis, M. A. (Eds.). *Current medical diagnosis and treatment*, 37th ed. (pp. 479-533). Stamford, CT: Appleton and Lange.

Little, D. (1999). Ambulatory management of common forms of anemia. *Am Fam Physician, 59*(6), pp. 1598-1604.

Ludwig, H., & Fritz, E. (1998). Anemia in cancer patients. *Semin Oncol, 25*(3), pp. 2-6.

Nail, L. M. (2000). Fatigue. In Nevidjon, B. M., & Sowers, K. W. (Eds.). *A nurse's guide to cancer care* (pp. 373-383). Philadelphia: Lippincott Williams & Wilkins.

Okuda, T., Kurokawa, K., & Papadakis, M. A. (1998). Fluid and electrolyte disorders. In Tierney, L. M., McPhee, S. J., & Papadakis, M. A. (Eds.). *Current medical diagnosis and treatment*, 37th ed. (pp 824-849). Stamford, CT: Appleton and Lange.

Pearson, L. J. (2000). Nurse practitioner's drug handbook, 3rd ed. (p. 679). Springhouse, PA: Springhouse Corporation.

Singer, G. G. (1998). Fluid and electrolyte management. In Carey, C. F., Lee, H. H., & Woeltje, K. F. (Eds.). *The Washington manual of therapeutics* (pp. 39-55). Philadelphia: Lippincott Williams & Wilkins.

Worrall, L. M., Tompkins, C. A., & Rust, D. (1999). Recognizing and managing anemia. *Clin J Oncol Nurs, 3*(4), pp. 153-160.

15 Oncologic Emergency: Case 1

Leslie Mathews

Peggy Princeton is a 39-year-old white woman who was diagnosed 18 months ago with non-Hodgkin's lymphoma. She was treated with six cycles of CHOP (cyclophosphamide, doxorubicin, oncovin, prednisone) chemotherapy. She returns today with complaints of an enlarged node in the right side of her neck and back pain that she characterizes as a tight, burning pain going around the chest; the pain is aggravated by lying down. Fine-needle aspirate of the enlarged supraclavicular lymph node demonstrates recurrence of Mrs. Princeton's lymphoma, and a chest radiograph reveals a bony lesion at T10 that is suspicious for epidural involvement.

QUESTIONS

1. What would you anticipate as the primary and initial management strategy for Mrs. Princeton?
   a. Resumption of CHOP chemotherapy until back pain can be further evaluated
   b. Use of second-line chemotherapy for lymphoma because the back pain will resolve as the primary tumor is treated
   c. Order for a magnetic resonance image (MRI) of the entire spine
   d. Order for a computed tomography (CT)-guided biopsy of the extradural lesion for histology

ANSWERS

1. Spinal cord compression (SCC) is a true neurologic emergency that develops in approximately 10% of patients with cancer (Bucholtz, 1999). It is a medical emergency because prompt intervention may prevent permanent neurologic disability. The therapy for the recurrent lymphoma will be put on hold until the potential SCC is stabilized. The outcome of treatment is directly related to how quickly symptoms are manifested and the patient's pretreatment neu-

rologic status. Without prompt treatment, the patient may sustain partial or complete paralysis, which can be nonreversible. Ambulatory patients have the best prognosis and are most likely to maintain their functional status. Any new or worsening back pain in a patient with cancer demands urgent radiographic evaluation. *Answer 1:* **c.**

QUESTIONS

2. Before initiation of treatment, what is the most critical prognostic factor in SCC?
   a. Type and histologic grade of the primary tumor
   b. Location of the tumor within the spinal cord
   c. Degree of neurologic deficit
   d. Level of tumor and degree of compression on the spinal cord

ANSWERS

2. Neurologic status before treatment is the single most critical prognostic factor in SCC. This argues for prompt recognition and treatment of SCC. Rehabilitative potential depends on the patient's pretreatment status and response to treatment. Of ambulatory patients, 80% remain ambulatory after treatment; however, only 30% of those with significant motor dysfunction are ambulatory after treatment (Bucholtz, 1999). *Answer 2:* **c.**

QUESTIONS

3. Mrs. Princeton's husband, Patrick, says, "I've only heard of spinal cord injuries in the neck, so isn't this rare to have this problem in the back?" Based on your knowledge of spinal involvement, in which area of the spine do most epidural metastases occur?
   a. Cervical
   b. Thoracic
   c. Lumbar
   d. Sacral

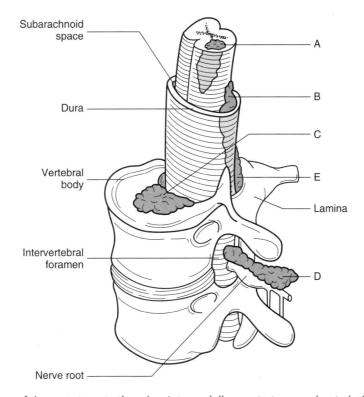

Subarachnoid space

Dura

Vertebral body

Intervertebral foramen

Nerve root

A

B

C

E

Lamina

D

Figure 15-1 Locations of the metastases to the spine. Intramedullary metastases are located within the spinal cord *(A)*. Leptomeningeal metastases are in the subarachnoid space *(B)* and are extramedullary and intradural. Epidural metastases arise from the extension of metastases located in the adjacent vertebral column *(C)*, in the paravertebral spaces throughout the intervertebral foramina *(D)*, or rarely, in the epidural space itself *(E)*. As these epidural metastases grow, they compress adjacent blood vessels, nerve roots, and the spinal cord, resulting in local and referred pain, radiculopathy, and myelopathy. (From Byrne, T. N. [1992]. Spinal cord compression from epidural metastases. *N Engl J Med, 327,* p. 614. Copyright 1992 Massachusetts Medical Society.)

ANSWERS

3. The thoracic spine is the most common site for epidural metastases, accounting for 70% of all occurrences; the next most common sites are the lumbosacral spine (20%) and the cervical spine (10%) (Held & Peahota, 1993). The most common solid tumors that cause SCC are breast, lung, prostate, kidney, and melanoma; hematologic malignancies that may cause SCC are multiple myeloma and lymphoma. SCC can occur at any time during the disease course, and in 10% of patients, it is the initial presenting symptom of the cancer. The onset of SCC may be prolonged, but once cord damage begins, the process can move along very quickly.

Most malignant lesions cause SCC by direct extension of tumor in the vertebral column, which invades the epidural space. This accounts for 95% of all SCC. The physiologic response to this mechanical compression injury is edema and inflammation. This is caused by obstruction of the venous plexus, which supplies the spinal cord. The extent and severity of neurologic symptoms depend on the rate and degree of compression (Ruckdeschel, 2000). See Figure 15-1. *Answer 3:* **b.**

QUESTIONS

4. You need to evaluate the extent of Mrs. Princeton's pain. The most common presenting symptom of SCC includes all of the following descriptions of pain *except:*
   a. Worsening back pain
   b. Bilateral lower extremity pain
   c. Pain while coughing
   d. Pain while having a bowel movement

5. What other findings would you expect when examining Mrs. Princeton?
   a. Respiratory difficulty
   b. Diarrhea
   c. Immobility
   d. Tenderness to spinal percussion

6. Mrs. Princeton tells you that she was moving some heavy furniture in her living room when the pain in her back started. Then she asks, "Couldn't this all be from muscle strain or a slipped disc?" The best response to her is that back pain in metastatic cord compression:
   a. Is aggravated by activity
   b. Is worsened with recumbency
   c. Progresses in a stocking-glove distribution
   d. Develops in a cephalocaudal manner

7. Mrs. Princeton's initial presenting symptom was back pain. What is the usual order for the development of the signs and symptoms of SCC?
   a. Pain, weakness, autonomic dysfunction, sensory loss
   b. Pain, weakness, sensory loss, autonomic dysfunction
   c. Weakness, sensory loss, pain, autonomic dysfunction
   d. Sensory loss, weakness, autonomic dysfunction, pain

––––––––––––––––––––––––––– **ANSWERS**

4-5. Worsening back pain is the most common presenting symptom of SCC, occurring in approximately 96% of patients. It may occur weeks or months before the compression takes place. The pain may be localized or radicular. Localized pain occurs over the area of involvement and is usually found within one or two vertebrae of the compression. Radicular pain is caused by compression of the nerve roots and is found in the dermatome of the affected area (Henson & Posner, 1993). The pain may be exacerbated by movement, change in position, cough, any act resulting in a Valsalva maneuver or physical strain, and on straight leg lifting. Back pain is often accompanied by tenderness to percussion at the affected site. *Answer 4:* **c.** *Answer 5:* **d.**

6. The main description of pain that distinguishes benign disc disease from SCC caused by cancer is that the pain is worse on recumbency. Metastatic SCC is not aggravated by activity but is sometimes improved with it. Often, a coincidental strain may occur. This situation still needs very close attention and follow-up. In the setting of known metastatic disease or in patients with lung, breast, or prostate cancer; myeloma; or lymphoma with high risk of developing metastasis, the tenet is to rule out SCC first. *Answer 6:* **b.**

7. The signs and symptoms of SCC are well known and usually occur in a stepwise, progressive manner if diagnosis and treatment are delayed.

The first symptom after the development of back pain at the affected site is usually weakness. This is followed by sensory loss in the affected dermatome distribution, which most often occurs before actual motor loss. Autonomic dysfunction with urinary retention, constipation, and loss of bowel and bladder control is a later and ominous finding because full paraplegia can quickly follow (Ruckdeschel, 2000). *Answer 7:* **b.**

QUESTIONS –––––––––––––––––––––––––

8. You ask Mrs. Princeton to perform heel-toe walking. What is it that you are trying to assess?
   a. Motor strength
   b. Sensory function
   c. Autonomic function
   d. Performance status

––––––––––––––––––––––––––– **ANSWERS**

8. Evaluating motor weakness includes assessment of muscle strength, paralyses, atrophy, involuntary movements, convulsions, gait or incoordination, and reflexes. Various approaches may be used to evaluate muscle strength, including performing deep knee bends, walking on heels, and walking on toes. The weakness is most obvious in the proximal muscles of the lower extremities. The patient may report difficulty rising from low chairs or a toilet seat or when climbing stairs. This information can be used to determine the level of compression and the total extent of impairment. *Answer 8:* **a.**

QUESTIONS –––––––––––––––––––––––––

9. Mrs. Princeton questions why you are sticking her with a pin up her legs. You explain that you are evaluating loss of feeling and sensations. What is this particular test called?
   a. Stereognosis
   b. Vibratory sense
   c. Romberg test
   d. Point localization

––––––––––––––––––––––––––– **ANSWERS**

9. It is important to evaluate the extent of involvement of the spinal tracts controlling the senses of temperature, touch, position sense, and vibratory sense. You should assess for sensations and symptoms of sensory loss, including numbness, tingling, paresthesia, and feelings of coldness in the affected area. Sensory levels to light touch and pinprick are landmarks for dermatome involvement. The location of the sensory loss helps pinpoint the site of the sensory damage. Deficits are described in relation to the dermatome distribution, which is the area of skin innervated by the sensory nerve root of a spinal segment. Vibratory sense is evaluated by placing a tuning fork on a bony prominence. Stereognosis is another test used to evaluate sensory function; it tests the ability to distinguish forms by placing objects in the patient's hands while his or her eyes are closed. The Romberg test evaluates stance and sense of balance. The test is performed by asking the patient to stand with feet together, eyes open, and then eyes closed (Bates, 1995). *Answer 9:* **d.**

QUESTIONS

10. What is the diagnostic test of choice for SCC confirmation in the cancer patient?
   a. Plain radiographs
   b. CT scans
   c. MRI
   d. Myelogram

ANSWERS

10. Plain films, CT scans, and bone scans are sometimes used initially for evaluating SCC, but they are generally regarded as not sufficiently sensitive; use of myelography or MRI is most preferred. Myelography has been found to be equal to MRI in accuracy of diagnosis. However, myelography is an invasive procedure and may be dangerous to patients with increased intercranial pressure or thrombocytopenia. MRI tends to be the diagnostic test of choice because it can give information concerning the presence of early metastasis elsewhere; it can also show if lesions are epidural, intradural, or intramedullary. The disadvantage of MRI is that patients need to lie still for 1 to 2 hours. In these cases myelography is a useful alternative. *Answer 10:* **c.**

QUESTIONS

11. In working with Mrs. Princeton, what are your goals of treatment for SCC?
   1. Preservation of neurologic function
   2. Palliation of pain
   3. Prevention of regional recurrence
   4. Preservation of spinal stability
      a. 1, 2, & 4
      b. 2, 3, & 4
      c. 1, 2, & 3
      d. All of these

ANSWERS

11. The intent of treatment is generally palliative but is mainly directed at recovery and maintenance of normal neurologic function, stabilization of the spine, and pain control. The choice of treatment depends on (1) the histology of the tumor; (2) the level, speed of onset, duration, and degree of block; (3) the site of presentation of the spinal involvement—anterior versus posterior; (4) the patient's functional level; and (5) prior therapy and available treatment modalities (Bucholtz, 1999). See Figure 15-2. *Answer 11:* **d.**

QUESTIONS

12. Mrs. Princeton tells you that she really does not want to take steroids because she knows she will get pudgy and does not want her husband to think she is getting fat. What major point about dexamethasone will you *strongly* emphasize when responding to Mrs. Princeton?
   a. It can shrink the tumor.
   b. It can be stopped if side effects occur.
   c. High-dose nonsteroidal antiinflammatory drugs (NSAIDs) are as effective.
   d. It may not be necessary if the radiation therapy starts immediately.

ANSWERS

12. Corticosteroids are used to relieve compression as rapidly as possible to prevent further damage to the spinal cord. Steroids have an oncolytic effect in that they may relieve SCC by shrinking tumors, especially in lymphoma and breast cancer, while also reducing the edema surrounding the tumor. The use of corticosteroids is definitive; the dosage is controversial. Based on the patient's signs and symptoms and a high index of suspicion for developing SCC, steroid administration may be started before the completion of the necessary diagnostic tests. Steroid-related side effects are common, requiring specific monitoring. The most commonly used regimens of dexamethasone are listed as follows:

   Loading dose of 100 mg intravenously followed by 24 mg orally four times a day
   10 mg to start, followed by 4 mg every 6 hours

The duration of steroid therapy is based on the patient's response to treatment. Tapering is done during radiation therapy (Bucholtz, 1999; Fuller, Heiss, & Oldfield, 1997). *Answer 12:* **a.**

QUESTIONS

13. What is the most commonly used treatment modality for SCC?
   a. Radiation therapy
   b. Surgery
   c. Surgery followed by radiation therapy
   d. Chemotherapy

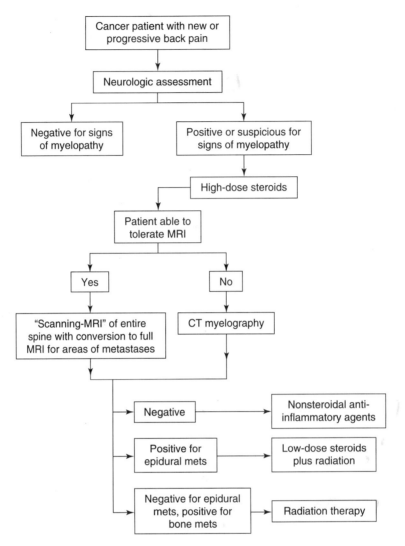

Figure 15-2 Myelography treatment algorithm. *CT,* Computed tomography; *MRI,* magnetic resonance imaging. (From Abeloff, M. D., Armitage, J. O., Lichter, A. S., & Niederhuber, J. E. [Eds.]. [2000]. *Clinical oncology,* 2nd ed. [p. 815]. Philadelphia, Churchill Livingstone.)

ANSWERS

13. Radiation therapy is the most commonly used treatment for patients with SCC. The general approach is to identify the site of the compression by MRI and to design a radiation portal that includes the site of compression and two vertebral bodies above and below the lesion. The dosage range varies slightly but is generally 30 to 50 Gy over 2 to 4 weeks. Steroids are usually tapered during radiation therapy (Fuller, Heiss, & Oldfield, 1997). If steroids are withdrawn prematurely or if the patient experiences increased neurologic deterioration, the steroid dosage will need to be increased. If the patient continues to experience symptoms while taking dexamethasone or if the patient has a highly unstable condition, surgery may be indicated.

Surgery is used in patients who develop SCC at sites that have already been irradiated, if the neurologic deficits are worsening while the patient is taking steroids and receiving radiation therapy, or when spinal instability results from vertebral destruction or collapse. It includes laminectomy for a posterior compression or vertebral body resection for an anterior compression.

Unfortunately, many patients in this situation are not candidates for aggressive surgery because of multiple vertebral body metastases and/or narrow life expectancies from advanced cancer. In these cases radiation therapy is offered with limited expectation of neurologic recovery. See Figure 15-3. *Answer 13:* **a.**

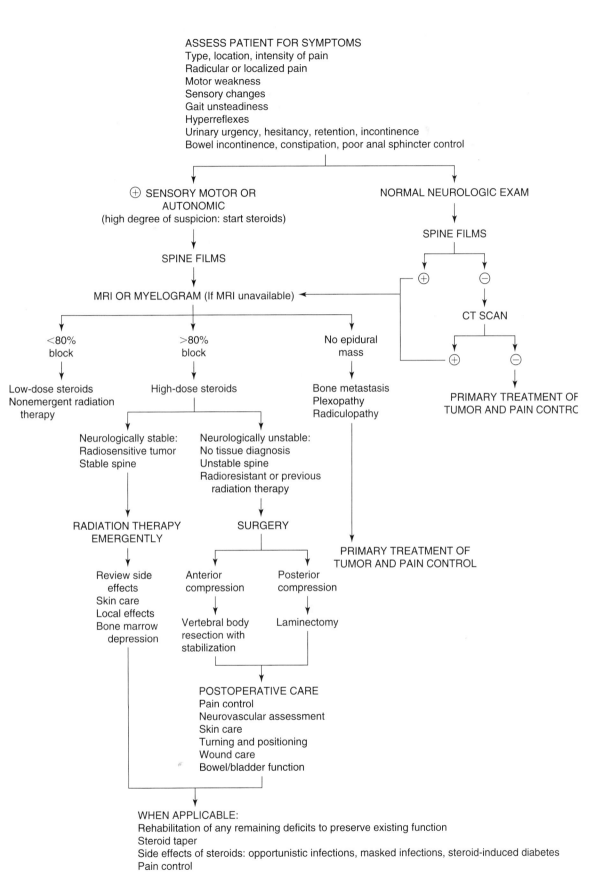

Figure 15-3 Clinical pathway for spinal cord compression. *CT,* Computed tomography; *MRI,* magnetic resonance imaging. (From Yarbro, C. H., Frogge, M. H., Goodman, M., & Groenwald, S. L. [2000]. *Cancer nursing: Principles and practice,* 5th ed. [p. 894]. Boston: Jones and Bartlett.)

Case Study continued

Mrs. Princeton was started on a course of dexamethasone and has been receiving radiation therapy to the affected area. She presents today with difficulty walking, foot drop, and complaints of urinary incontinence.

QUESTIONS

14. Evaluation of autonomic impairment requires evaluation of all of the following *except:*
  a. Bowel function and rectal sphincter tone
  b. Bladder function
  c. Ability to swallow and dysphagia
  d. Sexual function

ANSWERS

14. Patients experiencing difficulty walking should be maintained on bed rest until further evaluation. Bowel and bladder alterations need to be defined in terms of urgency, frequency, level of control of function, retention, and incontinence. Rectal sphincter tone should be evaluated by a rectal examination. Sexual function may also be impaired. It is important to evaluate patterns of dysfunction, recent changes, and associated signs and symptoms. Women may have normal sexual function, but genital sensation may be absent; with men, the impairment depends on prior function, the level and duration of the compression, and the status of the sacral reflex paths (Wilkes, 1996). Swallowing problems and dysphagia are not often associated with autonomic dysfunction. *Answer 14:* **c.**

Case Study conclusion

Mrs. Princeton had an anterior decompression, which involves resecting the vertebral body along with the tumor, followed by spinal stabilization with metal rods. Her postoperative period is uneventful, her spine is stable, and she is now ready to be discharged. You are called in to assist in making the home care arrangements.

Orders and recommendations include the following:
1. Provide adequate pain control as needed.
2. Provide rehabilitation of any remaining deficits to preserve existing function.
3. Consult with occupational and physical therapists.
4. Perform range-of-motion and isometric exercises after physical therapy evaluation.
5. Evaluate motor and sensory deficits and autonomic function.
6. Encourage independence within the limitations of the neurologic deficits.
7. Encourage patient and family to express concerns about the residual limitations.

To promote the return to normalcy, rehabilitation goals should be determined early in the treatment plan and reevaluated periodically.

REFERENCES

Bates, B. (1995). *A guide to physical examination*, 2nd ed. Philadelphia: Lippincott.

Bucholtz, J. D. (1999). Metastatic epidural spinal cord compression. *Semin Oncol Nurs, 15*, pp. 150-159.

Fuller, B. G., Heiss, J., & Oldfield, E. H. (1997). Spinal cord compression. In Devita, V. T., Hellman, S., & Rosenberg, S. (Eds.). *Cancer: Principles and practice of oncology*, 5th ed. Philadelphia: Lippincott-Raven.

Held, J. L., & Peahota, A. (1993). Nursing care of the patient with spinal cord compression. *Oncol Nurs Forum, 20*, pp. 1507-1514.

Henson, J. W., & Posner, J. B. (1993). Neurological complications. In Holland, J. F., Frei, E., Bast, R. C., et al. (Eds.). *Cancer medicine*, 3rd ed. Philadelphia: Lea & Febiger.

Ruckdeschel, J. C. (2000). Spinal cord compression. In Abeloff, M. D., Armitage, J. O., Lichter, A. S., & Niederhuber, J. E. (Eds.). *Clinical oncology*, 2nd ed. New York: Churchill Livingstone.

Wilkes, G. M. (1996). Neurological disturbances. In Groenwald, S. L., Goodman, M., Frogge, M. H., & Yarbro, C. H. (Eds.). *Cancer symptom management*. Boston: Jones and Bartlett.

16 Oncologic Emergency: Case 2

Esther Muscari Lin

Jenny Hayes is a 47-year-old woman status post an autologous bone marrow transplant for relapsed Hodgkin's disease. Key to Jenny's long health history is initial treatment with MOPP-ABVD upon relapse and, once clear of disease, a course of mantle radiation consolidation. The cytoablative regimen consisted of high-dose cyclophosphamide and etopside. Within days of her reinfusion, she developed an oral mucositis and the skin over her chest desquamated (Figure 16-1).

QUESTIONS

1. What is the most likely cause of her skin desquamation?
  a. Acute effects of the chemotherapy
  b. Delayed effects of mantle radiation therapy
  c. Acute effects of mantle radiation therapy
  d. Radiation recall

2. What life-threatening risk does the desquamation pose?
  a. Infection
  b. Bleeding
  c. Hypovolemia
  d. Electrolyte imbalance

3. What are three goals of care for Jenny while she experiences these skin changes?
  a. _____
  b. _____
  c. _____

4. Assessment of Jenny's oral cavity reveals open ulcerations, bleeding, pale and sloughing mucosa, and cream-colored patches on the tongue and palate. What assumption can you make about the mucositis that would contribute the *most* to your treatment plan for Jenny?
  a. The mucositis extends the entire length of the gastrointestinal tract.

  b. A candidal infection is present.
  c. The pain will resolve once the infection resolves.
  d. The salivary glands were affected by the radiation therapy, leading to a thicker, more difficult-to-manage saliva.

5. Which of the assumptions in question 4 has the highest chance of being incorrect and contributing the least, if anything, to a plan of care?

6. In intervening to provide pain relief, the resident hesitates to prescribe a continuous infusion and is unsure why oral as-needed morphine is inadequate. What characteristic of the advanced practice nurse (APN) role empowers the APN to advocate on the patient's behalf so that the plan can change?
  a. Knowledge of the research regarding around-the-clock pain control
  b. Ability to collaborate with all members of the health care team
  c. Expertise in pain management
  d. Ability to anticipate the bone marrow transplant course

ANSWERS

1. Certain chemotherapy agents can cause radiation recall. Radiation recall usually occurs within days of receiving the drug, and there is not a time limit from when the radiation was received in the past. The desquamation is contained to the skin within the mantle radiation field. The skin usually becomes inflamed, erythematous, friable, and tender to touch. Patients report feeling as if they have a terrible sunburn and may experience chills from the discomfort. *Answer 1:* **d.**

2. Because the skin is the initial barrier against infection, once the integrity is altered, the potential for superficial infection and bacterial entrance into the bloodstream is great. *Answer 2:* **a.**

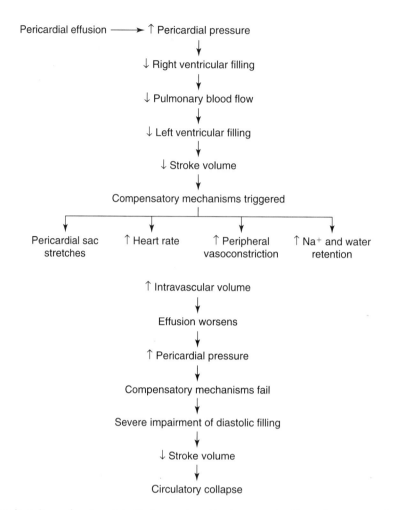

Pericardial effusion ⟶ ↑ Pericardial pressure

↓ Right ventricular filling

↓ Pulmonary blood flow

↓ Left ventricular filling

↓ Stroke volume

Compensatory mechanisms triggered

| Pericardial sac stretches | ↑ Heart rate | ↑ Peripheral vasoconstriction | ↑ Na⁺ and water retention |

↑ Intravascular volume

Effusion worsens

↑ Pericardial pressure

Compensatory mechanisms fail

Severe impairment of diastolic filling

↓ Stroke volume

Circulatory collapse

Figure 16-1 Pathophysiology of pericardial effusion and cardiac tamponade. (From Dragonette, P. [1998]. Malignant pericardial effusion and cardiac tamponade. In Chernecky, C. C., & Berger B. B. [Eds.]. *Advanced and critical care oncology nursing*. Philadelphia: WB Saunders.)

3. Goals of care include keeping the area clean, attempting to maintain any remaining skin integrity with a skin gel or topical barrier, and providing pain relief. If a venous access device is in the field, which in Jenny's case it is, an additional challenge is how to keep the device maintained without a traditional dressing. *Answer 3:* **See text.**

4-6. Expertise with any specialized patient population promotes identification of trends in patient and family responses as well as a repertoire of experiences from which to pull previous attempts at problem management, and so on. In this case, as with any patient receiving therapy, side effects of the drugs and their time of onset can be anticipated. Mucositis from the high dosages of etoposide is expected within days of drug infusion and neutropenia onset. The gastrointestinal tract, from mouth to anus lined continuously, with the highly

dividing cells within the mucosa, can be altered anywhere along the tract. It is safe to assume that Jenny's esophagus and oral cavity are involved. Knowing that the mucositis will persist until engraftment, you know she is going to be in pain until at least then, anywhere from 7 to 14 days, with the mucositis potentially worsening before improving. As long as Jenny is neutropenic, she will experience the pain from the mucositis. Anticipating the length of time she will have this severe sore throat as the mucosa is sloughed and her gastrointestinal tract remains raw also indicates how swallowing and potential nausea will make it difficult for Jenny to take any oral medications. Therefore the recommended pain regimen is inadequate for two reasons: There is an inability to take the prescribed regimen, and the peaks and valleys of intermittent drug administration will not achieve as great a comfort as with continuous drug infusion. It does not take into account that the severity and length of the pain expected from the symptom of mucositis. It is unreasonable to wait out the time of infection resolution. Even though there is a superimposed oral infection, most likely extending the length of the gastrointestinal tract as well, it is only contributing to the pain, not causing it. To assume treatment of the candida will resolve the pain reinforces the recommendation for intermittent, as-needed pain management in combination with oral fungal treatment. The desquamation must resolve and new tissue begin to form, the prerequisite being white blood cells before the pain will resolve. *Answer 4:* **a.** *Answer 5:* **c.** *Answer 6:* **d.**

QUESTIONS

7. Jenny's husband is concerned because she is unable to eat. As you contemplate the value of nutritional support in Jenny, what are contributors to nitrogen loss in her case?
  1. Increased metabolic rate of Hodgkin's disease
  2. Chemotherapy-induced cell destruction
  3. Skin desquamation
  4. Inadequate oral intake
  a. 1, 2, & 3
  b. 2, 3, & 4
  c. 1, 3, & 4
  d. All of these

8. What is the most accurate means for measuring Jenny's lean body mass loss?
  a. Nitrogen balance
  b. Creatinine clearance
  c. Triceps skinfold
  d. Resting energy expenditure (REE)

9. What is the most accurate means for measuring protein and calorie needs?
  a. Estimated energy expenditure
  b. REE
  c. Activity-associated energy expenditure
  d. 1-hour postprandial energy expenditure

ANSWERS

7-8. Nitrogen loss, the most accurate measurement of body mass loss, captures protein breakdown and loss. Any type of tissue breakdown, whether through trauma, surgery, open wounds, burns, or cell destruction, results in protein loss. Some cancers alter the metabolic rate, with the hematologic malignancies being associated with the higher rates, and therefore affect protein-calorie needs. However, Jenny does not have active disease because she was in complete remission be-

fore the transplant and her metabolic needs are influenced by what is physically occurring to her. The skin inflammation and tissue loss with the desquamation result in the need for new tissue, increasing Jenny's needs. As Jenny's inadequate intake remains consistently low, muscle breakdown occurs in the body in attempt to meet the body's protein needs. This also contributes to protein loss and urinary nitrogen. Protein loss is the nitrogen measured as urea in the urine. Lean body mass or skeletal mass is lost from organs such as the heart muscle, body muscles, respiratory muscles, and gastrointestinal mucosa (Tayek, 1995). Measuring the calorie needs of the patient can be done via an estimated measure or an REE measurement in which the amount of oxygen consumed and carbon dioxide produced is measured, determining the caloric needs (Bickston, 1995). *Answer 7:* **b.** *Answer 8:* **a.**

9. The most accurate but expensive method, the REE, requires specialized equipment, which is not available at every institution. The REE is measured when the patient has not eaten or had recent activity. To be in positive nitrogen balance means that the body is in an anabolic state, rather than a catabolic, negative nitrogen balance state. *Answer 9:* **b.**

Case Study continued

Jenny is begun on daily parenteral nutrition (1000 ml of D70) with an order for 20% lipid (500 ml) transfusion three times a week.

QUESTIONS

10. What does the lipid order suggest about Jenny's nutritional status?
  a. Carbohydrate needs are greater than those being met by the amino acid solution.
  b. Additional fat calories are needed each week.
  c. Jenny is slightly fluid overloaded.
  d. Jenny's resting blood glucose is most likely low.

11. What will be the earliest indicator of improved nutritional status?
  a. A negative nitrogen balance
  b. A positive nitrogen balance
  c. A weight increase
  d. An increased albumin level

ANSWERS

10. Standard lipid emulsions of 20% provide 2 kcal/ml, thereby providing an extra 1000 calories with each administration. This order suggests that Jenny's caloric needs are not quite met with the glucose calories (carbohydrate needs) in the parenteral nutrition, which are often written to provide 40% to 65% of calories. Caloric needs are met through a combination of amino acids (protein), lipid emulsions (fat), and dextrose (carbohydrates) (Bickston, 1995). *Answer 10:* **b.**

11. Albumin is a good indicator of somatic and visceral protein stores but has a 21-day half-life. Transferrin, with a 7-day half-life, responds more rapidly to nutritional support and can be a serial marker. Weight changes in the acutely ill patient are more reflective of fluid shifts than lean body mass. Once catabolism stops or is slowed, the nitrogen losses in the urine should decrease, with the nitrogen value moving toward the positive. A positive nitrogen balance is reflective of a state of nutritional recovery (Tayek, 1995). *Answer 11:* **b.**

Case Study continued

As the weeks progress following discharge, although maintaining her weight, Jenny complains of food sticking when she swallows. She is being followed by the Nutritional Support Service (NSS), which has worked closely with her to adjust her diet to accommodate her dysphagia.

QUESTIONS

12. Because you are the person obtaining the history of this present problem from Jenny, you recognize that she ate very little during her hospitalization. Which of the following questions must be asked and documented?
   1. What type of condition are your teeth in?
   2. Where does the difficulty in swallowing lie?
   3. Do you cough when you eat or drink?
   4. Do you have pain when you swallow?
      a. 1, 2, & 3
      b. 2, 3, & 4
      c. 1, 3, & 4
      d. All of these

13. What are risk factors for dysphagia in Jenny?
   1. Lengthy hospitalization and illness period
   2. History of candidal mucositis
   3. Cyclophosphamide-induced neuropathy
   4. Previous mantle radiation
      a. 1, 3, & 4
      b. 2, 3, & 4
      c. 1, 2, & 4
      d. All of these

14. Which of the following are signs and symptoms that Jenny is aspirating?
   1. Choking
   2. Fever
   3. Abnormal lung sounds
   4. Decreased oral intake
      a. 1, 3, & 4
      b. 2, 3, & 4
      c. 1, 2, & 3
      d. All of these

15. What are two potential differential diagnoses for Jenny's reports of dysphagia?
      a. _____
      b. _____

16. What diagnostic study would best reveal swallowing difficulties in Jenny?
      a. Esophagogastroduodenoscopy
      b. Esophageal manometry
      c. Bernstein test
      d. Barium swallow

ANSWERS

12. Assessment questions assist in identifying whether silent or obvious aspiration is occurring, if the insulting cause is increasing in size as the difficulty progresses from solids to liquids, and where along the swallowing stages the problem is occurring. Because swallowing begins in the mouth, dentition and oral structures need to be evaluated for their role in preparing the food bolus. If there is poor dentition or resected oral structures, swallowing will be impaired. In considering risk factors or possible causes for dysphagia in Jenny, it is realistic to consider impairment of oral intake with or without dysphagia because of emotional distress. She has been through a great deal of stress, is still dealing with side effects of an intense therapy, and may have the stress expressed in this fashion. Emotional distress can present in many somatic complaints. Despite it being a possibility, it is important to not limit the consideration of other possibilities. *Answer 12:* **d.**

13. Jenny, like many neutropenic patients, experienced an oral candidiasis, which most likely extended the length of the esophagus. Because of the common incidence of superficial candidiasis, endoscopy is often not performed because diagnosis is made based on the clinical picture and knowledge of the patient's disease and treatment course. Candidal treatment often occurs without tissue scraping/biopsy. Either continued candidal infection or some type of scarring from her previous experience places her at risk for stricture development. A neuropathy from an insulting agent is a possible cause of alterations in the swallowing stages, but cyclophosphamide is not a neurotoxic agent. The mantle radiation is definitely a factor to consider in Jenny or anyone's case as causing fibrosis and subsequent stricture. The advantage in this case is that you know firsthand Jenny's experience through treatment and are aware of the radiation recall she experienced, which is in the same field as the esophagus. Knowing the inflammation and desquamation of the skin that resulted from the radiation therapy causes one to consider the underlying structures and the inflammatory effect on them. *Answer 13:* **c.**

14. Signs and symptoms of aspiration include occasional or frequent choking, difficulty swallowing, fever, rales, or decreased breath sounds, often associated with pneumonia. Pain or odynophagia can be associated with infection, reflux esophagitis, abscess, or carcinoma (Chestnutt & Prendergast, 2001; Healey & Jacobson, 1994). *Answer 14:* **c.**

15. Potential differential diagnoses for Jenny include radiation fibrosis, infection, disease recurrence, and gastroesophageal reflux disease. *Answer 15:* **See text.**

16. Radiologic diagnosis with a barium swallow provides views of the barium-induced distended esophagus and pharynx (Nolan, 1998). Fluoroscopic and radiographic examination allow observation of the barium as it passes through the digestive tract, with spot films being taken (Healey & Jacobson, 1994). Barium swallow visualizes the entire length of the esophagus. With the esophageal stricture, the upper limit of the esophagus is distended and then narrows significantly. *Answer 16:* **d.**

Case Study continued

In the 6 months following Jenny's reinfusion, she has numerous complications, including gastrointestinal bleeding, an infected Hickman catheter, and an esophageal stricture. The ability for Jenny to receive the bulk of her care as an outpatient and remain in her home is largely because of the efforts of you, the APN, and the home care nurse, Holly, whom you work with closely. Jenny seems to have experienced a gamut of symptoms, often so general and nonspecific that identifying just one cause has been a challenge. Holly calls you Monday morning to report that Jenny is slightly more tachypneic than

the past week. She has been afebrile and seems a little short of breath, with an occasional cough upon walking through the house, but other than an accompanying tachycardia, she has no other profound signs or symptoms. Jenny refuses to come to the outpatient clinic and reassures Holly that she will call if she feels worse. Holly has drawn a complete blood count (CBC) and collected a urine sample for urinalysis (UA). After reviewing the normal results of the CBC and UA, you call Jenny at noon to check on her. You are struck by how short of breath Jenny sounds when she answers the telephone. Upon asking her where she was in the house when the phone rang, she answers "on the couch, next to the phone." Surprisingly, Jenny reports not feeling alarmed and would rather wait for her husband to come home from work before coming to the hospital.

QUESTIONS

17. Why should you not wait until the end of the day?

18. Which of the following diagnostic tests should be done first?
   a. Chest computed tomography (CT) scan
   b. Chest radiograph
   c. Pulmonary function tests (PFTs)
   d. Ventilation-perfusion ($\dot{V}/\dot{Q}$) scan

ANSWERS

17. Because of Jenny's complex history, the first possible problems for consideration are those she has experienced before: aspiration pneumonia, gastrointestinal bleeding, and infection. The laboratory tests drawn earlier in the day can be reviewed and compared with previous results so that the aforementioned problems can be ruled out rather quickly. In addition to the fact that Jenny's laboratory tests just ruled out earlier problems suggesting a new potential emergency, Jenny sounds as if her breathing pattern has worsened since Holly's earlier visit. She could be experiencing a pulmonary embolus, acute respiratory distress syndrome, pulmonary fibrosis, or cardiac failure requiring immediate evaluation. *Answer 17:* **See text.**

18. The fact that Jenny's shortness of breath is so striking and of an acute nature, immediate pulmonary evaluation is indicated. Insight and direction into pulmonary problems, whether cardiac or pulmonary in nature, can be quickly gained with a chest radiograph. A radiograph is often easier and quicker to obtain than a CT scan. It will be a good screening tool that can lead to more extensive diagnostic tests such as a CT, PFTs, and ($\dot{V}/\dot{Q}$) scan. *Answer 18:* **b.**

QUESTIONS

19. What finding on chest radiography would result in PFTs being ordered?
a. Diffuse pulmonary infiltrates with honeycomb-like appearance
b. Bilateral white out extending from the lung bases to midlung
c. Air space opacities with vascular redistribution
d. Right-sided atelectasis with a pleural effusion

20. What would you expect on physical examination of Jenny's lungs if she were experiencing pulmonary fibrosis?
a. Decreased lung expansion, increased breath sounds, wheezes
b. Decreased lung expansion, decreased breath sounds, rales
c. Increased lung expansion, decreased breath sounds, rhonchi
d. Increased lung expansion, increased breath sounds, wheezes

21. What might be found on a room air blood gas that would be consistent with pulmonary fibrosis?
a. Normal bicarbonate level, normal Po_2, elevated Pco_2
b. Low bicarbonate level, normal Po_2, elevated Pco_2
c. Elevated bicarbonate level, low Po_2, elevated Pco_2
d. Normal bicarbonate level, normal Po_2, normal Pco_2

22. PFTs in a person with pulmonary fibrosis are consistent with which of the following results?
a. Reduced lung volumes, increased forced vital capacity, increased diffusing lung capacity of oxygen (DLco)
b. Reduced lung volumes, reduced forced vital capacity, reduced DLco
c. Increased lung volumes, increased forced vital capacity, reduced DLco
d. Increased airway resistance, reduced forced vital capacity, increased DLco

ANSWERS

19-22. Radiation-induced pulmonary fibrosis tends to develop 2 to 4 months after treatment,

with patients presenting with cough, dyspnea, and pleuritic chest pain. The chest radiograph may show pulmonary infiltrates because of diffuse alveolar damage with interstitial fibrosis (Walsh & Flower, 1998). Classic symptoms include dyspnea, anxiety, and restlessness. Presenting signs include a dry cough with decreased breath sounds and decreased thoracic expansion, rales, and the use of accessory muscles. PFTs determine lung function. Because of the capillary damage/fibrosis, the tissue is being ventilated but not perfused. As lung volumes and vital capacities are reduced, so is lung expansion and the distance your hands spread when placed on the patient's back during inspiration. DLco will be low because the diffusing capacity of helium, carbon monoxide, oxygen, and nitrogen is affected by the disease states (Timmerman, 1998). *Answer 19:* **a.** *Answer 20:* **b.** *Answer 21:* **d.** *Answer 22:* **b.**

Case Study continued

Jenny's chest radiograph reveals lungs absent of infiltrates, effusions, or lesions. The notable and questionable area is an enlarged cardiac silhouette with hilar adenopathy, prompting an emergent follow-up study.

QUESTIONS

23. Why would an echocardiogram be ordered instead of a chest CT scan?
a. The echocardiogram differentiates between tumor and fluid better than CT.
b. The echocardiogram will identify the substance as being an exudate or transudate that is creating the shadow.
c. CT takes longer to schedule and duplicates the information that can be obtained from an echocardiogram.
d. CT does not provide hemodynamic information.

ANSWERS

23. An echocardiogram will show the presence of fluid between the heart and pericardium and will provide mitral valve flow and hemodynamic information. An MRI could provide more information by displaying the myocardial wall in addition to the cardiac chamber cavities. Also, an MRI may be an advantageous approach when the two-dimensional echocardiogram cannot delineate the extent of cardiac chamber wall involvement. CT would not be able to provide the hemodynamic details (Hackworth & Lipton, 1998). *Answer 23:* **d.**

Case Study continued

The two-dimensional echocardiogram performed on Jenny's heart finds changes in the size of the ventricles with inspiration, approximately 500 ml fluid in the pericardial sac, and an increased ejection fraction. The diagnoses of pericardial effusion and tamponade are made.

QUESTIONS

24. What finding on echocardiogram confirms tamponade?
- **a.** Chamber pressures equal to intracardial pressures
- **b.** Large pericardial effusion
- **c.** Tachycardia
- **d.** Increased ejection fraction

25. On review of Jenny's vital signs, her blood pressure is stable at 110/70 mm Hg. How is it that her blood pressure is maintained in light of the diagnosis of pericardial effusion and cardiac tamponade?
- **a.** She is well hydrated.
- **b.** Her stroke volume is supported by an increased ejection fraction.
- **c.** She leads a sedentary lifestyle.
- **d.** She maintains an upright position.

26. What is a hallmark vital sign finding for cardiac tamponade?
- **a.** The systolic pressure is auscultated only during inspiration.
- **b.** The systolic pressure is auscultated only during expiration.
- **c.** Orthostatic charges are seen in systolic measurements and pulse rate.
- **d.** The difference between the systolic and diastolic measurements increases as tamponade progresses.

27. Based on the pathophysiology associated with cardiac tamponade, during tamponade when ventricular filling is at its maximum, the ventricles are:
- **a.** Overfilled
- **b.** Highly excitable
- **c.** Underfilled
- **d.** Flaccid

28. With florid tamponade, what is the underlying pathophysiology for cardiac arrest?
- **a.** Intrapericardial chamber pressures equal to the left atrial and ventricle end-diastolic pressures
- **b.** Atrial filling during diastole in excess of ventricular contraction
- **c.** Increased pulmonary pressures that exceed right ventricular pressure
- **d.** α-Adrenergic stimulation resulting in massive peripheral vasoconstriction and an increased blood return to the right side of the heart

29. What is the value of performing an electrocardiogram?
1. The subxiphoid approach for pericardiocentesis can be monitored.
2. Ischemia can be managed pharmacologically.
3. The size of the effusion can be quantified.
4. Electrical alternans can be documented.
   - **a.** 1 & 2
   - **b.** 2 & 3
   - **c.** 1 & 4
   - **d.** 2 & 4

ANSWERS

24. Assessment for cardiac tamponade includes the clinical signs and symptoms noted in Table 16-1. Chest radiograph performed on a

TABLE 16-1	Clinical Features along the Continuum of Cardiac Tamponade	
MILD	**MODERATE**	**SEVERE**
General malaise	Tachycardia	Restlessness
Dyspnea	Muffled heart sounds	Hypoxia
Vague chest pain/palpitations	Elevation of jugular venous pressure/distended neck veins	Marked jugular venous pressure
Orthopnea		Increasing pulsus paradoxus
Dizziness/light-headedness	Pulsus paradoxus	Hypotension
Cough	Progressive dyspnea	Confusion
	Atrial arrhythmias*	Obtundation
	Low-grade fever*	Cardiac arrest
		Death

From Knoop, T., & Willenberg, K. (1999). Cardiac tamponade. *Semin Oncol Nurs, 15*(3), pp. 168-173.
*Possible, but atypical.

routine basis or in response to a changing physical status might show an increased cardiac silhouette with hilar adenopathy and increased mediastinal width. In combination with reviewing the clinical presentation and the patient's history with the chest radiograph, a two-dimensional echocardiogram is used for an ultrasound of the heart. This can determine the heart size, quantify the amount of pericardial fluid, and document the movements of the valves and chambers (Knoop & Willenberg, 1999; Shepherd, 1997). Electrical alternans, which is an alteration in QRS voltage, is specific for tamponade (Ball & Morrison, 1996). *Answer 24:* **a.**

25. Jenny's vital signs upon arrival are consistent with a gradual fluid accumulation. As the fluid in the pericardial sac increases slowly from the usual amount of 15 to 50 ml, the heart is capable of accommodating. The ventricular stroke volume increases the ejection fraction in the early stages (Ball & Morrison, 1996; Spodnik, 1998). With increases volumes and/or speedier fluid accumulation, the pericardial compression increases, reducing cardiac chamber compliance and limiting the amount of chamber filling. The body compensates with tachycardia and peripheral vasoconstriction to improve venous filling. Over time, the pericardial pressures' constant constriction on heart chamber refilling results in an equilibration of chamber pressures with the intracardiac pressures (Spodnik, 1998). Cardiac tamponade is at the point of heart chambers approaching equilibration with exaggerated fluctuation and measurements to inspiration. During peak inspiration, filling in the left side of the heart is minimal, is below pericardial pressure, and may refill only slightly with mitral valve opening during expiration. Thus volumes and pressures vary continuously during the cardiac cycle as chamber filling volumes vary with respiration (Spodnik, 1998). Because of increasing pericardial pressures, ventricular pressures are high during diastole and resist filling, further decreasing the filling volumes and cardiac output. This is reflected in dropping blood pressures resulting from the falling stroke volumes (see Figure 16-1). *Answer 25:* **b.**

26. Pulsus paradoxus, the hallmark abnormal finding for pericardial tamponade, is when the pulse during systole becomes weaker during inspiration. Pulsus paradoxus can be assessed via sphygmomanometry, palpation, and arterial waveform (Dragonette, 1998). *Answer 26:* **b.**

27. With worsening tamponade, the ventricles are at minimal volume, yet their ability to fill is at their maximum because of the overbearing intrapericardial pressure; therefore the ventricles remain critically underfilled relative to their capacity (Spodnik, 1998). *Answer 27:* **c.**

28-29. At the point of equilibration, cardiac arrest occurs as the heart is unable to pump. An electrocardiogram, in addition to documenting electrical alternans, also demonstrates the approach necessary for catheter insertion from the subxiphoid route (Ball & Morrison, 1996). *Answer 28:* **a.** *Answer 29:* **c.**

Case Study continued

On physical examination, Jenny's lungs are auscultated for some fluid but her dyspnea appears to be the same. Upon cardiac examination, sluggish capillary refill, cool extremities, and most notably muffled heart sounds are noted.

QUESTIONS

30. What is the *main* reason that cardiac tamponade is often not suspected until routine chest radiography raises suspicion or the patient experiences cardiovascular collapse?
   a. Cardiac tamponade commonly occurs in newly diagnosed patients who are experiencing numerous other side effects and complications.
   b. Nurses are undereducated in the signs and symptoms of tamponade.
   c. Cardiac tamponade is not a common occurrence.
   d. Early symptoms are often nonspecific and are respiratory in nature.

ANSWERS

30. The incidence of malignant pericardial effusions has been reported to range from 1% to 40% and are usually not suspected until a grossly outward clinical sign occurs (Ball & Morrison, 1996). The most common symptom on presentation is dyspnea, often leading to the consideration of many other potential causes (Ball & Morrison, 1996; Shepherd, 1997). Therefore, although a high index of suspicion is required and nurses require frequent education and discussion about the emergency, it should be understood that it is not an easy complication to pick up on. Staff are entitled to support in learning about the complication as well as how to assess for it. *Answer 30:* **d.**

Case Study conclusion

Management of tamponade is immediate intravenous fluid support, electrocardiographic monitoring, and pericardiocentesis. Removing the fluid via a percutaneous catheter provides immediate symptom relief and hemodynamic restabilization (Ball & Morrison, 1996). Because fluid reaccumulates quickly, plans for permanent fluid removal are required. Options include sclerotherapy, surgery, balloon pericardiotomy, and an indwelling catheter, all of which are dependent on the cause of the effusion. In Jenny's case, the pericardial constriction is caused by fibrosis and would therefore require consideration of pericardial stripping. Surgery is often not a strong first-line option in oncology patients because of their debilitated or unstable conditions (Shepherd, 1997).

REFERENCES

Ball, J. B., & Morrison, W. L. (1996). Cardiac tamponade. *Postgrad Med J, 73*(857), pp. 141-145.

Bickston, S. J. (1995). Nutritional therapy. In Ewald, G. A., & McKenzie, C. R. (Eds.). *Manual of medical therapeutics*, 28th ed. Boston: Little, Brown.

Chestnutt, M. S., & Prendergast, T. J. (2001). Lung. In Tierney, L. M., McPhee, S. J., & Papadakis, M. A. (Eds.). *Current medical diagnosis & treatment*, 40th ed. (pp. 263-351). New York: Lange Publishing.

Dragonette, P. (1998). Malignant pericardial effusion and cardiac tamponade. In Chernecky, C., & Berger, B. (Eds.). *Advanced and critical care oncology nursing* (pp. 425-433). Philadelphia: WB Saunders.

Hackworth, C. A., & Lipton, M. J. (1998). The cardiovascular system. In Curati, W. L., Cosgrove, D. O., Lipton, M.J., & Allison, D. J. (Eds.) *Imaging in oncology* (pp. 189-202). Great Britain: Oxford University Press.

Healey, P. M., & Jacobson, E. J. (1994). Respiratory disorders. In *Common medical diagnoses: An algorithmic approach*, 2nd ed. (pp. 12-22). Philadelphia: WB Saunders.

Knoop, T., & Willenberg, K. (1999). Cardiac tamponade. *Semin Oncol Nurs, 15*(3), pp. 168-173.

Nolan, D. J. (1998). The esophagus, stomach, duodenum, and small intestine. In Curati, W. L., Cosgrove, D. O., Lipton, M. J., & Allison, D. J. (Eds.). *Imaging in oncology* (pp. 79-98). Great Britain: Oxford University Press.

Shepherd, F. A. (1997). Malignant pericardial effusion. *Curr Opin Oncol, 9*, pp. 170-174.

Spodnik, D. H. (1998). Pathophysiology of cardiac tamponade. *Chest, 113*, pp. 1372-1378.

Tayek, J. A. (1995). Nutrition. In Bongard, F. S., & Sue, D. Y. (Eds.). *Critical Care Diagnosis and Treatment* (pp. 343-359). Stamford, CT: Appleton and Lange.

Timmerman, P. (1998). Pulmonary fibrosis. In Chernecky, C. C., & Berger, B. B. (Eds.). *Advanced and critical care oncology nursing* (pp. 512-535). Philadelphia: WB Saunders.

Walsh, G., & Flower, C. D. (1998). The lung and mediastinum. In Curati, W. L., Cosgrove, D. O., Lipton, M. J., & Allison, D. J. (Eds.). *Imaging in oncology* (pp. 47-62). Great Britain: Oxford University Press.

17 Oncologic Emergency: Case 3

Esther Muscari Lin

Maggie Lancaster, a 34-year-old mother of two young children, is newly diagnosed as having acute promyelocytic leukemia (APML). She was admitted 2 days ago straight from her physician's office after a workup that included a bone marrow aspirate and biopsy.

Yesterday Maggie had a double-lumen Hickman catheter placed, and last night her chemotherapy regimen of Ara-C (cytosine-arabinoside) and daunorubicin was begun. As of this morning, her counts were within low-normal ranges, except for a total white blood cell count of 28,000/mm³.

At 8 AM, Maggie requests a nurse because she feels something wet underneath her and is having difficulty moving because of stiffness from the surgery. As she is rolled onto her side, the nurse helping her freezes when she sees the blue pad underneath filled with blood. The nurse caring for Maggie requests input from the advanced practice nurse (APN) about what is "going on with Maggie."

QUESTIONS

1. What would be the quickest indicator while providing a good deal of information regarding Maggie's physical stability?
  a. Blood pressure and pulse
  b. Blood pressure and central venous pressure (CVP)
  c. Urine output and lung perfusion
  d. Urine output and neurologic status

2. What is an initial and early piece of information needed?
  a. Source of bleeding
  b. Medications that are presently infusing

  c. Neurologic changes
  d. Emotional status

3. Which system assessment would lend the most information in attempt to begin to identify what is occurring?
  a. Cardiac
  b. Respiratory
  c. Integumentary
  d. Renal

ANSWERS

1. Because hemorrhage is a medical emergency, the nurse needs to ascertain that hemodynamic instability as a result of a large volume loss has not occurred. With volume losses, the blood pressure decreases, so the heart compensates by increasing the rate so that stroke volume can attempt to be maintained. The CVP is a great measure of fluid status and can contribute to the picture but would follow an initial set of vital signs. *Answer 1:* **a.**

2. Maintaining an adequate circulatory volume is essential; therefore quick identification of volume loss and the source of bleeding should be the initial response. *Answer 2:* **a.**

3. It is because of all of the aforementioned factors that the cardiac system is an important system for early assessment and repeated monitoring as interventions are instituted. Integumentary assessment is crucial because early signs of bleeding are often evident on the skin and mucous membranes. Assessment for petechiae, bruising, hematomas, bleeding gums, conjunctival bleeding, and other areas of spontaneous bleeding can be warning signs of a coagulopathy. *Answer 3:* **c.**

Case Study continued

Laboratory work is performed on blood drawn via the Hickman. Stat results of the complete blood count (CBC) are as follows:

Hemoglobin (Hgb):	7 g/dl
Hematocrit (Hct):	22.3%
White blood cell (WBC) count:	15,000/mm^3
Absolute neutrophil count (ANC):	2000/mm^3
Platelets:	25,000/mm^3

As the nurse provides you with a description of what she has found since starting her day, you consider what the possibilities for the bleeding are. You mention to your nursing colleague that based on what you have heard so far, you wonder if Maggie is experiencing disseminated intravascular coagulation (DIC).

QUESTIONS

4. The nurse, looking somewhat surprised, asks how you could arrive at a possible diagnosis without any further assessment. Which of the following allowed you to make your diagnosis?

   a. Knowing Maggie's diagnosis and the fact that her bone marrow is filled with abnormalities

   b. Knowing Maggie's diagnosis and the fact that Ara-C is metabolized in the liver

   c. Knowing that Ara-C contributes to the activation of factor XII

   d. Knowing Maggie's diagnosis and what day it is in her treatment plan

ANSWERS

4. DIC assessment focuses on screening for signs of active bleeding as well as signs of excessive coagulation as demonstrated by clotting (Figure 17-1). Unless coagulation is occurring to a greater extent than fibrinolysis, bleeding is usually the more dominant sign. The spontaneous bleeding associated with acute DIC is often first noted at a previous wound or venipuncture site. It is the spontaneous bleeding that leads the health care provider to search for the source and other potential body sites. Acute DIC develops rapidly, and the skin manifestations of petechiae, nose bleeds, ecchymoses, hematomas, bleeding gums, conjunctiva bleeding, and bleeding from previously healed sites are common (Murphy-Ende, 1998). Chronic abnormal coagulation presents as a thrombotic complication such as thrombophlebitis, pulmonary embolus, or an infarct to a major organ. Because hemorrhage is the result of DIC, clotting factors and blood volume are quickly consumed or lost. This is reflected not only in laboratory values but also in hypovolemic

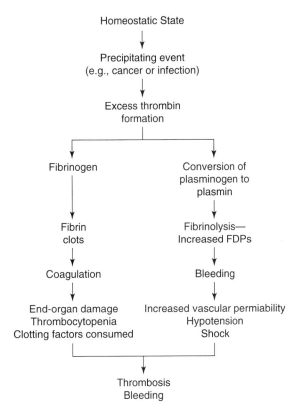

Figure 17-1 The process of disseminated intravascular coagulation. *FDPs,* Fibrin degradation products. (Modified from Gobel, B. H. [1999]. Disseminated intravascular coagulation. *Semin Oncol Nurs, 15,* pp. 174-182.)

vital signs. No matter where the blood is originating from, decreased blood, central venous, and pulse pressures will be evident. Therefore systems assessments, in particular the integumentary system, should be conducted regularly to monitor for bleeding or the effects of blood loss; vital signs should be measured much more frequently (Table 17-1).

DIC is always a result of another underlying problem. In the oncology patient, infection, hemolysis from a transfusion reaction, malignancy, pancreatitis, or a fat embolism can result in DIC. In Maggie's case, her diagnosis of leukemia is associated with triggering DIC. In particular, the best-known association is the DIC-triggering capability of APML during induction chemotherapy; however, it can also be triggered by other mucin-producing adenocarcinomas such as lung, pancreatic, gastric, and prostate cancer (Murphy-Ende, 1998). A large chemotherapy-induced cell kill or a procoagulant material released from the

TABLE 17-1 | Disseminated Intravascular Coagulation Body Systems Assessment

BODY SYSTEM	SYMPTOMS	SIGNS
Cardiac	Dizziness	Syncope
	Fatigue	Tachycardia
	Chest Pain	Orthostatic hypotension
Respiratory	Dyspnea	Epistaxis (nose bleed)
	Chest Pain	Hemoptysis
		Tachypnea
		Cough
Gastrointestinal	Nauea	Vomiting—heme+
		Melena
		Rectal bleeding
		Increased abdominal tenderness and girth
Genitourinary	Back, flank pain	Urine—heme+
		Decreased urine output
Neurologic	Confusion, "slow" or "muttled" thinking	Mentation changes
	Anxiety	Consciousness changes
	Restlessness	
	Headache	
Integumentary	Feeling cold	Bruises, hematomas
		Spontaneous oozing from previous IV or wound sites
		Pale, cool skin
		Petechiae
		Digital ischemia

TABLE 17-2 | Common Causes of Disseminated Intravascular Coagulation in Cancer

Infections	
Gram-negative bacteria	Meningococcus, *Salmonella, Pseudomonas* species, Enterobacteriaceae, *Hemophilus*
Gram-positive bacteria	*Pneumococcus,* staphylococci, hemolytic streptococci
Viremias	Hepatitis, varicella, cytomegalovirus, human immunodeficiency virus
Neoplasms	
Leukemias	Acute promyelocytic, acute myelogenous, acute lymphocytic, chronic myelogenous
Solid tumors	Adenocarcinomas (lung, breast, stomach, pancreas, prostate), ovary, colon, melanoma (rarely)
Hepatic complication	
Obstructive jaundice	
Fulminant hepatic failure	
Transfusion reactions	
Acute hemolytic transfusion	
Multiple transfusions of whole blood	
Prosthetic devices	

From Gobel, B. H. (1999). Disseminated intravascular coagulation. *Semin Oncol Nurs, 15,* pp. 174-182.

promyelocyte triggers tissue factor release. Tissue factor, a cofactor to coagulation, begins the process of platelet activation and clotting. *Answer 4:* **d. See Table 17-2.**

QUESTIONS

5. In response to the nurse's request for guidance, your best approach would be to:

    a. Suggest that she observe you as you complete a physical assessment

    b. Offer to look after the nurse's other patients so that she can do a focused, thorough assessment on Maggie

    c. Tell her to complete the assessment and relay the findings to you

    d. Coordinate the nurse's assessment with Maggie's physician's

6. The cardiac assessment of a person with DIC can reflect which of the following?

a. Decreased CVP and symptoms of chest heaviness
b. Normal rhythm on electrocardiogram
c. Consistent, steady pulse
d. Decreased CVP and increased mean arterial pressures

ANSWERS

5. Because DIC can be overwhelming to even the most experienced nurse, it is important to assess where the nurse managing the crisis is in her learning curve, other patient responsibilities, and the stability of the critically ill patient. It is possible that the nurse caring for the patient focuses only on the visible bleeding and excretions that can be tested for heme. However, hemostasis is a risk with potential infarcts or bleeding anywhere in the body, including the major organs. The risk of a life-threatening event occurring internally can be overlooked because there are so many tasks and observations to be performed.

Stepping in to conduct an aspect of assessment on Maggie minimizes the learning that can occur for the nurse and also sending a message of inadequacy. Acting without assessing the nurse's learning needs raises the possibility of doing something that does not help the nurse nor contributes to the care the nurse is planning to provide to Maggie and her family. Once learning what the nurse's needs are, the two colleagues can decide together what would work best for the nurse and the patient. It is possible that the nurse just wants to bounce her plan for assessment and care off of the APN to make sure nothing is being missed. For future consultations, collaborations, and involvement with that nurse and on that unit, the APN needs to be aware to not "take responsibilities away" from the staff and to be especially aware of not sending unspoken messages of condescension or inadequacy. *Answer 5:* **b.**

6. The cardiac assessment of a patient with DIC will likely reveal decreased CVP and symptoms of chest heaviness. *Answer 6:* **a.**

QUESTIONS

7. Once learning that Maggie's cardiovascular status is not unstable, what would your next approach be?
a. Repeat the cardiovascular assessment to be sure that she does not need to be transferred to an intensive care unit
b. Support the nurse in her explanation to the family that DIC is suspected
c. Wait for confirmation of DIC and then approach Maggie and her family

d. Knowing that Maggie's cardiovascular status is stable, continue on with finding potential other sources of bleeding

8. Why is it important that you explain to Maggie's family that DIC is not just a bleeding disorder?

9. Maggie's husband requests that the chemotherapy be discontinued immediately so that the bleeding will stop. What is the *best* response?
a. The underlying problem of excessive clotting will be controlled with pharmacologic agents that interfere with thrombin formation.
b. The underlying problem of excessive clotting is short lived, and Maggie will be at risk for only another few days.
c. The underlying problem of APML needs to be irradicated to end the risk of hemorrhage.
d. Replenishment of clotting factors normally made by the liver will stop the bleeding.

ANSWERS

7. In addition to being frightening, it is also a difficult complication to manage. The flurry of activity and health care providers that DIC results in contributes to the anxieties, fears, and misperceptions that patients and families experience. Waiting to give the patient or family information on what they are seeing contributes to the anxiety but also can lead to misperceptions and mistrust because they may believe "something has gone wrong" and that there is an iatrogenic cause they are not being informed about. Once the patient's stability is ensured for the moment, updating and educating the patient and family about DIC, the purpose of the laboratory tests, and the goals of care is critical (Murphy-Ende, 1998). *Answer 7:* **b.**

8-9 DIC is extremely frightening to the patient and family because of the uncontrolled bleeding. However, because so many of the assessment and monitoring behaviors focus on potential internal injury, patients and families need to understand that it is the initiation of the clotting cascade that has resulted in DIC. When it is explained that DIC is the result of some other problem and it is the APML triggering the abnormalities, the patient and family can begin to grasp the role the leukemia is playing and the importance of treating the disease to bring the coagulopathy under better control. *Answer 8:* **See text.** *Answer 9:* **c.**

10. During your consultation with Maggie's nurse, what other body systems will you guide her in assessing? How should they be assessed?

11. Maggie, although frightened by what she is experiencing, is adamant about maintaining her independence and autonomy. Therefore what are the *main* reasons for ordering a bedside commode and mandating that Maggie call for a nurse's assistance when she needs to use it?
1. A fall could result in bleeding.
2. Urine output volumes require monitoring.
3. All excretions can be tested for blood.
4. Less risk of tension on the IV lines and new Hickman can be accessed easier.
   a. 1, 2, & 3
   b. 2, 3, & 4
   c. 3 & 4
   d. All of these

12. A new onset of pain reported by Maggie should be managed in what fashion?
a. Initiation of an intravenous analgesic as needed because the intravenous route avoids having to deal with the potential interference from nausea and vomiting
b. Determination of the cause of the pain because thrombosis or infarct can present as pain
c. Advocation for an oral analgesic because you want to start with the least invasive route and lowest dosage
d. Recheck of the chemotherapy administration schedule, ascertaining that the infusion is on time, because the pain is most likely an indication of leukemic infiltrates

13. Maggie's nurse thanks you for your participation. In signing off to the next nurse, you hear her tell the next nurse a number of times how to observe for bleeding and which body sites to observe for bleeding. What of the following misperceptions might require clarification based on what you are hearing?
1. Hemorrhage is the only consequence of DIC.
2. The consequences of DIC are always visible.
3. Bleeding from DIC is iatrogenic.
4. DIC assessment requires the expertise of an experienced practitioner.
   a. 1 & 2
   b. 1 & 3
   c. 2 & 4
   d. All of these

10. Because coagulation is activated to a greater extent than fibrinolysis, signs of bleeding are observed via the integumentary system. Neurologic changes can be reflected in alterations of level of consciousness, blurred vision, and headaches. Peripheral vascular changes may be reflected in decreased or absent pulses, distal edema, or pain. Urinary output will drop if the renal system is affected by loss of blood or thrombosis (Linker, 2001).

11. Because spontaneous bleeding can occur without trauma, the goals of care include precautions that minimize the risk of accidental bleeding. A fall or bump, or even minor tear in skin integrity, can result in significant bleeding. Because hemostasis is altered and volume status is static, the patient can become orthostatic, dizzy, and unstable without notice. Maintaining bed rest or close control over ambulation is an attempt at keeping the patient safe. Urine output can drop because of a thrombus and renal cortical necrosis or because of decreased blood flow to the kidney as the body shunts blood to vital organs in the case of severe hypotension. Monitoring and heme testing of the urine output are means for monitoring for these risks. *Answer 11:* **a.**

12-13. Signs of thrombosis are similar to those associated with deep vein thromboses of the lower extremities, with phlebitis, redness, or warmth along the vein or pain if it occurs in the fingers or toes. Low back pain might indicate renal infarction, whereas a headache could signal central nervous system (CNS) bleeding or thrombosis. Chest pain might suggest pulmonary embolus, but chest pains or feelings of heaviness can be present in the anemic patient as well. Because DIC is a simultaneous loss of control in coagulation as well as fibrinolysis, any report of pain should be investigated before treating with an analgesic. *Answer 12:* **b.** *Answer 13:* **d.**

Case Study continued

As Maggie's nurses transition care, the results of the laboratory work drawn earlier are called to the unit. The results confirm the diagnosis of DIC.

14. Based on the DIC confirmation, complete the following table based on what you would expect the laboratory results to look like, (1) noting whether the blood products are elevated (↑) or diminished (↓) and (2) noting the reasons for the changed levels as either consumed, lost through bleeding, or the product of fibrinolysis.

Components	↑ or ↓	Reason for Change
Platelets	_____	_____
Fibrinogen	_____	_____
Fibrin degradation products	_____	_____
Hgb	_____	_____
Hct	_____	_____
Prothrombin time (PT)	_____	_____
Partial thrombo-plastin time (PTT)	_____	_____

ANSWERS

14. Blood components are consumed or lost through bleeding. *Answer 14:* **See Table 17-3.**

QUESTIONS

15. The laboratory results are called to the unit at the change of shift. Upon learning the results, new orders are written. Knowing Maggie's new nurse is transitioning into her care, what approach might you take next?

a. Offer to spend some time with Maggie and possibly teach a relaxation exercise
b. Offer to work and care for the nurse's other patients

c. Ask the nurse if she has a few moments so that you might share your perspective on Maggie's care in attempt to meet Maggie's needs
d. Now that the diagnosis is confirmed, leave the unit and wait until you are needed again

ANSWERS

15. For many of the reasons cited, the APN might be able to contribute the most at this point by supporting Maggie emotionally. Helping Maggie gain some control over her anxiety meets one of Maggie's needs. However, it also gives the nurse transitioning into Maggie's care some added time to organize herself and respond to the changes in Maggie's plan of care. *Answer 15:* **a.**

QUESTIONS

16. Maggie's new nurse asks you why a low-molecular-weight heparin (LMWH) is being used instead of unfractionated heparin. A suitable response would be all *except:*

a. LMWHs can be administered only once daily.
b. LMWHs have a more predictable anti-thrombotic effect.
c. LMWHs require very little laboratory monitoring.
d. LMWHs have been proven superior over unfractionated heparin.

TABLE 17-3 Adult Serum Laboratory Values During Disseminated Intravascular Coagulation

PRODUCT	NORMAL LEVEL	PROLONGED OR ELEVATED	REASON
Hemoglobin			
Male	13-18 g/dl		
Female	12-16 g/dl	Decreased	Bleeding
Hematocrit			
Male	40%-52%		
Female	35%-47%	Decreased	Bleeding
Platelets	150-440 × 10³/ml	Decreased	Consumed
Fibrinogen	200-400 mg/dl	Decreased	Consumed and fibrinogenolysis
Prothrombin time (PT)	11-15 sec	Increased	Insufficient number of vitamin K–dependent factors
Activated partial thromboplastin time (aPTT)		Increased	Consumption of clotting factors
Reticulocyte count	0.5%-1.5% of all red blood cells	Increased	Blood loss
Fibrin degradation products	2-10 mg/L	Increased	Fibrinolysis
International Normalized Ratio	?		
D-Dimer		Increased	
Thrombin		Increased	

Adapted from Murphy-Ende, K. (1998). Disseminated intravascular coagulation. In Berger, C. C., & Berger, B. J. (Eds.). *Advanced and critical care oncology nursing.* Philadelphia: WB Saunders; and Lin & Beddar.

17. What are the goals of care?
  1. Blood product repletion
  2. Circulatory volume support
  3. Eradication of underlying cause
  4. Comfort and reassurance
  5. Normalized PT and PTT times
      a. 1, 2, 3, & 4
      b. 1, 2, 3, & 5
      c. 2, 3, 4, & 5
      d. All of these

ANSWERS

16. LMWHs are a relatively new class of antico-agulants that are still being compared with unfractionated heparin. LMWHs have higher bio-availability, a longer half-life, and a more predictable antithrombotic effect. Because of these properties, they are prescribed in fixed-weight adjusted dosages and administered once or twice daily subcutaneously, without laboratory monitoring (Dolovich, Ginsberg, Douketis, et al., 2000). There is some suggestion that they are safer and more effective than unfractionated heparin, particularly in venous thrombosis and pulmonary embolus; however, these assumptions have not been proven. The advantage appears to be in use with an outpatient population because of its safety and less stringent monitoring requirements. In the inpatient population and in patients with DIC, the superiority of LMWHs over unfractionated heparin is unfounded to date. *Answer 16:* **d.**

17. The ultimate goal of care is to achieve hemostasis, and in order to do so, the primary focus is on treating the underlying cause or trigger of the DIC. When DIC is resulting in serious consequences, as is seen in the bleeding with Maggie, and successful treatment of the underlying cause is not immediate, anticoagulation may be the only way to control what is occurring. Anticoagulation is performed routinely, and then repletion of consumed blood components occurs. Interference with the production of thrombin prolongs the bleeding times, but it is easier for the health care professional to manage DIC. Thrombin interference ultimately decreases the number of clots that are formed. Replacement therapy with platelets and red blood cells is in direct response to the volume and component losses. Replenishment with cryoprecipitate, clotting factors, fresh frozen plasma, and vitamin K is controversial because the concern is an overabundance of thrombus production or increased levels of fibrin degradation products,

possibly impairing hemostasis further (Gobel, 1999). *Answer 17:* **a.**

QUESTIONS

18. As you leave the unit passing Maggie's room, Maggie's husband reaches out for you. He tells you that he is concerned about Maggie being so drowsy that she cannot stay awake when he arouses her. The nurse caring for her during the day had done a wonderful job explaining all that she is at risk for with excessive clotting and bleeding. He notices that the health care team keeps checking her neurologic status, and he wonders if "you think she might be having a stroke"? How might you respond to him?
  a. "Neurologic checks are a standard of practice instituted with the person experiencing DIC, and it is rare for patients to experience an intracranial event."
  b. "Not to worry, she will be fine once she has received her course of chemotherapy."
  c. "This is a worrisome sign of a cerebrovascular accident and requires a quick health care team response."
  d. "A drop in blood volume results in a fatigue that is difficult to comprehend to outsiders, yet is reflected in shortness of breath, tired muscles, irritability, lowered mental status, malaise, and sleepiness."

ANSWERS

18. It is no surprise that frightened significant others look for the signs of the dangerous possibilities they have been educated about. In addition to the factual information, reassurance is very important to the patient and family. Supporting loved ones in their efforts at care provision involves not placing more responsibility on them than they are capable of managing. It is also a fine balance to not dismiss their observations either. Because of the frequent neurologic assessments, the health care team is in a position to observe subtle changes. Although the husband's concerns will be considered, the sleepiness being observed is most likely a result of the sudden drop in blood volume and oxygenation. The fatigue that accompanies low Hgb and Hct can be profound and shows itself in a variety of ways, including slight confusion or disorientation. *Answer 18:* **d.**

REFERENCES

Dolovich, L. R., Ginsberg, J. S., Douketis, J. D., et al. (2000). A meta-analysis comparing low-molecular-weight heparins with unfractionated heparin in the treatment of venous thromboembolism. *Arch Intern Med, 160*, pp. 181-188.

Gobel, B. H. (1999). Disseminated intravascular coagulation. *Semin Oncol Nurs, 15*, pp. 174-182.

Lin, E. M., & Mitchell, S. (1996). Abnormalities in hemostasis and coagulation. In McCorkle, R., Grant, M., Frank-Stromborg, M., & Barid, S. (Eds.). *Cancer nursing: A comprehensive textbook* (pp. 979-1009). Philadelphia: WB Saunders.

Linker, C. A. (2001). Blood. In Tierney, L. M., McPhee, S. J., & Papdakis, M. A. (Eds.) *Current medical diagnosis & treatment*, 40th ed. (pp. 505-558). New York: Lange Medical Books.

Murphy-Ende, K.(1998). Disseminated intravascular coagulation. In Berger, C. C., & Berger, B. J. (Eds.). *Advanced and critical care oncology nursing.* Philadelphia: WB Saunders.

18 Oncologic Emergency: Case 4

Deborah Boyle

Mrs. Darlene Sanders is a 55-year-old woman who was diagnosed with stage IIB invasive breast cancer 3 years ago. She underwent a lumpectomy with axillary lymph node dissection. In addition, she completed a course of adriamycin/Cytoxan chemotherapy. Approximately 3 months ago, she began experiencing soreness in her right upper arm. This continued for 2 months, but she attributed it to overuse of that arm associated with readying her house for the Christmas holidays. She repeatedly reassured her daughter that this was the cause because she had breast cancer in her left breast and it was her right arm that was bothering her. When the pain became so pronounced that she found herself unable to hold the telephone receiver up to her ear, she decided to call her medical oncologist. A bone scan subsequently revealed metastases but no fracture to her right humerus and asymptomatic metastases to the sternum. Two months ago, she completed a 10-day course of radiation therapy to her right humerus.

Today's visit is for follow-up and consideration of further treatment. Mrs. Sanders is accompanied to the office by her 24-year-old daughter, who has temporarily moved home to help care for her mother. She is brought to the office reception area in a wheelchair but insists on walking back to the examination room without assistance. She has a steady, slow gait but easily maneuvers herself up to the examination table. When you take her hand in yours to greet her, you notice her forearm appears thin with the appearance of muscle wasting and she has poor skin turgor.

You remember that immediately following completion of her radiation, Mrs. Sanders, her husband, and her daughter traveled to California for her son's wedding. You ask her about the

wedding, and she tells you how wonderful the event was. When asked how she is feeling now, she replies, "The pain in my arm is almost totally gone, but as long as I take my pain medicine, I'm OK. Other than that, I feel great." She denies new pain in other sites. You check the staff nurse's recording of vital signs. Mrs. Sanders's temperature is 99° F, her pulse is 96 beats/min, and her blood pressure is 90/54 mm Hg. Her weight has dropped from 124 pounds to 116 pounds since her last visit. When you ask if she needs help getting into a gown, she replies, "No, I can do it," and similarly dismisses her daughter's offering of assistance.

Medications
Tamoxifen 20 mg every day
MS Contin 30 mg orally two times a day
Naproxen 250 mg orally two times a day
Senokot 2 tablets daily
Colace 100 mg every morning
Restoril 15 mg daily

Social History
Mrs. Sanders lives with her husband of 26 years, a U.S. Foreign Service executive who travels extensively. Mrs. Sanders has lived in Belgium, Pakistan, and Singapore. She quit smoking 3 years ago, at the time of her breast cancer diagnosis. She was a social drinker up until that time as well.

QUESTIONS

1. Based on your initial observations and queries, for which problems is Mrs. Sanders most at risk?
  a. Spinal cord compression and dehydration
  b. Pathologic fracture and hypercalcemia
  c. Deep vein thrombosis and spinal cord compression
  d. Pathologic fracture and brain metastases

2. The results of the chemistry panel are now available. You note that the serum calcium is 11.4 mg/dl. With this new finding, which symptoms would not be consistent with a diagnosis of hypercalcemia?

  a. Jaundice, lymphedema, dyspnea
  b. Weakness, lethargy, fatigue
  c. Nausea, anorexia, constipation
  d. Polydipsia, polyuria, dehydration

3. In addition to patient report of complaints, what physical finding would heighten your suspicion for hypercalcemia?

  a. Slight weight gain
  b. Elevated blood pressure
  c. Hyperactive bowel sounds
  d. Diminished deep tendon reflexes

ANSWERS

1. Bone is one of the three most favored sites of solid tumor metastasis, suggesting that the skeletal microenvironment affords fertile terrain for the evolution of human tumors (Mundy, 1997). Because bones are the major repository of calcium, compromise to bone structure, such as bone metastases, is the most common cause of hypercalcemia in cancer patients (Fisher, Mayer, & Struthers, 1997). Because of the predominance of bone metastases in breast cancer, hypercalcemia is common in this patient population. At least one third of patients with breast cancer develop hypercalcemia, usually late in their disease course. Hence, hypercalcemia was immediately considered acknowledging Mrs. Sanders's history of bony metastases. In addition, her history of bone metastases makes the likelihood of pathologic fracture a major concern. *Answer 1:* **b.**

2. It is important to note that humoral hypercalcemia of malignancy (HHM) can evolve from a complex paradigm unrelated to osseous metastases. Numerous factors released from or induced by malignant cells can promote increased osteoclastic activity and calcium absorption (Kaplan, 1994). These factors include parathyroid hormone–related protein (PTH-rP) and transforming growth factor-α (TGF-α), which interface to enhance osteoclastic activity, inhibit bone formation, and increase renal tubulin reabsorption of calcium. Other humoral factors that act synergistically with PTH-rP and TGF-α include osteoclast-activating factors (OAFs), hematopoietic colony-stimulating factors (CSFs), prostaglandin E series, and 1,25-dihydroxyvitamin D (vitamin D). Although hypercalcemia may evolve from processes distinct from bone resorption, in primary renal cell carcinoma (not primary breast cancer), hypercalcemia often mimics hyperparathyroidism. Primary nonmalignant hyperparathyroidism is the most common cause of hypercalcemia in the general population and is commonly a disease of older women. *Answer 2:* **a.**

3. Nonspecific symptoms characterize the early presentation of hypercalcemia and are easily attributed to other cancer-related phenomena. A history of bone metastases increases risk for subsequent skeletal involvement. Despite the fact that Mrs. Sanders denies new pain, evolving bone destruction and resultant hypercalcemia could be manifested by her general symptoms of weakness, lethargy, and fatigue. Her slightly elevated temperature and pulse and her low systolic blood pressure are also potential indications of hypercalcemia. Gastrointestinal implications of hypercalcemia often include anorexia, nausea, constipation, and even adynamic ileus. These symptoms occur as a result of impaired nerve impulse transmission and muscle hypotonicity, as do diminished deep tendon reflexes. Jaundice, lymphedema, and dyspnea would be associated with liver, axillary, and pulmonary metastases, respectively.

Polydipsia and polyuria result from elevated calcium ion concentration, which interferes with the action of antidiuretic hormone (ADH) on the collecting tubules in the kidney. This tubular deficit then impairs glomerular filtration and urine concentration ability, promoting a polyuric state with subsequent dehydration. Poor skin turgor, as noted during the initial greeting in the office with Mrs. Sanders, could be a manifestation of dehydration. *Answer 3:* **d.**

QUESTIONS

4. What laboratory value must be considered when analyzing serum calcium levels?

  a. Phosphorous
  b. Creatinine
  c. Albumin
  d. Calcitonin

5. What physical findings must be considered when analyzing serum calcium levels?

  a. Volume status and nutritional status
  b. Level of consciousness and urine output
  c. Sites of metastases and medication list
  d. Oral intake and chemotherapy history

ANSWERS

4. Calcium is a critical ion for numerous metabolic processes, including sustainment of bone and teeth, enhancement of enzyme cofactors in blood clotting, nerve impulse transmission, hormone secretion, muscle contraction, and cellular permeability (Meriney & Reeder, 1998). The pathophysiology of calcium regulation has been elucidated by Kaplan (1994, p. 1040):

> In normal calcium homeostasis, the rate of bone formation is equivocal to the rate of bone resorption. Similarly, calcium absorption from the gut parallels the urinary excretion of calcium. Normal calcium homeostasis is governed by a sensitive negative feedback loop that is controlled by the concentration of serum-ionized calcium and the action of three hormones: parathyroid hormone, vitamin D and calcitonin. *Answer 4:* **c.**

5. The majority of calcium (99%) is found in bone, where it combines with phosphate to give bone structure and rigidity. The remainder of calcium is intracellular and in plasma. Hence, the proportion of serum calcium is minimal. Of this serum calcium, 50% is ionized calcium, the physically active form that must be maintained within narrow limits to facilitate optimal neuromuscular activity and hormone secretion. Protein-bound (specifically, albumin-bound) calcium represents 40% of serum calcium and is not biologically active. However, in the presence of anorexia/cachexia with resultant catabolic wasting, less calcium is protein bound. Fluid overload can have a dilutional effect on albumin. Because it requires approximately 10 to 15 days for an albumin to reflect visceral protein changes, a series of albumin measurements should be reviewed in light of the patient's fluid status. Evidence of hypoalbuminemia (less than 4.0 g/dl) mandates quantification of serum ionized calcium or calculation of a corrected calcium. This then provides a more accurate picture of circulating serum calcium. A small fraction (10%) of serum calcium is neither ionized nor protein bound but is configured to the anions citrate, phosphate, and sulfate. *Answer 5:* **a.**

QUESTIONS

6. Mrs. Sanders's serum calcium is 11.4 mg/dl and her albumin level is 1.9 g/dl. Calculate the corrected serum calcium.
- **a.** $4.0 - 1.9 = 2.1$
- **b.** $2.1 \times 0.8 = 1.7$
- **c.** $11.4 + 1.7 = 13.1$
- **d.** The ionized calcium level is 13.1 mg/dl, which indicates moderate hypercalcemia; this is significantly higher than the uncorrected serum calcium level of 11.4 mg/dl.

TABLE **18-1**	Degrees of Hypercalcemia
CORRECTED SERUM CALCIUM LEVEL	**DEGREE OF HYPERCALCEMIA**
8.5-10.5 mg/dl	Normal
10.5-12.0 mg/dl	Mild
12.0-13.5 mg/dl	Moderate
>13.5 mg/dl	Severe

Renal function is an important clinical parameter particularly as treatment of hypercalcemia is considered.

ANSWERS

6. Although investigation of weight loss in conjunction with low albumin was in order for Mrs. Sanders, hypoalbuminemia is common in cancer patients because of catabolism. Thus the predominance of the anorexia/cachexia syndrome often mandates adjustment in serum calcium levels (Table 18-1). *Answer 6:* **c.**

Case Study continued

Mrs. Sanders's daughter pulls you aside and says, "My mother is putting on a big front for you. She put on her make-up this morning and insists on walking back here, but let me tell you, she's a lot worse since we came back from my brother's wedding. She's been on the couch for the last 3 days and hasn't eaten anything since yesterday morning." You ask Mrs. Sanders's daughter about her mental acuity, specifically whether there has been evidence of confusion or disorientation. She replies, "Well, now that you mention it, she had her friends from church over yesterday, and she kept getting their names mixed up. She kept apologizing and laughing it off as menopause and old age. I didn't think much more of it. And you know, she was a bit off while we were out in California. She was having problems remembering even little things. My dad and I just attributed it to her pain medications, jet lag, and everything she's been through. Why are you asking about that? What do you think is going on?"

QUESTIONS

7. You are concerned about confusion, which is often a corollary of hypercalcemia. The best assessment question to ask Mrs. Sanders to determine mental status change is:
- **a.** Do you know where you are right now?
- **b.** Who is the president?
- **c.** Have you had problems with your memory and things getting mixed up lately?
- **d.** Can you subtract 7 from 100 and continue counting down?

ANSWERS

7. Patients with early signs of metabolically induced confusion and disorientation are often aware of cognitive changes (Weinrich & Sarna, 1994). However, they may minimize or defer them to nonmalignant sources. Still many patients harbor ongoing concern over the nature of these changes. Some patients become offended when confronted with a formal mental status examination. Acknowledging Mrs. Sanders's attempts at maintaining independence and her need to discount the intensity of her symptoms, a less-threatening measure to determine problems with memory and mentation might encourage her revelation of cognitive change rather than investing in efforts at symptom concealment. You tell Mrs. Sanders's daughter that you need to do more investigation into her symptoms and look at her blood work but that she may be having some problems related to the bone involvement from her cancer. You reassure her that you will explain your findings once you have a better idea of what may be evolving. *Answer 7:* **c.**

Case Study continued

When you reenter the room, you ask Mrs. Sanders about her nutritional intake. She states that she has no desire to eat and that she thinks it is because she is constipated. In fact, she is sure her bowel problems are making her nauseated. She states that she feels thirsty but does not want to drink too much because she has had to repeatedly get up during the night to urinate and then she feels tired during the day because she has not slept well. She tells you, "My daughter doesn't realize how it affects you when you don't get a good night's sleep." Mrs. Sanders admits that she has had problems with her memory and she gets mixed up at times. You explain to her that this may be caused by too much calcium in her blood. She then states, "Oh, that makes me feel better. For a while there, I thought I was losing it."

With a serum albumin of 1.9 g/dl, Mrs. Sanders's corrected calcium is 13.1 mg/dl (Box 18-1). You inform Mrs. Sanders and her daughter that her serum calcium is elevated, which is probably responsible for many of her current symptoms. You state that consideration must now be made about appropriate therapy because there is concern about further problems when high calcium levels are not treated. Mrs. Sanders promptly states, "I don't care what you do, but I'm not going into the hospital and I'm not staying

---

BOX 18-1 Calculating Ionized Calcium

The corrected serum calcium is obtained by adjusting the calcium level upward by 0.8 mg for every gram of albumin under 4 g/dl or downward by 0.8 mg for every gram of albumin over 4 g/dl.
1. Subtract the albumin level from 4.0.
2. Multiply the difference by 0.8.
3. If the result is a positive number, add it to the serum calcium; if it is a negative number, subtract it.
4. The answer is the corrected calcium.

From Jensen, G. (1997). Hypercalcemia of malignancy. In Gates, R. S., & Fink, R. M. (Eds.). *Oncology nursing secrets* (pp. 336-341). Philadelphia: Hanley & Belfus.

---

here all afternoon. I've had enough of these places."

QUESTIONS

8. Your best response to Mrs. Sanders would be:
   a. "Mrs. Sanders, this is an emergent situation that requires hospitalization. You could have heart and kidney problems, and I am concerned about your safety."
   b. "Let me explain why we're worried about your high calcium."
   c. "I understand your concern, but we need to treat the underlying cause of your high calcium. We need to consider giving you more chemotherapy. You won't need to be hospitalized for that."
   d. "Let's talk about what we need to do to get your calcium down."

9. In treating hypercalcemia, the primary goal is to:
   a. Treat the underlying malignancy
   b. Inhibit bone resorption
   c. Promote calcium excretion
   d. Minimize potential cardiac and renal damage

10. For Mrs. Sanders to go home after this visit, you would assess whether she and her family could do all the following *except:*
   a. Take her furosemide (Lasix) and temazepam (Restoril) as ordered
   b. Monitor her urine output
   c. Walk up and down stairs every 3 hours
   d. Push her oral intake over the next 24 hours

11. What is the rationale for reviewing the 24-hour urine for creatinine clearance and her serum blood urea nitrogen (BUN) and creatinine?

1. The glomerular filtration rate (GFR) can be decreased because hypercalcemia interferes with ADH secretion.
2. The GFR is only an estimate when calculated from serum chemistries.
3. Dehydration is a common presentation in patients newly diagnosed as having hypercalcemia.
4. Hypercalcemia-induced diarrhea aggravates fluid loss.
    a. 2, 3, & 4
    b. 1, 2, & 3
    c. 1 & 3
    d. All of these

ANSWERS

8. There are two pieces of information that guide the appropriate response. First, Mrs. Sanders has moderate (versus severe, emergent) hypercalcemia. Second, she has made her wishes clear that she does not want to be hospitalized. These two variables must be considered in the context of patient safety and the likelihood of achieving desired outcomes. Can the hypercalcemia be managed at home? What measures would ensure an optimal outcome regardless of the setting of care? How invested are the patient and her family in taking on added responsibilities in the home setting to facilitate Mrs. Sanders's wishes? Engaging the patient in the contemplation of what would need to be done gives control to Mrs. Sanders and makes her a partner in her treatment regimen. This is particularly important in the case of cancer recurrence (Coward & Wilkie, 2000). However, because of the patient's subtle confusion and memory impairment, there needs to be reinforcement of the necessary requirements to implement the therapeutic regimen at home. The family must also be invested in this effort. In addition, criteria must be set to determine whether the home care regimen fails. This needs to be agreed on at the outset. *Answer 8:* **d.**

9. The potential systemic effects of unchecked hypercalcemia could result in renal failure, seizure, coma, and cardiac arrest. Once the serum calcium has been reduced to normal range, secondary efforts should focus on methods to inhibit bone resorption, and this is usually achieved by treating the underlying malignancy. Hence, treatment approaches are often biphasic: First, the potentially life-threatening symptom of hypercalcemia needs to be managed, then the root cause of the calcium imbalance, the metastatic breast cancer, can be addressed. *Answer 9:* **c.**

10. The ability to push oral fluids comparable with intravenous (IV) volumes would be necessary. Mrs. Sanders's output would need to be monitored to establish adequate calcium excretion with hydration efforts. An activity regimen would negate the deleterious effects of immobilization and should include weight-bearing exercise, which prevents bone resorption. One of the consequences of maintaining a diuresis at home is that Mrs. Sanders could not enjoy long periods of uninterrupted sleep because fluid intake, urine output, and monitoring of both would be required even at night. Hence, the sleep medication Restoril would not be indicated because hydration and output monitoring would be required during night hours similarly to the day hours. *Answer 10:* **a.**

11. Because hydration, activity, and calcium excretion are the mainstays of hypercalcemia management, renal function must be intact. Without adequate renal function, the calcium would continue to climb, further resulting in altered ADH secretion and a decreased GFR. Inhibition of ADH action on kidneys leads to a diabetes insipidus–type picture with large urine output and subsequent dehydration. The destruction of glomeruli from dehydration leads to a decreased GFR, which can result in renal failure. The dehydration in turn compounds bowel problems with constipation as a consequence, rather than diarrhea. *Answer 11:* **b.**

Case Study continued

It is decided that Mrs. Sanders can go home, but she must comply with a series of self-care instructions. The clinic nurses give Mrs. Sanders a bolus of fluids. You instruct the patient and her daughter about taking her oral antiemetics and determine that they have some prochlorperazine suppositories at home as well. You write down a schedule for pushing oral fluids and keeping track of her urine output; you also include an activity regimen and a list of symptoms they must call in to the physician if any evolve during the night. Mrs. Sanders is given an appointment to return late tomorrow morning. She returns with her daughter the next morning and has samples drawn for laboratory tests. Her BUN, creatinine, and potassium are normal, and her corrected calcium is down to 11.5 mg/dl.

QUESTIONS

12. You evaluate how the regimen worked and decide on which of the following priority steps?

a. Discussion of calcitonin therapy
b. Scheduling of another bolus of IV fluids
c. Determination of whether she can continue the current home regimen
d. Discussion with her daughter about Mrs. Sanders's symptoms

13. In telling Mrs. Sanders the results, she states, "Well, I guess I'm fine now." You talk to her about the need for further treatment of her hypercalcemia. If she were to receive pamidronate, what symptom would be worrisome to you if she called the office 2 days after treatment?
a. Low-grade fever
b. Obvious phlebitis at the injection site
c. Muscle cramps
d. Myalgias

14. Mrs. Sanders's daughter asks you, "What do I need to look for at home to know my mom is in trouble? She can't die from this can she?" Your best response would be:
a. "I don't want to scare you, but high calcium is considered an emergency situation in cancer care. Let me write down for you what you should look for."
b. "Serious symptoms would be if she had a seizure or you couldn't arouse her at all."
c. "We hope that this treatment we're giving her will keep her calcium under control. Here is a booklet that lists signs of high calcium."

d. "It's a big responsibility to take care of your mom at home and a scary one too. I can see why you'd be worried. Let's talk about all this."

15. Common signs and symptoms of rising calcium include which of the following?
a. Polyuria, polyphagia, polydipsia
b. Anorexia, polyuria, polydipsia
c. Confusion, heart palpitations, weight gain
d. Personality changes, bradycardia

ANSWERS

12. Mrs. Sanders has had a good response to the home regimen. However, the optimal desired outcome would be for the serum calcium to decrease 2 to 3 mg/dl within 24 to 48 hours. The first priority would be for evaluation of Mrs. Sanders's ability and willingness to continue her regimen at home. She could then continue this and return to the office tomorrow for further follow-up. In addition, discussion with her daughter about the symptoms at home would help assess overall adherence to the regimen. If Mrs. Sanders stated that she could not or did not want to continue this regimen, IV fluids would be in order along with consideration of hospitalization. Calcitonin is a hypocalcemic agent, which is generally used to treat severe hypercalcemia (Table 18-2). Although it has a rapid onset of action, it has minimal long-term effects. It is usually used for more emergent serum calcium levels and in conjunction with other longer-acting hypocalcemic agents. *Answer 12:* **c.**

TABLE 18-2 Hypocalcemia Agents		
DRUG	**ACTION**	**COMMENTS**
Calcitonin (SC, IM)	Inhibits bone resorption	Nontoxic; rapid onset and short duration of action; tachyphylaxis quickly develops; useful in decreasing calcium initially while more potent, longer-acting agents are taking effect
Plicamycin (Mithramycin) (IV)	Inhibits bone resorption	One of the first recognized hypocalcemia agents; may cause nephrotoxicity, hepatotoxicity, and platelet defects; potent irritant, avoid extravasation

Adapted from Meriney, D. K., & Reeder, S. J. (1998). Hypercalcemia. In Chernecky, C. C., & Berger, B. J. (Eds.). *Advanced and critical care oncology nursing* (pp. 254-269). Philadelphia: WB Saunders; Body, J. J., Bartl, R., Burckhardt, P., et al. (1998). Current use of bisphosphonates in oncology. *J Clin Oncol, 16*(12), pp. 3890-3899; Hillner, B. E., Ingle, J. N., Berenson, J. R., et al. (2000). American Society of Clinical Oncology guidelines on the role of bisphosphonates in breast cancer. *J Clin Oncol, 18*(6), pp. 1378-1391; and Lipton, A. (1997). Bisphosphonates and breast cancer. *Cancer, 80*(8 suppl), pp. 1668-1673.

Continued

TABLE **18-2** Hypocalcemia Agents—cont'd

DRUG	ACTION	COMMENTS
Gallium nitrate (IV)	Increases bone formation	Potent; hypocalcemia effect is sustained; causes dose-related nephrotoxicity
Phosphate (IV)	Inhibits bone resorption	May cause skeletal and potentially fatal soft tissue precipitation and is therefore not recommended
Bisphosphonates	Inhibit osteoclastic bone resorption	Lower serum calcium gradually over several days; do not affect the renal component of hypercalcemia and therefore have limited efficacy in the patients with elevated serum PTH-rP levels
First generation: Etidronate (IV, PO) *Second generation:* Pamidronate (IV) Clodronate (PO) *Third generation:* Alendronate (IV, PO) YM175 BM21.0955	Exhibit an affinity for bone and are selectively delivered to site of increased bone formation or resorption	*First generation:* etidronate has little advantage over other therapies *Second generation:* pamidronate currently is the most effective therapy because of its noticeable reduction and short-term and long-term efficacy; clodronate may be an effective adjuvant therapy in breast cancer; low-grade fever; phlebitis, nausea are common *Third generation:* presently these agents are under investigation

Adapted from Meriney, D. K., & Reeder, S. J. (1998). Hypercalcemia. In Chernecky, C. C., & Berger, B. J. (Eds.). *Advanced and critical care oncology nursing* (pp. 254-269). Philadelphia: WB Saunders; Body, J. J., Bartl, R., Burckhardt, P., et al. (1998). Current use of bisphosphonates in oncology. *J Clin Oncol, 16*(12), pp. 3890-3899; Hillner, B. E., Ingle, J. N., Berenson, J. R., et al. (2000). American Society of Clinical Oncology guidelines on the role of bisphosphonates in breast cancer. *J Clin Oncol, 18*(6), pp. 1378-1391; and Lipton, A. (1997). Bisphosphonates and breast cancer. *Cancer, 80*(8 suppl), pp. 1668-1673.

13. The most common side effects of pamidronate are transient fever, myalgias, and an infusion site reaction (Rugo, 2001). The development of muscle cramps after taking pamidronate could suggest an excess of calcium loss and possibly a concurring hypomagnesemia or hyperphosphatemia (because of inverse relationship). *Answer 13:* **c.**

14. Assisting the patient and family with adaptations required in the home setting is an important nursing responsibility (Mayer, Struthers, & Fisher, 1997). Some anxiety with assimilating new care demands in the home should be anticipated, and it is crucial that you listen attentively to messages relayed by Mrs. Sanders's daughter. First, she needs information about what to expect in the home setting in terms of emergent symptoms. Second, she is asking for validation about the ultimate seriousness of her mother's situation and is verbalizing underlying anxiety about the progressive nature of her mother's breast cancer. Responses other than choice d address only one part of her query. They respond to her need for factual information but do not address her worry about the fact that her mother may be dying. The best response relays to Mrs. Sanders's daughter that her fear is acknowledged, it is normal because hypercalcemia is a bad prognostic sign, and more discussion is warranted. In light of the fact that the daughter has shared her concerns, the door has been opened for further communication about Mrs. Sanders and this new phase in her cancer trajectory. *Answer 14:* **d.**

15. Common signs and symptoms of rising calcium include anorexia, polyuria, and polydipsia, confusion, and weakness. *Answer 15:* **b.**

REFERENCES

Body, J. J., Bartl, R., Burckhardt, P., et al. (1998). Current use of bisphosphonates in oncology. *J Clin Oncol, 16*(12), pp. 3890-3899.

Coward, D. D., & Wilkie, D. J. (2000). Metastatic bone pain: Meanings associated with self-report and self-management decision-making. *Cancer Nurs, 23*(2), pp. 101-108.

Fisher, G., Mayer, D. K., & Struthers, C. (1997). Bone metastases: Part I—Pathophysiology. *Clin J Oncol Nurs, 1*(2), pp. 29-35.

Hillner, B. E., Ingle, J. N., Berenson, J. R., et al. (2000). American Society of Clinical Oncology guidelines on the role of bisphosphonates in breast cancer. *J Clin Oncol, 18*(6), pp. 1378-1391.

Jensen, G. (1997). Hypercalcemia of malignancy. In Gates, R. S., & Fink, R. M. (Eds.). *Oncology nursing secrets* (pp. 336-341). Philadelphia: Hanley & Belfus.

Kaplan, M. (1994). Hypercalcemia of malignancy: A review of advances in pathophysiology. *Oncol Nurs Forum, 21*(6), pp. 1039-1046.

Lipton, A. (1997). Bisphosphonates and breast cancer. *Cancer, 80*(8, suppl), pp. 1668-1673.

Mayer, D. K., Struthers, C., & Fisher, G. (1997). Bone metastases: Part II—Nursing management. *Clin J Oncol Nurs, 1*(2), pp. 37-44.

Meriney, D. K., & Reeder, S. J. (1998). Hypercalcemia. In Chernecky, C. C., & Berger, B. J. (Eds.). *Advanced and critical care oncology nursing* (pp. 254-269). Philadelphia: WB Saunders.

Mundy, G. R. (1997). Mechanisms of bone metastasis. *Cancer, 80*(8, suppl), pp. 1546-1556.

Rugo, H. S. (2001). Cancer. In Tierney, L. M., McPhee, S. J. & Papadakis, M. A. (Eds.). *Current medical diagnosis & treatment* (pp. 62-108). New York: Lange Medical Books.

Weinrich, S., & Sarna, L. (1994). Delirium in the older person with cancer. *Cancer, 74*(7), pp. 2079-2091.

Suggested Reading

Clayton, K. (1999). Cancer-related hypercalcemia: How to spot it, how to manage it. *Am J Nurs, 97*(5), pp. 42-49.

Cowap, J., Hardy, J. R., & A'Hern, R. (2000). Outcome of malignant SCC at a cancer center: Implications for palliative care services. *J Pain Sympt Manage, 19*(4), pp. 257-264.

19 Oncologic Emergency: Case 5

Esther Muscari Lin

Mr. Joseph Richard, a 57-year-old man, has been receiving cyclophosphamide and etoposide for recurrent non-Hodgkin's lymphoma for the last 4 concurrent days. He is admitted to the oncology inpatient unit because he has become neutropenic and febrile. Despite being uncomfortable with the fever, Mr. Richard complains more about the frequent diarrhea he has had since the chemotherapy onset. On admission, a clearly defined circular area to the left of his hilum is noted on chest radiograph. His admission note lists the area as a previous problem with aspergillus and has been managed with amphotericin.

Medication Profile

Vancomycin	Amitriptyline
Gentamycin	Furosemide
Ticarcillin	Omeprazole
Amphotericin	Iron

Outpatient laboratory tests taken yesterday are unremarkable with the exception of his serum sodium, noted at 129 mmol/L.

QUESTIONS

1. Upon noting the sodium level, what is the rationale for assessing orthostatic vital signs?
   a. Consideration of the possibility of renal dysfunction
   b. Volume status evaluation
   c. Evaluation of Mr. Richard's ability to compensate for decreased cardiac output
   d. Determination of the cause of the hyponatremia

2. What laboratory analysis is absolutely necessary to evaluate the serum sodium?
   a. Complete blood count
   b. Urinalysis for electrolytes
   c. Serum potassium
   d. Arginine vasopressin level

3. Which organ systems must be evaluated first before the syndrome of inappropriate antidiuretic hormone secretion (SIADH) is considered a possibility?
   1. Renal
   2. Adrenal
   3. Thyroid
   4. Circulatory
      a. 1, 2, & 3
      b. 2, 3, & 4
      c. 1, 3, & 4
      d. All of these

4. What evaluation can you instruct Mr. Richard's primary nurse to do that would contribute the *most* to the SIADH evaluation?
   a. Lung assessment for rales
   b. Weight measurement
   c. Urine specific gravity
   d. Personality changes

ANSWERS

1. Hyponatremia, as noted on the admitting laboratory values, is usually a dilutional effect. There is an alteration in the sodium:water ratio. For some reason, to be determined, there is excess water in relation to the sodium. Baroreceptors and osmoreceptors respond to changes in blood pressure and plasma osmolality. When the pressures drop, baroreceptors stimulate the release of antidiuretic hormone (ADH) in the hypothalamus. ADH then acts on the renal tubules and collecting ducts to reabsorb water. Once sufficient water has been reabsorbed and pressures increase, ADH stimulation stops and water is not reabsorbed any further. Osmoreceptors respond to increased osmolality or increased solutes, such as sodium in the plasma with ADH stimulation and fluid reabsorption. Again, fluid is reabsorbed until the negative feedback occurs to shut the ADH off. The continued release of

ADH with continued renal excretion of sodium despite the feedback mechanisms is considered abnormal and the cause of SIADH (Hirshberg & Ben-Yehuda, 1997). *Answer 1:* **b.**

2. With this in mind, when reviewing sodium, the first thought is usually one of fluid overload. Therefore consideration needs to focus on this possibility. In Mr. Richard's case, intake and output (I&O) plus comparative weights will provide this information. Because there are no weights to compare, the admitting weight will need to serve as a baseline. The urine specific gravity will indicate whether the fluid is concentrated with a high osmolality. To be fluid overloaded, one would expect the specific gravity to be low. Although an arginine vasopressin level would provide a direct response to the question of whether there is inappropriate ADH secretion, it is a costly and impractical test (Kamoi, Kurokawa, Kasai et al., 1998). The urinalysis will be the most critical test to perform next. *Answer 2:* **b.**

3. A plasma osmolality will tell the level of solutes present because an elevated level would trigger ADH secretion and fluid reabsorption. These results will provide the information necessary to determine the presence of SIADH. *Answer 3:* **a.**

4. Hypovolemia needs to be evaluated with skin turgor assessment and orthostatics because Mr. Richard could be hypovolemic from the diarrhea he has been experiencing, and his SIADH may have had only a recent onset. Therefore, even though fluid excess is the cause of the hyponatremia, he may not yet be fluid overloaded, which needs to be evaluated as well. Before SIADH is considered a possibility, proper renal, thyroid, and adrenal function need to be ensured. *Answer 4:* **c.**

Case Study continued

Urinalysis Results
Osmolality: 450 mmol/kg
Sodium: 158 mmol/kg
Plasma osmolality: 215 mmol/kg
Plasma sodium: 120 mmol/kg

QUESTIONS

5. What are the confirming results for a diagnosis of SIADH? Place the words *high* or *low* in the appropriate places.

_____ Serum Na   _____ Urine Na
_____ Serum osmolality _____ Urine osmolality

6. Which of the following factors from Mr. Richard's history place him at risk for SIADH?
  1. Amitriptyline
  2. Furosemide
  3. Amphotericin
  4. Aspergillous pneumonia
  5. Cyclophosphamide
  6. Etoposide
  7. Elderly age
    a. 1, 2, 3, 4, & 5
    b. 3, 4, 5, & 7
    c. 1, 4, 6, & 7
    d. 1, 2, 4, & 5

7. Because signs and symptoms of SIADH are vague and nonspecific, with the abnormality usually being picked up during routine laboratory work, what would you look out for in Mr. Richard that reflects worsening SIADH?
  a. Cardiac failure
  b. Seizures
  c. More than 1 L of diarrhea per day
  d. Falling specific gravity

8. Which factors place Mr. Richards *most* at risk for negative sequelae of hyponatremia?
  1. Rate of change in sodium values
  2. The actual level of sodium
  3. Mr. Richard's elderly age
  4. Hydration necessary for cyclophosphamide administration
    a. 1, 2, & 3
    b. 3 & 4
    c. 2 & 4
    d. 1 & 2

9. If Mr. Richard's ADH secretion is unchecked, what other objective measure can *best* document his worsening condition?
  a. Weight
  b. Blood pressure
  c. Level of orientation
  d. Respiratory status

ANSWERS

5. The diagnosis of SIADH is made on the presence of high urine sodium and osmolality and low serum sodium and osmolality in light of normal renal and adrenal function. The diagnosis is often made once an abnormal serum sodium is noted on routine laboratory work. See Table 19-1. *Answer 5:* **See text.**

6. The connection to the possibility of SIADH tends to be made quicker in the patient more likely to be at risk, which in the case of the oncology population, is the patient with small cell lung cancer, occurring in approximately 15% of cases (Sorensen, Andersen, & Hansen, 1995). Other risk factors in the oncology population include cyclophosphamide administration or the

---

TABLE **19-1**   **Diagnostic Criteria for SIADH**

Laboratory tests
  Serum sodium <135 mEq/L (hyponatremia)*
  Plasma osmolality <275 mOsm/kg
    (hypoosmolality)*
  Urine osmolality >300 mOsm/L*
  Specific gravity >1.015
  Blood urea nitrogen >30 mmol/L
  Creatinine <0.5 mg/dl
  Uric acid <2.4 mg/dl
Physical findings
  Euvolemia*
  Absence of edema
Differential diagnosis
  Exclude hypovolemia (orthostatic
    hypotension, tachycardia, poor skin turgor,
    dry mucous membranes)
  Exclude hypervolemia (edema, increased
    jugular venous distension)
Workup
  Normal thyroid, adrenal, cardiac, hepatic,
    and renal function*
  No recent or current use of diuretics

From Keenan, A. M. (1999). SIADH. *Semin Oncol Nurs,*
15(3), pp. 160-167.
*Absolute criteria.

---

use of thiazide diuretics, nonmalignant pulmonary disease, lung abscesses, use of tricyclic antidepressants, and use of medications associated with other major medical problems (Andersen & Sorensen, 1997; Keenan, 1999). See Box 19-1. *Answer 6:* **d.**

7-8. Because the symptoms of SIADH are nonspecific and can suggest numerous problems experienced by the oncology patient, the potential consequences of hyponatremia and SIADH are the specifics upon which the nurse can focus assessment efforts. Fluid overload signs include jugular venous distension, weight gain, bounding pulses, S_3 heart sound, and possibly signs of congestive heart failure (Maxson, 1998). With inappropriate and unchecked ADH secretion, the water retention that results can lead to a body weight increase of 5% to 10% (Gill & Leese, 1998). The dangers of an abnormally low serum sodium level are neurologic in nature with intracellular brain swelling, with the possibility of seizures (Keenan, 1999). Changes in mentation can be difficult to assess objectively because of the numerous sedating pharmacologic agents a patient may receive while hospitalized. *Answer 7:* **b.** *Answer 8:* **d.**

9. The ability and stimuli necessary to arouse a person may be more helpful than reports of weakness, lethargy, or sleepiness. Mr. Richard's risk for the negative consequences of hyponatremia

---

BOX **19-1**   **Causes of SIADH Associated with Malignancy**

Neoplastic	Central nervous system
Bronchogenic	Meningitis, encephalitis, abscess
Small cell lung	Pharmacologic
Non–small cell lung	Chemotherapeutic agents
Extrapulmonary small cell	Cyclophosphamide
Head and neck	Vincristine
Hodgkin's and non-Hodgkin's lymphomas	Vinblastine
Leukemia	Cisplatin
Ewing's sarcoma	Melphalan
Neuroblastoma	Analgesics
Prostate	Acetaminophen
Pancreatic	Opioids
Breast	Antidepressants
Bladder	Tricyclic
Duodenal	Selective serotonin reuptake inhibitors
Esophageal	Other
Thymoma	Azithromycin, barbiturates, carbamazepine,
Carcinoid	chlorpropamide, clofibrate, isoproterenol,
Mesothelioma	nicotine, thiazides
Infectious	Miscellaneous
Pulmonary	Head trauma
Pneumonia, aspergillosis, tuberculosis,	Intracranial hemorrhage
abscess	Positive pressure ventilation

From Keenan, A. M. (1999). SIADH. *Semin Oncol Nurs, 15*(3), pp. 160-167.

are directly related to the rate of hyponatremia onset and how low the level of serum sodium is. See Box 19-2. *Answer 9:* **c.**

QUESTIONS

10. What would be the initial intervention for Mr. Richards at this time?
   a. Fluid restriction and demeclocycline
   b. Hypertonic (3%) solution
   c. Fluid restriction
   d. Demeclocycline

11. What is the underlying principle of SIADH correction?
   a. Treat the underlying problem
   b. Treat the SIADH first
   c. Replenish the sodium first
   d. Put the patient on fluid restriction

12. While responding to the hyponatremia, what is the management principle that guides the choice of intervention or interventions?
   a. Correct the hyponatremia slowly
   b. Correct the hyponatremia quickly
   c. Maintain a urine output that is slightly less than the oral intake
   d. Maintain a urine output that is slightly greater than the oral intake

---

BOX **19-2** | **Clinical Signs and Symptoms of Hyponatremia**

Mild
   Anorexia
   Difficulty concentrating
   Fatigue
   Headache
   Muscle cramps
   Weakness
   Weight gain
Moderate
   Confusion
   Depressed deep tendon reflexes
   Impaired taste
   Incontinence
   Lethargy
   Nausea, vomiting, diarrhea
   Oliguria
   Personality changes
   Thirst
Severe
   Coma
   Seizure activity

From Keenan, A. M. (1999). SIADH. *Semin Oncol Nurs,* *15*(3), pp. 160-167.

13. Which of the following are indicators of successful intervention for SIADH?
   1. 2- to 3-kg weight loss over 3 to 4 days
   2. 2-kg weight loss in 24 hours
   3. Decreasing specific gravity
   4. Increasing specific gravity
   5. Stable sodium in the first 2 to 3 days of taking demeclocycline
      a. 1 & 4
      b. 2 & 3
      c. 2, 4, & 5
      d. 1, 3, & 5

ANSWERS

10-11. Although interventions are aimed at increasing the serum sodium level to prevent neurologic complications from fluid shifts within the brain, the underlying principle for SIADH correction is irradication of the cause (Gill & Leese, 1998). Therefore, if the underlying cause is a malignancy, treatment will focus on eradicating the cancer. In Mr. Richard's case, he has a number of risk factors. Time away from cyclophosphamide administration will provide a clue as to whether that was the cause because the risk decreases as the time from administration increases. The other risk factors, such as the medications, need to be changed and a possible aspergillosis pneumonia is a possible factor for SIADH recurrence. *Answer 10:* **d.** *Answer 11:* **a.**

12. Correction needs to be gradual, with sodium correction not to exceed 0.5 mEq/L/hr or 10 to 15 mEq/L/24 hr (Gill & Leese, 1998; Soupart & Decaux, 1996). Rapid correction of severe hyponatremia has been associated with osmotic demyelination syndrome within the brain, a life-threatening condition (Gill & Leese, 1998). Drug doses are subject to adjustment based on the patient's sodium level and neurologic status. If the sodium is slightly lower than normal, restricting fluids to 500 to 1000 ml/24 hr is a reasonable approach to increase the plasma sodium within a few days. For lower levels or in patients in whom fluid restriction is not a possibility, demeclocycline, which inhibits the fluid reabsorption at the renal tubules by blocking ADH, is the drug of choice. Of note, the benefits of this drug are not seen for 3 to 5 days, with effects persisting beyond drug completion. Fluid restriction does not need to be ordered or maintained when the patient is receiving demeclocycline (Keenan, 1999). Hypertonic (3%) saline solution is controversial because there is a possibility of inducing the osmotic demyelination syndrome (Gill & Leese, 1998). If it is used, it is done so with extreme caution and is recommended by some to be administered with a loop diuretic such as furosemide (Gill & Leese, 1998). *Answer 12:* **a.**

13. Fluid excretion is evidenced by a falling specific gravity, and more dilute urine is an indication of successful SIADH intervention. Weight loss should accompany the pace of the rising serum sodium, with 2 to 3 kg occurring over 3 to 4 days. Because demeclocycline does not have an onset for 3 to 5 days, sodium increases may not be noted immediately. However, even maintaining a sodium level, rather than having it fall further, is progress in SIADH management. Other management issues surround the effects and severity of the fluid overload and the person's ability to manage the fluid. *Answer 13:* **d.**

References

Andersen, M. K., & Sorensen, J. B. (1997). Development of syndrome of inappropriate secretion of antidiuretic hormone during progression of metastatic breast cancer. *Acta Oncologica, 36,* pp. 535-537.

Gill, G., & Leese, G. (1998). Hyponatremia: Biochemical and clinical perspectives. *Postgrad Med, 74,* pp. 516-523.

Hirshberg, B., & Ben-Yehuda, A. (1997). Syndrome of inappropriate antidiuretic hormone secretion in the elderly. *JAMA, 103,* pp. 270-273.

Kamoi, K., Kurokawa, I., Kasai, H., et al. Asymptomatic hyponatremia due to inappropriate secretion of antidiuretic hormone as the first sign of a small cell lung cancer in an elderly man. *Intern Med, 37*(11), pp. 950-954.

Keenan, A. M. (1999). Syndrome of inappropriate secretion of antidiuretic hormone in malignancy. *Semin Oncol Nurs, 15*(3), pp. 160-167.

Maxson, J. L. H. (1998). Syndrome of inappropriate antidiuretic hormone secretion. In Chernecky, C. C., & Berger, B. J. (Eds.). *Advanced and critical care oncology nursing: Managing primary complications* (pp. 622-636). Philadelphia: WB Saunders.

Sorenson, J. B., Andersen, M. K., & Hansen, H. H. (1995). Syndrome of inappropriate secretion of antidiuretic hormone in malignant disease. *J Intern Med, 238,* pp. 97-110.

Soupart, A., & Decaux, G. (1996). Therapeutic recommendations for management of severe hyponatremia: Current concepts on pathogenesis and prevention of neurologic complications. *Clin Nephrol, 46,* pp. 149-169.

20 Oncologic Emergency: Case 6

Esther Muscari Lin

Robin Novick has been treated for newly diagnosed acute myelogenous leukemia (AML) and has been neutropenic for almost 10 days in the inpatient unit. She has done quite well, defervescing within 24 hours of her only fever. She is receiving broad-spectrum intravenous (IV) antibiotics for gram-positive and gram-negative coverage, as well as vancomycin for the indwelling triple-lumen Hickman catheter.

As you are leaving the unit at the end of the day, you hear shift report and are surprised to note that Robin has not been out of bed into the hall nor has she been as talkative as you know this 24-year-old woman to be. Yet, you also hear that she received 2 units of packed red blood cells (PRBCs) and single-donor platelets with premedications. You decide to stick your head into her room just to tease her a little bit as you are heading to your office. Robin is curled up on her side with her head under a blanket sleeping soundly. Her mother, who looks up from her reading, comments to you that "it hasn't been a good day. Robin just hasn't been her normal self." You explain that her counts are low, and anyone with a low hemoglobin and hematocrit feels fatigued. You wish her a good night and start to leave the room. As you reach the door, you hear Robin call you a name of someone with whom you are unfamiliar. As you turn, you see her looking at you from under the sheet and mumbling something inaudible. You approach the bed to make close contact when she swears at you and accuses you of lying to her. At this point, Robin's mother stands up, comes around the bed, and firmly explains to Robin who you are. After staring blankly at you, she groggily focuses in and says she realized it was you but was thinking of someone else. She tries to explain that she felt like she knew she was confused when she was talking to you but felt unclear in her head. Donna, the evening shift nurse, comes in at that point and takes Robin's temperature. She informs Robin's mother that Robin does not have a fever (temperature of 36° C). Donna continues her routine, checking the IV fluids and so on.

QUESTIONS

1. What finding is *most* alarming for a potential hemodynamic instability in this situation?
- **a.** Robin's temperature
- **b.** Robin's disorientation
- **c.** Donna's nonchalant attitude
- **d.** The day shift nurse's description of Robin's behavior

2. What available data from Robin's recent history could assist your diagnostic reasoning at this point?
- **a.** Previous temperature
- **b.** Blood pressure (BP) and pulse readings from the last 24 hours
- **c.** Time of blood transfusion
- **d.** Time of last acetaminophen dose

3. Considering the possibility of sepsis, what further inquiry might contribute the most to your assessment of Robin?
- **a.** Robin's mother's perception
- **b.** Robin's description of confusion
- **c.** Donna's interpretation of the temperature
- **d.** Vital signs from past 24-hour bedside chart

4. What critical data could you extrapolate from Robin's antibiotic profile at this point that would contribute to her risk of hemodynamic instability?
- **a.** That drug levels are adequate
- **b.** That the renal function is sufficient for the chosen antibiotics

c. That the specificity of the antibiotics match the culture results

d. Which organisms the antibiotics do not cover

5. Why would you choose to conduct a cardiovascular assessment at this point?

ANSWERS

1. By the cues received from the change of shift nursing staff, the mother, and Robin's interactions with you, your antenna has gone up that something is wrong with Robin. At this point, your reaction is to figure out whether there is something wrong with Robin resulting in disorientation and fatigue. Because Robin was quickly reoriented to person, the chances of a serious primary neurologic problem are small. Being 10 days out from treatment, chances are that Robin has been anemic before, which has resulted in transfusions, so why should she be "more fatigued" or not herself today because of anemia? Hearing that Robin's temperature is 36° C should raise concern because an abnormally low temperature is just as alarming as a fever. *Answer 1:* **a.**

2. Hypothermia (lower than 36° C) in the neutropenic patient can signal sepsis (Balk, 2000). Reviewing the previous temperature provides a comparison but is only an addition of one reading. The early stages of sepsis can last for hours. However, the previous 24 hours' worth of pulse and pressure readings can give the most amount of information regarding Robin's hemodynamic status. If Robin is in the early stage of sepsis, a nonclassic presentation of infection could still be reflected in her hemodynamic status, in particular her diastolic pressure. Because of decreased vascular resistance in the early stage of sepsis, blood return to the right side of the heart is decreased and the diastolic volume and pressure are lower (Shelton, 1999). The heart compensates to maintain the stroke volume by increasing the rate at which it pumps. Early in the course of sepsis, this results in an increased cardiac output. Reviewing Robin's baseline vital signs promotes a comparison with other values as opposed to interpreting the information in isolation of other physical data. One or two measurements may not appear to be remarkable or a significant finding, yet a declining or increasing *trend* is a much more credible and significant finding. Although every organ system is affected by the sepsis, the effect on the cardiovascular system is more obvious in the early stage, with physical signs quicker to evaluate and subtle signs picked up on before any outward sign becomes profound. Recognizing that hypothermia is a rare but serious indicator of systemic inflammatory response syndrome (SIRS), one other clinical manifestation is required to meet the criteria (Box 20-1). Therefore an elevated heart or respiratory rate in combination with the low temperature would confirm some type of SIRS response. *Answer 2:* **b.**

3. Robin's mother, knowing her the best, may have witnessed or sensed abnormalities in her daughter that would serve as clues to you as to what is occurring with Robin. Because the assumption that "Robin was not being herself" means that she was fatigued from a low circulation blood volume, further inquiry into what Robin's mother meant by her perception was stifled. Had Robin not awoken, obviously disoriented, the opportunity to witness signs of potential clinical problems might have been missed. Family members often provide information by which health care members can compare their current findings. It would be important to learn what Donna's interpretation of the low temperature is because she should be aware of the serious problem hypothermia can signal. Direct discussion with the day staff might identify clues or other signs of sepsis that had occurred but had been too subtle or nonspecific to be picked up. If the abnormal vital signs persist in the face of a documented infection, the diagnosis becomes sepsis, with it progressing to severe sepsis or severe SIRS in the event of hypotension. *Answer 3:* **d.**

4-5. Recognizing a temperature of 36° C as a potential sign of infection causes you to stop and consider what could cause Robin to become infected while taking antibiotics. Broad-spectrum antibiotics and vancomycin cover the general risks of a gram-negative and gram-positive infection, with additional particular attention to the inherent risks and common infections associated with an indwelling venous access device. Although it is part of the care to ascertain adequate drug levels and renal function, review of the drugs provides the most information. A review not only points out what organisms are covered by the prophylaxis but also reveals which ones are not being covered. In the neutropenic patient taking antibiotics, the risk of a fungal infection increases with time (Shelton, 1999). The expertise of anticipating the body's response to the disease and treatment course places the advanced practice nurse (APN) in the position to anticipate what Robin is at risk for at this particular point. *Answer 4:* **d.** *Answer 5:* **See text.**

ACCP/SCCM Consensus Conference Definitions of Sepsis, Severe Sepsis, and Septic Shock

Systemic Inflammatory Response Syndrome (SIRS): The systemic inflammatory response to a wide variety of severe clinical insults, manifested by two or more of the following conditions:
1. Temperature >38° C or <36° C
2. Heart rate >90 beats/min
3. Respiratory rate >20 breaths/min or $Paco_2$ <32 mm Hg
4. White blood cell count >12,000/mm^3, <4000/mm^3, or >10% immature (band) forms

Sepsis: The systemic inflammatory response to a documented infection. In association with infection, manifestations of sepsis are the same as those previously defined for SIRS. It should be determined whether they are a direct systemic response to the presence of an infectious process and represent an acute alteration from baseline in the absence of other known causes for such abnormalities. The clinical manifestations would include two or more of the following conditions as a result of a documented infection:
1. Temperature >38° C or <36° C
2. Heart rate >90 beats/min
3. Respiratory rate >20 breaths/min or $Paco_2$ <32 mm Hg
4. White blood cell count >12,000/mm^3, <4000/mm^3, or >10% immature (band) forms

Severe Sepsis/SIRS: Sepsis (SIRS) associated with organ dysfunction, hypoperfusion, or hypotension. Hypoperfusion and perfusion abnormalities may include, but are not limited to, lactic acidosis, oliguria, or an acute alteration in mental status.

Sepsis (SIRS)-Induced Hypotension: A systolic blood pressure <90 mm Hg or a reduction of ≥40 mm Hg from baseline in the absence of other causes for hypotension.

Septic Shock/SIRS Shock: A subset of severe sepsis (SIRS) and defined as sepsis (SIRS)-induced hypotension despite adequate fluid resuscitation along with the presence of perfusion abnormalities that may include, but are not limited to, lactic acidosis, oliguria, or an acute alteration in mental status. Patients receiving inotropic or vasopressor agents may no longer be hypotensive by the time they manifest hypoperfusion abnormalities or organ dysfunction, yet they would still be considered to have septic (SIRS) shock.

Multiorgan Dysfunction Syndrome (MODS): Presence of altered organ function in an acutely ill patient such that homeostasis cannot be maintained without intervention.

From Bone, R. C., Balk, R. A., Cerra, F. B., et al. (1992). American College of Chest Physicians/Society of Critical Care Medicine Consensus Conference: Definitions for sepsis and organ failure and guidelines for the use of innovative therapies in sepsis. *Chest, 101,* pp. 1644-1655.

QUESTIONS

6. Upon suspicion of sepsis, what should the immediate next course of action be?
   a. Volume repletion/maintenance
   b. Multiorgan system assessment
   c. Blood, urine, throat, and stool cultures
   d. Dopamine drip at renal perfusion doses to maintain urine output

7. Upon confirmation of severe sepsis/SIRS-induced hypotension, as defined by the American College of Chest Physicians/Society of Critical Care Medicine Consensus Conference (ACCP/SCCM), what should the immediate next course of action be?
   a. Volume repletion/maintenance
   b. Multiorgan system assessment
   c. Blood, urine, throat, and stool cultures
   d. Dopamine drip at renal perfusion doses to maintain urine output

8. What is the *most* common reason for infections to occur?
   a. Glucose-containing IV fluids
   b. Preexisting risk factor such as diabetes, elderly age, and so on
   c. Penetration of the epithelial barrier
   d. Protein malnutrition

9. Which organs are most commonly colonized by bacteria?
   a. Respiratory, genitourinary, circulatory
   b. Circulatory, genitourinary, respiratory
   c. Genitourinary, circulatory, gastrointestinal
   d. Gastrointestinal, genitourinary, respiratory

10. Which of the following organisms are *most* commonly identified with infections that often lead to sepsis in the oncology patient?
   1. *Escherichia coli*
   2. *Staphylococcus aureus*

3. *Pseudomonas aeruginosa*
4. Mucormycosis
   a. 1, 2, & 3
   b. 2, 3, & 4
   c. 1, 2, & 4
   d. All of these

ANSWERS

6. Because mediators such as endotoxins are released from microorganisms, they stimulate the release of macrophage-derived cytokines, such as tumor necrosis factor (TNF), interleukin (IL)-1, and IL-8. The effects are those associated with sepsis-induced hypotension: low cardiac index, low BP, low pulmonary artery pressure, and low systemic vascular resistance (SVR). The low SVR is the result

of peripheral vasodilation with venous pooling and low return to the right side of the heart. *Answer 6:* **b.**

7. Because of the hemodynamic instability that can result from SIRS or severe sepsis, every organ system is affected. Ongoing and consistent assessment is necessary to evaluate for the body's systemic response to infection (Table 20-1). The most common initial clues to infection are the vital signs, and in particular, a change in temperature, with an elevation being the most common occurrence. Hypothermia, occurring in only a small percentage of patients, is associated with an increased mortality rate (Balk, 2000). The effects of a systemic inflammatory response are evident in

TABLE 20-1	Risk Factors for Infection in the Immunocompromised Patient
PATIENT CHARACTERISTICS	**PHYSIOLOGIC MECHANISM OF INFECTIOUS RISK**
Host characteristics	
Elderly	Slowed phagocytosis: increased bacterial infection, more rapid dissemination of infection
	Slowed macrophage activity: more fungal infection, more visceral infection
	Atrophy of thymus: increased risk of viral illness
	Decreased antigen-specific immunoglobins: diminished immune memory
Frequent hospitalizations	Frequent exposure to environmental organisms other than own normal flora
	Potential exposure to resistant organisms
	Potential exposure to other people's organisms via equipment, supplies, transport, person-to-person exposure
Malnutrition	Inadequate WBC count: infection
	Reduced neutrophil activity: bacterial infection, risk of infection dissemination
	Impaired phagocytic function: bacterial infection
	Impaired integumentary/mucosal barrier: general infection risk
	Decreased macrophage mobilization: increased risk of fungal or rapidly disseminating infection
	Decreased lymphocyte function: increased risk of viral and opportunistic infection
Disease processes	
Cardiovascular disease	Inadequate tissue perfusion slows WBC response to tissue with pathogenic organism
Diabetes mellitus	Decreased numbers of neutrophils
	Hyperglycemia causes decreased phagocytic activity and immunoglobin defects
	Neuropathy and glycosuria predispose to decreased bladder emptying and urinary tract infections
Gastrointestinal disease	Decreased bowel motility allows normal flora to translocate across the gastrointestinal wall to the blood stream
Hepatic disease	Decreased neutrophil count and phagocytic activity
	Altered antibody responses
Pulmonary disease	Inadequate oxygenation suppresses neutrophil activity
Renal disease	Decreased neutrophil activity
	Decreased immunoglobin activity

From Shelton, B. K. (1999). Sepsis. *Semin Oncol Nurs*, *15*(3), pp. 209-221.
WBC, White blood cell.

every organ system. Identifying the different signs contributes to early SIRS or sepsis identification and early antibiotic institution, thereby decreasing the mortality and morbidity of sepsis (Simon & Trenholme, 2000; Teplick & Rubin, 1999).

Diagnosis of severe sepsis/SIRS means that there is organ dysfunction, hypoperfusion, or hypotension and can include a range of clinical findings. Sepsis-induced or SIRS-induced hypotension means that the systolic BP has fallen below 90 mm Hg with circulatory collapse and further hypoperfusion a possibility. Therefore maintaining a circulating blood volume and perfusion to vital organs is the priority. The first line of response is to support the intravascular volume, either by repletion or by maintenance. *Answer 7:* **a.**

8. The epithelia, consisting of the skin and lining of internal organs, is a person's physical barrier between the body's internal milieu and bacteria. Bacterial colonization or penetration of the epithelial barrier results in infection. Although protein malnutrition, high glucose concentrations, and some preexisting conditions increase a person's risk of an infection and life-threatening sepsis, it is the skin that is the first line and most important barrier (Casey, 2000). *Answer 8:* **c.**

9. The most common areas for bacteria to enter and/or colonize are the respiratory, genitourinary, and gastrointestinal tracts. Many bacteria result in infections that eventually overwhelm the body's immune defenses. The longer a person is neutropenic, the greater the risk of infection (Pizzo, 1993). There are multiple risk factors for infection and sepsis, and they require a knowledge of the patient's medical history, age, and present treatment plan (see Table 20-1). *Answer 9:* **d.**

10. Organisms that are naturally within the gastrointestinal tract or on the skin such as *E. coli* or *S. aureus* are commonly seen in the oncology patient. *P. aeruginosa* is the most feared pathogen for nosocomial pneumonia. Previous antibiotic use, advanced age, and immunosuppressive therapy combined are multiple risk factors (Simon & Trenholme, 2000). *Candida*, a fungal infection, is the most commonly occurring systemic infection, with aspergillosis, an endemic fungal pneumonia. Mucormycosis is not commonly seen. *Answer 10:* **a.**

Case Study continued

Donna records the following findings: 4 PM: occasional disorientation, "picking" in the air and pulling at pieces of her pajamas, drowsy but easily arousable, seems irritated with her mother; oral intake is minimal, with nutrition limited to parenteral nutrition; urinary output = 250 ml/hr (100 ml/hr greater out than in); BP, 118/90 mm Hg; pulse, 98 beats/min.

QUESTIONS

11. Which of the following signs correlate with the phase of SIRS just exemplified?
a. Extremities cool to touch, bowel ileus
b. Decreased bowel sounds, respiratory acidosis
c. Metabolic acidosis, arrhythmias
d. Hyperglycemia, respiratory alkalosis

12. Review each of the following organ systems, noting expected findings during the later stage of severe sepsis.

Cardiovascular
Cardiac output _____
Quality of pulse _____
Pulse rate _____
BP _____

Genitourinary
Urine output _____
Creatinine _____
Blood urea nitrogen (BUN) _____

Laboratory Values
Potassium _____
Glucose _____
Serum bicarbonate _____
Hepatic transaminases ____
Increased bilirubin _____
Oxygen saturation _____

ANSWERS

11. The physical findings documented by Donna at 4 PM are consistent with early sepsis; therefore the cardiac output is still high, with adequate perfusion of organs. As sepsis progresses, it can be viewed as a continuum with increasing severity of organ dysfunction, increased mortality, and multisystem end-organ failure (Balk, 2000). The skin is warm to touch, with brisk capillary refill, as systemic peripheral vascular resistance is decreased (Balk, 2000). As perfusion to the kidneys decreases with progressive sepsis, altered urine output can occur with the potential for acute tubular necrosis and acute renal failure occurring in the face of hypotension and nephrotoxic antibiotics. Gastrointestinal abnormalities can begin with abdominal discomfort or nausea and progress to decreased bowel sounds, abdominal distension, and possible ileus as the patient experiences septic shock/SIRS shock. With septic shock/SIRS shock, hypotension persists despite fluid resuscitation. The metabolic and electrolyte abnormalities include altered glucose metabolism and insulin resistance, with hyperglycemia during the early stress response stage and hypoglycemia later in severe sepsis (Mizock, 2000). Respiratory alkalosis tends to occur early in sepsis as the patient is tachypneic (blowing of carbon dioxide). As resistant hypoxemia occurs, lactic acidosis and metabolic acidosis with hypokalemia, hyponatremia, hypocalcemia, hypomagnesemia, hypophosphatemia, thrombocytopenia, and altered coagulation result (Balk, 2000; Mavrommatis, Theodoridis, Orfanidou, et al., 2000; Mizock, 2000). Multiorgan dysfunction syndrome is a possible end to the spectrum of sepsis/SIRS when there is multiorgan dysfunction and hemodynamic instability resists inotropic or vasopressor therapy. *Answer 11:* **d.** *Answer 12:* **See Box 20-2 and Table 20-2.**

BOX **20-2** | Calculation of Mean Blood Pressure

Hemodynamic assumptions:
1. BP comprises vessel tone and circulating volume.
2. Vessel tone (amount of vasodilation or vasoconstriction) is evidenced by the diastolic BP.
   a. Vasodilation causes the diastolic BP to decrease.
   b. Vasoconstriction causes the diastolic BP to increase.
3. Circulating blood volume is reflected in systolic BP.
   a. High systolic pressure often indicates high circulating blood volume.
   b. Low systolic pressure often indicates low circulating blood volume.
4. Organ perfusion is the result of a pressure that reflects both systolic and diastolic BPs and is called the MAP.
   a. The brain requires an MAP of 65-70 mm Hg.
   b. The kidneys require an MAP of 60-65 mm Hg.

Formula for MAP:
$$(2 \times diastolic) + Systolic \div 3$$
Example of vasodilation: BP = 96/40 mm Hg
$$(2 \times 40) + 96 \div 3 = 58 \text{ mm Hg}$$
Example of decreased volume: BP = 90/68 mm Hg
$$(2 \times 68) + 90 \div 3 = 75 \text{ mm Hg}$$

From Shelton, B. K. (1999). Sepsis. *Semin Oncol Nurs,* *15*(3), pp. 209-221.
Abbreviations: *BP,* Blood pressure; *MAP,* mean arterial pressure.

Case Study continued

At 6 PM, Donna records a temperature of 104° F with BP the same as earlier but the pulse rate slightly increased. Robin is returning to bed from the bathroom; she appears a little perkier but is visibly short of breath. Upon lung auscultation, rales are heard bilaterally in the bases.

QUESTIONS

13. What other pulmonary findings would you expect to find upon further examination of Robin at this time?
  1. Use of accessory muscles
  2. Pleural effusions on chest radiograph
  3. Oxygen saturation less than 90%
  4. Orthopnea
     a. 1, 2, & 4
     b. 2 & 3
     c. 1 & 4
     d. All of these

14. How is acute respiratory distress syndrome (ARDS) association with sepsis *best* described?
  a. ARDS is a pulmonary manifestation of a systemic inflammatory response.
  b. ARDS is the only pulmonary insult in multiorgan dysfunction syndrome resulting in respiratory failure.
  c. ARDS is the result of a direct injury to the lung.
  d. ARDS is a separate disorder that commonly results in SIRS.

15. ARDS is the result of what type of injury to the lung parenchyma?
  a. Indirect
  b. Direct

16. Because of the pathophysiologic occurrences during ARDS, which of the following events occur?
  1. Decreased alveolar size
  2. Decreased lung compliance
  3. Decreased functional residual capacity
  4. Arterial hypocapnia
     a. 1, 2, & 3
     b. 2 & 3
     c. 3 & 4
     d. All of these

ANSWERS

13. *Acute lung injury* (ALI) is a "syndrome of inflammation and increased alveolar capillary permeability associated with a constellation of clinical, radiologic, and physiologic abnormalities that cannot be explained by left atrial or pulmonary capillary hypertension. ARDS is in that subset of patients at the severe end of the spectrum of ALI" (Fein & Calalang-Colucci, 2000, p. 291). ARDS is the result of an indirect injury and the systemic inflammatory response to infection. *Answer 13:* **c.**

14. The frequency of ARDS ranges from 18% to 38% of patients with bacteremia or sepsis, with 18% to 25% of these patients developing gram-negative sepsis (Fein & Calalang-Colucci, 2000). The risk of ARDS is higher in the patients who have a systemic hemodynamic response, impaired perfusion, and multiorgan dysfunction (Fein & Calalang-Colucci, 2000). *Answer 14:* **a.**

15. In ARDS, the alveolocapillary unit is injured indirectly in the case of sepsis, resulting in increased permeability. The endothelial cells swell, with intercellular junctions widening, the membrane being disrupted, and edema forming. Alveolar flooding is associated with arterial hypoxemia resistant to oxygenation, decreased lung compliance as the alveoli stiffen and fibrose, and decreased functional residual capacity (Fein & Calalang-Colucci, 2000). *Answer 15:* **a.**

16. Upon physical examination, the patient's respiratory rate increases as the edema worsens. Patients sit further upright, using accessory muscles in attempt to breathe, and they describe feelings of dyspnea as "not being able to catch their breath or take a deep breath in." Serial chest radiographs will show infiltrates along the bases, usually bilaterally, with whitening out of the lungs as the fluid rises. Pleural effusions are not hallmark characteristics of ARDS because the SIRS effects to an infection are within the lung parenchyma. Dullness to percussion is consistent with areas of fluid, and frequent auscultations depict the increase in fluid as rales progress up the lungs. *Answer 16:* **b.**

Case Study continued

At 8 PM, the following vital signs are recorded for Robin:
Temperature: 98° F
Pulse: 90 beats/min
Respirations: 28 breaths/min
BP: 80 mm Hg/palpation
Arterial blood gases: 7.32/40/80%; HCO_3-15 mEq/L on 40% oxygen

QUESTIONS

17. What are the potential results of aggressive fluid hydration in Robin?

TABLE 20-2 Clinical Presentation of Sepsis

EARLY/COMPENSATORY	LATE/REFRACTORY
Signs and Symptoms	
Blood pressure <90 or >40 mm Hg below baseline	Profound hypotension
High cardiac output	Low cardiac output
Low systemic vascular resistance	High systemic vascular resistance
Urine output <0.5 ml/kg/hr	Anuria
Warm, flushed, dry skin	Cold, pale, clammy skin
Increased heart rate	Tachycardia, arrhythmias
Bounding pulses	Weak, thready pulse
Fever	Decreased core body temperature
Decreased level of consciousness	Decreased level of consciousness
Increased respiratory rate	Shortness of breath
Decreased respiratory depth	Decreased respiratory depth
Crackles	Crackles, wheezes
Diagnostic tests	
Increased WBCs	Increased or decreased WBCs
Hyperglycemia	Hypoglycemia
	Increased serum amylase, lipase
Metabolic acidosis/respiratory alkalosis	Metabolic/respiratory acidosis
Hypoxemia: Svo_2 >80% (tissue extraction increased)	Refractory hypoxemia: Svo_2 <60% (tissue extraction decreased)
Thrombin time prolonged	Decreased clotting factors
Decreasing clotting factors	Increased hepatic transaminases
Increased fibrin split products	Increased bilirubin, blood urea nitrogen, creatinine

From Shelton, B. (1999). Sepsis. *Semin Oncol Nurs, 15*(3), pp. 209-221.
WBCs, White blood cells.

a. Normal filling pressures, high SVR
b. Low cardiac index, high filling pressures, pulmonary edema
c. High cardiac index, low SVR, pulmonary edema
d. Low cardiac index, low filling pressures, low SVR

18. In the face of increasing oxygen concentrations, Robin's Po_2 remains low and appears to be falling further. What is this called?
a. Pulmonary fibrosis
b. Refractory hypoxemia
c. Fluid overload
d. Increased venous capacitance

19. What are possible reasons for hypovolemia in Robin?
1. Venous pooling
2. Increased insensible losses
3. Capillary leak
4. Lack of oral intake
   a. 1, 2, & 3
   b. 2, 3, & 4
   c. 1, 3, & 4
   d. All of these

20. What is the major challenge you face in aggressive volume resuscitation with Robin?
a. Prevention of pulmonary edema
b. Accentuation of high pulmonary pressures
c. Potentiation of the endotoxin effect on the blood vessels
d. Compounding of the problem of high SVR

21. What are the indications for vasopressor therapy in Robin?
a. Increased stroke volume
b. Increased cardiac contractility
c. Persistent peripheral vasoconstriction
d. Persistent hypotension despite adequate volume therapy

22. Which of the following are clinical signs of volume overload?
1. Decreased oxygen saturation on pulse oximetry
2. Steady level of jugular venous pressure
3. S_3
4. Auscultation of rales
   a. 1, 2, & 3
   b. 2, 3, & 4
   c. 1, 3, & 4
   d. All of these

23. What are clinical signs of response to volume and vasopressor therapy?

ANSWERS

17-18. A hyperdynamic cardiovascular state is the hoped-for result with aggressive volume resuscitation in the patient with sepsis shock. Because, by definition, septic shock is accompanied by hypotension and a systolic arterial pressure less than 90 mm Hg, it is critical to stabilize the patient's circulation and simultaneously manage the patient's airway and breathing (Jindal, Hollenberg, & Dellinger, 2000). A high cardiac index, normal filling pressures, and low SVR are the goals of fluid and vasopressor resuscitation. Because mediators such as endotoxins are released from microorganisms, they stimulate the release of macrophage-derived cytokines, such as TNF, IL-1, and IL-8. The effects are those associated with sepsis-induced hypotension: low cardiac index, low BP, low pulmonary artery pressure, and low SVR. *Answer 17:* **c.** *Answer 18:* **b.**

19. The low SVR is caused by peripheral vasodilation with venous pooling and low return to the right side of the heart. Hypovolemia is compounded in Robin with the insensible losses of sweating, tachypnea, and capillary leak. Although her oral intake is low, her intake and volume has been artificially managed with total parenteral nutrition. Losses also occur with vomiting, diarrhea, bleeding, and the decreased venous return. *Answer 19:* **a.**

20. ARDS handicaps the clinician's ability to institute aggressive volume hydration because fluid extravasation limits how much can be infused without resulting in pulmonary edema. Low colloid osmotic pressure, high hydrostatic pressure, and the capillary leak associated with septic shock–related ARDS compound the challenge of fluid resuscitation (Jindal, Hollenberg, & Dellinger, 2000). *Answer 20:* **a.**

21. The rule of thumb is that the volume of fluid necessary is that which maintains an optimal cardiac output for tissue perfusion without inducing the noncardiogenic pulmonary edema (Abraham, Matthay, Dinarello, et al., 2000). Because of these limitations, vasopressors and inotropic agents are initiated in light of hypotension in the face of adequate volume resuscitation (Jindal, Hollenberg, Dellinger, 2000). A combination of agents are aimed at improving the mean arterial pressure (Table 20-3) and increasing the SVR with improvement in the preload volumes and heart contractility. Bedside clinical signs of response and circulatory adequacy include improved mentation, urine output restoration, improved BP, falling

| TABLE 20-3 | The American-European Consensus Committee Recommended Criteria for Acute Lung Injury (ALI) and Acute Respiratory Distress Syndrome (ARDS) |

CRITERIA	TIMING	OXYGENATION	CHEST RADIOGRAPH	PULMONARY ARTERY WEDGE PRESSURE
ALI	Acute onset	Pao_2/Fio_2 ≤300 mm Hg (regardless of PEEP level)	Bilateral infiltrates seen on frontal chest radiograph	≤18 mm Hg when measured or no clinical evidence of left atrial hypertension
ARDS	Acute onset	Pao_2/Fio_2 ≤200 mm Hg (regardless of PEEP level)	Bilateral infiltrates seen on frontal chest radiograph	≤18 mm Hg when measured or no clinical evidence of left atrial hypertension

From Bernard, G. R., Brigham, K. I., & Artigas, A. (1994). The American-European Consensus Conference on ARDS: Definitions, mechanisms, relevant outcomes, and clinical trial coordination. *Am J Respir Crit Care Med, 149*, pp. 818-824. *PEEP*, Positive end-expiratory pressure.

heart rate, and skin perfusion with the temperature increasing and capillary refill returning. *Answer 21:* **d.**

22-23. Volume overload is very obvious because the person's breathing ability worsens with increased rate, coughing, signs of dyspnea, and decreased oxygen saturation on pulse oximetry. An elevated jugular venous pressure and S_3 gallop will be noted on examination. *Answer 22:* **c.** *Answer 23:* **See text.**

Case Study continued

In discussion with Robin and her mother, it is explained that Robin's pulmonary edema is worsening, requiring institution of mechanical ventilation. It is also explained that ventilatory support can improve gas exchange, minimize high airway pressures, and promote healing. Robin's mother is visibly shaken, yet Robin is quick to agree, requesting the health care team to hurry.

QUESTIONS

24. Which of the following are additional benefits and goals of ventilatory support?
1. Robin's workload to breathe is reduced.
2. Lung tissue healing is promoted.
3. Deflation of collapsible alveoli is prevented.
   a. 1 & 2
   b. 2 & 3
   c. 1 & 3
   d. All of these

25. Robin's mother, standing outside her daughter's room as she is intubated, repeatedly asks why her daughter was so eager to be ventilated. She is worried that she is giving up fighting. What can you share with her?

ANSWERS

24. Refractory hypoxemia, a potential consequence of ARDS because of the ALI to the alveolar capillary membrane, may require ventilation. By the time ventilatory support occurs, the patient has been working very hard to breathe and has been frightened by the air hunger he or she has experienced. Most patients are exhausted by the time they are placed on a ventilator because they have been using their accessory muscles, breathing very fast with deep breaths, and have been deprived of sleep because of their deteriorating condition. Ventilatory support has a number of goals, all with lung protection, systemic oxygenation, and improved survival in mind. There are a number of approaches with mechanical ventilation, including efforts to prevent deflation of collapsible alveoli at the end of expiration, improve alveolar ventilation, and minimize the number of alveoli undergoing repetitive recruitment and collapse (Fein & Calalang-Colucci, 2000). *Answer 24:* **d.**

25. Seeing a loved one on a ventilator is a terrifying experience, requiring support and ongoing explanation as to what is occurring and why. It may be helpful to explain to Robin's mother that Robin has been working hard while being frightened and that this is a chance for her to rest while the ventilator works for her. Also, being able to have control over the oxygenation allows clinicians to narrow their focus to hemodynamic support and eradication of the insulting organisms. Despite advances in mechanical ventilation strategies, mortality still remains high and patients and their families deserve a considerable amount of support. This can be difficult to achieve when patients are transferred to an intensive care unit. Families often feel lost or abandoned, returning to the oncology unit for support, explanations, and guidance. These are often excellent opportunities for the APN to maintain continuity with the patient and family, connect them with helpful resources, facilitate communication between the intensive care unit staff and family, and provide ongoing concern. *Answer 25:* **See text.**

REFERENCES

Abraham, E., Matthay, M. A., Dinarello, C. A., et al. (2000). Consensus conference definitions for sepsis, septic shock, acute lung injury, and acute respiratory distress syndrome: Time for a reevaluation. *Crit Care Med, 28*(1), pp. 232-235.

Balk, R. A. (2000). Severe sepsis and septic shock. Definitions, epidemiology, and clinical manifestations. *Crit Care Clin, 16*(2), pp. 179-191.

Casey, L. C. (2000). Immunologic response to infection and it's role in septic shock. *Crit Care Clin, 16*(2), pp. 193-209.

Fein, A. M., & Calalang-Colucci, M. G. (2000). Acute lung injury and acute respiratory distress syndrome in sepsis and septic shock. *Crit Care Clin, 16*(2), pp. 289-317.

Jindal, N., Hollenberg, S. M., & Dellinger, R. P. (2000). Pharmacologic issues in the management of septic shock. *Crit Care Clin, 16*(2), pp. 233-246.

Mavrommatis, A. C., Theodoridis, T., Orfanidou, A., et al. (2000). Coagulation system and platelets are fully activated in uncomplicated sepsis. *Crit Care Med, 28*(2), pp. 451-457.

Mizock, B. A. (2000). Metabolic derangements in sepsis and septic shock. *Crit Care Clin, 16*(2), pp. 319-336.

Pizzo, P. A. (1993). Management of fever in patients with cancer and treatment-induced neutropenia. *N Engl J Med, 328*, pp. 1323-1332.

Shelton, B. K. (1999). Sepsis. *Semin Oncol Nurs, 15*(3), pp. 209-221.

Simon, D., & Trenholme, G. (2000). Antibiotic selection for patients with septic shock. *Crit Care Clin, 16*(2), pp. 215-226.

Teplick, R., & Rubin, R. (1999). Therapy of sepsis: Why have we made such little progress? *Crit Care Med, 27*(8), pp. 1682-1683.

CHAPTER

21

Oncologic Emergency: Case 7

Deborah Boyle

Mr. Stuart Jackson is a 72-year-old man with small cell carcinoma of the right lung. At the time of his initial diagnosis, he was noted to have mild uptake at T8 on his bone scan, suggestive of early bone metastases. However, he was asymptomatic, and it was decided to proceed with chemotherapy.

He was admitted 2 days ago to the oncology unit for neutropenic fever. He is now 8 days postcompletion of his second course of chemotherapy (cisplatin, etoposide). He is currently receiving antibiotics and growth factors. His granulocytopenia is improving, and he is hopeful he will be discharged over the next few days. He is a deacon in his church and very much wants to be home to attend this Sunday's Easter service.

Weekly interdisciplinary rounds take place this morning, and the staff nurse reviews what is transpiring for Mr. Jackson. She states his white blood cell (WBC) count is $1.1/mm^3$, his granulocyte count is $800/mm^3$, platelets are $90,000/mm^3$; his hemoglobin and hematocrit are normal, and he has not spiked a temperature over the last 48 hours. He is scheduled to finish his intravenous (IV) antibiotics tomorrow, and teaching has begun about administering his growth factors at home upon discharge.

Medications
Neupogen 300 µg subcutaneously (SC) every day
Acetaminophen as needed for fever
Ceftazidime (Fortaz) 2 g intravenously every 8 hours
Docusate (Colace) 100 mg twice a day
Milk of Magnesia 30 to 60 ml at bedtime
Fentanyl patch 25 µg every 72 hours
Oxycodone hydrochloride (Percocet) 1 to 2 tablets
   every 6 hours as needed

Mr. Jackson has been widowed for 7 years and lives alone but has three grown daughters who live in his neighborhood and are involved in his

care. He is a retired postal worker. He was a heavy smoker up until his diagnosis of lung cancer last month, he does not drink, and he is active socially in his church.

The staff nurse states, "He's chomping at the bit to leave. Can we get home care to check on him after he's discharged?"

QUESTIONS

1. As you determine issues that require attention before discharge, what response from a team member would solicit the most concern?
   a. Physical therapist states, "I can't get him to work with me. He'd rather do it himself."
   b. Pharmacist relates, "Maybe we should switch him to Oxycontin to manage his pain."
   c. Oncologist shares, "We may need to reevaluate his chemotherapy."
   d. Dietitian comments, "He's still quite nauseous, and his intake is poor."

2. What inferences can you make inferring from the pharmacist's comment?

ANSWERS

1. The advanced practice nurse (APN) must help staff assess the global nature of the patient's problems associated with antineoplastic therapies and metastatic cancer. When a patient is hospitalized, the chief reason for his or her admission may become the sole focus of the staff's concern, and other related sequelae may go unrecognized. In Mr. Jackson's case, awareness of the patterns of metastases related to his primary small cell lung cancer, should facilitate inquiry into prodromal signs of a worsening disease course. *Answer 1:* **b.**

2. What was the impetus for the pharmacist's comment? Was this stated because of increasing needs for breakthrough pain medications? The pharmacist's comment about optimal narcotic dosing should solicit query about the patient's medication requirements, particularly acknowledging the predominance of pain. A review of pain medication consumption over the past 2 days could reveal increasing requirements for Percocet, which would promote the need for a more in-depth pain assessment. The physical therapist's comment may not necessarily relate to mobility impairment, a potential corollary of evolving spinal cord compression, but rather to overall weakness, depression, or struggle for independence. The oncology fellow's statement could stem from concern about the degree of neutropenia after Mr. Jackson's first course of chemotherapy. Although important and requiring attention, the dietitian's comment would be a somewhat secondary concern in conjunction with the overall assessment of comfort. *Answer 2:* **See text.**

QUESTIONS

3. What components of your pain assessment would lead to a diagnosis of spinal cord compression?
   a. Usually occurs in conjunction with bowel and bladder dysfunction
   b. Most often occurs in the lumbosacral spine
   c. Often follows other symptoms by days
   d. Often worsens with recumbency

4. Which of the following neurologic deficits would alert you to potential spinal cord compression?
   a. Hyperreflexia, decreased rectal tone, erectile dysfunction
   b. Increased rectal tone, decreased pain, hyporeflexia
   c. Distended bladder, loss of proprioception, bowel incontinence
   d. Erectile dysfunction, overflow incontinence, dermatomal pain

ANSWERS

3. Spinal cord compression is a neurologic oncologic emergency, which may result in varying levels of sensory, motor, and autonomic deficits (Abrahm, 1999; Camp-Sorrell, 1998). Lung, breast, and prostate tumors account for nearly 60% of primary neoplasms associated with this problem (Loblaw & Lapierriere, 1998). Other malignancies associated with this complication of metastatic cancer include kidney and thyroid tumors, myeloma, melanoma, lymphoma, and sarcoma. Cord compression evolves from either direct or indirect impingement on the spinal cord, producing edema with resultant ischemia, neural damage,

and ultimately spinal cord infarction (Figure 21-1). The most common site of compression occurs adjacent to the anterior spinal cord or nerve roots. Vertebral collapse or metastatic disease evolving from the vertebral body extends into the epidural space. A paraspinal mass extending through the intervertebral foramen may also cause impingement.

Pain is the hallmark symptom in spinal cord compression, occurring in more than 95% of cases (Mayer, Struthers, & Fisher, 1998; Sitton, 1998). It is thought to evolve from periosteum expansion. Depending on the level of involvement, back pain usually precedes other symptoms by weeks to months. It is often described as constant and dull. A tendency for the pain to worsen with recumbency (in contrast with pain from disc prolapse or osteoarthritis, which tends to improve when the patient lies down) often points to pain with a malignant origin. Pain can be local or radicular. Radicular pain stemming from a thoracic vertebral site usually starts from the back and circles ventrally, causing a bilateral constricting sensation (Schiff, Batchelor, & Wen, 1998). Radicular pain usually signifies nerve root compression. The thoracic level of the axial spine is the most common site of bone involvement (70% of cases) (Petersen-Rivera & Watters, 1997). Spinal cord compression is considered fatal when diagnosed in the cervical spine with respiratory paralysis. Early versus late signs indicate the degree of progression in the metastatic cascade (Box 21-1). *Answer 3:* **d.**

4. Hyperreflexia, decreased rectal tone, distended bladder, and erectile dysfunction are all examples of neurologic deficits that typically evolve below the level of cord compression, and their presence signifies autonomic dysfunction. Other sensory signs include decreased sensation of pain, temperature, and light touch; paresthesias; and numbness and tingling in the lower extremities. In addition to hyperreflexia, other motor signs of spinal cord compression include gait changes and ataxia. Percussion of the involved spinal processes often reveals tenderness and localized pain. In osseous metastases, this discomfort is usually more prominent in the thoracic region. In contrast, the pain of degenerative spinal disease is more often cervical or lumbosacral (Newton, 1999). *Answer 4:* **a.**

QUESTIONS

5. You ask the staff nurse about Mr. Jackson's bladder and bowel status, and she states, "Oh, he's already on a bowel prophylaxis regimen. He's

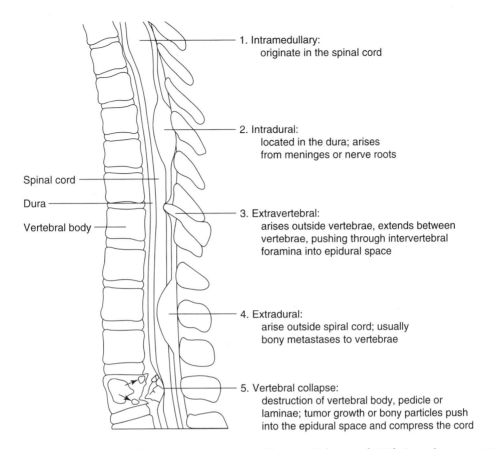

1. Intramedullary:
   originate in the spinal cord

2. Intradural:
   located in the dura; arises
   from meninges or nerve roots

Spinal cord

Dura

Vertebral body

3. Extravertebral:
   arises outside vertebrae, extends between
   vertebrae, pushing through intervertebral
   foramina into epidural space

4. Extradural:
   arise outside spiral cord; usually
   bony metastases to vertebrae

5. Vertebral collapse:
   destruction of vertebral body, pedicle or
   laminae; tumor growth or bony particles push
   into the epidural space and compress the cord

Figure 21-1 Malignant invasion of the spinal cord. (Adapted from Bucholtz, J. D. [1998]. Central nervous system metastases. *Semin Oncol Nurs, 14*[1], pp. 61-72.)

had cisplatin and is on pain medications."
Your next appropriate response might be:
  a. "That's great you've thought ahead."
  b. "What has his bowel and bladder output been over the past 48 hours?"
  c. "How much fluid is he taking?"
  d. "The reason I'm asking is because I'm concerned about spinal cord compression."

──────────────────────────────── **ANSWERS**

5. Although the staff nurse acknowledged the need to proactively treat bowel function when patients are taking medications that have peripheral neurotoxic effects, the APN's assessment in conjunction with mentoring responsibilities should foster the staff nurse's critical thinking ability. Determination of recent bowel and bladder symptoms could raise suspicion about early signs of neurologic compromise. Autonomic dysfunction can manifest as urinary retention, constipation, or incontinence. Assessing these symptoms will help determine the level of spinal tract involvement. In

| BOX 21-1 | Signs and Symptoms of Spinal Cord Compression |

TIME FRAME	SIGN/SYMPTOM
Early	Pain
	Sensory loss: numbness, tingling, sensory changes
⬇	Motor weakness or gait change
	Autonomic disturbances: bowel (constipation) and/or bladder retention dysfunction
Late	Bowel and/or bladder incontinence
	Paralysis

Adapted from Held, J. L., & Peahota, A. (1993). Nursing care of patients with spinal cord compression. *Oncol Nurs Forum, 21*(10), pp. 1507-1514.

addition, even in the absence of these symptoms, there must be ongoing evaluation of the efficacy of a bowel prophylaxis regimen. *Answer 5:* **b.**

Case Study continued

You say to the staff nurse, "After rounds, let's evaluate Mr. Jackson together." Having reviewed his narcotic requirements for the past 48 hours, you and the staff nurse speak with him. You suggest that he is having increasing pain in his lower back, but he tells you, "I think it's because I'm in bed so much lately." In further assessing his pain, Mr. Jackson states, "It feels like I have a belt on that's too tight." You ask him about his bowel and bladder function and his mobility. He says timidly, "I'm still having some problems with constipation and my legs feel so weak and heavy." You decide to assess Mr. Jackson further. You evaluate all vertebral spinous processes using gentle percussion.

QUESTIONS

6. Which of the following findings would most likely result in ordering magnetic resonance imaging (MRI)?

1. Localized pain on percussion at T8-T9
2. A band of numbness at T8-T9 extending around Mr. Jackson's body
3. Negative Romberg's test
4. Increased muscle tone and reflexes of lower extremities
   a. 1, 2, & 3
   b. 2, 3, & 4
   c. 1, 3, & 4
   d. 1, 2, & 4

7. The MRI reveals a worsening lesion at T8 with epidural extension, cord impingement, and early T9 vertebral collapse. Steroids are prescribed for Mr. Jackson. He receives an IV bolus dose of dexamethasone 10 mg and soon after starts dexamethasone 4 mg orally every 6 hours for 48 hours. What symptom would *not* be an untoward effect of steroid use?

a. Hemoccult-positive stool
b. Hyperglycemia
c. Mild forgetfulness
d. Mild hunger

8. Mr. Jackson will start radiation therapy this afternoon. His daughters ask about his going home for Easter this weekend. When considering discharge, what is the priority health issue?

a. Pain management
b. Safety

c. Bowel control
d. Emotional state

9. What factors, consistent with principles of radiation therapy, most likely led Mr. Jackson to agree to radiation therapy?

1. Can be conducted as an outpatient
2. Has minimal toxicities because of limited dose
3. Provides rapid pain relief
4. Preserves sexual function
   a. 1 & 3
   b. 1 & 2
   c. 2 & 3
   d. 3 & 4

10. Mr. Jackson is concerned about the effects of radiation therapy over the Easter weekend. In teaching Mr. Jackson about what to expect, you tell him he could experience:

a. Worsening fatigue
b. Improved back pain
c. Problems with upset stomach
d. Problems with diarrhea

ANSWERS

6. The physical examination in someone at high risk for spinal cord compression is critical in determining which diagnostic tests are indicated. Examination helps pinpoint the level of compression. There can be localized pain at the spinal column with lancinating pain, paresthesias, and numbness in the distribution of the dermatome. The muscles innervated by the affected nerves can be weaker and have decreased tone and reflexes. However, with slowly progressing lesions, the muscle tone and reflexes can be increased.

MRI is the diagnostic tool of choice for spinal cord compression. It is noninvasive and has distinct advantages in that it can determine both the nature and extent of the spinal lesion, which also aids in treatment planning. *Answer 6:* **d.**

7. Gastrointestinal bleeding, hyperglycemia, and hunger are symptoms associated with steroid use. Steroid-induced psychosis is usually an acute syndrome with dramatic changes in personality and activity levels, with delusions and paranoia. Mild forgetfulness may be an early sign of an evolving delirium. A pattern can often be discerned between symptom presentation and steroid administration.

The exact mechanism of steroid efficacy in treating spinal cord compression is unclear (Cowap, Hardy, & A'Hern, 2000). Steroids decrease edema and the mass effect responsible for pain, which is thought to promote neurologic improvement (Walsh, Doona, Molnar, & Lipnickey, 2000). Enlarging epidural tumors may cause early obstruction of the epidural venous plexus, resulting in venous edema. The beneficial action of steroids may be most obvious in this scenario (Schiff, Batchelor, & Wen, 1998). However, controversy remains about optimal steroid dosages and their use in ambulatory patients without compromised motor function (Kovner, Spigel, Rider, et al., 1999). *Answer 7:* **c.**

8. In the context of home care planning and evaluation of readiness for discharge, safety is always the priority concern. Anticipation of possible safety issues is often best deliberated within a team forum. Physical and occupational therapists, along with nursing staff, can anticipate barriers to safety and plan preventive interventions, which require communication with the family and the patient. Effective symptom management is a corollary of discharge planning and should always be considered in tandem with overall safety evaluation. Severe motor impairment or paraplegia necessitates many adaptations in the home. In addition, these patients may also require long-term venous embolism prophylaxis. *Answer 8:* **b.**

9. Radiation therapy is usually the treatment of choice for spinal cord compression. With transportation support from home, it can be completed as an outpatient. Although effective in managing pain, it often takes three to five treatments for its benefits to be recognized. When the osseous metastases are cervical or when there is an acute loss of motor function, radiation therapy is administered emergently.

Radiation therapy has comparable efficacy to surgical intervention. However, there are some unique indications for surgery in the management of spinal cord compression. The generally accepted indications are as follows (Kovner, et al., 1999; Loblaw & Laperriere, 1998):

- The level of the spinal cord compression in an area previously irradiated (i.e., relapse postirradiation or prior radiation to that area of the spinal cord)
- Neurologic deterioration during radiation therapy
- Evidence of spinal instability or bony compression of the spinal cord
- Need for tissue diagnosis
- Intractable pain
- Spinal cord compression in a patient with no history of cancer or a remote history of cancer

End results from therapy for spinal cord compression depend on both the rapidity of symptom presentation and neurologic status at the time of diagnosis. The more rapid the onset of symptoms and the more severe the neurologic deficit, the more unfavorable the outcomes. In addition to pain relief, reversibility of neurocompromise is the ultimate goal of treatment. Stability of deficit or prevention of further impairment is a secondary goal. Classification systems that predict outcome from therapy are the focus of recent investigation and address functional status at the time of spinal cord compression diagnosis. Categories of ambulatory, paraparetic nonambulatory, and paraplegic correlate with treatment outcomes. Generally, 80% of ambulatory patients at diagnosis of spinal cord compression remain ambulatory after treatment. For patients who are paraplegic at diagnosis, fewer than 10% will regain mobility. *Answer 9:* **a.**

10. Mr. Jackson's lower thoracic vertebrae involved with bone metastases will be radiated within a posterior spinal field. This field will encompass two vertebrae above and below the involved T8-T9 lesions. Toxicities depend on field size, dose fractions, and total dose delivered. Because of the anatomic focus of the radiation beam to T6-T11, some component of the gut will be in the radiation field. Hence, Mr. Jackson will most likely experience problems with nausea. Pretreatment medication with an antiemetic often reduces the intensity of this potential problem.

For spinal cord compression, treatment length averages from 8 to 12 days. Pain relief occurs in more than 85% of patients, but it often takes at least three to five treatments for some symptom relief to be noted. In addition, a pain flare phenomenon may occur early in the treatment course. This is thought to be the result of acute edema prompted by the onset of radiation therapy. Like nausea, fatigue is associated with cumulative doses of radiation therapy. It often presents beyond the midpoint of treatment and is more severe at the end of the week rather than at the beginning. Diarrhea is associated with pelvic radiation therapy fields. *Answer 10:* **c.**

Case Study continued

Three weeks later, Mr. Jackson's daughter calls you for advice. Her father has finished his radiation therapy and is functioning fairly well. However, he is having ongoing problems with constipation and is embarrassed to tell anyone about this. He eats bran every morning and takes Colace twice a day. However, he has not had a bowel movement in 4 days. You discuss options with Mr. Jackson's daughter for a regimen to promote timely bowel evacuation over the next 24 hours. Now you need to decide on a bowel prophylaxis regimen for him.

QUESTIONS

11. What are the potential causes of Mr. Jackson's constipation?

12. In considering a bowel regimen for Mr. Jackson, an ideal *initial* program might include:
   a. Docusate sodium 100 mg + Senokot 2 tablets orally twice a day
   b. Docusate sodium 100 mg + Senokot S 2 tablets orally twice a day
   c. Senokot S 2 tablets orally twice a day + glycerin suppository every morning
   d. Lactulose 30 ml every morning + bisacodyl 10 mg orally every evening

ANSWERS

11. Constipation is the most common opioid-induced side effect (Komurcu, Nelson, Walsh, et al., 2000). In addition, it does not resolve with time. In Mr. Jackson's case of progressive cancer, opioid-induced constipation is exacerbated by poor oral intake (i.e., fluids and fiber), history of neurotoxic drug therapies, immobility, and spinal cord compression. Advanced age and other common corollaries of growing old, such as diabetes, use of contrast materials in diagnostic procedures, inactivity, hypothyroidism, depression, and polypharmacy, are other factors to consider when the cancer patient is elderly. In addition to opioid use, anticholinergics, diuretics, antacids, phenothiazines, and antihypertensive drugs must be contemplated in prescription and over-the-counter formulations because of potential offending agents. *Answer 11:* **See text.**

12. Medications to manage constipation are often prescribed without consideration of their mechanisms of action. Like many other drug regimens, multimodality therapy works best in managing chronic constipation by altering different causative mechanisms (Table 21-1). For example, docusate sodium (Colace) softens stool by promoting water entry into feces. However, it does not affect

TABLE 21-1	Constipation Medications: Laxatives and Cathartics	
DRUG	**MECHANISM OF ACTION**
BULK FORMERS Psyllium (Metamucil) Methylcellulose (Cologel, Citrucel) Polycarbophil Onset of effect: 12 hr-3 days	Nondigested plant cell walls absorb water in feces; softens, increases stool size, thus increasing peristalsis; acts in small and large intestines

BOWEL STIMULANTS
Diphenylmethanes
   Phenolphthalein (in Ex-lax, Feen-a-mint, Correctol, Doxidan)
   Bisacodyl (Dulcolax): 5 mg enteric-coated tablet orally 1-3 times/day; 10-mg suppository (single dose as needed)
Onset of effect: 6-10 hr; rectally: 15-60 min
	Directly stimulates nerve plexus of colon
	Irritates smooth muscle of intestine, stimulating peristalsis
	Phenolphthalein and Bisacodyl first metabolized in liver, then colon; effect may be prolonged

Arthraquinones
   Senna (Senekot, X-Prep): 187-mg tablet; daily maximum of 8 tablets or 4 tsp granules (326 mg)/day
   Cascara Sagrada (aromatic): 5 ml or 1 tablet (325 mg) at bedtime as needed
   Casanthranol (cascara derivative): 30 mg, usually in combination with docusate
Onset of effect: 6-12 hr
	Exact mechanism unknown; may stimulate colon and myenteric plexus
	Senna stimulates submucosal nerve plexus and peristalsis in transverse and descending colon, decreases sodium and water absorption; produces semiliquid or formed stool
	Cascara directly irritates intestinal mucosa, results in motility and changes in fluid and electrolyte secretion

From Tuchmann, L. (1997). Constipation. In Gates, R. S., & Fink, R. M. (Eds.). *Oncology Nursing Secrets.* Philadelphia: Hanley & Belfus.

stool motility. Senna derivatives increase peristalsis and thus stimulate bowel evacuation. Hence, they are very effective in combination but rarely work in isolation as in cases of chronic constipation such as Mr. Jackson's.

For Mr. Jackson, Colace and Senna derivatives, such as Senokot, would be the optimal first choice for the prevention of constipation (Levy, 1996). Senokot S has senna plus Colace; hence, additional Colace would be redundant. Similarly, Peri-Colace is a stool softener with a cascara derivative, which acts as a stimulant; hence, Senokot may not be required or smaller doses may be in order. Significant effort should be made to devise a regimen via the oral route as an initial effort. Glycerin suppositories, although very effective, would be a second choice after titrating senna and Colace, optimally with constipation still occurring. Lactulose is difficult to tolerate, and knowing Mr. Jackson's recent problems with nausea, any agent that could potentiate this symptom should be avoided. Bisacodyl (Dulcolax) should be reserved as a stimulant when no bowel movement has occurred over 24 to 48 hours. It should not be taken daily. It commonly is associated with gastrointestinal cramping. All bowel evacuation regimens require reconsideration in the event of a suspicious bowel obstruction.

Regimens for chronic constipation must be consumed daily rather than as needed because the underlying causes remain constant in the case of advanced cancer (Robinson, Fritch, Hullett, et al., 2000). Patients experiencing paralysis will require an aggressive bowel regimen similar to those used in rehabilitation settings for paraplegics. Dietary maneuvers to increase fiber and the establishment of a routine for elimination help retrain the bowel in conjunction with medication support. Fluid intake is critically important as an adjunct to any dietary/drug regimen. A simple recipe that can be used at home to manage constipation is illustrated in Box 21-2. *Answer 12:* **a.**

BOX 21-2 Power Pudding

Mix equal parts of prune juice, applesauce, and bran (fine bran works better than bran flakes). Blend together and keep in freezer; take 1 to 2 tablespoons every morning before breakfast.

Modified from Tuchmann, L. (1997). Constipation. In Gates, R. S., & Fink, R. M. (Eds.). *Oncology nursing secrets* (pp. 216-225). Philadelphia: Hanley & Belfus.

CONTRAINDICATIONS	ADVERSE EFFECTS	DRUG INTERACTIONS
Intestinal strictures, partial or total bowel obstruction or fecal impaction, phenylketonuria Advanced cancer with early satiety, nausea, anorexia Caution in diabetics due to sugar content	Flatulence, erratic habits, abdominal discomfort or initiation	May decrease effects of tetracycline, anticoagulants, digitalis glycosides or salicylates, nitrofurantoin
Bowel obstruction Phenolphthalein less suitable in cancer patient because major gastrointestinal peristaltic effect difficult to predict and control Bisacodyl: abdominal pain	Phenolphthalein: diarrhea, cramps, skin reactions, photosensitivity, hypersensitivity-type encephalitis Bisacodyl: cramps, urgency, incontinence	Bisacodyl decreases effect of warfarin
Bowel obstruction	Cathartic colon, may result in intestinal atony Fluid and electrolyte disturbances	Cascara decreases effect of oral anticoagulants

Continued

TABLE 21-1 Constipation Medications: Laxatives and Cathartics—cont'd	
DRUG	**MECHANISM OF ACTION**
OSMOTIC LAXATIVES	

Lactulose
  Cephulac: 30-45 ml 3 or 4 times/day or hourly
    to induce rapid effect in initial phase
  Chronulac: 15-30 ml/day; may increase to
    60 ml/day
Sorbitol: 3-150 ml/day (70% solution)
	Lactulose/Sorbitol: nonabsorbable sugars; exert
	  osmotic effect mostly in large bowel
	Lactulose also used in hepatic encephalopathy to
	  lower serum ammonia

Polyethylene glycol electrolyte solution
  (Colyte, Golytely); 8 oz orally every 15 min
  as tolerated over 3-4 hr until 1 L taken or
  diarrhea results
Onset of effect:
  Lactulose: 24-48 hr
  Polyethylene glycol: first bowel movement
    within 1 hr
	Polyethylene glycol: catharsis by strong electrolyte
	  and osmotic effects

Glycerin: rectal suppositories, 1-2/day as needed,
  or 5-15 ml as enema
Onset of effect: within 30 min of use
	Lubricates and softens
	Stimulates defecation osmotically; sodium
	  stearate in suppository may irritate rectal
	  membranes

LUBRICANTS	

Mineral oil: 15-40 ml/day orally (once or in divided
  doses): as retention enema: 60-150 ml/day as
  single dose
Onset of effect: within 8 hr
	Lubricates intestinal mucosa and feces; softens
	  stool by preventing loss of water from feces

DETERGENT LAXATIVES	

Docusate: 50-500 mg/day in 1-4 doses
Docusate sodium = Colace
Docusate calcium = Surfak
Onset of effect: 24-72 hr
	Decreases surface tension and allows water and fat
	  penetration of hard stool
	Mucosal contact effect decreases electrolyte and
	  water reabsorption in small and large intestines

SALINE LAXATIVES	

Magnesium (Mg) salts
  Mg citrate: ½-1 full bottle (120-300 ml) orally as
    needed
  Mg hydroxide (e.g., Milk of Magnesia Regular
    Strength): 30-60 ml/day orally or in divided
    doses
	Mg increases gastric, pancreatic, small intestine
	  secretion and motor activity of small and large
	  intestines
	Mg and Na salts are poorly absorbed and draw
	  water into lumen, thus increasing stool water
	  content and frequency

Sodium (Na) salts
  Sodium phosphate
    Fleet Phospho-soda: 20-30 ml as single dose
    Fleet enema: 4.5-oz enema; may repeat
Onset of effect:
  Mg citrate: 30 min-6 hr, depending on dose
  Mg hydroxide: 4-8 hr
  Sodium phosphate: Oral: 3-6 hr
                Rectal: 2-5 min	

From Tuchmann, L. (1997). Constipation. In Gates, R. S., & Fink, R. M. (Eds.). *Oncology Nursing Secrets*. Philadelphia: Hanley & Belfus.

CONTRAINDICATIONS	ADVERSE EFFECTS	DRUG INTERACTIONS
Lactulose/Sorbitol: avoid with fecal impaction or intestinal obstruction Caution with severe cardiopulmonary and renal impairment (contraindicated in anuria) May cause elevations in blood glucose levels in diabetics	Lactulose: cramps, flatulence, nausea, vomiting; excessive use may cause electrolyte losses, diarrhea Chronulac: gas from bacterial degradation Sorbitol: edema, nausea, vomiting, diarrhea, abdominal discomfort, potential fluid and electrolyte loss	Decreases effect of neomycin, other antiinfectives, and antacids
Golytely: do not give with bowel obstruction (high risk for perforation), toxic colitis, megacolon, gastric retention, bowel perforation	Polyethylene glycol: nausea, abdominal fullness, bloating, cramps	Do not give oral medications within 1 hr of Golytely
Abdominal pain, nausea, vomiting	May cause rectal irritation if used too frequently; headache	
Known reflux, dysphagia (risk of lipid pneumonia or aspiration pneumonitis, especially in elderly)	Excessive use may lead to anal leakage and irritation Chronic use reduces absorption of fat-soluble vitamins Lipid pneumonitis with aspiration	Docusate sodium increases absorption and risk of lipid granuloma of gut wall Alters absorption of antibiotics, anticoagulants, oral contraceptives, digitalis glycosides
Intestinal obstruction, acute abdominal pain, nausea, or vomiting	Diarrhea, abdominal cramps Prolonged use may lead to dependence or electrolyte imbalance	Increases mineral oil absorption Decreases effect of warfarin and aspirin
Fecal impaction, intestinal obstruction, nausea, vomiting, abdominal pain Avoid Mg salts in renal failure, myocardial damage, heart block, hepatitis, ileostomy, colostomy	Mg salts: excessive use may cause electrolyte losses, hypermagnesemia, diarrhea, cramps, gas	Effects of Mg counteracted by aluminum salt in many antacids Milk of Magnesia decreases absorption of tetracyclines, digoxin, indomethacin, or iron salts
Avoid Na salts in cardiac or renal disease, hyperphosphatemia, hypernatremia, hypocalcemia; use with caution if diet is sodium-restricted	Na salts: nausea, vomiting, diarrhea, edema, hypotension; excessive use may cause dependence	Na phosphate: do not give with Mg or aluminum-containing antacids or sucralfate; they may bind with phosphate

REFERENCES

Abrahm, J. L. Management of pain and spinal cord compression in patients with advanced cancer. *Ann Intern Med, 131*(1), pp. 37-46.

Bucholtz, J. D. (1998). Central nervous system metastases. *Semin Oncol Nurs, 14*(1), pp. 61-72.

Camp-Sorrell, D. (1998). Spinal cord compression. *Clin J Oncol Nurs, 2*(3), pp. 112-113.

Cowap, J., Hardy, J. R., & A'Hern, R. (2000). Outcomes of malignant spinal cord compression at a cancer center: Implications for palliative care services. *J Pain Sympt Manage, 19*(4), pp. 257-264.

Held, J. L., & Peahota, A. Nursing care of patients with spinal cord compression. *Oncol Nurs Forum, 20*(10), pp. 1507-1514.

Komurcu, S., Nelson, K. A., Walsh, D., et al. (2000). Common symptoms of advanced cancer. *Semin Oncol, 27*(1), pp. 24-33.

Kovner, F., Spigel, S., Rider, I., et al. (1999). Radiation therapy of metastatic spinal cord compression. *J Neuro-Oncol, 42*, pp. 85-92.

Levy, M. H. (1996). Pharmacologic treatment of cancer pain. *N Engl J Med, 335*(15), pp. 1124-1132.

Loblaw, D. A., & Laperriere, N. J. (1998). Emergency treatment of malignant extradural spinal cord compression: An evidence-based guideline. *J Clin Oncol, 16*(4), pp. 1613-1624.

Mayer, D., Struthers, C., & Fisher, G. (1998). Nursing management of the patients with bone metastases. *Semin Oncol Nurs, 14*(3), pp. 199-209.

Newton, H. B. (1999). Neurologic complications of systemic cancer. *Am Fam Physician, 59*(4), pp. 878-886.

Petersen-Rivera, L., & Watters, M. R. (1997). Spinal cord compression. In Gates, R. S., & Fink, R. M. (Eds.). *Oncology nursing secrets* (pp. 352-355). Philadelphia: Hanley & Belfus.

Robinson, C. B., Fritch, M., Hullett, L., et al. (2000). Development of a protocol to prevent opioid-induced constipation in patients with cancer: A research utilization project. *Clin J Oncol Nurs, 4*(2), pp. 79-84.

Schiff, D., Batchelor, T., & Wen, P. Y. (1998). Neurologic emergencies in cancer patients. *Neurol Clin North Am, 16*(2), pp. 449-481.

Sitton, E. (1998). Central nervous system metastases. *Semin Oncol Nurs, 14*(3), pp. 210-219.

Tuchmann, L. (1997). Constipation. In Gates, R. S., & Fink, R. M. (Eds.). *Oncology nursing secrets* (pp. 216-225). Philadelphia: Hanley & Belfus.

Walsh, D., Doona, M., Molnar, M., & Lipnickey, V. (2000). Symptom control in advanced cancer: Important drugs and routes of administration. *Semin Oncol, 27*(1), pp. 69-83.

CHAPTER

22 Oncologic Emergency: Case 8

Nancy Jo Bush

Michael Polanski is a 37-year-old white man who presented to the emergency room complaining of a severe headache for 2 days, which was unrelieved by analgesics. After borrowing two tablets of sumatriptan succinate (Imitrex) from a friend and finding no relief, he decided to seek help. Michael's laboratory results reveal an elevated white blood cell (WBC) count with increased monocytes and decreased platelets. The presence of blasts is noted in his peripheral smear. Further laboratory data reveal elevated lactic dehydrogenase (LDH) and uric acid levels. A bone marrow biopsy confirms acute monocytic leukemia, and Michael is admitted for induction chemotherapy consisting of high-dose Ara-C (cytosine-arabinoside) and idarubicin. Treatment to prevent tumor lysis syndrome (TLS) is initiated.

QUESTIONS

1. TLS occurs when:
   a. Tumor cell kill results in the release of intracellular components
   b. Tumor cell kill causes bacterial release of endotoxins
   c. Tumor cells invade vital organs
   d. Tumor cells invade interstitial spaces during antineoplastic therapy

2. TLS results in an increase in serum:
   a. Sodium, potassium, calcium
   b. Potassium, phosphorus, uric acid
   c. Potassium, calcium, albumin
   d. Magnesium, phosphorous, calcium

3. TLS is most often associated with all of the following *except:*
   a. Lymphoproliferative disorders
   b. Elevated LDH
   c. High WBC counts
   d. Solid tumors

4. TLS-associated hypocalcemia is caused by:
   a. The release of intracellular calcium into the bloodstream
   b. The release of calcium from the bone
   c. The inverse relationship between calcium and phosphorous
   d. The exchange of calcium and magnesium

ANSWERS

1-4. TLS is a metabolic disorder characterized by the rapid release of intracellular contents (potassium, phosphorus, and nucleic acid) into the bloodstream upon rapid tumor cell kill. This results in four metabolic abnormalities:
   1. Hyperkalemia
   2. Hyperphosphatemia
   3. Hyperuricemia
   4. Hypocalcemia

Because of the inverse relationship between calcium and phosphorous, hypocalcemia results from increased phosphorous binding to the calcium in the bloodstream, forming calcium phosphate salts (Finley, 1998).

TLS is most commonly associated with diseases that have a rapid cellular proliferation and large tumor burden (e.g., lymphoproliferative disorders) as evidenced by high WBC counts and elevated LDH. TLS may occur in patients with both acute myelogenous leukemia (AML) and acute lymphocytic leukemia (ALL), but it is seen more often in patients with ALL. In AML, TLS is most common in patients diagnosed with monocytoid leukemia, as in Michael's case (Dietz, 1999). The acute and blast crisis of chronic myelogenous leukemia (CML) is also associated with TLS and is the most common oncologic emergency associated with Burkitt's lymphoma (Oksenholt & Seelig, 1999). Small cell lung cancer also has a high growth fraction, placing the patient at risk for TLS (Finley, 1998). TLS is rare in patients with solid tumors because these tumors respond more slowly to chemotherapy, yet in addition to a slight risk in small cell lung cancer, TLS has been observed in a subset of patients with breast cancer (Drakos, Bar-Ziv, & Catane, 1994; Sklarin & Markham, 1995). *Answer 1:* **a.** *Answer 2:* **b.** *Answer 3:* **d.** *Answer 4:* **c.**

Case Study continued

Michael and his wife are anxious to get treatment started. Although the diagnosis confronting them was shocking, both of them are looking forward to Michael feeling relief from his excruciating headache.

Michael's Treatment Orders

Ara-C 200 mg/m^2 for 7 days
Idarubicin 12 mg/m^2 for 3 days
Zofran 32 mg intravenously
Decadron 10 mg intravenously 30 minutes before idarubicin
D$_5$ ½-NS at 150 ml/hr with 50 mEq sodium bicarbonate each liter
Allopurinol 600 mg orally on days 1 through 3; then 300 mg orally every day

A neurologist has been called in to administer intrathecal methotrexate (MTX) to Michael on day 2 of treatment.

QUESTIONS

5. What knowledge motivates you to conduct a focused TLS assessment?
   a. Certain conditions place patients at higher risk for TLS.
   b. Pharmacologic management of TLS requires confirmation of healthy organs.
   c. Dosages of antineoplastic therapy may be adjusted for TLS risk factors.
   d. AML treatment is delayed 12 hours after TLS prophylaxis is begun.

6. Your focused assessment of Michael's clinical condition will look for which of the following risk factors?
   a. Elevated magnesium level
   b. Renal insufficiency
   c. Bladder outlet obstruction
   d. Elevated calcium level

7. What signs and symptoms alert you to the presence of TLS after Michael's induction treatment has begun?
   a. Muscle cramps, constipation, paresthesias
   b. Lethargy, diarrhea, nausea
   c. Paresthesias, hypotension, vomiting
   d. Weight gain, weakness, constipation

| BOX **22-1** | **Risk Factors for Tumor Lysis Syndrome** |

> High white blood cell count
> Impaired renal function
> Hyperuricemia
> Sepsis
> Elevated lactate dehydrogenase
> Dehydration

From DiBella, N. J. (1994). Acute myelogenous and lymphocytic leukemia. In Wood, M. E., & Bunn, P. A. (Eds.). *Hematology oncology secrets* (pp. 115-118). Philadelphia: Hanley & Belfus.

ANSWERS

5. A focused TLS assessment must be carried out during induction chemotherapy because certain medical conditions place patients at higher risk than others. *Answer 5:* **a.**

6. The metabolic abnormalities of TLS can be exacerbated if the patient is dehydrated, has renal insufficiency, or has azotemia before therapy. Other risk factors include sepsis, high WBC counts at diagnosis, and an elevated LDH (Box 22-1). *Answer 6:* **b.**

7. Early signs of TLS include diarrhea, lethargy, muscle cramps, nausea and vomiting, weakness, and paresthesias (Dietz & Flaherty, 1993). *Answer 7:* **b.**

Case Study continued

Michael is starting the first day of induction therapy. He is feeling slight relief from his headache but feels waves of nausea controlled by ondansetron (Zofran) 8 mg orally every 8 hours. His oral intake is poor, and he appears withdrawn. After reviewing Michael's chart, you express your concern that he is at higher risk for TLS because of his large tumor burden.

QUESTIONS

8. The staff nurse caring for Michael wonders how you can assume that he has a large tumor burden. What findings in your assessment support your assumption?
   a. Bone involvement
   b. Severe, uncontrolled pain
   c. Elevated pretreatment LDH and uric acid
   d. Presence of blasts in the peripheral smear

9. The staff nurse inquires about TLS. You explain that all of the following interventions have

been included in Michael's protocol to prevent TLS *except:*
   a. Hydration
   b. Sodium bicarbonate
   c. Dietary restriction of calcium and phosphorous
   d. Allopurinol

10. What is the role of allopurinol in the treatment of TLS?
   a. Decreases uric acid production
   b. Prevents calcium-phosphorous binding
   c. Binds with potassium to prevent hyperkalemia
   d. Alkalinizes the urine

--- **ANSWERS**

8. TLS is anticipated before oncologic treatment in high-risk tumors such as Michael's. His symptom of sudden-onset, intense headache reflected rapid tumor proliferation. He also presented with an elevated LDH and hyperuricemia, indicative of high tumor burden and rapid cell turnover, which occurs with leukemia (Tracey & Kruger, 1996). *Answer 8:* **c.**

9. The principal treatment for TLS is prevention. One of the major goals is to prevent uric acid crystallization in the kidney tubules. Pretreatment of TLS begins with pharmacologic interventions using allopurinol (Zyloprim) and sodium bicarbonate ($NaHCO_3$) with vigorous hydration before and after treatment. Alkaline hydration increases the solubility of uric acid. *Answer 9:* **c.**

10. Allopurinol is a xanthine oxidase inhibitor that decreases uric acid production metabolically. The role of allopurinol before and during initial chemotherapy is to decrease uric acid concentration to prevent uric acid neuropathy. Allopurinol acts by decreasing both the serum and urine levels of uric acid (Zobec, 1997). Uric acid is highly soluble in alkaline urine and intravenous fluids are given to hydrate the patient, flush the kidneys, and prevent uric acid crystal formation. If hyperphosphatemia occurs, alkalinization should be avoided in these patients to prevent calcium phosphate deposition (Miller & Parnes, 1994; Oksenholt & Seelig, 1999). The urine pH should be maintained at higher than 7 to 7.5, with specific gravity less than 1.010 (Heffner & Polman, 1998). Other pharmacologic management may include the use of diuretics to maintain adequate urinary output, aluminum hydroxide to bind dietary phosphate from the small bowel, and exchange resins such as sodium polystyrene sulfonate (Kayexalate) to

BOX 22-2 | **Medical Management of Tumor Lysis Syndrome**

NONPHARMACOLOGIC INTERVENTIONS
Intravenous hydration
Dialysis
Potassium/phosphorous restrictions

PHARMACOLOGIC INTERVENTIONS
Allopurinol
Sodium bicarbonate
Diuretics
Aluminum hydroxide
Kayexalate

MONITORING
Serum electrolytes (potassium, phosphorous, calcium)
Uric acid levels
Blood urea nitrogen and creatinine
Electrocardiography

From Finley, J. D. (1998). Metabolic emergencies. In Itano, J. K., & Taoka, K. N. (Eds.). *Core curriculum for oncology nursing* (3rd ed.) (pp. 315-339). Philadelphia: WB Saunders.

decrease potassium levels (Finley, 1998). An overview of pharmacologic and nonpharmacologic measures used in the treatment of TLS is presented in Box 22-2. *Answer 10:* **a.**

Case Study continued

On day 2 of induction chemotherapy, physical assessment reveals rales in the lower lung fields. You note that Michael's urinary output over the past 8 hours is only 200 ml.

Michael's Laboratory Data on Day 4

Urine pH	6.0
$NaHCO_3$, serum	20 mEq/L
Uric acid, serum	8.4 mg/dl
Potassium, serum	5.7 mEq/L
Phosphorous, serum	7.4 mg/dl
Calcium, serum	6.8 mg/dl
Blood urea nitrogen (BUN), serum	54 mg/dl
Creatinine	1.9 mg/dl

QUESTIONS

11. What organ systems are most affected by TLS and demand your thorough assessment at this stage of Michael's induction therapy?
   a. Liver, lungs, kidneys, gastrointestinal (GI) system
   b. Kidneys; cardiac, neuromuscular, GI systems
   c. Kidneys, gallbladder, GI system, liver
   d. Cardiac system, lungs, kidneys, bone marrow

BOX 22-3 | Clinical Manifestations of Tumor Lysis Syndrome

RENAL PROBLEMS

Decreased urine output
Elevated blood urea nitrogen and serum
   creatinine
Elevated serum uric acid
Uric acid crystallization in renal tubules
Acute renal failure

CARDIAC ARRHYTHMIAS

Atrioventricular blocks
Ventricular tachycardia
Cardiac arrest

NEUROMUSCULAR IRRITABILITY

Tetany
Carpopedal spasm
Muscle cramps
Confusion, delirium, hallucination
Seizures
Digital and perioral paresthesias

GASTROINTESTINAL EFFECTS

Nausea and vomiting, anorexia
Intestinal colic
Diarrhea
Hyperphosphatemia

From Zobec, A. (1997). Tumor lysis syndrome. In Gates, R. A., & Fink, R. M. (Eds.). *Oncology nursing secrets* (pp. 367-369). Philadelphia: Hanley & Belfus.

12. Assessment of Michael's laboratory data leads you to first suspect that he is experiencing:
   a. Acute TLS
   b. Resistance to chemotherapy
   c. Acute renal failure
   d. Metabolic acidosis

13. What is the differential diagnosis for Michael's present fluid status?
   a. Dehydration
   b. Fluid overload
   c. Renal failure
   d. Renal obstruction

14. Which of the following diuretics may be ordered for Michael?
   1. Furosemide (Lasix)
   2. Mannitol
   3. Hydrochlorothiazide
      a. 1 & 2
      b. 1, 2, & 3
      c. 1 & 3
      d. 2 & 3

ANSWERS

11. Those organ systems most at risk with TLS are the cardiac, neurologic, renal, and GI systems. Clinical manifestations of TLS related to dysfunction in these systems are outlined in Box 22-3. On day 2 of induction therapy, Michael's laboratory data indicate acute TLS. Pertinent laboratory data that support this diagnosis are presented in Table 22-1. Serious renal complications are likely to occur when serum uric acid levels exceed 15 mg/dl (Heffner & Polman, 1998). *Answer 11:* **b.**

12. Assessment of Michael should focus on prevention and early detection of metabolic abnormalities related to TLS. This includes assessment

TABLE 22-1 | Pertinent Laboratory Values and Tumor Lysis Syndrome

Elevated uric acid	>8.0 mg/l
Elevated potassium	>5.5 mEq/L
Elevated phosphorous	>7.0 mg/dl
Low calcium	<7.0 mg/dl
Elevated blood urea nitrogen	>50 mg/dl
Elevated creatinine	>1.6 mg/dl
Elevated lactate dehydrogenase	>1500 IU/L
Arterial blood gas	Low in metabolic acidosis

From Robinson, J. G. (1998). Tumor lysis syndrome. In Chernecky, C. C., & Berger, B. J. (Eds.). *Advanced and critical care oncology nursing* (pp. 637-659). Philadelphia: WB Saunders.

of both laboratory data and symptoms related to hypokalemia, hypophosphatemia, hypocalcemia, and hyperuricemia. Close monitoring of metabolic parameters includes serum electrolytes (potassium, phosphorous, and calcium), uric acid, LDH, and renal function studies, including BUN and creatinine. Monitoring of laboratory values should take place every 6 to 8 hours during the first 72 hours after induction chemotherapy. *Answer 12:* **a.**

13. Your physical assessment of Michael revealed bilateral rales and a urine output of less than 30 ml/hr. To prevent hyperuricemia, the fluid hydration ordered for Michael is $D_5W/0.45NS$ with sodium bicarbonate 50 to 60 mEq/L at 150 ml/hr (Dietz & Flaherty, 1993). *Answer 13:* **b.**

14. Close monitoring for fluid overload must be carried out by evaluating intake and output and daily weights and by assessing for edema. The need for diuresis may be demonstrated by distended neck veins, shortness of breath, cough, and rales on auscultation. Nonthiazide diuretics, such as furosemide or mannitol, may be given intravenously to promote urine flow in cases such as Michael's. For patients with preexisting evidence of fluid retention with marked edema, ascites, or oliguria, low-dose dopamine can be initiated with diuretics (Dietz & Flaherty, 1993). Thiazide diuretics should be avoided because they block tubular reabsorption of uric acid, as do other drugs such as probenecid and aspirin (Heffner & Polman, 1998). *Answer 14:* **d.**

Case Study continued

Michael's LDH level persists at greater than 1500 IU/L. Upon further evaluation of Michael's laboratory data, you note a low urine pH and a low $NaHCO_3$. A urinalysis reveals a high specific gravity and urate crystals. You are also concerned about the elevated levels of serum potassium, phosphorous, BUN, and creatinine.

QUESTIONS

15. These data support the finding that $NaHCO_3$ is ineffective for urinary alkalinization. What other drug may be substituted?
  a. Bethanechol chloride (Urecholine)
  b. Acetazolamide (Diamox)
  c. Phenazopyridine (Pyridium)
  d. Flavoxate (Urispas)

16. Acute renal failure from TLS may be caused by:
  1. Hyperuricemia
  2. Hyperphosphatemia
  3. Hyperkalemia
  4. Hypercalcemia
    a. 1 & 2
    b. 1, 2, & 3
    c. 1, 3, & 4
    d. 1 & 3

17. What complication is Michael most at risk for if he develops acute renal failure?
  a. Seizure
  b. Disseminated intravascular coagulation (DIC)
  c. Respiratory failure
  d. Cardiac arrhythmia

18. Clinical manifestations and laboratory data associated with renal failure would be:
  a. Metabolic acidosis with decreased serum calcium, pH, and bicarbonate

  b. Metabolic alkalosis with increased serum calcium, pH, and bicarbonate
  c. Metabolic acidosis with increased glomerular filtration rate (GFR)
  d. Metabolic alkalosis with decreased GFR

ANSWERS

15. Because the kidneys are the primary mechanism to eliminate potassium, phosphorous, and uric acid, renal failure and death can result if TLS is not treated aggressively (Oksenholt & Seelig, 1999). Hyperuricemia is the major disorder of metabolism leading to acute renal failure in TLS. Even with TLS prophylaxis, approximately 10% of patients treated for leukemia or lymphoma will experience some degree of renal deterioration as a result of hyperuricemia (Heffner & Polman, 1998).

Uric acid nephropathy is a major, life-threatening complication. It is caused by the formation of uric acid crystals in the distal tubules and collecting ducts of the kidneys. Ensuing obstructive uropathy results in decreased urine output, increased hydrostatic pressure, and decreased GFR (Stucky, 1993). The risk of acute renal failure from TLS can be compounded by hyperphosphatemia-forming calcium phosphate crystals, also causing obstructive uropathy. The ensuing decreased GFR in renal failure causes metabolic acidosis related to an increase in BUN and serum creatinine associated with a decrease in serum calcium, pH, and bicarbonate (Stucky, 1993). *Answer 15:* **b.**

16. If Michael were to go into acute renal failure, cardiac arrhythmias would be another sequelae related to hyperkalemia or hypocalcemia. *Answer 16:* **d.**

17. In addition to allopurinol and hydration, urinary alkalinization is important to prevent uric acid crystals by maximizing its solubility in urine (Heffner & Polman, 1998). In Michael's case, his urine pH is not being maintained at higher than 7.0 with the addition of the $NaHCO_3$ to each liter of intravenous fluid. Therefore acetazolamide (Diamox) is a secondary choice for urinary alkalinization, and it has a diuretic effect as well. *Answer 17:* **d.**

18. After evaluating Michael's laboratory data and physical findings, a forced diuresis is planned to maintain his urine output at greater than 150 ml/hr by increased hydration, alkalinization, and diuretic therapy. This simultaneous hydration and diuresis should promote further excretion of potassium and phosphorous, which are both elevated. Once the hyperuricemia has been corrected, urinary alkalinization should be stopped for two reasons: (1) to prevent phosphate precipitation in the renal tubules because phosphates are not soluble in alkaline urine and (2) to prevent alkalosis, which may also predispose the patient to neuromuscular irritability by exacerbating hypocalcemia (Dietz & Flaherty, 1993; Stork, 1994). As you evaluated Michael's laboratory data, you would continue to monitor intake and output and assess Michael for hematuria, crystalluria, and flank pain caused by renal calculi occluding the ureters. *Answer 18:* **a.**

Case Study continued

Michael becomes restless and complains of body aches and not being able to find a comfortable position. You take the time to assess for metabolic abnormalities.

QUESTIONS

19. What diagnostic sign can you assess for in hypocalcemia?
    a. Trousseau's sign
    b. Chvostek's syndrome
    c. Homan's sign
    d. Both a and b

20. Which of the following symptoms would alert you to the possibility of hypocalcemia?
    a. Muscle weakness and cramping
    b. Diarrhea
    c. Nausea and vomiting
    d. Anorexia

21. A patient with hypocalcemia and hyperkalemia would have what type of deep tendon reflexes?
    a. Hyperactive
    b. Hypoactive
    c. Flaccid
    d. Spastic

22. In addition to neuromuscular effects, what system is most affected by hypocalcemia and hyperkalemia?
    a. Pulmonary
    b. Cardiac
    c. Renal
    d. Hematologic

ANSWERS

19-22. The metabolic effects of hypocalcemia and hyperkalemia are both neurologic and cardiac. The cardiac effects of hypocalcemia may be severe: arrhythmias, 2:1 heart block, and cardiac arrest (Zobec, 1997). The neurologic effects of hypocalce-

mia include muscle weakness, cramping, twitching, tetany, and carpopedal spasm. Two physical assessment signs are indicative of hypocalcemia. Chvostek's sign is positive for facial twitching when the examiner taps at a site near the tragus nerve. Trousseau's sign, carpopedal spasm after occlusion of blood flow in the arm with a sphygmomanometer, is also positive in hypocalcemia. As a result of both hyperkalemia and hypocalcemia, the patient's deep tendon reflexes will be hyperactive. Late symptoms of hypocalcemia include laryngospasm, paresthesias, seizures, confusion, and delirium.

Hyperkalemia is the most dangerous immediate consequence of TLS. Hyperkalemia results in cardiovascular, neuromuscular, and GI irritability. Hyperkalemia leads to delayed cardiac conduction and slowed repolarization. These changes can lead to atrioventricular block, ventricular tachycardia, ventricular fibrillation, or asystole (Robinson, 1998; Zobec, 1997). The cardiac effects of hyperkalemia can be exacerbated by hyponatremia and hypocalcemia. The neuromuscular effects of hyperkalemia include muscle weakness and irritability, cramps, twitching, and paresthesias in the form of tingling and burning. Finally, the GI effects of hyperkalemia are the result of increased peristaltic movement, causing nausea, diarrhea, and intestinal colic (Robinson, 1998; Zobec, 1997). *Answer 19:* **d.** *Answer 20:* **a.** *Answer 21:* **a.** *Answer 22:* **b.**

Case Study continued

By day 4 of induction therapy, treatment for Michael is focused on correcting the metabolic imbalances caused by TLS and managing the adverse effects of the chemotherapy regimen. In addition to antiemetic therapy, lorazepam (Ativan) is ordered for Michael as needed for his acute anxiety. You also notice a maculopapular rash on his trunk and forearms.

QUESTIONS

23. What are the probable causes for Michael's rash?
    a. Leukemic infiltrates
    b. Urate crystals
    c. Allopurinol treatment
    d. Redman's syndrome

24. What pharmacologic measure is initiated for hyperkalemia greater than 7 mEq with electrocardiographic (ECG) changes?
    1. Calcium gluconate
    2. Kayexalate
    3. Sodium bicarbonate
    4. Furosemide

a. 1 & 2
b. 1 & 3
c. 2 & 3
d. 3 & 4

25. You can anticipate all of the following interventions for hyperphosphatemia *except:*
   a. Administration of Amphojel
   b. Restriction of soft drinks
   c. Hypertonic glucose and insulin
   d. Kayexalate

26. What nursing intervention is most important for Michael if he develops hypocalcemia?
   a. Hydration
   b. Dietary restrictions
   c. Seizure precautions
   d. Urinary catheterization

27. What is your best intervention to assist Michael in handling his anxiety?
   a. Informing Michael that once the TLS is under control, he will never be at risk for this complication again
   b. Educating Michael about the signs and symptoms of TLS so that he can become an active participant in his own care
   c. Telling Michael that you are doing everything possible to ensure his best care and that he should leave the worrying to you
   d. Letting Michael know that it is certainly understandable that he is anxious in light of the serious nature of his disease and treatment

_____ **ANSWERS**

23. The resolution of TLS depends on several factors, including the tumor's response to treatment and whether adequate renal function has been maintained. Cytolysis usually occurs within 7 days of treatment, and TLS most often resolves within this time frame if appropriate measures are undertaken to ensure renal function and correct metabolic abnormalities (Dietz & Flaherty, 1993). *Answer 23:* **c.**

24. In addition to treating hyperuricemia as discussed, an initial treatment for hyperkalemia is ordering intravenous furosemide because this diuretic wastes potassium. Mannitol is second-line treatment as an osmotic diuretic (forced diuresis) and is used to treat the oliguric phase of acute renal failure. Other interventions for Michael could include stopping any dietary intake of potassium or stopping any drugs that promote

potassium retention (e.g., potassium-sparing diuretics). For potassium levels lower than 7 mEq and no ECG changes, such as in Michael's case, cation-exchange resins, such as Kayexalate with sorbitol, can be given by mouth or via retention enema to bind the potassium and promote excretion via the GI system. For potassium levels higher than 7 mEq and ECG changes, calcium gluconate can be administered intravenously in conjunction with cardiac monitoring. Calcium gluconate antagonizes the action of potassium on the heart muscle (Stucky, 1993). Other interventions for hyperkalemic-induced metabolic acidosis include the administration of sodium bicarbonate as a bolus intravenously to alkalinize the plasma by shifting potassium into the cells. Finally, for oliguric renal failure, an intravenous solution of 50% glucose with insulin may be ordered to raise plasma insulin levels, causing an intracellular shift of potassium (Dietz & Flaherty, 1993; Stucky, 1993). *Answer 24:* **d.**

25. Certain medications that may be needed to treat TLS (e.g., furosemide, mithramycin, certain anticonvulsants) may increase the occurrence of both hyperphosphatemia and hypocalcemia (Ezzone, 1999). The administration of phosphate-binding antacids, such as Amphojel or Basaljel, are used to treat the hyperphosphatemia. Stool softeners or laxatives are recommended to prevent constipation with the use of these agents. Dietary intake of phosphates (e.g., soft drinks) and phosphate-containing medications (e.g., Phos-Tabs) should be discontinued (Robinson, 1998). Hypocalcemia can be treated with calcium supplements or, in severe cases, with a calcium gluconate infusion. *Answer 25:* **d.**

26. Patients with severe hypocalcemia must be placed on seizure precautions (Robinson, 1998). If acute uric acid or phosphate nephropathy occurs, dialysis may be initiated to treat the severe metabolic derangements such as hyperkalemia, acidosis, hypocalcemia, or azotemia. The type of dialysis used will depend on the patient's status but may include hemodialysis, hemofiltration, or peritoneal dialysis. Other treatments for acute renal failure may include leukopheresis, exchange transfusions, and low-dose steroids. *Answer 26:* **c.**

27. Michael's care should include patient education regarding TLS, its manifestations, and self-care to prevent relapse (Box 22-4). Michael will need to continue on allopurinol at 300 mg/day indefinitely. The maculopapular rash on his trunk and forearms is a possible side effect of allopurinol

BOX **22-4** | **Patient Instructions Regarding Signs and Symptoms of Tumor Lysis Syndrome**

Notify your primary care provider if you notice any of the following signs:
- Nausea, vomiting, lack of appetite
- Watery stools
- Muscle cramps, spasms, twitching, or weakness
- Numbness or tingling
- Increased fatigue
- Decreased frequency of urination
- Side pain
- Cloudy urine or blood in urine
- Weight gain or swelling
- Shortness of breath
- Pain and swelling at joints
- Change in mental status
- Seizure activity

Adapted from Robinson, J. G. (1998). Tumor lysis syndrome. In Chernecky, C. C., & Berger, B. J. (Eds.). *Advanced and critical care oncology nursing* (pp. 637-659). Philadelphia: WB Saunders; and Oksenholt, N., & Seelig, F. (1999). Burkitt's lymphoma. In Miaskowski, C., & Buchsel, P. (Eds.). *Oncology nursing: Assessment and clinical care* (pp. 1353-1372). St. Louis: Mosby.

that may occur within the first 7 days of treatment. It will resolve over time and can be treated with hydrocortisone cream or diphenhydramine lotion. A hypersensitivity to allopurinol may also present as fever, eosinophilia, or an exfoliative dermatitis (Dietz & Flaherty, 1993; Stucky, 1993).

Continuation of a high fluid intake is necessary in addition to dietary restrictions of potassium and phosphorous. Phosphorous-containing foods, such as milk, cheese, meat, eggs, poultry, fish, nuts, legumes, breads, cereals, and carbonated beverages, are encouraged (Ezzone, 1999). In addition to the drugs that are contraindicated (thiazide diuretics, probenecid, and aspirin), phosphate- and potassium-containing medications (e.g., clindamycin, sodium-potassium phosphate) should also be avoided (Ezzone, 1999). Radiographic contrast dye studies are contraindicated because the dye may block tubular reabsorption of uric acid (Zobec, 1997). You are in a pivotal position to educate Michael about the rationale behind the frequency of blood draws, the need for vigorous hydration, and the special attention to monitoring daily weights and intake and output. By providing instructions on what signs and symptoms to watch for, Michael can become an active participant in his care. This knowledge will also help allay Michael's anxiety. *Answer 27:* **b.**

REFERENCES

DiBella, N. J. (1994). Acute myelogenous and lymphocytic leukemia. In Wood, M. E., & Bunn, P. A. (Eds.). *Hematology oncology secrets* (pp. 115-118). Philadelphia: Hanley & Belfus.

Dietz, K. (1999). Acute leukemia. In Miaskowski, C., & Buchsel, P. (Eds.). *Oncology nursing: Assessment and clinical care* (pp. 1223-1237). St. Louis: Mosby.

Dietz, K. A., & Flaherty, A. M. (1993) Oncologic emergencies. In Groenwald, S. L., Frogge, M. H., Goodman, M., & Yarbro, C. H. (Eds.). *Cancer nursing: Principles and practice* (3rd ed.). (pp. 800-839). Boston: Jones and Bartlett.

Drakos, P., Bar-Ziv, J., & Catane, R. (1994). Tumor lysis syndrome in nonhematologic malignancies. *Am J Clin Oncol, 17*, pp. 502-505.

Ezzone, S. A. (1999). Tumor lysis syndrome. *Semin Oncol Nurs, 15*, pp. 2-8.

Finley, J. P. (1998). Metabolic emergencies. In Itano, J. K., & Taoka, K. N. (Eds.). *Core curriculum for oncology nursing* (3rd ed.). (pp. 315-339). Philadelphia: Saunders.

Heffner, M., & Polman, L. S. (1998). Hyperuricemia. In Chernecky, C. C., & Berger, B. J. (Eds.). *Advanced and critical care oncology nursing* (pp. 314-325). Philadelphia: Saunders.

Miller, J., & Parnes, H. L. (1994). Metabolic problems & emergencies. In Cameron, R. B. (Ed.). *Practical oncology* (pp. 84-90). Norwalk, CT: Appleton and Lange.

Oksenholt, N., & Seelig, F. (1999). Burkitt's lymphoma. In Miaskowski, C., & Buchsel, P. (Eds.). *Oncology nursing: Assessment and clinical care* (pp. 1353-1372). St. Louis: Mosby.

Robinson, J. G. (1998). Tumor lysis syndrome. In Chernecky, C. C., & Berger, B. J. (Eds.). *Advanced and critical care oncology nursing* (pp. 637-659). Philadelphia: Saunders.

Sklarin, N. T., & Markham, M. (1995). Spontaneous recurrent tumor lysis syndrome in breast cancer. *Am J Clin Oncol, 18*, pp. 71-73.

Stork, L. (1994). Childhood acute lymphoblastic leukemia. In Wood, M. E., & Bunn, P. A. (Eds.). *Hematology/oncology secrets* (pp. 342-345). Philadelphia: Hanley & Belfus.

Stucky, L. A. (1993). Acute tumor lysis syndrome: Assessment and nursing implications. *Oncol Nurs Forum, •*, pp. 49-59.

Tracey, L., & Kruger, S. (1996). Leukemia. In Gates, R. A., & Fink, R. M. (Eds.). *Oncology nursing secrets* (pp. 96-107). Philadelphia: Hanley & Belfus.

Zobec, A. (1997). Tumor lysis syndrome. In Gates, R. A., & Fink, R. M. (Eds.). *Oncology nursing secrets* (pp. 367-369). Philadelphia: Hanley & Belfus.

23 Oncologic Emergency: Case 9

Nancy Jo Bush

Steven Bloomberg is a 46-year-old white man who was brought to the emergency room by ambulance after experiencing a seizure. This occurred after spending the day at the beach playing volleyball. Steven remembered only a feeling of "spaceyness," followed by a witnessed seizure, loss of consciousness, and tonic-clonic activity. Steven denies a history of seizures, epilepsy, or recent trauma. He denies any previous loss of consciousness, dizziness, or vertigo. Further review of systems was positive for complaints of headache for approximately a few months' duration. Steven's medical history was also positive for hypertension and hyperlipidemia managed by atenolol, furosemide (Lasix), and Lipitor. Steven denies a history of smoking or alcohol or drug abuse. His vital signs are 120/60-92-24. His weight is 260 pounds, and he is 5 feet, 9 inches tall.

QUESTIONS

1. Assessment of Steven's seizure should begin with which of the following?
   a. A thorough neurologic examination
   b. Computed tomography (CT) scan of the brain
   c. Identification of behavior or personality changes
   d. Administration of an anticonvulsant medication

2. The neurologic examination on Steven must include assessment of which of the following?
   a. Cerebellar function (the finger-to-nose test)
   b. Deep tendon reflexes
   c. Sensory examination (pinprick and vibration)
   d. All of these

3. Seizure activity is best captured by:
   a. Patient recall
   b. Lactic acid production
   c. Family members
   d. Anticonvulsant drug levels

ANSWERS

1. A thorough neurologic examination must be carried out on any patient presenting with a seizure. This first includes a description of the seizure activity, including any symptoms of impending seizure or aura (e.g., dizziness, a sense of dread, olfactory disturbances, aphasia, circumoral numbness) (Kernich, 1998). The type of seizure—partial or generalized—is often determined by the motor and sensory activity of the seizure and is important in identifying the cause. Partial seizures may be simple or complex and result from the activation of one hemisphere of the brain. Generalized seizures are caused by activation of both hemispheres, resulting in petit mal, myoclonic, or tonic-clonic seizures. Subjective data needed to evaluate seizure activity are summarized in Table 23-1. Patient history must include seizures, epilepsy, recent head trauma, or cancer or radiation therapy to the brain. *Answer 1:* **a.**

2. The neurologic examination should begin with assessment of the patient's mental status, including level of consciousness, mood states, affect, memory, attention, and judgment. The neurologic examination must also include assessment of cranial nerve function, sensory and motor function, reflexes, and cerebellar function (Belford & Gargon-Klinger, 1999). Cranial nerves III, IV, and VI are tested by checking the pupils for size, regularity, equality, light reaction, and accommodation and also by checking extraocular movements (EOMs). Ophthalmoscopic examination should be done to check for papilledema, which, in some patients, may be the first sign of increased intracranial pressure (ICP) if the pressure

TABLE 23-1	Assessment of Seizure Activity
History	History of seizures or convulsions?
	Age of onset?
	Diagnosis/treatment for epilepsy?
	Time/date of last seizure?
Precipitating factors	Activity?
	Fatigue?
	Stress?
Aura	Auditory, visual, or motor?
	Dizziness?
	Impending doom?
Motor activity	Body part(s) involved in seizure?
	On one side of the body or both?
	Muscles tense or limp?
	Jerking of the extremities?
Associated features	Color change in face or lips?
	Automatisms (e.g., lip smacking, biting of tongue)?
	Eyes rolling?
	Incontinence?
Mental status	Loss of consciousness?
Duration	How long did seizure activity last?
Postictal phase	Confusion?
	Weakness?
	Sleepiness?
	Headache?
	Muscle aches?
Current medications	Anticonvulsants? When/how long?
	New medications? When/how long?
	Medications with seizure risk (e.g., antidepressants)?

From Jarvis, C. (1996). *Physical examination and health assessment.* Philadelphia: Saunders.

has developed gradually over time (Hickman, 1998). Sensations of touch and pinprick validate cranial nerve V involvement (Jarvis, 1996). Testing of motor function should include evaluation of deep tendon reflexes and extremity strength and weakness. Transient focal weakness or sensory changes after a generalized seizure indicate a focal brain lesion (Kernich, 1998). Evaluation of cerebellar function is also important and includes neurologic tests such as the finger-to-nose test, observation of gait, and the Romberg test (Jarvis, 1996). *Answer 2:* **d.**

3. Family members or witnesses to the seizure activity are often important participants in gather-

ing the pertinent information needed to adequately assess seizure activity. *Answer 3:* **c.**

Case Study continued

Steven's neurologic examination was significant for occasional mild headaches that had been increasing in frequency and duration over the last several weeks. Steven described his headaches as occurring most frequently in the early morning upon arising, lasting a few hours and then resolving. Recently, the headaches had awakened him from sleep, and he had a few bouts of projectile vomiting. Self-prescribed analgesics did not provide relief. The headaches were not associated with any visual or auditory changes. Steven had attributed the headaches to stress at work and family pressures. His wife stated, "Steven has been very irritable and not himself lately."

QUESTIONS

4. Assessment of Steven's recent headaches would most likely reveal all of the following *except:*
  a. The location of the pain
  b. The time of day of recurrent headaches
  c. Hypotension
  d. The duration of headaches

5. The most important laboratory data ordered in the emergency room would be:
  a. Complete blood count
  b. Chemistry panel
  c. Arterial blood gases
  d. Cholesterol level

6. Diagnostics in the emergency room most likely would include:
  a. CT of the brain
  b. Lumber puncture
  c. Magnetic resonance imaging (MRI) of the brain
  d. Single-photo emission computed tomography (SPECT) of the brain

7. Differential diagnoses for Steven include all of the following *except:*
  a. Hyponatremia
  b. Epilepsy
  c. Obesity
  d. Primary brain tumor

ANSWERS

4. In the emergency room an electrocardiogram (ECG) should be performed to rule out cardiovascular causes of seizure activity such as syncope or hypotension. In Steven's case, the neurologic assessment must also include his history of hypertension and medication treatment. Although rare, headaches can be associated with hypotension (Robinson, 1998). Assessment of Steven's headaches must include the location, time of day, duration, and the precipitating and aggravating factors. The possibility of hypotension related to his antihypertensive medications must also be evaluated because syncope—a temporary loss of consciousness from a lack of cerebral blood flow—may also cause seizure activity. *Answer 4:* **c.**

5. Any person presenting with a primary seizure and who has a history of headaches, including nausea and vomiting, should be evaluated for a possible CNS lesion (Sheidler & Bucholtz, 1996). Malignant tumors of the CNS can be primary in nature (20%) or most often occur from metastases from cancers such as breast, lung, colon, prostate, kidney, and thyroid (Hickman, 1998). Differential diagnoses such as fluid or electrolyte imbalances and epilepsy will also guide diagnostic studies. Laboratory data pertinent to diagnosis include a chemistry panel. An underlying disease state or metabolic imbalance can predispose a person to seizure activity. Dilutional hyponatremia related to syndrome of inappropriate antidiuretic hormone secretion (SIADH) by a primary tumor of the lung or brain may lead to convulsions caused by water retention and edema of the brain (McDermott, 1997). Severe hypoglycemia related to excess insulin may also manifest in convulsions. This may occur in the diabetic patient or in the case of pancreatic islet cell tumors or insulinomas (McDermott, 1997). *Answer 5:* **b.**

6. Follow-up studies may also include an electroencephalograph (EEG) to rule out epilepsy. For young persons presenting with a seizure and a history of drug abuse (e.g., alcohol, cocaine) or trauma must be considered. For older persons, common causes of seizure may include alcoholism and cardiovascular or metabolic abnormalities. In any person presenting with an isolated seizure, the possibility of brain tumor must be ruled out. Two major diagnostic tools used to rule out primary or metastatic brain tumors include CT and MRI. In the emergency room, a CT scan of the brain would be ordered to identify any soft tissue changes, bone abnormalities, or space-occupying lesions. Follow-up studies include MRI scanning for more definitive diagnosis. MRI has surpassed CT scanning because of its ability to differentiate cyst versus tumor and because it is capable of providing high definition of areas of cerebral edema and the responsible lesions (Strickler & Phillips, 2000; Wilkes, 1999). More specific imaging studies may include positron emission tomography (PET) scan or SPECT after tumor diagnosis or treatment. Lumbar puncture should not be performed if increased ICP is suspected because the induced pressure changes can cause brainstem herniation (Wilkes, 1999). *Answer 6:* **a.**

7. Seizure activity has been defined as an irritation of the central nervous system (CNS) resulting in excessive and abnormal neuronal discharges within the brain (Kernich, 1998). Differential diagnoses for a seizure must rule out fluid and electrolyte imbalances such as hyponatremia, epilepsy, and a primary or metastatic brain tumor. A seizure may be an isolated event without any other neurologic symptoms or it may be indicative of increased ICP or encephalopathy. An isolated seizure must be considered a medical emergency and demands a thorough investigation (Kernich). *Answer 7:* **c.**

Case Study continued

The CT scan revealed a left frontal mass. Phenytoin (Dilantin) 400 mg/day was ordered. After his initial emergency room examination, Steven was referred to a neurologist for further evaluation. Upon further assessment, Steven described difficulties in concentrating at his job as a certified public accountant, which was causing him to feel pressured and moody. He states that he feels like his "world is falling apart." During his neurologic examination, he was anxious and restless. An MRI of the brain demonstrated a large, infiltrating frontal lobe lesion—$3.8 \times 2 \times 3$ cm, multicystic, with peritumoral edema, increased mass effect, and vascular changes. Steven consented to an open biopsy, which allowed diagnosis of a grade IV astrocytoma, which was responsible for Steven's seizure as a direct result of increased ICP. Steven and his wife were informed of the prognosis and the postoperative possibilities of radiation and chemotherapy.

QUESTIONS

8. Which of the following statements is *false* regarding a grade IV astrocytoma?

   a. An astrocytoma is a primary brain tumor deriving from cells called *astrocytes.*
   b. The prognosis for a grade IV astrocytoma is very poor.
   c. A grade IV astrocytoma is a well-differentiated, benign tumor.

d. An astrocytoma is also known as a *glioblastoma multiforme*.

9. Primary or metastatic brain lesions contribute to increased ICP by:
   a. Direct tumor growth increasing brain volume
   b. Associated edema of brain tissue
   c. Obstruction of cerebrospinal fluid (CSF)
   d. All of these

10. Increased ICP is best defined as:
    a. The buildup of toxic substances within the brain that occurs with encephalopathy or fluid and electrolyte imbalances
    b. The blockage of circulation within the blood-brain barrier related to obstruction, as in the case of a space-occupying lesion
    c. Acid-base imbalances causing a retention of carbon dioxide and acidosis
    d. The expansion of brain tissue, the vascular bed, or CSF with concomitant failure of compensatory compliance

11. The normal pressure range for intracranial pressure is:
    a. 0 to 15 mm Hg
    b. 15 to 30 mm Hg
    c. 30 to 45 mm Hg
    d. <45 mm Hg

ANSWERS

8. Primary tumors of the CNS are classified by the type of cell from which they arise. Most are made up of glial cells that provide the supportive structure to the neurons in the brain and spinal cord. Glial tumors are further classified according to specific cell type: (1) astrocytes, (2) oligodendrocytes, (3) ependymal cells, and (4) Schwann cells (Schnell & Maher de Leon, 1998). Astrocytomas are tumors that arise from astrocytes, and they are one of the most common primary brain tumors (Strickler & Phillips, 2000). Astrocytes are starlike projections that cover the exposed surfaces of the CNS, such as the neurons. As the malignancy develops, clusters of budding tumors invade surrounding tissue, causing mild, transient symptoms in the early stages of development. More ominous symptoms such as Steven presented with (headache, seizure, nausea, vomiting, and sensory changes) carry a poorer prognosis and signify advanced disease (Strickler & Phillips, 2000). Astrocytomas are classified as grades I to IV according to the degree of cellular differentiation and malignant characteristics. A grade IV astrocytoma is also termed *glioblastoma multiforme* and

consists of poorly differentiated cells, is highly malignant, has areas of necrosis, and has a prognosis of 12 to 18 months. *Answer 8:* **c.**

9. The neurologic symptoms that present with any primary or metastatic tumor are directly related to the location of the space-occupying lesion within the closed system of the brain and spinal cord. Local effects are caused by the infiltration, invasion, and destruction of brain tissue (Strickler & Phillips, 2000). Changes causing Steven to feel stress (e.g., difficulty concentrating with his work) can be directly attributed to the malignant invasion of the frontal lobe. In addition, behavior changes such as irritability can be attributed to tumor location within the brain and the primary functions that are disrupted. Often, these symptoms may be insidious in nature, and the patient may be unaware that his or her behavior has changed or has become inappropriate (Schnell & Maher de Leon, 1998). Rapidly growing tumors with associated edema can cause the early symptoms that Steven experienced related to both direct tumor invasion and increased ICP because of changes and expansion in brain volume. *Answer 9:* **d.**

10-11. Symptoms of increased ICP are caused by a disruption of the normal physiology of brain function and CSF circulation. The skull is a rigid, closed system; therefore an increase in volume increases ICP. Under normal conditions, ICP is maintained within a normal range of 0 to 15 mm Hg by autoregulatory mechanisms of vasodilation and vasoconstriction. This balance is maintained despite transitory fluctuations in arterial and venous pressure. For the pressure to remain normal, an increase in any of the three brain components—the brain tissue, the vascular bed, and the CSF—must be compensated for by a decrease in another. This mechanism is termed *compensatory compliance.* In early shifts or changes in ICP, a decrease in cerebral blood flow, a decrease in CSF absorption, or brain fluid shifting from the head to the spinal cavity can maintain normal pressure.

In the case of metastatic or primary brain tumors, disruption of normal autoregulation or compensatory compliance may be caused by (1) displacement of brain tissue, (2) edema of brain tissue, (3) obstruction of CSF, or (4) increased vascularity by tumor growth (Hunter, 1998). A tumor will produce symptoms of increased ICP based on how rapidly the tumor grows, the ability of the brain volume and space to compensate for the expanding lesion, and the tumor location

(Hickman, 1998). Slow-growing tumors allow adaptability of the CNS to accommodate space occupation up to a critical-mass threshold. Fast-growing tumors such as Steven's do not allow ample time for accommodation, and the result is more pronounced symptoms (e.g., seizures, headaches with projectile vomiting). *Answer 10:* **d.** *Answer 11:* **a.**

Case Study continued

On initial diagnosis and following tumor biopsy, two of the major goals of Steven's treatment were to minimize the risk of increased ICP and to control symptoms. This included prescribing a corticosteroid in addition to the previously prescribed anticonvulsant phenytoin.

QUESTIONS

12. Which corticosteroid is the most commonly prescribed for the treatment of increased ICP?
   a. Methylprednisolone
   b. Dexamethasone
   c. Prednisolone
   d. Any of these

13. The direct effect of a corticosteroid on increased ICP is best described as:
   a. Reducing focal cerebral edema
   b. Enhancing the effect of the anticonvulsant
   c. Minimizing cognitive and motor changes
   d. Causing cerebral vasoconstriction

14. A major side effect of corticosteroids that is often overlooked but that affects the patient's quality of life is:
   a. Nausea and vomiting
   b. Overwhelming fatigue
   c. Muscle weakness in the proximal extremities
   d. Excessive diuresis

15. What could be considered an anaphylactic reaction to phenytoin precipitating you to discontinue the drug?
   a. Dyspnea
   b. Headache
   c. Skin rash
   d. Palpitations

ANSWERS

12-13. Patients with brain tumors commonly present with symptoms related to increased ICP (e.g., nausea, vomiting, headache, seizure) resulting from both the mass effect of the tumor plus the surrounding edema. Abnormal blood

| TABLE 23-2 Side Effects of Corticosteroids ||
BODY IMAGE CHANGES	MEDICAL CHANGES
Fluid retention	Increased susceptibility to infection
Weight gain	Gastric irritation
Flushed face	Mood changes and irritability
Abdominal striae	Muscle weakness in proximal extremities
Growth of facial/ body hair	Adrenal insufficiency syndrome

Based on information from Owens B., & Lillehei, K. (1997). Brain tumors. In Gates, R. A., & Fink, R. M. (Eds.). *Oncology nursing secrets* (pp. 135-141). Philadelphia: Hanley & Belfus.

vessels within the tumor allow fluid to leak from the intravascular spaces into surrounding brain tissue. Corticosteroids directly improve the adherence of endothelial cells within the tumor blood vessels, decreasing the leakage of fluid that is responsible for the symptoms of increased ICP (Owens & Lillehei, 1997). Therefore the direct effect of corticosteroids in the treatment of increased ICP is to reduce focal cerebral edema (Hickman, 1998).

Dexamethasone is the most commonly prescribed corticosteroid for its fast-acting effects on increased ICP at dosages ranging from 0.25 to 40 mg/day; the maximal effective dosage is 40 mg/day (Owens & Lillehei, 1997). *Answer 12:* **b.** *Answer 13:* **a.**

14. Significant side effects of corticosteroids are outlined in Table 23-2. An often overlooked side effect that affects the patient's quality of daily life includes the development of muscle weakness in the proximal extremities. This effect can make it difficult for the patient to carry out simple activities such as rising from a sitting position in a chair or raising one's self off the toilet seat. The weakness in the proximal muscles may also compound previous motor and sensory dysfunctions related to increased ICP (e.g., impaired balance or gait). Other significant side effects of corticosteroids that may be difficult to differentiate from symptoms of increased ICP include mood changes and irritability. Any steroid taken for longer than 7 to 14 days must be gradually tapered to prevent rebound effects related to adrenal insufficiency syndrome. A rule of thumb is that the longer the patient has taken the steroid and the higher the dosage, the longer and slower the tapering must be carried out (Owens & Lillehei, 1997). *Answer 14:* **c.**

15. Anticonvulsants are often prescribed for the treatment of increased ICP not to control cerebral edema but to control the seizure activity (Hickman, 1998). This is the case if the patient has experienced a previous seizure, as in Steven's case, but also if the patient is to undergo biopsy or surgery. Patients may be prescribed anticonvulsants before craniotomy and for a few days postoperatively. Patients who have experienced a seizure may continue anticonvulsant therapy indefinitely. In either case, it is recommended that an anticonvulsant such as corticosteroids be tapered slowly to decrease the risk of severe seizure when the drug is discontinued (Owens & Lillehei, 1997). Side effects of anticonvulsants (e.g., drowsiness, confusion, irritability, headache, depression, tremor, slurred speech) may also compound those of increased ICP or be difficult to differentiate. Phenytoin is the most commonly prescribed anticonvulsant and must be taken for 7 to 10 days before a therapeutic blood level is reached. Any type of rash—measleslike, maculopapular, or urticarial—may be an allergic and even life-threatening reaction to phenytoin, so the drug should be discontinued (Owens & Lillehei, 1997). Second-line anticonvulsants include carbamazepine, clonazepam, gabapentin, and valproic acid. *Answer 15:* **c.**

Case Study continued

Following surgical biopsy, radiation therapy is ordered for Steven with the goal of reducing tumor size before attempting surgical resection. A dose of 6000 cGy was ordered to be administered over a 7-week period. The radiosensitizer tripazamine was also ordered. Patient and family education is carried out to help Steven and his wife become aware of recurring symptoms of increased ICP and to help them cope with the demands of illness and treatment. As treatment progresses, Steven begins to show further signs of mood disturbances and personality changes. He expresses anger related to his inability to work and is becoming progressively fatigued with daily activities. His wife begins to also express difficulty dealing with his mood swings.

QUESTIONS

16. An early sign of recurrent increased ICP may include all of the following *except:*
  a. Decreased attention span, short-term memory loss, difficulty concentrating
  b. Anxiety, restlessness, irritability

  c. Increased blood pressure, decreased pulse, widening pulse pressure
  d. Blurred vision, diplopia, decreased visual acuity

17. A legal and ethical issue surrounding Steven's diagnosis includes:
  a. Appropriate follow-up care
  b. Driving
  c. Behavioral outbursts
  d. Medical leave of absence

18. Which of the following is important to include in patient and family education for increased ICP?
  a. Safety issues in the home environment
  b. Regular exercise
  c. Adequate nutrition
  d. Anxiolytics as needed

ANSWERS

16. As Steven's disease and treatment progress, continual assessment for signs and symptoms of recurrent increased ICP are an integral part of care planning and follow-up. The addition of radiation therapy may compound the risk of cerebral edema (Hickman, 1998). Early signs and symptoms of recurrent increased ICP are outlined in Table 23-3. *Answer 16:* **c.**

17. A legal and ethical issue that can be very disruptive is the concern regarding driving privileges. This must be addressed if the patient has experienced seizures or when cognitive deficits become apparent. As sensory-motor changes become more evident, safety issues surrounding the patient's home environment must also be investigated. Continuity of care includes planning for rehabilitation needs, home nursing visits, or hospice care if needed. *Answer 17:* **b.**

18. Changes in mental status may range from irritability to disorientation. Often, these changes can be insidious in nature and recognized only by a family member and not by the patient. It is important to educate the family to recognize that subtle changes in personality or disposition may be indicative of changing ICP. Changes in vital signs or increased somnolence are late, not early, signs of increased ICP (Hickman, 1998). With the progression of either metastatic or primary brain lesions, the emotional reactions related to issues of cognitive impairment may become difficult to differentiate from signs of increased ICP. Expressions of anger and hostility that alarm the family may be a common reaction to the serious diagnosis

TABLE 23-3 Clinical Manifestations of Increased Intracranial Pressure

SIGNS	PATIENT SYMPTOMS
Mental status changes	Irritability, confusion, decreased cognition
Alterations in level of consciousness	Restlessness, disorientation, lethargy
Headaches	Associated with early morning awakening
	May be sharp, dull, or throbbing
	Commonly frontal or occipital
	Aggravated by Valsalva maneuver
	May be associated with vomiting
Vomiting	Unrelated to food ingestion
	Sudden and projectile in nature
Visual changes	Blurring, diplopia, decreased acuity
Sensory-motor	Weakness
	Lethargy
	Ataxia
	Contralateral hemiparesis
Late changes	Somnolence, stupor, coma
	Cushing's triad: hypertension, bradycardia, irregular respirations
	Papilledema

Based on information from Hickman J. L. (1998). Increased intracranial pressure. In Chernecky, C. C., & Berger, B. J. (Eds.). *Advanced and critical care oncology nursing: Managing primary complications* (pp. 371-381). Philadelphia: Saunders.

but an uncommon coping mechanism for the patient. Feelings of hopelessness and despair may peak, requiring emotional support both for the patient and family. Approaching the patient in a calm, comforting, and consistent manner helps build trust and enables the patient to express feelings of fear and anxiety (Strickler & Phillips, 2000). Changes resulting from cognitive impairment affect all areas of quality of life—family functioning, work, and safety issues. These mental status changes often prove the most challenging to the patient and family as the disease progresses (Owens & Lillehei, 1997). Both the patient and family commonly feel powerless to control behavior, personality changes, and ensuing deficits. Changes in reasoning and judgment and difficulty in concentration may make occupational demands impossible. Short-term memory loss may cause the patient to ask repeated questions and make following through on simple tasks impossible. A lack of awareness of inappropriate behaviors may also challenge the patience of family members and strain interpersonal relations (Owens & Lillehei, 1997). *Answer 18:* **a.**

Case Study continued

Steven's condition continues to deteriorate. He is admitted to the hospital one morning after his wife is unable to arouse him from sleep. She becomes frightened and calls 911. Upon admission, Steven is unresponsive, exhibiting slow, irregular respirations. He is admitted to the

intensive care unit for treatment of increased ICP. Vital signs are 180/60-48-8.

QUESTIONS

19. Immediate treatment of Steven's increased ICP may include administration of which of the following?
   a. Mannitol
   b. Furosemide
   c. Phenobarbital
   d. All of these

20. A significant change in Steven's vital signs indicative of irreversible increased ICP would be:
   a. Tachycardia
   b. Hypotension
   c. Widening pulse pressure
   d. Tachypnea

21. The most dangerous risk of untreated increased ICP is:
   a. Cerebral herniation
   b. Cerebral hypoxia
   c. Uncontrolled seizures
   d. Permanent brain damage

ANSWERS

19. Numerous critical care therapies are available to normalize ICP and maintain adequate cerebral perfusion. These include (1) hyperventilation to reduce intracerebral blood volume, (2) CSF drainage to reduce the intracerebral CSF volume, (3) the

administration of pharmacologic agents to induce diuresis or sedation, and (4) surgery (Hudak, Gallo, & Morton, 1998). Osmotherapy is initiated to pull water from edematous brain tissue into the vascular system and also to decrease total body fluid.

Mannitol is used as an osmotic diuretic, and furosemide is used both as a systemic diuretic and to decrease CSF production. Barbiturates such as phenobarbital are administered to reduce cerebral blood flow and volume by vasoconstriction and to inhibit seizures (Hickman, 1998; Hudak, Gallo, & Morton, 1998; Wilkes, 1999). Surgical procedures may include the insertion of a ventriculostomy catheter to drain CSF, resulting in the immediate reduction of ICP or, in Steven's case, tumor resection and debulking (Hickman, 1998). *Answer 19:* **d.**

20-21. When normal compensatory mechanisms fail and medical interventions do not take place, intracranial tension increases rapidly until herniation (displacement of brain tissue into adjacent areas of the brain or outside the cranial vault) (Hudak, Gallo, & Morton, 1998) occurs and the blood supply to the medulla is cut off. A change in a patient's vital signs occurs in the very late stages of increased ICP. A widening pulse pressure is a grave sign of increasing ICP and is caused by hypoxia from compression of the arteries supplying oxygen to the brain. In response, sympathetic stimulation increases the systolic blood pressure in an effort to increase oxygenation and diastolic pressure drops, thereby widening the pulse pressure. Bradycardia results from parasympathetic stimulation of the heart, and the respiratory center in the medulla responds with slow, irregular respirations. The occurrence of these three significant changes in vital signs is termed *Cushing's triad* (Hickman, 1998; Wilkes, 1999). When this classic triad occurs, it is sign of severe decompensation, with brain damage and death imminent (Hudak, Gallo, & Morton, 1998). *Answer 20:* **c.** *Answer 21:* **a.**

REFERENCES

Belford, K., & Gargon-Klinger, R. (1999). Astrocytoma. In Miaskowski, C., & Buchsel, P. (Eds.). *Oncology nursing: Assessment and clinical care* (pp. 493-541). St. Louis: Mosby.

Hickman, J. L. (1998). Increased intracranial pressure. In Chernecky, C. C., & Berger, B. J. (Eds.). *Advanced and critical care oncology nursing: Managing primary complications* (pp. 371-381). Philadelphia: Saunders.

Hudak, C. M., Gallo, B. M., & Morton, P. G. (1998). *Critical care nursing.* Philadelphia: Lippincott-Raven.

Hunter, J. C. (1998). Structural emergencies. In Itano, J. K., & Taoka, K. N. (Eds.). *Core curriculum for oncology nursing* (pp. 340-354). Philadelphia: Saunders.

Jarvis, C. (1996). *Physical examination and health assessment.* Philadelphia: Saunders.

Kernich, C. A. (1998). Seizures. In Chernecky, C. C., & Berger, B. J. (Eds.). *Advanced and critical care oncology nursing* (pp. 536-548). Philadelphia: Saunders.

McDermott, M. T. (1997). Endocrine cancers. In Gates, R. A., & Fink, R. M. (Eds.). *Oncology nursing secrets* (pp. 157-161). Philadelphia: Hanley & Belfus.

Owens, B., & Lillehei, K. (1997). Brain tumors. In Gates, R. A., & Fink, R. M. (Eds.). *Oncology nursing secrets* (pp. 135-141). Philadelphia: Hanley & Belfus.

Schnell, S., & Maher de Leon, M. E. (1998). Anatomy of the central nervous system. *Semin Oncol Nurs, 14,* pp. 2-7.

Sheidler, V. R., & Bucholtz, J. D. (1996). Central nervous system tumors. In McCorkle, R., Grant, M., Frank-Stromberg, M., & Baird, S. B. (Eds.). *Cancer nursing: A comprehensive textbook* (pp. 826-839). Philadelphia: Saunders.

Strickler, R., & Phillips, M. L. (2000). Astrocytomas: The clinical picture. *Clin J Oncol Nurs, 4,* pp. 153-158.

Wilkes, G. M. (1999). Neurologic disturbances. In Yarbro, C. H., Frogge, M. H., & Goodman, M. (Eds.). *Cancer symptom management* (pp. 344-381). Boston: Jones and Bartlett.

24 Oncologic Emergency: Case 10

Esther Muscari Lin

While covering for your advanced practice nurse (APN) colleague who is on vacation, you are called by a member of the inpatient nursing staff. She is worried about a patient who appears to be having some difficulty with his breathing. Jack Morrison is a 42-year-old man who was admitted 6 days ago for sepsis after receiving high-dose chemotherapy for a malignant glioblastoma.

QUESTIONS

1. Knowledge about which of the following organ systems will contribute the *most* to his history in assessment of the current situation?
　　1. Cardiac
　　2. Pulmonary
　　3. Neurologic
　　4. Renal
　　　　a. 1, 2, & 4
　　　　b. 2 & 4
　　　　c. 1, 2, & 3
　　　　d. All of these

2. Is learning the cancer diagnosis and stage critical to the assessment of this patient?
　　a. It is not critical because you have not even learned what symptoms Jack is experiencing.
　　b. It is critical because this information contributes to development of a list of possibilities for his signs and symptoms.
　　c. It is critical. If Jack has a cancer disease unfamiliar to you, you could call someone else to care for him.
　　d. It is not critical because that information will contribute more toward the development of interventions.

3. Which of the following characteristics about the onset of signs and symptoms is *true* and contributes to a comprehensive assessment?

a. Jack could have a longstanding medical problem that really does not warrant your involvement.
b. Signs and symptoms lasting more than 48 hours tells you that Jack has already accommodated for whatever changes are going on in his body, and interventions at 48 hours are not as successful as an earlier intervention.
c. Onset of symptoms less than 24 hours suggests an acute process.
d. Time of symptom onset dictate which diagnostic tests are needed.

4. What is the rationale behind inquiring into the amount of carmustine (BCNU) that Jack has received and the date of the last dose?
　　a. Pulmonary toxicity from BCNU occurs within the first month of high-dose drug administration.
　　b. BCNU is associated with pulmonary hemorrhage.
　　c. Pulmonary fibrosis is a delayed side effect of BCNU.
　　d. If administered within the last 7 to 10 days, BCNU could be causing myelosuppression and adult respiratory distress syndrome.

ANSWERS

1. Your initial response to a report of shortness of breath and possible dyspnea is to learn the specifics of the symptoms and signs. Because tachypnea can be compensatory for hypercapnia or reflective of hypoxia, evaluating possible causes of altered oxygen and carbon dioxide levels is the initial approach. Because cardiovascular, pulmonary, and renal dysfunction are the most common causes of altered oxygenation, evaluation of these systems begins the assessment. Cardiovascular or pulmonary disease as part of the medical history has numerous etiologies, such as congestive heart failure, ischemia, atherosclerosis, and chronic obstructive pulmonary disease. Knowing this information provides the APN with a baseline of what to expect in this patient's organ functioning while also contributing to the initial differential diagnostic list. *Answer 1:* **a.**

2. The cancer diagnosis is crucial because it provides the APN with potential causes of altered oxygenation directly related to primary or metastatic disease. Oncology APNs have disease site–specific knowledge that frames many of their assessments and interventions. The site-specific expertise contributes to identifying possible sites for metastasis and potential high problem areas associated with Jack's diagnosis. Even though the APN may be unfamiliar with a particular cancer diagnosis, responding to the nurse's request for help is consistent with the clinical support APNs provide. The in-depth assessment skills of the APN place the APN in the position of mentoring and guiding the nurse toward accurate identification, assessment, and management of the problem that is causing the "breathing problems." *Answer 2:* **b.**

3. Identifying subjective symptoms such as dyspnea, anxiety, chest pain, and nausea further contributes in identifying possible causes and developing a differential diagnosis list. Onset of symptoms, duration, and contributing and alleviating symptoms provide the means for ruling out as well as "ruling in" possibilities. An onset of longer than 48 hours does not guarantee compensation from other organ systems. A lengthy duration raises the question in the APN's mind of how long the patient will be able to keep up a rapid respiratory rate or endure one or more symptoms for a lengthy period. Regardless of symptom duration, a response to the consult is indicated, and only after an initial assessment indicates a problem beyond the APN's role, scope, or responsibilities should the APN request to not be involved. *Answer 3:* **c.**

4. BCNU at conventional doses does not usually result in myelosuppression at 7 to 10 days but is known more for the risk of pulmonary fibrosis. A later effect of BCNU, pulmonary fibrosis, begins with inflammatory changes of the alveoli, and the progression leads to the signs and symptoms at least 6 weeks after drug administration (Timmerman, 1998). *Answer 4:* **c.**

Case Study continued

Upon arriving in Jack's room, you note the head of the bed is elevated almost 90 degrees and Jack has one hand placed on his sternum and the other on the handrail. Jack anxiously describes a

2-hour onset of feeling short of breath and having chest heaviness. He cannot remember a history of feeling like this.

Lung auscultation reveals bilateral rales in the bases, a respiratory rate of 34 breaths/min, use of accessory muscles with respiration, and pain on inspiration. His temperature is 100° F, and he is diaphoretic. Heart rate is 110 beats/min and regular.

QUESTIONS

5. Which diagnostic tests should be ordered first to provide expedient and vital information?
1. Electrocardiogram (ECG)
2. Arterial blood gas
3. Chest radiograph
4. Blood cultures
   a. 1 & 3
   b. 2 & 4
   c. 1, 2, & 3
   d. All of these

6. What is the rationale for ordering an ECG as an initial test?
   a. Because of the possibility of a myocardial infarction (MI), chest pain needs to be evaluated immediately upon presentation.
   b. Cardiac tamponade, a possible diagnosis, will be reflected in intraventricular conduction disturbances.
   c. Significant pleural effusions (quantities greater than 150 ml) contribute to atrioventricular conduction blocks.
   d. Performing an ECG is in anticipation of Jack potentially becoming critically ill and having a recent baseline study.

7. Jack's blood gas results are 7.48/30/92 with an HCO_3 of 20 mmol/L. Which of the following is an appropriate initial intervention?
   a. Administration of an anxiolytic
   b. Administration of oxygen through a rebreather mask
   c. Change of intravenous fluids to include bicarbonate
   d. Controlled intubation

ANSWERS

5-6. A sudden onset of shortness of breath and dyspnea, with or without chest pain, requires cardiac and pulmonary assessment. An ECG can provide immediate answer as to whether cardiac ischemia or injury is occurring. ST elevation with or without inverted peaked T waves is indicative of a myocardial injury. Q-wave development indicates an MI but can occur with prolonged ischemia. Q waves present at baseline suggest a previous MI (Winters & Eisenberg, 1998). The ECG changes associated with cardiac tamponade include tachycardia and, classically, electrical alternans (Ewald & Rogers, 1998). Pleural effusions do not contribute to atrioventricular (AV) blocks. AV blocks are the result of a delay or block in the conduction of an atrial impulse to the ventricle and are usually associated with bradycardia (Botteron & Smith, 1998). *Answer 5:* **c.** *Answer 6:* **a.**

7. Jack's arterial blood gas reveals respiratory alkalosis, which results from the excessive removal of CO_2 via hyperventilation. Classic findings of respiratory alkalosis are an elevated pH (alkaline) and a decreased P_{CO_2}. Administration of an anxiolytic will not resolve the hyperventilation or feelings of dyspnea and may worsen the situation by causing respiratory depression. The cause of Jack's signs and symptoms needs to be identified first. Because Jack's arterial blood gas is altered because of a respiratory problem and abnormal renal function has not been noted, his kidneys are able to compensate in this acid-base disturbance. Before a mixed acid-base disturbance is suspected, Jack's current compensatory renal response should be assessed. The normal compensatory renal response to a respiratory alkalosis is a slowly decreasing HCO_3 in an acute situation and a more dramatic drop in HCO_3 in chronic situations (Singer, 1998).

Hemoglobin, hematocrit, and coagulation studies are also reasonable and appropriate initial tests. Hemorrhage can be signaled by the sudden onset of dyspnea, chest pain (if significant), tachycardia, and hypotension (Lin & Mitchell, 1996). *Answer 7:* **b.**

Case Study continued

In addition to the ABG results, the other test results are as follows:

Chest radiograph:	atelectasis and a few nonspecific infiltrates bilaterally
Hemoglobin/hematocrit:	low normal, stable over the past 24 hours
ECG:	tachycardia and nonspecific ST-T wave changes

QUESTIONS

8. Based on the test results, what differential diagnoses remain on your list?
1. Infection
2. Pleural effusions
3. Late-stage pulmonary fibrosis

4. Pulmonary embolus (PE)
- **a.** 1, 2, & 3
- **b.** 2, 3, & 4
- **c.** 1, 3, & 4
- **d.** All of these

ANSWERS

8. Although infection remains on the differential diagnoses list, it is low in possibility for a number of reasons. Jack remains hemodynamically stable and has no local or systemic signs of infection. If he was experiencing an acute lung injury from infection, it would most likely be accompanied by other signs and symptoms such as fever, hypotension, increased "whitening out" of the lung bases bilaterally, and a much more significant hypoxemia.

Pleural effusions, often accompanied by pain on inspiration, would be noted by dullness on percussion and be clinically evident on chest radiograph. Jack's chance of a pleural effusion causing his symptoms is essentially ruled out with the preliminary chest radiograph.

Pulmonary fibrosis is still a possibility because BCNU, a pulmonary toxic agent, is in Jack's history.

PE has not been ruled out. The symptoms of chest pain, dyspnea, and apprehension/anxiety are seen in people experiencing a PE as well as in those with pulmonary fibrosis and infection resulting in acute lung injury. *Answer 8:* **c.**

QUESTIONS

9. After narrowing down the differential list, which of the following is a realistic intervention that would contribute to addressing the potential problem of infection?
- **a.** Review of antibiotic medication profile to ensure adequate broad-spectrum coverage
- **b.** Change of the gram-negative coverage to a third-generation cephalosporin
- **c.** Addition of amphotericin to ensure fungal coverage
- **d.** Blood, urine, stool, and sputum cultures

10. Which of the following data result in pulmonary fibrosis being removed from the differential diagnoses list?
1. The BCNU total dose is 250 mg/m^2.
2. BCNU was administered only in the past month.
3. A combination of mitomycin and cyclophosphamide was the previous drug regimen received by Jack.
4. Pulmonary function tests reveal reduced lung volumes.

a. 1 & 2
b. 3 & 4
c. 1 & 3
d. All of these

d. Pulmonary emboli occur as a result of deep venous thromboses, often resulting after a period of prolonged nonambulation or bed rest.

ANSWERS

9. Causes of respiratory alkalosis include hypoxemia from pulmonary disease (pneumonia, edema, emboli, interstitial fibrosis), anemia, heart failure, or respiratory center stimulation.

Changing the antibiotic profile, either by adding or deleting a drug, would be presumptuous until there was information supporting the change. If clinical signs of infection are lacking and the patient is hemodynamically stable, the first thing to do is to become familiar with the patient's medication profile and documentation of past infections. Unless previous culture results indicated inadequate coverage, you would be hard pressed to prove why you changed a regimen that has been successful to this point. *Answer 9:* **a.**

10. Pulmonary fibrosis is usually a late effect of BCNU, occurring at least months after administration. Inflammatory changes of the alveoli progress to fibrosis, with connective tissue replacement and restrictive lung disease resulting (Timmerman, 1998). Often, patients report and clinicians observe an increasing intensity and worsening of the signs and symptoms as opposed to an acute, severe episode, as depicted by Jack.

Contributing risk factors include a total dose greater than 1500 mg/m^2 and a young age at the time of treatment. In addition, a number of chemotherapy combinations contribute to the toxicity potential, of which mitomycin and cyclophosphamide are included (Timmerman, 1998). When abnormal pulmonary function tests reveal a reduction in lung volumes, forced vital capacity, and total lung capacity, altered lung tissue or vascular abnormality is suspected. Hypoxemia becomes more evident as the complication progresses. *Answer 10:* **a.**

QUESTIONS

11. Zeroing in on ruling out a PE, why do you inquire into a recent history of major surgery, paralysis as a result of the brain tumor, and whether Jack has an indwelling central venous catheter?

a. Indwelling catheters can release particles of debris into the bloodstream.
b. Brain tumors are known to release a fibrin-type material.
c. If recent surgery has occurred, you can pinpoint the signs and symptoms to be a result of fluid overload.

ANSWERS

11. Prolonged immobilization, either after surgery or because of paralysis, predisposes patients to thromboembolic disease. Peripheral vascular disease, heart failure, certain cancers, and indwelling venous access devices are other contributors to thromboembolic disease. Deep venous thromboses and PE should be considered one entity because treatment is indicated if either one is established. The preceding questioning is seeking out the presence and probability of risk factors. Hypercoagulable states are associated with some malignancies, increasing the risk of thromboembolic disease and PE (Reid, 1999). *Answer 11:* **d.**

Case Study *continued*

Because the chest radiograph and ECG have both ruled out primary cardiopulmonary problems, such as MI or heart failure, lung scanning is indicated. A ventilation-perfusion ($\dot{V}/\dot{Q}$) scan is ordered for Jack.

QUESTIONS

12. The results of the $\dot{V}/\dot{Q}$ scan are reported as intermediate probability for PE. Based on this result, what would the next step be in assessment and management of Jack?

a. Blood draws for bleeding times are conducted.
b. The $\dot{V}/\dot{Q}$ scan is repeated in 12 hours.
c. Low-molecular-weight heparin is begun.
d. Jack undergoes pulmonary angiography.

ANSWERS

12. $\dot{V}/\dot{Q}$ scans can have varying probability for the presence of PE. They are reported as normal, low or intermediate, and high probability. The test is mainly useful in final diagnosis if the result is normal or high probability. A "normal" $\dot{V}/\dot{Q}$ scan definitively rules out a PE. A result of "high probability" in conjunction with clinical signs is definitive for immediate treatment of a PE. A report of "low or intermediate probability" requires further evaluation. Because a PE arises from the infemoral venous system, a noninvasive ultrasound or lower extremity venography can be performed. However, if the results of these two tests are negative and there is a high clinical suspicion for PE, a pulmonary angiography is

Pulmonary Embolus Signs and Symptoms

Symptoms:
Chest pain (anginal type)
Dyspnea (sudden onset)
Syncope
Anxiety/apprehension
Nausea
Cough
Back pain
Abdominal pain
Signs:
Fever
Thrombophlebitis
Second heart sound accentuation
Right-sided gallop
Tachypnea
Rales
Hemoptysis
Hemodynamic instability

reasonable because angiography is highly sensitive, although expensive (Reid, 1999). The combination of an indeterminate $\dot{V}/\dot{Q}$ scan and a negative lower extremity venous ultrasound does not exclude the presence of a PE (Daniel, Jackson, & Kline, 2000).

Because PE can be difficult to diagnose via tests, the clinical presentation is important in guiding assessment and management approaches. Stein (2000) reported PE as the unsuspected antemortem in approximately 70% of patients in whom PE was shown to contribute to death. A large number of deep vein thromboses are silent, contributing to "silent" PE (Meignan, Rosso, Gauthier, et al., 2000). It is the characteristics of PE, based on components of the history and physical, that lead to confident suspicion of a PE. See Box 24-1. *Answer 12:* **d.**

QUESTIONS

13. What is the mechanism for a PE as the cause of cardiac arrest in a patient like Jack?
   a. Cardiac ischemia
   b. Overload of the right ventricle
   c. Increased peripheral vascular resistance
   d. Inadequate venous return

ANSWERS

13. Pulmonary obstruction from a PE leads to increased right ventricular afterload. An increase in the right ventricle leads to decreased left ventricular diastolic filling and end-diastolic volume. This results in a significantly decreased preload. Inadequate volume is able to be pumped out at the same time that the right ventricle is failing, causing right atrial pressure to rise and

cardiogenic shock to ensue (Kurkciyan, Meron, Sterz, et al., 2000). *Answer 13:* **b.**

QUESTIONS

14. If you are concerned about Jack's cardiac stability, what test would provide you with the most information about his cardiac status?
   a. Echocardiogram
   b. ECG
   c. Swan catheter
   d. High-resolution computed tomography (CT) scan

ANSWERS

14. Patients with echocardiographic right ventricular dysfunction are at risk for a PE associated death (Grifoni, Olivotto, Cecchini, et al., 2000). A standard two-dimensional echo Doppler examination provides a report on the functioning of the right ventricle. Grifoni reported on 31% of patients experiencing a PE who were clinically normotensive but presented with right ventricular dysfunction, having a 10% rate of PE-related shock and a 5% mortality rate. This study underwrites the need for early detection of echocardiographic right ventricular dysfunction. *Answer 14:* **a.**

Case Study conclusion

Because of a high clinical suspicion, Jack is begun on intravenous heparin as he is being scheduled for the pulmonary angiography.

REFERENCES

Botteron, G. W., & Smith, J. M. (1998). Cardiac arrhythmias. In Carey, C. F., Lee, H. H., & Woeltje, K. F. (Eds.). *The Washington manual of medical therapeutics*, 29th ed. Philadelphia: Lippincott Williams & Wilkins.

Daniel, K. R., Jackson, R. E., & Kline, J. A. (2000). Utility of lower extremity venous ultrasound scanning in the diagnosis and exclusion of pulmonary embolism in outpatients. *Ann Emerg Med, 35*(6), pp. 547-554.

Ewald, G. A., & Rogers, J. G. (1998). Heart failure, cardiomyopathy, and valvular heart disease. In Carey, C. F., Lee, H. H., & Woeltje, K. F. (Eds.). *The Washington manual of medical therapeutics*, 29th ed. Philadelphia: Lippincott Williams & Wilkins.

Grifoni, S., Olivotto, I., Cecchini, P., et al. (2000). Short-term clinical outcome of patients with acute pulmonary embolism, normal blood pressure, and echocardiographic right ventricular dysfunction. *Circulation, 101*, pp. 2817-2822.

Lin, E., & Mitchell, S. (1996). Abnormalities in hemostasis and coagulation. In McCorkle, R., Grant, M., Frank-Stromborg, M., & Baird, S. (Eds.). *Cancer nursing. A comprehensive textbook* (pp. 979-1009). Philadelphia: WB Saunders.

Kurkciyan, I., Meron, G., Sterz, F., et al. (2000). Pulmonary embolism as cause of cardiac arrest. *Arch Intern Med, 160,* pp. 1529-1535.

Meignan, M., Rosso, J., Gauthier, H., et al. (2000). Systematic lung scans reveal a high frequency of silent pulmonary embolism in patients with proximal deep venous thrombosis. *Arch Intern Med, 160,* pp. 159-164.

Reid, E. (1999). Pulmonary embolism: an overview of treatment and nursing issues. *Br J Nurs, 8*(20), pp. 1373-1378.

Singer, G. G. (1998). Fluid and electrolyte management. In Carey, C. F., Lee, H. H., & Woeltje, K. F. (Eds.). *The Washington manual of medical therapeutics,* 29th ed. Philadelphia: Lippincott Williams & Wilkins.

Stein, P. D. (2000). Silent pulmonary embolism. *Arch Intern Med, 160,* pp. 145-146.

Timmerman, P. (1998). Pulmonary fibrosis. In Chernecky, C. C., & Berger, B. J. (Eds.). *Advanced and critical care in oncology nursing. Managing primary complications.* Philadelphia: WB Saunders.

Winters K. J., & Eisenberg, P. R. (1998). Ischemic heart disease. In Carey, C. F., Lee, H. H., and Woeltje, K. F. (Eds.). *The Washington manual of medical therapeutics,* 29th ed. Philadelphia: Lippincott Williams & Wilkins.

Administrator/ Coordinator Role

25 Administration

Constance Engelking

CASE STUDY

You have just been employed by a network of three hospitals to establish a networkwide oncology program with participation in clinical trials. Two of the hospitals in the network have 100 to 200 beds, and the third is a 550-bed facility. State-mandated reporting of cancer data is the responsibility of the Medical Records Departments in all three hospitals. There are four medical oncology and hematology practices in the region. Physicians from each group have admitting privileges at all three hospitals, but each practice is aligned with a different member institution of the network. The network's decision to create the new advanced practice nurse (APN) position is in response to the demands of the strongest and largest medical oncology private practice, which has ties to the 550-bed hospital. Although there is no dedicated oncology unit or nursing staff in any of the three hospitals, each practice has identified a preferred patient care unit for admissions and has developed relationships with the nursing staff of that particular unit. The extent of nurse preparation is on-the-job instruction by physicians. A few staff members have attended some oncology nursing workshops and seminars. Two other APNs are on staff at the large hospital: a cardiology nurse practitioner who works exclusively with the cardiology private practice and a psychiatric clinical nurse specialist who has housewide responsibility.

QUESTIONS

1. The administrator role requires knowledge of a variety of management processes that make up the role. Match the activities listed with the appropriate management process identified.

a. Outlines competencies required for registered nurse (RN) assignment to patients undergoing chemotherapy

b. Recommends chairperson and core members to establish a cancer committee

c. Monitors chemotherapy administration practices in accordance with established institutional standards

d. Prepares a budget for the operation of the oncology unit

e. Mobilizes oncology staff interest in participating in cancer screening outreach program

f. Forecasts resource needs for incorporating a new radiation medicine procedure

g. Conducts multidisciplinary discussion addressing resistance to use of a newly introduced pain control algorithm

h. Evaluates proposed cancer clinical trials for impact on institutional resources

i. Delegates responsibility for palliative care performance improvement initiative to tenured oncology nurse with OCN

Planning
Coordinating
Staffing
Directing
Controlling

j. Develops job description for the new bone marrow transplant (BMT) nurse coordinator position

k. Prepares for American College of Surgeons Commission on Cancer site survey

l. Meets with director of medical oncology to discuss concerns about staff practice

m. Compares previous month's admissions, discharges, and transfers to the oncology unit with current statistics

---

ANSWERS

1. Management has been defined in a variety of ways. Although the focus may differ in those definitions, key themes remain the same. Management is working with and through others to meet established goals and to accomplish the objectives of an organization and its members in an ever-changing environment (Montana & Charnov, 1993). Management relies on the activities of procurement and coordination of material and human resources needed to achieve the goals of the organization. Management is a dynamic rather than static process (Hellriegel & Slocum, 1989).

Within the context of nursing, *management* has been defined as "the process of working through nursing staff to provide care, cure and comfort to patients" (Gillies, 1989). Like the nursing profession, management is both a science and an art. In both cases a scientific foundation underlies the primary processes of the profession. Those processes are carried out in accordance with a set of principles and methods that, in conjunction with an individual manager's personal style in selecting and applying those principles and methods, constitutes the artistry. The primary processes associated with management include planning, organizing, staffing, directing, coordinating, and controlling (Douglass, 1996; Marriner-Tomey, 1996; Montana & Charnov, 1993). Descriptions and key functions affiliated with each process and examples of applications in oncology nursing are detailed in Table 25-1. *Answer 1:* **a: staffing; b: coordinating; c: controlling; d: directing; e: planning; f: directing; g: planning; h: directing; i: staffing; j: coordinating; k: controlling; l: controlling; m: planning.**

| TABLE 25-1 | Management Processes and Their Applications to Oncology Nursing |

MANAGEMENT PROCESSES	DESCRIPTION OF FUNCTIONS	RELEVANCE TO NURSING	ONCOLOGY APPLICATION
Planning	Forecasting future events or trends that will affect the business and projecting the most effective future activities on behalf of the organization within a particular division or service area. Involves decision-making processes and tools to identify and "live" the purpose of the organization; define goals and objectives; prepare budgets and effectively manage the time and resource expenditures of the organization dedicated to achieving the desired outcomes. Involves both strategic (long range, 3 to 5 years), and operational plans (short-term dealing with day-to-day maintenance).	Planning for: • Delivering nursing care to patients and families • Operating a patient care unit or clinic including staffing, equipment/supplies, physical plant/environment; compliance with regulatory agency requirements • Implementing new treatment and care technologies • Modifying, merging, or modifying patient care service offerings	Planning for: 1. Providing specific care to patients undergoing cancer therapies 2. Operating an inpatient oncology unit or outpatient ambulatory facility dedicated to a specific population of cancer patients (e.g., tumor-, treatment-, or symptom-specific patient groups) 3. Implementing new drug or drug regimens 4. Transitioning selected components of a BMT/stem cell service from inpatient to outpatient setting

BMT, Bone marrow transplant; *RN,* registered nurse.

TABLE 25-1	Management Processes and Their Applications to Oncology Nursing—cont'd		
MANAGEMENT PROCESSES	**DESCRIPTION OF FUNCTIONS**	**RELEVANCE TO NURSING**	**ONCOLOGY APPLICATION**
Organizing/ coordinating	Establishing a formal structure that provides for coordination of resources to accomplish objectives; develop policy and procedure, create position qualifications/descriptions, and determine the methods by which authority and responsibility for various aspects of the business are delegated to identified managers.	Coordinate plans to launch a specialty patient care unit within the context of established framework for clinical units under the auspices of the nursing department organizational table, reporting structure, and operations plan.	Establish a cancer committee; select chairman and core members; establish four subcommittees, each with responsibility for various aspects of decision-making as it relates to cancer care at the institution: • Cancer quality management • Clinical resource management • Public awareness and outreach • Professional education
Staffing	Establishing personnel selection/assignment systems and mechanisms by which staffing schedules are determined and modified.	• RN job descriptions • Nurse recruitment • Retention strategies • Patient assignment	• Distinguish between general and oncologic specialty RN practice in job description. • Determine additional qualifications for assignment to oncology specialty practice areas in job specifications. • Recruit oncology-experienced RNs via Oncology Nurses Society national or local chapters. • Establish criteria for assigning RNs with oncology experience to patients with cancer on general medical-surgical units.
Directing/ leading	Employing methodologies for accomplishing work through others, which involves recognizing, addressing, and resolving conflict; motivating and disciplining staff; and engaging in suitable delegation of work through effective communication and assertive behavior.		
Controlling	Setting standards by which to measure performance, reporting results, taking corrective action, monitoring overall clinical and financial outcomes.		Review and apply elements of established oncology practice standards developed by cancer-related national organizations (e.g., ONS, ASCO, ACoS Commission on Cancer, FAHCT) to institution cancer program or center.

BMT, Bone marrow transplant; *RN*, registered nurse.

QUESTIONS

2. Many techniques exist. Which of the following would you select to evaluate productivity and resource use?
   a. Nominal group process
   b. Gantt charting
   c. Fishbone diagramming
   d. Retrospective chart review

3. Your quarterly report reflects an emphasis on which of the following?
   a. Time studies
   b. Productivity
   c. Administrative goals
   d. Professional advancement

ANSWERS

2-3. Today's management approaches are based on the evolution of management theory during the past century, and they incorporate elements of the various schools of management thought that have evolved during the past century. *Scientific management,* the earliest construct, focuses on determining the best method for accomplishing a task. It is from this theoretical construct that management tools such as time-and-motion studies have been adopted (Taylor & Gilbreth). The Gantt chart depicts the relationship of planned or completed work to the amount of time needed or used, the value of evaluating the cost of input against the resulting output (Cook), and the principles of efficiency including standardization and documentation (Emerson). *Classic organization-administration* thought perceives the organization as a whole rather than focusing solely on the production dimension, and it incorporates the concepts of span of control, accountability of line-staff relationships, specialization, decentralization, and departmentalization. The *human relations* school of management focuses attention on the impact of individuals on the success or failure of organizations. It is from this management construct that concepts of group process, interpersonal relations, leadership, and communication are identified as elements essential to successful management. Required for success is cooperation between management and labor (Barnard), coordination of the psychologic and sociologic aspects (Follett), the effects of establishing group norms (Hawthorne), force-field analysis as an element of planning for change (Lewin), and sociometrics (including role-playing, psychodrama, sociodrama techniques) for analyzing interpersonal relations. Current-day management thought has arisen from the *behavioral science* approach and incorporates hierarchy of needs model (Maslow), critical incident review

methods (Herzberg), theory X (goals of the organization)/theory Y (goals of the individual) approaches (McGregor), the models of participative management (Likert), and management by objectives (Drucker) both of which invest the individual with responsibility and accountability for his or her own performance (Marriner-Tomey, 1996; Montana & Charnov, 1993).

The hallmarks of contemporary corporate management are the movement away from autocratic to democratic leadership with greater emphasis on the individual within the organization and on results and productivity rather than on the particular activities of the individual within the organization. In addition, there is a growing recognition of the benefits of achieving outcomes that simultaneously satisfy both an employee's personal objectives and organizational goals. Many of the management principles and methods used today in the field of nursing have been borrowed from corporate management theory and modified to fit the health care model. Within the context of nursing, management behaviors can be further categorized as patient care management, operational management, and human resources management (Genovich-Richards & Carissimi, 1986). *Answer 2:* **b.** *Answer 3:* **b.**

QUESTIONS

4. Following orientation to the hospital, what would be the best initial activity you could engage in?
   a. Selecting the patient care unit that would be best suited to become a dedicated oncology unit
   b. Developing a basic oncology nursing education program for staff to minimize the risk for medication incidents
   c. Gathering data to profile physician/nurse practices, patient profiles, existing policy/procedure relevant to cancer care at the three institutions
   d. Getting acquainted with the other two APNs on staff and establishing a regular meeting time to explore interface opportunities

5. How will you *best* assess the formal structure of the institutional environment?
   a. Review the philosophy, mission, and values of the system
   b. Determine the volume and flow of information in the system
   c. Compare leadership styles of the APNs and administrators
   d. Identify systems issues that are potential political land mines

6. Planning for the implementation of a new investigational combination chemotherapy regimen will entail which of the following actions?

    a. Delivering an in-service education program addressing the new regimen

    b. Projecting volume and special needs of patients who will be eligible

    c. Orienting the pharmacists to protocol details and reporting requirements

    d. Measuring clinical and financial outcomes associated with the regimen

4-6. Although it is the tendency to immediately initiate problem-solving action, it must be recognized that successful implementation of a change project relies on having a sound plan that draws from information gathered during a focused evaluation. The first step in program planning is to conduct a situational assessment designed to determine need while profiling the environment within which new programs will be integrated or existing programs modified. Knowledge of the philosophy, mission, and values of each of the three institutions in the network will provide insights regarding the priorities for and design of the cancer program as well as your APN position within the organizational structure (Krumm, 1996). Understanding the current profile of patients, physicians, and institutional infrastructure, as well as patient flow, work processes, clinical practice patterns, staff and consumer preferences, and past performance, is essential to the creation of a solid plan for programmatic change that meets the needs of the population to be served. *Answer 4:* **c.** *Answer 5:* **a.** *Answer 6:* **b.**

QUESTIONS

7. Critical early coordinative activities you need to undertake when charged with building a network cancer program includes which of the following?

    a. Cultivating relationships with the oncologists from the four private practices and the staff from the units to which they admit patients

    b. Recruiting and selecting appropriate candidates for staff positions on the oncology units in each of the participating institutions

    c. Developing a program of professional development for all employees who will staff the cancer program

    d. Creating the links necessary to connect the information systems of each institution to achieve a common cancer database

7. It is well accepted that successful implementation of a planned change relies on organizational efforts that incorporate strategies to obtain "buy in" from those influencing individuals who are most invested in project outcomes.

Prematurely initiating actions such as staff recruitment or assignment, professional education, and database development will likely result in resistance from leaders who have been excluded from the process and in the establishment of mechanisms that do not meet the users' needs. Rather, identifying and developing interpersonal relationships with key stakeholders and involving them in the process on the front end often helps ensure smooth and therefore successful execution of the elements of a plan as it unfolds. This approach can facilitate achievement of the established endpoints for the project. *Answer 7:* **a.**

Case Study continued

As you continue to gather data about the existing infrastructure within which the new cancer program must fit and the individuals who constitute the key stakeholder group, you learn that there are conflicting opinions about who should have responsibility for chemotherapy admixture and administration. Some believe it is a physician function with pharmacy backup. Others believe that nursing should take on the responsibility for both admixture and administration.

QUESTIONS

8. Which of the following would be the *best* way to handle this issue?

    a. Advise the appropriate network hospital administrator and request a resolution compatible with institutional mission, values, and resources

    b. Draw on expert knowledge of chemotherapeutics, establish a new policy incorporating all three disciplines, and distribute a memo apprising those involved

    c. Present the issue at the newly convened cancer committee for discussion and development of a recommendation for resolution to be submitted to network hospital administration

    d. Delegate responsibility for resolution conflicts associated with this issue to the nurse managers of patient care units on which the majority of chemotherapy administration takes place.

9. You are aware that achieving national regulatory agency approval can be one step in ensuring quality care and building visibility for the network cancer program. Approval from which of the following national regulatory agencies would be most appropriate for you to pursue as a goal for the developing cancer program?

  a. Joint Commission on Accreditation of Healthcare Organizations (JCAHO)
  b. American Cancer Society Clinical Practice Review Group (ACS CPRG)
  c. Foundation for the Accreditation of Hematopoietic Cell Therapy (FAHCT)
  d. American College of Surgeons Commission on Cancer (ACoS CoS)

ANSWERS

8-9. Conflict arises in an environment characterized by competition for scarce resources, ambiguous jurisdiction, and the absence of mechanisms to achieve consensus among those involved in a particular endeavor or specialty. It occurs when the involved individuals do not share the same information or have different pieces of information, when they define or value problems or aspects of a problem differently, and when there are divergent perceptions of power and authority (Marriner-Tomey, 1996; Northouse & Northouse, 1992). Often, it is conflict that initiates and drives program development as a resolution strategy. In this scenario, in addition to the desire to improve the quality and efficiency of cancer care, network cancer program development is a resolution to expressed physician dissatisfaction. Establishing the network cancer committee is a vehicle to multidisciplinary and interinstitutional communication. Using this vehicle for problem identification and resolution is a win-win strategy because it allows the group to concentrate on goals, processes, and outcomes rather than focusing on the negative aspects of the problem and individual power issues, neither of which are productive activities. Group process emphasizes a collaborative approach to decision making, thus enriching the experience by allowing for the contribution of each group member and shifting attention away from a single policy maker. Moreover, a functional cancer committee clearly engaged in a planned program of performance improvement is required for approval by the American College of Surgeons Commission on Cancer as a cancer program. This national regulatory agency, which grants approval at five levels associated with organizational size and patient care complexity, has recently finalized a reciprocity agreement with JCAHO that states that approval by one of the two regulatory agencies will be accepted by the other without the need for duplicating the review process. *Answer 8:* **c.** *Answer 9:* **d.**

QUESTIONS

10. Which of the following is a viable option to pursue for integrating clinical research as a component of cancer program service offerings for the hospital network?

  a. NCI designation as a Comprehensive Cancer Center
  b. NCI designation as a Cooperative Group Outreach Program
  c. NCI designation as a Community Clinical Oncology Program
  d. NCI designation as a Community Cancer Advisory Board

ANSWERS

10. During the 1970s, the National Cancer Institute (NCI) established its Cancer Centers Program and Cooperative Group Outreach Program (CGOP) infrastructure. Comprehensive cancer center status denotes centers that have demonstrated success in basic, clinical, and epidemiologic studies; that engage in interdisciplinary collaboration; and that provide cancer information, education, and outreach activities in the service catchment area. Currently, 58 centers meet the criteria for comprehensive cancer center status. The intent in creating the CGOP structure was to facilitate patient accrual and the conduct of clinical research through an outreach initiative that would familiarize community physicians with cancer clinical trials and permit their involvement. Currently, there are 14 national and regional CGOPs (e.g., Gynecologic Oncology Group [GOG], National Surgical Adjuvant Breast and Bowel Project [NSABBP], Radiation Therapy Oncology Group [RTOG], Eastern Cooperative and Southwest Oncology Groups [ECOG and SWOG]). Academic centers are the core institutions, comprising the CGOP with community facility affiliates. The 59 Community Clinical Oncology Programs (CCOP) currently in existence receive support from cancer centers but are more loosely structured and function more independently than the CGOP affiliates. The CCOPs lend themselves to phase IV community integration projects and cancer prevention trials (Wujcik & Fraser, 2000). *Answer 10:* **c.**

QUESTIONS

11. A decision is made to concentrate oncology patients on one unit of the largest hospital in the network. In preparation for implementing that strategic plan, needed staffing resources must be determined. Which of the following variables reflect the most critical data set needed to develop an appropriate staffing plan for the new oncology unit?

a. Staff availability, scheduling method, shift preferences
b. Patient types and volumes, acuity, complexity of care to be delivered
c. Staff educational background, experience, credentials, OCN certification
d. Patient length of stay, incidence of complications, readmission rates

ANSWERS

11. Adequately projecting the number, level, and mix of personnel required to staff a patient care unit relies primarily on knowing the amount, level, and type of care patients will require. Defining the needed care requires description not only of the anticipated number of patients to be admitted but also of the following:

• Subpopulations that will make up the group to be served (e.g., age range, tumor types, cultural background)
• Extent of disease and presence of comorbid conditions in the predominant subgroups (e.g., incidence of local or newly diagnosed versus advanced disease)
• Presence of accompanying chronic conditions (e.g., cardiac, pulmonary, and renal diseases; chronic pain syndromes)
• Planned conventional and investigational treatment regimens (e.g., multimodal versus single-approach therapies, dose-intensive versus conventional-dose regimens, use of phase I to III clinical trials, incorporation of intensive regimens such as stem cell transplantation)

By providing the descriptive details associated with the populations to be served and therapeutic services to be delivered, the oncology APN can be especially helpful to hospital administrators and nurse managers as they plan for staffing the new unit. Patient acuity can be projected using the patient classification system used by the institutions involved. Staff workload projections can be further detailed by establishing time standards (i.e., through the conduct of time and motion studies) for high-frequency activities and procedures that will be performed on the new oncology unit. *Answer 11:* **b.**

QUESTIONS

12. Performance appraisals are conducted primarily for which of the following reasons?

a. To establish the reporting structure within the institution
b. To validate the span of control for a specific clinical area
c. To meet regulatory agency and state health department requirements
d. To identify accomplishments and areas for professional growth

13. Which of the following methodologies is best suited for appraisal of the oncology APN's performance?

a. Criterion ranking
b. SWOT analysis
c. Management by objectives (MBO)
d. Force-field analysis

ANSWERS

12. Performance appraisal is a periodic formal evaluation to analyze the level and quality of employee performance within a specified time frame. Employee performance appraisals (EPAs) serve many purposes, including determining job competence, providing professional development opportunities, discovering an individual's aspirations and recognizing achievements, improving communications between managers and staff associates, developing mutual agreement as to the established performance objectives, taking inventory of talent within the organization and reassessing assignments, selecting qualified individuals for advancement and salary increases, and identifying unsatisfactory employees (Marriner-Tomey, 1996). The APN can take advantage of the EPAs to grow professionally, to make the manager aware of special interests and talents, and to explore opportunities for advancement compatible with personal aspirations. *Answer 12:* **d.**

13. MBO is a methodology used to enhance the effectiveness of program planning and performance appraisal. Rather than focusing attention on subjective aspects such as personality characteristics, MBO emphasizes the achievement of predetermined objectives. Thus this approach addresses an individual's accomplishments on behalf of the organization and measures results against the defined standards within a specified period rather than on the specific activities engaged in by the individual. Developing objectives entails a delineation of major job responsibilities that can be culled from an existing job description coupled with an analysis of daily practice and personal perception of what the job should entail. Once major job responsibilities are identified, expected levels of accomplishment and productivity can be determined and consensus regarding their appropriateness obtained. From these mutually agreed-upon expectations, realistic, measurable, and results-oriented criteria for evaluation of employee effectiveness are developed and serve as a guide (Marriner-Tomey, 1996; Montana & Charnov, 1993). The newly hired APN can generate clear objectives related to the charge of developing an oncology network program. Such parameters as marketshare percentages, number of oncology admissions and discharges, or staff validated in oncology-related competencies may serve as objectives for year 1. Achievement of ACoS Commission on Cancer approval and integration of clinical trials may be measures in following years. Direct care measures may include number of patients admitted with a cancer diagnosis consulted by the APN within 24 hours of admission or the incidence of avoidable complications and readmission rates. *Answer 13:* **c.**

QUESTIONS

14. Which data set contains the parameters for performance measurement most applicable to justification of a newly created APN position?

   a. Demonstrated clinical competencies, collaboration, and leadership
   b. Participation and skill in committee, board and task force activities
   c. Quality of documentation, level of communication, presentation skill
   d. Quantifiable cost savings, revenues generated, clinical outcomes

ANSWERS

14. Significant economic pressures imposed for the past decade on health care institutions by the prospective payment system, the managed care trend, and the intensification of government regulation associated with the delivery and reimbursement of health care (e.g., ambulatory payment classification [APCs]) have left hospitals and private practices struggling to meet their operating margins. Positions perceived to be nonrevenue generating are often eliminated or downsized as a cost-saving measure. Under these circumstances, APNs are faced with the challenge of concretizing their financial worth to the employing organization. Although clinical competency, interpersonal skills, and the ability to present are important when evaluating the *individual* who occupies a position, these data do little to justify the *position* within the organization. Rather, outcomes of the APN's interventions rather than the particular interventions are more important measures of the effectiveness of the position. Impact on revenue saved and generated, if positive, can demonstrate that the APN position "pays for itself" or at least contributes to underwriting the cost of the position. Revenue-generating programs, successful grant proposals, cost-saving projects, and services receiving third-party reimbursement (e.g., establishment of a consultation service for symptom management) should all be included as part of the performance appraisal. These measurable outcomes quantify the value of the APN position in fiscal terms (Ferraro-McDurrie, Chan, & Jerome, 1993). In addition, positive patient outcomes such as customer satisfaction scores, improved symptom control, and reduced complication and readmission rates attributable to APN intervention should always be documented. *Answer 14:* **d.**

CASE 2 STUDY

Hospital X, a 650-bed tertiary care university-affiliated institution, has made the strategic decision to engage in a reengineering effort. An external consulting group has been contracted to guide the organization through the process. The goals of the redesign project are formidable and include increasing customer satisfaction, enhancing patient outcomes, and reducing costs by the "stretch goal" of 25%. The redesign process selected is a team-based approach in which 42 groups of employees representing all disciplines and levels are organized along the lines of hospital functions. The work of the teams is to analyze processes for their specific areas, formulate a plan, and seek review of the executive team. The plan must redesign systems in such a way as to achieve the stated goals of the project. The executive team then gives approval based on the ability to successfully implement the approved version. As the APN, you have been appointed team leader for the cancer services redesign team. Your team consists of an interdisciplinary group including oncology nurses from the inpatient medical oncology unit and radiation medicine service, oncology social worker, the BMT nurse coordinator, the clinical trials coordinator, the cancer registry administrator, radiation therapy technologist, and a supervising pharmacist. The members of this group have different reporting relationships within the organization, including the departments of nursing, social services, pharmacy, and the cancer center. In addition, two physicians, the chief of oncology and the clinical director of the radiation medicine service, have been asked to serve in an advisory capacity as an adjunct to core members of the team.

QUESTIONS

1. A group or team that includes interdisciplinary membership in which members have different reporting relationships and focuses on the customer being served is known as:
- **a.** Function-oriented/department-based team
- **b.** Formal task-oriented/centralized team
- **c.** Systems-oriented/patient-centered team
- **d.** Informal outcome-oriented/decentralized team

2. Successful groups form:
- **a.** Because of the leader
- **b.** Spontaneously
- **c.** Because of the members
- **d.** In phases over time

3. The most effective way for you to open the first meeting of the cancer services redesign team is to:
- **a.** Distribute instructional handouts, record contact information, and assign team members to required tasks outlined by the consultants
- **b.** Discuss a complex patient care incident involving several team members to maximize time together
- **c.** Ask team members to introduce themselves, identify their role in cancer services, and explain their perceptions of their contributions to the project
- **d.** Provide an opportunity for socializing among the team members for an identified period as an icebreaker

4. Which of the following *best* exemplifies why you emphasize team-building over meeting mechanics during the initial meeting of the redesign group?
- **a.** To provide an opportunity for building the personal self-confidence needed to actualize the role of team leader
- **b.** To establish in members the sense of group belonging essential for their full participation
- **c.** To gain the group member acceptance required by the leader to move the agenda forward
- **d.** To communicate the message that rules and regulations are not as important as relationships

1-2. Different types of groups may be convened to serve different purposes and reflect different organizational structures. Function-centered/department-based groups typically focus on tasks or functions performed exclusively by a particular department or service. Generally, membership of this group type has a common reporting structure. Staff meetings are an example of this type of group. In contrast, a system-based/patient-centered group is more decentralized and includes members from various disciplines across departments or service lines. Typically, members of systems-based groups have different reporting relationships and roles in the delivery of service to the population of patients that is the focus of this group. A performance improvement team is an example of this type of group. The development of successful teams or groups relies on the interactions among and between the leader and the members. Groups evolve over time and occur in phases, including (1) orientation, or "forming"; (2) conflict, or "storming"; (3) cohesion, or "norming"; (4) working, or "performing"; and (5) termination phases (Tuckman, 1956; Yalom, 1975). *Answer 1:* **c.** *Answer 2:* **d.**

3-4. During the "orientation phase," members seek to define the degree to which they are considered a part of the group, specifically what team membership entails, how they were chosen to be part of the group, how open they can be in the group, the level of commitment necessary, and whether they possess the requisite skills or attributes for inclusion (Yalom, 1975). This phase has also been referred to as the *mutual acceptance stage* because it is the time during which team members become acquainted; learn about the knowledge, skills, capabilities, and interests of each team member; and develop the trust and confidence levels needed to permit reliance upon one another (Montana & Charnov, 1993). Leadership during this phase is focused on assisting individual members to "satisfy their needs for belonging" and feel embraced as a team member, while at the same time ensuring a sense of independence and privacy for each member (Northouse & Northouse, 1992). Although the provision of instructions and the completion of assigned tasks are ultimately important to goal achievement, focusing on meeting mechanics and group tasks at the outset does not permit the level of interaction needed to establish the sense of group belonging required by members to fully participate. Spending time socializing or discussing patient care issues can distract group members from the purpose at hand. Instead, an approach that recognizes the need for trust-building and mutuality within the context of the group's overarching mission is the most effective way to launch the team. *Answer 3:* **c.** *Answer 4:* **b.**

QUESTIONS

5. When forming a new group, what key assessments do you need to make to avoid or minimize deterrents to productive team function?
   a. Group characteristics, individual member roles, interaction styles, communication patterns within the group
   b. Member relationships with health team members outside the group, personal agendas, past team performance of each group member
   c. Individual member workload and schedules, specific clinical skills and interests, key alignments within the organization
   d. External and internal perceptions of group potential for success, expressed commitment to productivity, outcomes identified as high priority

---
ANSWERS

5. APNs often find themselves involved as leaders in the implementation of new services or technology, in the revision of existing programs, or in the initiation of change projects designed to improve outcomes and enhance revenues or marketshare. Team-building is an essential skill for the APN because successful implementation in all of these cases relies heavily on acceptance and investment in the proposed plan by the key stakeholders. This is especially true when the desired outcome is service integration, as is the case in this scenario. Assessment of group or team characteristics, individual member group roles and interaction styles, and group communication patterns is critical to formulating a leadership approach that will minimize barriers to team coalescence and productivity and subsequently facilitate success during the implementation phases of the project. *Answer 5:* **a.**

QUESTIONS

6. During the first team meeting, you observe that the physician member of the group does most of the talking, outlining his vision for the redesign and assigning group members to specific tasks. You recognize that this individual is assuming which of the following group roles?
   a. Dysfunctional individual role of aggressor
   b. Task role of initiator-contributor
   c. Dysfunctional individual role of dominator
   d. Task role of coordinator

7. During this initial meeting, you further observe that team members are subgrouping according to their service departments and are submissive to the direction of the physician who has integrated himself as a core member of the team. This is in direct opposition to the original role laid out as advisory by the hospital's chief executive officer (CEO) at the outset of the project. What would be the most effective leadership strategies for you could use in this situation?
   a. Apprise the physician that meetings are open only to core members
   b. Organize team tasks around the natural member subgroupings
   c. Openly share your views and expectations about group function
   d. Engage the team in establishing a clear set of group norms and goals

8. List four potential barriers to the successful development of a functional team or group.
   a. _____
   b. _____
   c. _____
   d. _____

9. List four leader behaviors that will promote the development of a functional team or group.
   a. _____
   b. _____
   c. _____
   d. _____

ANSWERS

6. Group task roles, team-building and maintenance roles, and dysfunctional group member roles are listed for review in Table 25-2 (Marriner-Tomey, 1996; Northouse & Northouse, 1992). The dominator role, naturally assumed by the physician advisor in this case, is a dysfunctional role that can quickly undermine the purpose of the group, stifle creative thought, and redirect the group's focus to the physician's agenda. However, exclusion of the physician advisor from group participation could alienate this key stakeholder, creating a potential barrier to future implementation of the elements of the redesign plan related to his sphere of control. Therefore rigid exclusion criteria for participation or closing off team meetings to physicians would not be the best approach in this situation because physician buy-in will be necessary to effect change in the future. *Answer 6:* **c.**

7. Subgrouping is a natural group occurrence arising from interpersonal comfort shared by individual group members through previously

TABLE 25-2 Functional and Dysfunctional Group Roles

TASK ROLES	TEAM-BUILDING AND MAINTENANCE ROLES	DYSFUNCTIONAL INDIVIDUAL ROLES
Initiator-contributor	Gatekeeper	*Aggressor:* satisfies own personal needs at the expense of other team members by exhibiting disapproval or disdain to deflate others' status
Orienter/recorder/ procedural technician	Encourager	*Dominator:* asserts own personal authority/superiority by flattering, disrupting, and giving authoritative direction
Information giver/seeker	Harmonizer	*Recognition seeker:* calls attention to self through boasting or behaving in an unusual manner
Opinion giver/seeker	Compromiser	*Special-interest pleader:* speaks for a particular group and addresses issues that best meet the needs of that group
Energizer	Follower	*Self-confessor:* uses the group as a vehicle to express personal feelings that may be unrelated to the task
Elaborator	Group observer	*Help/seeker:* expresses insecurity, personal confusion, depreciation to elicit sympathy for self
Coordinator	Standard setter	*Playboy/playgirl:* disinterested in the group, appears disconnected and nonchalant
Evaluator-critic		*Blocker:* negative, resistant, disagreeable without reason; raises issues after group has rejected them

developed relationships and functional familiarity. Left unchecked, however, subgrouping early on in the group maturation process can interfere with building a "groupthink" context within which member integration can take place. Thus steering team members away from clustering in familiar groups at the outset will promote cohesion and help build a strong team. In addition, leaders must engage in behaviors that strike balance between building the team and stifling critical thinking. Avoiding behaviors such as stating personal preferences and expectations in favor of encouraging members to play devil's advocate during the early stages of group development are leader behaviors that will assist in striking the balance.

Effective leadership in groups also requires awareness of the other potential barriers to successful team development. Obstacles can arise in relation to goal setting, establishment of group norms, the degree of cohesiveness, and leader and member behaviors. Problems associated with goal setting include the development or existence of noncompatible goals among team members, the setting of overly ambitious or unachievable goals, the development of restrictive rather than empowering group norms, submission to scenarios that threaten cohesiveness, and negative leader or member behaviors (Northouse & Northouse, 1992). Incompatible goals can produce competition among team members, which disrupts communication flow, interferes with collaboration, and prevents consensus-building, all elements necessary for successful achievement of team goals. Setting unrealistic goals undermines team func-

tion by overwhelming or frustrating team members when they are unable to attain the established goals, thus creating a sense of personal failure and subsequent disinterest in group participation. Similarly, a lack of clarity regarding the nature of the goals and the plan for their achievement confuses, frustrates, and produces anxiety among team members as they struggle to interpret the substance of the team's goals, the timeline, and their respective roles in effecting those goals. In contrast, setting feasible clearly defined goals contributes to the success of the team provided the goals are not so simplistic that team members loose interest and motivation to participate in the activities necessary for goal achievement.

Another dimension in which barriers to successful team development can arise is group norms. Norms are the ground rules established for group behavior. Norms prescribe acceptable group behaviors and are needed to ensure a level of consistency and predictability that facilitates the trust necessary for open participation by all team members. Group behavior occurs within a range of acceptable performance levels from lowest to highest. Empowering norms include expecting team members to complete assigned tasks, coming to meetings prepared for the agenda, and offering constructive feedback. Restrictive norms are characterized by their inhibiting influence on group function and include permission to engage in behaviors such as chronic lateness or inconsistent attendance, lack of preparation, and verbal attacks by group members. Successful leaders attend early to the development and shaping of norms, which will facilitate productive team function and the achievement of established goals (Marriner-Tomey, 1996; Montana & Charnov, 1993; Northouse & Northouse, 1992). *Answer 7:* **d.**

8. Potential barriers to successful team or group development include (1) the setting of noncompatible, unachievable, or unclear goals; (2) establishment of restrictive group norms; (3) evolution of subgroups or splinter groups; and (4) negative leader or member behaviors. *Answer 8:* **See text.**

9. Leader behaviors that promote successful team or group development include (1) facilitative rather than authoritative style, (2) early establishment of group norms and goals, (3) awareness of member interaction styles and roles, and (4) encouragement of team members to express divergent views. *Answer 9:* **See text.**

QUESTIONS

10. Which of the following actions is likely to interfere with the development of a successful cancer services redesign team?
  a. Providing for alternate or substitute members to cover for core team members when they are involved in unanticipated patient care issues
  b. Permitting conflicting views and hostility to be openly expressed in accordance with varying opinions among team members
  c. Putting the team on "automatic pilot" once group cohesiveness has been achieved and members work through their tasks
  d. Summarizing the team's work activities, goal achievement, team relationships, and personal feelings about the group

ANSWERS

10. Hallmarks of successful team-building include behaviors designed to facilitate open communication among team members; group self-management; and awareness of the purpose, plan, and progress of the group. A leader seeking to bring together a solid productive team does well to stimulate the open expression of divergent views among team members because it is from these differing opinions that new and innovative ideas can emerge. Dissent and critique stimulate the development of creative ideas and quality decision making and are therefore healthy group behaviors. Leaders are busy during this phase, first facilitating the dialog and then assisting the group

to establish consensus about ideas that have been put forth. Generally, this occurs during the "storming" phase of group development. Once the group has reached consensus, it progresses to the cohesion, or "norming," stage. Leadership during this stage is focused on providing guidance and direction on an as-needed basis, thus allowing for self-management. In addition to group deviants, subgrouping, and leadership problems, a primary threat to establishing cohesion is unstable membership. Avoiding transient inconsistent membership or participation is key to achieving the level of cohesion necessary to permit self-management. *Answer 10:* **a.**

QUESTIONS

11. Members of the design team decide to eliminate the bereavement program of the adjoining hospital because it is not economically beneficial. Another APN has developed this program over the past few years and is very proud of the outcomes achieved. You are distressed by the group's recommendation that the program be eliminated. Which of the following ethical principles guides your initial actions in this case to deter the group from eliminating the bereavement program?
  a. Professional integrity
  b. Distributive justice
  c. Right to health care
  d. Autonomy

12. Based on adherence to your moral code, which of the following actions is indicated?
  a. Support the employer's efforts to reduce costs by eliminating programs that do not generate revenue
  b. Advocate for client and family needs for a bereavement program
  c. Schedule an appointment with her boss to discuss the elimination of this program and the group's lack of support
  d. Assist team members to find a compromise position that reduces team conflict

ANSWERS

11-12. Professional integrity is a fundamental value underlying ethical behavior. APNs are often asked to balance multiple obligation to patients, colleagues, employers, their profession, and self, and at times, these multiple obligations may conflict. Yeo and Ford (1991) have identified four components of the concept of professional integrity: moral autonomy, fidelity to promise, steadfastness, and wholeness. Moral autonomy is the gradual development of our own moral code, shaped by our family, church, profession, and own reflection. As we develop moral autonomy, we are guided more fully by our own moral sense, rather than being guided by others. Professional integrity also includes holding to the promises we make to our patients, our colleagues, and our own moral principles. Steadfastness obliges us to adhere to our moral code and to our promises, even when doing so involves difficulties or sacrifices. Wholeness requires us to integrate our values, principles, and ideals into all of the situations and roles in which we find ourselves. In other words, in aspiring to wholeness we avoid taking a moral stance in one situation that is actually a betrayal of the promises made in another situation or dimension of our life or professional roles. Yeo and Ford (1991) argue that moral integrity is a more fundamental value than even confidentiality, autonomy, and truthfulness.

Although the APN has an obligation to her employer, she also has an obligation to advocate for client needs, and in fact, one could argue that such advocacy is her highest professional responsibility. Assisting team members to find a compromise position that reduces team conflict might be helpful; however, it is helpful only if that compromise still preserves the best interests of patients and families. Meeting with her boss to discuss the elimination of the program removes the discussion from the group, where the final recommendation is going to be made, and further deflects the APN from her obligation to adhere to her responsibility to advocate for patient and family needs. *Answer 11:* **a.** *Answer 12:* **b.**

QUESTIONS

13. Which of the following types of leadership and power base explains the group's deference to the physician in this group?
 a. The physician is the informal leader with an expert power base.
 b. The physician is the formal leader with a legitimate power base.
 c. The physician is natural leader based on education and position.
 d. Physician leadership supersedes APN leadership based on licensure.

14. Following a brief review of the redesign project goals by yourself, discussion among team members grows negative. Team members express their disapproval of the project because it takes them away from their work and because of their mistrust in management and their disbelief in the project goals stating that "this is management's way of cutting staff positions." What

forms of power and influence are most applicable for you in this situation?
 a. *Power:* coercive; *influencing actions:* sanctioning, exchange
 b. *Power:* expert, legitimate; *influencing actions:* rationality, ingratiation
 c. *Power:* informational; *influencing actions:* assertiveness, coalition
 d. *Power:* reward, referent; *influencing actions:* upward appeal, blocking

15. Your response to the "negative talk" situation that is most likely to move the group to more productive behavior would be:
 a. "Time is evaporating. Let's move on to the first item on the agenda so we don't go over our time."
 b. "Tell me more about the concerns you are having about management's redesign plan."
 c. "Everyone seems to have concerns. Let's go around the table and get some of those ideas on the flip chart."
 d. "If you are so concerned about this, why haven't you made an appointment to talk to administration?"

ANSWERS

13. Leaders are either formal or informal. A formal leader is chosen and granted official authority to direct others, whereas an informal leader is chosen by the group based on a variety of factors, including age, seniority, expertise, and perceived position in an organization. Informal leaders are not officially sanctioned to act and can be a positive or negative influence in the group depending on the level of congruency with the organization's goals. A leader's power base and ability to influence others play a large role in her or his effectiveness. APNs find themselves involved in a spectrum of administrative activities requiring leadership every day. These activities range from overseeing the delivery of patient/family care to managing clinical and financial operations. Understanding the sources and types of power held by an individual ANP, as well as influencing actions that may be used to effect change or move an agenda forward, helps strategize for success in different situations. Five sources of power (Table 25-3) and eight influencing actions have been delineated (Douglass, 1996; Marriner-Tomey, 1996). *Answer 13:* **a.**

14. *Legitimate, reward,* and *coercive power* are granted by organizations, whereas *expert* and *referent* power arise from the personal character-

TABLE **25-3** **Forms of Leader/Manager Power**

TYPE OF POWER	DESCRIPTION	APPLICATION
Legitimate power	Accompanies the position in the organization's hierarchy; sanctioned through titles	Nurse manager has authority to hire/terminate, approve schedules, direct staff
Reward power	Derived from leader's access and ability to control/provide rewards For compliance with orders or requests; response based on desire; authorized by organization	Rewarding project leadership with promotion, praise, access to resources, etc.
Coercive power	Derived from leader's ability to use punishment/discipline for noncompliance with orders or requests; response based on fear of consequences; authorized by organization	Punishing lack of compliance with reprimand, isolation, blame, harassment behaviors
Informational power	A benefit of possessing exclusive information; overlaps with expert power	Knowledge of an appointment that has not yet been announced
Expert power	Emerges from demonstration of specialized abilities, skill, or knowledge; response based on need for information to perform	OCNS knowledgeable about new chemotherapeutic agents in phase I clinical trials
Referent power	Arises from charismatic personal style or relationship with another powerful individual	ONP in partnership with the chief of oncology is sought after to establish connection with service physician leader

Adapted from Douglass, L. M. (1996). *The effective nurse: leader and manager,* 5th ed. St Louis: Mosby; and Marriner-Tomey, A. (1996). *Guide to nursing management and leadership.* St Louis: Mosby.

istics of the individual. *Informational power* crosses both arenas, with some information being officially released to select individuals and some acquired through the personal skills of the individual. A variety of influencing actions are used in conjunction with an individual's power, depending on the situation. In the cancer services redesign scenario, the physician member of the group is rendered the informal leader based on the group's view of his expertise and position in the organization. With regard to the APN, the use of *coercive* or *reward power* sources is not an option because the APN, in a staff position, is not typically granted the authority to control those organizational resources, unless he or she is in an administrative role. However, APNs do possess *expert power* based on advanced knowledge and skills in oncology and *legitimate power* through official appointment as team leader for this project. Inappropriate influencing actions in this situation include s*anctioning* (controlling pay or benefits), because the APN is typically not granted such

power; *exchanging* favors, because the use of bribery would likely result in a failed long term outcome; and *blocking,* because threats would alienate the team being built. Because this project has been mandated by senior management, the *upward appeal* technique, in which support from a higher authority is requested, is unnecessary. In this instance, *rationality,* in which consensus is achieved through the use of a detailed plan, supporting documentation, reasoning, and logic, and *coalitioning* to encourage team members to join together and reach consensus in building their redesign plan would be appropriate actions. *Answer 14:* **b.**

15. Redirecting negativism through a coordinating approach such as using a flip chart to record each team members opinion about the project refocuses the group and turns nonproductive "gripe session" into a productive activity while simultaneously providing opportunities for controlled dialog among group members. *Answer 15:* **c.**

CASE 3 STUDY

Hospital X has gained IRB approval for and launched a new multimodality protocol in which patients with cervical cancer who are undergoing brachytherapy with cesium-137 receive simultaneous chemotherapy to potentiate radiation effects. Currently, chemotherapy administration is reserved for the oncology units where nursing staff has specialized skills and must satisfy related competencies. Brachytherapy patients requiring inpatient care are assigned to different patient care units throughout the hospital on a monthly rotational basis. This practice was adopted many years earlier because of nursing concerns regarding radiation exposure. Past attempts to concentrate brachytherapy patients to units where nursing staff have specialized oncology nursing skills have failed because of staff resistance and limited dedicated bed availability for oncology. Recently, a 21-bed medical-surgical unit was converted to surgical oncology, making available additional inpatient beds. In the absence of a plan for implementation of this new multimodal protocol, patient care problems have arisen, including treatment delays or omissions constituting protocol violations, inaccurate patient/family education, and patient/family complaints about fragmentation of care. The issue is raised by the oncology clinical nurse specialist at the cancer center operations team meeting. The specialist recommends resurrection of the proposal to concentrate brachytherapy patients on the oncology units.

QUESTIONS

1. At the outset of any project designed to introduce something new or to modify or alter an existing program, managers must recognize that change is a(n):
   a. Static event stimulated by equal driving and restraining forces
   b. Episodic negative event that should be recognized and avoided
   c. Dynamic process stimulated by unequal driving and restraining forces
   d. Episodic positive event that should be identified and encouraged

2. The change process is characterized by which of the following constructs?
   a. Preparation → initiation → exploration → termination

   b. Unfreeze → move → refreeze
   c. Antecedents → manifest behavior → conflict resolution → aftermath
   d. Input → throughput → output

3. Which of the following forces for change do you need to consider as the group plans for changes in response to the problems identified with the delivery of brachytherapy to inpatients?
   a. Marketing and public relations plan
   b. Policy/procedure and standing orders
   c. Leadership and organizational climates
   d. State legislation related to radiation handling

4. What are the first steps to be undertaken as you address the patient care issues associated with brachytherapy raised at the cancer center operations team meeting?
   a. Work with the chief physicist and nurse manager to revise the existing brachytherapy admission schedule and circulate an announcement describing the new plan
   b. Develop a patient/family education booklet with current information about brachytherapy procedures and potential side effects
   c. Convene a multidisciplinary performance improvement team that includes staff nurses from each of the oncology units to be used for brachytherapy patients
   d. Order film badges for all staff on the oncology units and offer an optional educational program regarding brachytherapy

ANSWERS

1. Change is natural and ever present in our lives. *Change* is variously defined as the process of becoming different, an adjustment in the status quo, a situation in which one thing is replaced by another, or an alteration in circumstances that results in differences or causes a transformation in how an individual or the entire organization currently acts from one set of behaviors to another. Change may be planned and systematic or unplanned and random (Douglass, 1996; Montana & Charnov, 1993). Change is closely associated with conflict. It is conflict that creates the need for change and, at the same time, can also be an effect of change. Internal and external forces drive the phenomenon of change. Lewin's force-field analysis theory postulates that when driving forces for change equal restraining forces against change, the status quo is maintained and that change occurs only when the relative strength of these two opposing forces becomes unbalanced (Newman, 1996). *Answer 1:* **c.**

2-4. Change occurs in three phases: unfreezing, moving, and refreezing. Awareness that a problem and therefore the need for change exist occurs during the *unfreezing phase.* If the group believes that change is feasible and will result in an improved circumstance, *movement* will occur. It is during this second phase in the change process that the problem is identified and described through data collection and analysis, that alternatives are explored, and that goals and objectives for planned change are developed and implemented. The refreezing phase follows and encompasses integration of the change into routine practice or operations and stabilization of the change.

The steps in the process of planned change are outlined in Figure 25-1. The APN, who responds to demands for change in the system by engaging a group consisting of those intimately familiar with the procedure or process, has a greater chance for achieving successful change because involvement

1. Nurse perceives a need for change

2. Group interaction
   a. Identify internal and external forces
   b. State the problem
   c. Identify constraints
   d. List change strategies or possible approaches to the problem
   e. Select the best change strategy or strategies
   f. Develop plan for implementation
   g. Select or develop tools for evaluation
3. Implement plan one step at a time, if possible Conduct evaluation sessions as changes are in progress

4. Evaluate overall results of the change Retain as is, alter, delete parts, or decide to discontinue the plan

Figure 25-1 The change process. (From Douglass, L. M. [1996]. *The effective nurse leader and manager,* 5th ed. St. Louis: Mosby.)

affords opportunities for unfreezing existing behavior patterns and facilitates willingness to accept new methodologies for achieving work (Jost, 2000). *Answer 2:* **b.** *Answer 3:* **c.** *Answer 4:* **c.**

QUESTIONS

5. You convene a group to address the issues raised at the operations team meeting regarding delivery of brachytherapy to the inpatient population. Which of the following techniques would be the *most* appropriate way to initiate performance improvement addressing this issue?
  a. Time and motion studies
  b. Work activity analysis
  c. Pareto diagramming
  d. Flow process analysis

6. In planning a corrective action as part of the performance improvement, which of the following is the *most* important step before implementation?
  a. Ensuring that every team member accepts the corrective action plan
  b. Establishing baseline data against which plan results can be compared
  c. Obtaining reliability and validity of the identified survey instrument
  d. Providing reassurance that job functions will not be jeopardized

ANSWERS

5-6. When problems, issues, or inefficiencies associated with the delivery of clinical care are identified, an opportunity for performance improvement is born. Understanding the problem at hand requires having detailed knowledge of existing care delivery processes. Involved parties and departments, steps in the process, pass-off points, and projected time needs versus actual time devoted overall and to each aspect in the process are all critical data points to be captured at the outset. Then and only then can the specific problematic areas be identified. Flow process analysis, or flow charting, is an effective and widely used problem identification tool that a working group can use to block out major pass-off points in a process and to systematically analyze each key step in the process identified for improvement. Often, a process is not carried out precisely in the way it is thought to work. Instead, additional steps have been built into the process because existing systems either have been poorly designed or do not work well enough to get the job done. Key steps in the flow charting technique are documenting each and every step of the process (e.g., use Post-It notes and poster board), incorporating wait times (i.e., routine and those produced by inefficiencies), and determining decision points (i.e., those points at which judgments regarding how to proceed need to be made). Once a profile of the process has been created, specific problems can be identified and a corrective action plan generated. Before implementing the plan, however, it is essential that baseline data associated with the "old way" be gathered so that the findings of follow-up monitors can be compared with the baseline, thus illustrating the level of effectiveness of the plan. *Answer 5:* **d.** *Answer 6:* **b.**

QUESTIONS

7. The corrective action plan for delivery of optimal care to patients undergoing concomitant brachytherapy and chemotherapy is to concentrate these patients on the three patient care units dedicated to oncology, where staff possess specialized skills. What is the most effective strategy for minimizing staff resistance to the new plan?

- **a.** Providing focused staff education and incrementalizing the change
- **b.** Issuing a memorandum from senior management directing the change
- **c.** Transferring staff uncomfortable with the new plan to other patient care units
- **d.** Arranging a meeting to provide staff the opportunity to express their concerns

ANSWERS

7. Change within organizations often produces conflict and resistance. People resist change because it alters the status quo, threatening that which is known to them and that which creates stability in their work world. Individuals defy change to preserve their comfort zone and often because there is an information gap. In the case of the brachytherapy scenario, the staff may be resistive because of misconceptions and fears about radiation exposures. Although it may represent the most rapid solution, having senior management mandate the change in the absence of information will merely inflame the resistance. On the other hand, dialog sessions generally prolong the process and often become nonproductive "gripe sessions." In this situation, an effective implementation plan would be to build in systematic staff education targeting information to assuage fears and to phase in the change over time to provide an opportunity for staff to develop their comfort level with the new care delivery process. *Answer 7:* **a.**

QUESTIONS

8. Your role as leader of the performance improvement team places you in an ideal position to engage in mentorship. List the seven characteristics most commonly associated with an ideal mentor.

- **a.** _____
- **b.** _____
- **c.** _____
- **d.** _____
- **e.** _____
- **f.** _____
- **g.** _____

9. List the seven roles identified as being within the scope of a mentor.

- **a.** _____
- **b.** _____
- **c.** _____
- **d.** _____
- **e.** _____
- **f.** _____
- **g.** _____

10. One of the oncology nurse members of the brachytherapy performance improvement working group has sought your recommendations for carrying out her assignment to gather staff input on the process analysis activity. In actualizing the role of mentor, which of the following would be your best response?

- **a.** "I think you can handle that on your own, don't you?"
- **b.** "Tell me what you were thinking about how to do this."
- **c.** "It's really simple. Just have your peers comment on the chart."
- **d.** "Glad you asked. Why don't I go up to the unit and do it with you."

ANSWERS

8. Qualities most commonly associated with the ideal mentor include (1) demonstrates clinical expertise and competency in patient/family care; (2) possesses high self-esteem and confidence; (3) has a deep sense of commitment and demonstrates concern for others; (4) has a high energy level; (5) is honest, reliable, and accountable for own actions; (6) leads and communicates effectively; and (7) can successfully coordinate human efforts and unit activities (Atwood, 1986). *Answer 8:* **See text.**

9. Mentor roles that have been delineated include (1) teacher/coach/trainer, (2) positive role model, (3) developer of talent, (4) door opener (ensures that opportunities are made available), (5) sponsor (provides visibility for the protégé), (6) protector, and (7) successful leader who will permit others to ride on his or her coattails (Atwood, 1986).

10. The term *mentor* is used in health care environments to describe an individual who serves as an advisor, an agent, or an experienced counselor to one who is younger and/or less experienced. Mentors generously commit their time, energy, and material support to teach, guide, assist, and inspire their protégés (Marriner-Tomey, 1996). The mentoring relationship is described as a noncompetitive nurturing connection between two individuals that promotes independence, autonomy, and self-actualization in the protégé while simultaneously fostering a sense of pride, fulfillment, and continuity, as well as a sense of being supported to grow professionally and personally (Douglass, 1996). The process of nurturing entails creating circumstances in which the protégé feels safe to attempt independent action. Often, the mentor can simply open the door for the less-experienced individual to explore his or her own ideas about how to shape a project or proceed with an activity. A pitfall for mentors is the urge to complete the project design or assignment for the protégé, thinking erroneously that this is the best way to assist. A successful mentor will hold back his or her own action and pave the way for the protégé to take the lead. *Answer 10:* **b.**

REFERENCES

Atwood, A. H. (1986). *Mentoring: a paradigm for nursing* (pp. 1-161). Los Altos, CA: NNR Publishing.

Douglass, L. M. (1996). *The effective nurse leader and manager*, 5th ed. St. Louis: Mosby.

Ferraro-McDurrie, A., Chan, J. S. L., & Jerome, A. M. (1993). Communicating the financial worth of the CNS through the use of fiscal reports. *Clin Nurse Special*, 7(2), pp. 91-97.

Genovich-Richards, J., & Cassimi, D. C. (1986). Developing nurses managerial competencies. *Nurs Mgmt*, 17(3), pp. 36-38.

Gillies, D. (1989). *Nursing management: A systems approach*, 2nd ed. Philadelphia: WB Saunders.

Hellriegel, D., & Slocum, J. (1989). *Management*, 5th ed. New York: Addison-Wesley.

Jost, S. G. (2000). An assessment and intervention strategy for managing staff needs during change. *J Nurs Admin*, 30(1), pp. 34-40.

Krumm, S. L. (1996). Administrative justification and support for advanced practice nurses. In Hamric, A. B., Spross, J. A., & Hanson, C. M. (Eds.). Advanced nursing practice: An integrative approach. Philadelphia: WB Saunders.

Marriner-Tomey, A. (1996). *Guide to nursing management and leadership*, 5th ed. St. Louis: Mosby.

Montana, P. J., & Charnov, B. H. (1993). *Management*, 2nd ed. Hauppauge, NY: Barron's Educational Series.

Newman, D. K. (1996). Program and practice management for the advanced practice nurse. In Hamric, A. B., Spross, J. A., & Hanson, C. M. (Eds.). *Advanced nursing practice: An integrative approach*. Philadelphia: WB Saunders.

Northouse, P. G., & Northouse, L. L. (1992). *Health communication: Strategies for health professionals*, 2nd ed. Norwalk, CT: Appleton and Lange.

Tuckman, B. W. (1956). Developmental sequences in small groups. *Psychol Bull*, 63(6), pp. 384-399.

Wujcik, D., & Fraser, M. C. (2000). The national cancer program. *Semin Oncol Nurs*, 16(1), pp. 65-75.

Yalom, I. D. (1975). *The theory and practice of group psychotherapy*, 2nd ed. New York: Basic Books.

Yeo, M., & Ford, A. (1991). Integrity. In Yeo, M. (Ed.). *Concepts and cases in nursing ethics*. Lewiston, NY: Broadview Press.

26 Professional Issues

Sandra A. Mitchell

CASE | STUDY

Jan Smith recently completed her master's degree and nurse practitioner (NP) requirements and is employed as a staff nurse at her local hospital while searching for an advanced practice job. One evening, she is caring for a patient in pain. She pages the resident on call to discuss changes to the patient's pain control regimen, but she does not receive a response to her page. Her patient remains in pain, so she writes the following order: Morphine 10 mg intravenously now. She signs the order: Jan Smith, NP.

QUESTIONS

1. You are the clinical nurse specialist (CNS) on the unit. Which of the following *best* captures the rationale why Jan should not be writing orders for her patients?

   1. Until she is employed as an advanced practice nurse (APN), she should not be writing orders.

   2. She does not have a specific practice protocol for ordering pain medications.

   3. Unless she is credentialed as an APN with specific privileges for ordering medications, Jan should not be writing orders.

   4. Until she receives her state license as an APN, she should not be writing orders.

   5. Until she receives her Drug Enforcement Agency (DEA) number she should not be writing orders.

   a. 1, 2, & 4

   b. 1 & 5

   c. 3 only

   d. All of these

2. Which of the following statements regarding credentialing is *not* accurate?

   a. Credentialing is the process of verifying and assessing the education, licensure, and certification of a health care practitioner to provide patient care services in or for a health care organization.

   b. Credentialing outlines the scope of service an individual practitioner can provide in

an organization and therefore also identifies the limits to his or her practice.

   c. A variety of structures, processes, and mechanisms have evolved to accomplish the goals of credentialing. Institutional structures for credentialing may include committees or specifically designated staff members or departments to whom these responsibilities are assigned.

   d. Elements of a credentialing application usually include proof of national certification, proof of education, evidence of state licensure, and summary of employment history.

ANSWERS

1-2. Unless Jan is credentialed as an APN in her institution with specific privileges for ordering medications, she is practicing outside of her scope. Licensure is the legal permission to practice within a specific scope of practice once educational requirements are met, and in some states, a national examination has been successfully completed. Receipt of a DEA number authorizes an individual to prescribe controlled substances but only when credentialed by the organization to do so. Credentialing and privileging consist of a series of activities designed to determine whether a person will be authorized to practice within a particular role within a health care organization and, if so, what specific activities the person will be authorized to perform within that setting. Jan's credentials as a registered nurse (RN) were verified by the department of nursing, and she has been granted the RN privileges identified in her RN job description. Although she has the necessary education and training as an APN, until she has been credentialed as an APN by an organization and has been granted privileges, she may not expand her scope of practice.

Privileging, not credentialing, outlines the scope of service an individual can provide and therefore defines the limits to a person's practice (Kamajian, Mitchell, & Fruth, 1999). As Hravnak, Rosenzweig, Rust, and Magdic (1998) point out in contrasting privileging and credentialing, a person may be capable by preparation, license, and practice history to perform certain tasks (credentialed); however, to provide these services to the agency's clients, they must be granted specific permission (privileged).

The elements commonly required during the credentialing process are listed in Box 26-1. It may

---

BOX 26-1 | Elements of Credentialing Application

Proof of education (transcripts and/or copies of diplomas may be required), including registered nurse (RN) education and advanced degrees

Evidence of state licensure as an RN and second licensure/certification as a nurse practitioner (if required in your state)

Drug Enforcement Agency (DEA) number, if applicable

Proof of national certification as a nurse practitioner, and in specialty field (if applicable)

Current life support certification

Summary of employment history, history of other locations at which you have held privileges

Membership in professional associations

References

Professional liability history, including proof of liability insurance

Written collaborative practice agreement between nurse practitioner and collaborating or supervising physician

Practice protocols

Privileges request form

Curriculum vitae

Photograph

Application fee (if not an employee of agency)

Proof of rubella immunity and negative tuberculosis testing

In addition to the above, you may also be required to provide information regarding the following:

Suspension or revocation of DEA license

Any physical, mental health, or chemical dependency problems that could affect ability to practice

Performance measures, including types and numbers of procedures performed, complication rates, readmissions within 30 days of prior hospitalization, clinical outcome data, and frequency of visits by diagnosis

Financial factors, including accessibility, appointment waiting times, visits per hour, and after-hours coverage arrangements

From Kamajian, M., Mitchell, S., & Fruth, R. (1999). Credentialing and privileging of advanced practice nurses. *AACN Clin Iss, 10*(3), p. 321.

---

take a significant amount of time to assemble the required elements for the first credentialing application. However, once developed, the credentialing portfolio should assist in providing the required information for each subsequent application. *Answer 1:* **c.** *Answer 2:* **b.**

QUESTIONS

3. The privileges a practitioner requests may be influenced by all of the following *except:*
   1. National standards for the nurse practitioner
   2. State nurse practice act
   3. Job description
   4. Clinical practice agreement
   5. Education, training, continuing education, and experience
   6. The APN's goal to acquire additional technical skills such as bone marrow aspirate and biopsy, skin biopsy, insertion of central venous catheters, and so on
   a. 1 & 2
   b. 1, 2, & 5
   c. All of these except 6
   d. All of these

ANSWERS

3. National standards, the state nurse practice act, the job description, and the clinical practice agreement will all shape the privileges a practitioner requests (Kamajian, Mitchell, & Fruth, 1999). Educational training, experience, and extent of supervision available in the role may also influence privilege requests. It is the practitioner's responsibility to prove that he or she has the necessary education, training, and experience to be granted the requested privileges and to prove competency in performing requested invasive procedures. Furthermore, the educational background, training, and continuing education undertaken by the APN should relate to the privileges requested. The privileges requested should be similar to those typically requested by other practitioners in the same specialty (Kinney, Hawkins, & Hudmon, 1997). The privileges requested may expand over time, based on the acquisition of additional training, evolution of clinical mastery, and an expansion in the scope of services provided by a clinical care team. APNs wishing to gain experience with the performance of an invasive procedure should first develop the necessary skills under carefully supervised practice and should have demonstrated safe performance before requesting privileges to perform the procedure. *Answer 3:* **c.**

QUESTIONS

4. Which of the following strategies would you recommend to facilitate the process of credentialing and privileging?

   a. Identify members of the credentialing committee who do not appear to understand or support the role of the APN and write them letters enclosing a copy of articles on the APN role and telling them that you are counting on their support.
   b. Submit the credentialing application as soon as you can complete it, and then send along the supporting documentation. This will allow you to assume temporary privileges immediately, rather than waiting for all of the details to be completed.
   c. Maintain a professional portfolio that includes evidence of continuing education; copies of the curriculum vitae, professional licenses, and national certifications; evidence of continuing education; peer evaluations; and patient and family comments and evaluations.
   d. Speak with staff physicians to learn what worked for them.

ANSWERS

4. Credentialing does not usually begin until all of the required supportive documents (including proof of licensure, educational transcripts, evidence of malpractice insurance, and so forth) have been assembled. Temporary practice privileges may be granted once a completed application package has been submitted to the credentialing body. Writing a letter informing someone that you are counting on his or her support may not address the need to develop that support through a discussion that allows the person with resistance to the role to share his or her concerns as well as allows the APN to provide information that is tailored to the person's concerns (Kinney, Hawkins, & Hudmon, 1997). Methods of building support may include sending a letter of introduction; asking to meet with an individual member of the committee or the chairperson; and enlisting the support of members of nursing administration, the physicians, or the departmental leader who is recruiting the APN. Although physician colleagues may be knowledgeable about the credentialing process, they may not be fully cognizant of the challenges the APN is likely to encounter in the process. Clinical organizations may be less familiar with how to manage the privilege and credentialing requests that are received from allied health care professionals.

APN colleagues can provide valuable information about their experiences with the credentialing process in a specific institution. Questions to ask that can gauge the degree of institutional support for credentialing of the APN include the following:

1. Is the application for privileges specifically tailored to reflect the qualifications of the APN and the standard applicable to their practice?
2. Have other APNs been credentialed by the organization?
3. What has been their experience with the process?
4. Is the APN role generally well understood and supported by nursing administration? by practicing physicians? by physician administration? by other groups, such as pharmacists, social workers, and physical therapists?
5. Is APN practice at the boundaries encouraged and supported, or is it feared and criticized?

Kamajian, Mitchell, and Fruth (1998) recommend that APNs develop and maintain a professional portfolio so that the necessary materials for credentialing and recredentialing are easily accessible. They recommend that that the portfolio contain documentation of participation in continuing education, committee participation, professional and community leadership activities, performance appraisals, peer evaluations, patient and family comments and evaluations, copies of progress notes, copies of specialty and national certifications, professional licenses, curriculum vitae, evidence of malpractice insurance, and DEA number. *Answer 4:* **c.**

QUESTIONS

5. Jan is seeking certification from the Oncology Nursing Society as an AOCN. All of the following are true with regard to national certification *except:*

   a. National certification in a specialty is required by all states for licensure as an APN.
   b. National certification acknowledges that a person has mastered a body of knowledge required for the practice of a particular specialty.
   c. Individual state practice acts designate whether certification is required for APN practice.

d. National certification provides the opportunity for acknowledgment by one's profession, by other health care professionals, and by patients.

5. State licensure as an APN is granted on the basis of education and, in some states, on the basis of national certification. Some states have incorporated voluntary national certification into the requirements for state recognition, thus essentially making certification equal to licensure. Individual state practice acts designate whether certification is required for APN practice (Pearson, 2000), although currently there is a trend toward the use of national certification as an APN licensing mechanism, rather than as a voluntary measure of competence. *Answer 5:* **a.**

Case Study continued

Jan has been working as an APN for about 1 year. The vice president of nursing has asked her and other APNs to establish a tool to evaluate the effectiveness of advanced nursing practice in the institution. The committee decides that monitoring of outcomes and role evaluation can be captured by three components that shape role effectiveness: (1) structure, including patient, APN, and organizational variables that influence (2) process, including what the APN does within the role components of clinician, educator, researcher, and administrator, and the way the role is enacted; and (3) outcomes, including patient and cost-related outcomes of intervention.

QUESTIONS

6. Categorize each of the following activities as either a structure (S), process (P), or outcome (O) measure.
   a. The number of workshops given for staff and the number of staff who attend each workshop
   b. Staff nurse satisfaction with the APN
   c. Peer review
   d. Improvements in patient symptom control
   e. Time spent in role components
   f. Patient education resources and critical pathways developed
   g. The number of patients seen in the clinic per hour
   h. Reduction of reasons for hospital readmission within a patient population
   i. Improvements in patient satisfaction with care

j. Reduction in the rate of hospital readmission and in the average length of stay
k. Degree to which the goals established for the APN by the organization have been met
l. Completeness and timeliness of APN documentation
m. Reduction in the incidence of chemotherapy medication errors on a unit

6. A number of authors have proposed frameworks for the evaluation of APN practice (Kleinpell-Nowell & Weiner, 1999; Shah & Sullivan, 1998; Sidani & Irvine, 1999). Although each of these evaluation frameworks varies somewhat in its definition and grouping of variables, most are based on a consideration of structure, process, and outcome variables. Structure variables consist of APN, patient, staff, and organization variables that influence the processes and outcomes of care. Process variables include how the APN role is implemented or performed, including both the technical and human aspects of care and service provision. Structure and process variables can be examined independently of outcomes to describe what the APN does in fulfilling his or her clinical, educational, administrative, consultative, and research roles. Outcomes evaluation involves the measurement of the effects of the APN role on patients. These outcomes may be clinical, functional, perceptual, or financial (Shah & Sullivan, 1998). The selection of outcome measures for APNs is challenging because traditional medical outcomes may not adequately capture the full contributions of advanced practice nursing care (Kleinpell-Nowell & Weiner, 1999). Because patient care is multidisciplinary, it is difficult to establish the true effect of advanced practice nursing in isolation. Evaluation of several dimensions of APN functioning, including structure, process, and outcome variables, may be needed to establish the impact of the APN's role. *Answer 6:* **a: S; b: P; c: P; d: O; e: S; f: P; g: S; h: P; i: O; j: O; k: P; l: P; m: O.**

QUESTIONS

7. One of Jan's APN colleagues is asked to chair a unit-based committee seeking to improve the provision of patient education. This is an example of:
   a. Consultative role
   b. Educator role
   c. Development of a critical pathway
   d. Continuous quality improvement or process improvement

7. As the chair of the committee, the APN has moved out of the consultant role and is now responsible for the effectiveness and outcomes of the committee. Continuous quality improvement, sometimes also called *process improvement,* is a formal program that attempts to improve the delivery of care by identifying a problem or issue, collecting sufficient data to accurately diagnose the problem, planning a change to address the problem, and then monitoring the change process to ensure that it is having the desired effect. A critical pathway contains key patient care activities and the time frames for those activities for a specific type of patient problem; it is therefore a blueprint for the delivery of care by all disciplines. *Answer 7:* **d.**

QUESTIONS

8. You are asked to consult on a patient with severe uncontrolled pain who the staff believe may also be involved in "drug-seeking behavior." The patient perceives that the staff is controlling how much medication he receives. Which of the following would *not* be a component of the consultant role?

   a. Assessing the patient's level of pain and writing orders for appropriate pain management strategies
   b. Clarifying with the staff their responsibilities and the responsibility of the APN in the consultation
   c. Gathering more data from the staff and patient regarding perception of the problem
   d. Sharing alternative perspectives on the problem and proposing possible solutions for effective pain management

8. Assessing the patient's level of pain and then writing orders for pain management would be an example of comanagement or collaboration with the staff in solving the problem rather than consultation. *Answer 8:* **a.**

QUESTIONS

9. All of the following may be helpful strategies in resolving territoriality between nurse colleagues or members of other health disciplines *except:*

   a. Firmly defining the role components and intervention approaches that are within the exclusive purview of each discipline

   b. Acknowledging that a certain amount of duplication and overlap will exist, while at the same time opening up an ongoing dialog about shared and distinct areas of responsibility
   c. Providing opportunities for shared practice and educational activities that enhance mutual understanding
   d. Engaging a resistant or threatened colleague as a partner on clinical projects, soliciting his or her advice and involvement

10. Collaboration among all providers is necessary for success of APNs in oncology. Which of the following *best* demonstrates a dimension of a collaborative practice model?

   a. In an effective collaborative practice, for a significant number of functions, one team member or type of provider should be able to substitute for another member of the team.
   b. The APN and physician both assess the patient and jointly implement and evaluate a plan of care for a specialty population.
   c. Shared decision making leading to better patient care tends to occur when all team members clearly define for themselves those pieces of care provision that they are uniquely trained to provide.
   d. The APN's role and scope of practice is determined based on the preferences, needs, and practice patterns of the collaborating physician.

9-10. With territoriality, the focus on the patient has been displaced, and the professionals and their perceptions of their role, knowledge base, or authority become the focal point of care. The process of resolving territoriality needs to acknowledge that a certain amount of duplication and overlap will exist, and the APN should provide opportunities for the development of a common purpose, recognition of divergent and complementary skills and contributions, and effective communication. Territoriality may actually be increased if one attempts to artificially define which role components or intervention approaches are the exclusive responsibility or expertise of any one discipline or role. Successful professional collaboration requires work, practice, and patience; however, at the same time, it reduces redundancy, enhances continuity, and contributes to the elimination of fragmentation in patient care (King & Baggs, 1998).

Baggs (1994) defined six critical elements for effective collaborative practice: trust, cooperation, assertiveness, shared decision making, communication, and coordination. Central to a collaborative practice model are the tenets that patient needs are the foremost priority in the provision of care (DeAngelis, 1994) and that patients require the abilities and expertise of different types of providers simultaneously during each encounter or hospital admission (King, Parrinello, & Baggs, 1995). It therefore follows that if an optimal outcome is to be achieved, one type of provider cannot substitute for the unique functions of another member of the team. However, simply defining pieces of care provision that individual team members are uniquely trained to provide is not consistent with a focus on the needs of the patient and does not contribute to coordination of care, cooperation, or shared decision making. In a successful collaborative practice, medical and nursing care plans for an individual patient are developed, implemented, and evaluated in a coordinated fashion, resulting in continuous, consistent, highest-quality care. By defining the APN's role and scope of practice solely based on the preferences, needs, and practice patterns of the collaborating physician, there is a risk that the APN role is seen as subordinate rather than as a true complementary partner. Such a stance has the disadvantage that the APN's scope of practice is defined only as that part that is a subset of the attending physician's scope (King & Baggs, 1998). With this approach, the unique and independent functions of the APN that contribute to patient outcomes may be minimized. In addition, this approach inadvertently supports the notion that physicians own the entire domain of health care and thus retain the right to apportion parts of care and tasks to fit their needs (King & Baggs, 1998). *Answer 9:* **a.** *Answer 10:* **b.**

REFERENCES

Baggs, J. G. (1994). Development of an instrument to measure collaboration and satisfaction about care decisions. *J Adv Nurs, 20,* pp. 176-182.

DeAngelis, C. D. (1994). Nurse practitioner redux. *JAMA, 271,* pp. 868-871.

Hravnak, M., Rosenzweig, M. Q., Rust, D., & Magdic, K. (1998). Scope of practice, credentialing and privileging. In Kleinpell, R. M., & Piano, M. R. (Eds.). *Practice issues for the acute care nurse practitioner* (pp. 41-65). New York: Springer.

Kamajian, M., Mitchell, S. A., & Fruth, R. (1999). Credentialing and privileging of advanced practice nurses. *AACN Clin Iss, 10*(3), pp. 316-336.

King, K., & Baggs, J. (1998). Collaboration: The essence of acute care nurse practitioner practice (p. 67-78). In Kleinpell, R. M., & Piano, M. R. (Eds.). *Practice issues for the acute care nurse practitioner* (pp. 67-78). New York: Springer.

Kinney, A., Hawkins, R., & Hudmon, K. S. (1997). A descriptive study of the role of the oncology nursing practitioner. *Oncol Nurs Forum, 24*(5), pp. 811-820.

Kleinpell-Nowell, R., & Weiner, T. M. (1999). Measuring advanced practice nursing outcomes. *AACN Clin Iss, 10*(3), pp. 356-368.

Pearson, L. J. (2000). Annual legislative update: How each state stands on legislative issues affecting advanced nursing practice. *Nurse Pract, 25*(1), pp. 16-68.

Shah, H. S., & Sullivan D. T. (1998). Evaluation of the acute care nurse practitioner's role. In Kleinpell, R. M., & Piano, M. R. (Eds.). *Practice issues for the acute care nurse practitioner* (pp. 111-143). New York: Springer.

Sidani, S., & Irvine, D. (1999). A conceptual framework for evaluating the nurse practitioner role in acute care settings. *J Adv Nurs, 30*(1), pp. 58-66.

27 Documentation of Service

Sandra A. Mitchell

CASE | STUDY

1. What are three reasons why documentation of advance practice nurse (APN) services is important?

    a. _____

    b. _____

    c. _____

ANSWERS

1. Quality documentation of APN services is important for at least five reasons. First, APN documentation of assessment and intervention with patients helps ensure coordination of care and achievement of desired clinical outcomes. Second, APN documentation reflects the value APNs bring to practice, especially focusing on comprehensive evaluation and holistic intervention. Third, quality APN documentation contributes to an image of the APN as a knowledgeable and effective member of the care team and reinforces the visibility of the APN role. Fourth, our participation in receiving direct reimbursement for our services requires that our documentation meet certain quality standards. Fifth, documentation allows appropriate utilization review and quality of care evaluation, as well as the collection of data that may be useful for research and education.

Components of APN documentation include history and physical examination, progress notes, consultations, discharge summaries, orders, and prescriptions. *Answer 1:* **See text.**

History and Physical

See Box 27-1.

QUESTIONS

2. In what way or ways should the progress note in Box 27-1 be improved?
1. Include a description of the findings of psychosocial assessment
2. Include a review of systems documenting positives and relevant negatives
3. Include an assessment or impression of the evaluation along with the plan
4. Document the plan only when all of the necessary data have been obtained
5. Avoid intermingling review of systems, physical examination, and laboratory data
    a. 1, 2, 4, & 5
    b. 1, 3, & 5
    c. 1, 2, 3, & 5
    d. All of these

3. Which of the following statements regarding documentation of the history and physical is *inaccurate*?
    a. The objective data are those that are measured in laboratory tests and diagnostic studies.
    b. The subjective data are those that are observed by the examiner.
    c. The review of systems includes information about the patient's subjective symptoms.
    d. For each impression or assessment of an abnormality documented, there should also be an identified plan.

BOX **27-1** | **Progress Note: John Doe**

John is admitted today for cycle 2 of consolidation chemotherapy in treatment of his AML. On examination, laboratory results are within normal limits, and he denies fever or chills, his lungs are clear, and heart rate is regular. He indicates that his energy level and appetite have been very good. The skin is without rashes, bruising, or petechiae. Vital signs are as follows: T: 37° C; pulse: 88 beats/min; respirations: 22 breaths/min; blood pressure: 130/77 mm Hg.

Plan: Proceed with chemotherapy if CBC normal.

AML, Acute myoblastic leukemia; *CBC,* complete blood count.

4. Match the following statements to the section of the history and physical examination where they should be placed:

- **a.** Female patient is seen in clinic today for continuing follow-up of her stage IIIB multiple myeloma; she is now status post two cycles of chemotherapy.
- **b.** Patient is married with two children. He works as a professor at the local community college. He drinks 1 to 2 drinks per week and is a nonsmoker. He denies a history of recreational drug use. He has no history of occupational exposure to chemicals or ionizing radiation.
- **c.** Patient denies fever, chills, cough, shortness of breath, dyspnea, and chest pain. He has no hemoptysis or sputum.
- **d.** Lungs clear to auscultation and percussion anteriorly and posteriorly. No wheezing, rales, or rhonchi.
- **e.** Pulmonary functions tests reveal an FEV_1 of 88%, forced vital capacity (FVC)/FEV of 76%, and a DLco of 61%.

1. Family history
2. Social history
3. Review of systems
4. Chief complaint
5. History of present illness
6. Review of systems: pulmonary
7. Physical examination: lungs
8. Laboratory and diagnostic test results
9. Assessment and plan

f. Afebrile, nonneutropenic male patient continuing on treatment of *Staphylococcus epidermidis* bacteremia with vancomycin 1 g intravenously every 12 hours. He will complete a 14-day course of therapy on March 5, 2002.

ANSWERS

2-4. The comprehensive history and physical examination may be completed using a standardized written institutional form or may be dictated. The components of the history and physical examination, however, remain the same. An outline of the history and physical examination format is given in Box 27-2.

Whatever format is used, organization and clarity are essential. The subjective data are those that the patient describes, whereas the objective data are those that are observed by the examiner, including the physical examination and laboratory and diagnostic tests. The review of systems includes information about the patient's subjective symptoms. The review of systems should also indicate whether any new symptoms or issues have developed since the previous patient encounter.

The findings of interim evaluations and clinic visits, as well as daily hospital visits, can be documented in a progress note. The progress notes document the pertinent findings, plan of care, and patient's progress; in addition, they serve as documentation of the history, examination, and complexity of medical decision making performed during the patient encounter. These elements—history, examination, and medical decision–making—are taken together in determining the level of service provided during the visit and thus the level at which the visit may be billed (Buppert, 1999). Progress notes may follow SOAP format, with the subjective being provided as a review of systems, objective findings the physical examination, laboratory and diagnostic tests, and the assessment and plan. In organizing your presentation of the plan, it may be helpful to express aspects of the plan that relate directly to the assessment and management of the disease itself, followed by an assessment and plan in relationship to organ systems and/or the high incidence problem areas in oncology, such as hematology, infection, fluids, electrolytes and nutrition, gastrointestinal system, dermatologic system, neurologic comfort, and rehabilitation. An example of a detailed progress note, with an assessment and plan, is given in Figure 27-2 at the end of the chapter.

BOX 27-2 | Outline Format of History and Physical Examination

Patient: Date of Admission/Service:
Age: Dictating Provider:

Current Complaint: history character, location, onset, radiation, intensity, duration, associated events, palliative and provocative factors

History of Present Illness: symptoms at presentation, disease stage, pathology, and metastatic evaluation at presentation; initial treatment(s), including agents, number of cycles, dosages, date of relapse/progression, salvage treatment(s)

Medical History: arthritis, asthma, blood diseases, bronchitis, cancer, diabetes, emphysema, epilepsy, infections, gout, hepatitis, heart disease, hypertension, liver disease, pneumonia, rheumatic fever, seizures, thyroid disease, ulcers

Surgical History:

Injuries:

Family History:

Family Cancer History:

Social History: where and with whom patient lives; occupation; history of cigarette, alcohol, over-the-counter medications, recreational drug use; occupational exposures; military history; travel outside North America

Allergies:

Current Medications:

REVIEW OF SYSTEMS

General: changes in weight, appetite, sleep, mood

HEENT: headache, blurred vision, diplopia, photophobia or vision changes; changes in auditory acuity, pain, discharge; sinus pain, pressure, drainage, epistaxis; oral cavity pain or lesions; sore throat, odynophagia, dysphagia; neck pain or stiffness; neck masses

Respiratory: cough, sputum, shortness of breath, dyspnea, inspiratory chest pain, hemoptysis, tachypnea

Cardiovascular: chest pain, palpitations, cyanosis, dizziness, exertional dyspnea, hypertension, palpitations, peripheral edema

Gastrointestinal: constipation, diarrhea, abdominal pain, change in quality of stools, hematemesis, hematochezia, hemorrhoids, rectal pain, indigestion, nausea, vomiting

Genitourinary: dysuria, hematuria, nocturia, frequency, hesitancy, incontinence, discharge, rhinolithiasis

Gynecologic: bleeding, discharge, dyspareunia

Breasts: nipple discharge, pain tenderness

Neuromuscular: anesthesias, paresthesias, arthralgias, myalgias, syncope, weakness, vertigo, limitations in range of motion, back pain, joint swelling

Skin: rashes, bruising, dryness, lesions/sores

Lymph/Heme: anemia, bleeding tendency, easy bruising, lymphadenopathy

Psychologic: altered mood, sleep disturbances, anxiety, depression, drug or alcohol problems

PHYSICAL EXAMINATION

Vital signs, pulse oximetry, weight, performance status

General: general appearance (pale, cachectic, frail), alopecia, well nourished, alertness, cooperation, level of distress

Head: atraumatic, normocephalic, symmetric and without deformities

Eyes: PERRLA, EOMI bilaterally; no conjunctival injection, ptosis, or scleral icterus; fundoscopic examination reveals no AV nicking, papilledema, retinal hemorrhages, or retinopathy

Ears: external ear examination reveals no abnormalities, external ear canals patent, TM intact with normal cone of light and no erythema

Mouth/Throat: gums pink and without bleeding, open lesions, mucosa moist, condition of teeth, pharyngeal or tonsillar hyperemia or exudates

Neck: carotid pulses equal and adequate bilaterally with no bruits auscultated; trachea midline, no JVD, thyroid not enlarged; no cervical, supraclavicular lymphadenopathy; no nuchal rigidity

Lungs: clear to auscultation and percussion; without wheezing, rales, rhonchi respirations normal/labored with good chest motion; tactile and vocal fremitus are equal in all areas

Heart: regular rate and rhythm without murmurs, clicks, gallop, rub or extra heart sounds; PMI is at fifth intercostal space, midclavicular line

Breast: normal symmetry, no discrete masses, scars, nipple discharge, dimpling, introversion or tenderness noted; no axillary lymphadenopathy

Abdomen: soft, rounded (flat, obese), nontender; no masses, organomegaly, or rebound tenderness; scars noted; active bowel sounds noted in all four quadrants; no pulsations, bruits or flank pain noted

Extremities: no clubbing, cyanosis edema, or varicosities noted; pulses equal and adequate; no cutaneous temperature difference bilaterally; strength 5+ and equal bilaterally in upper and lower extremities

Neurologic: oriented ×3, deep tendon reflexes equal and adequate in upper and lower extremities; good grip strength noted bilaterally, no involuntary movements, no tremor; sensation is intact to pain and light touch; cerebellar function intact with finger to nose, heel to shin and normal rapid alternating movements and with a normal gait; cranial nerves II-XII intact; Babinski reflex is downgoing

Genitalia: normal, no discharge, inflammation, or evidence of infection

Rectal: no masses, polyps, hemorrhoids palpated; sphincter tone adequate; hemoccult; prostate has no nodules and tenderness or enlargement

Skin: texture, rigor, pigmentation appear normal; no rashes, cyanosis, or petechiae; normal hair pattern for sex and age

Laboratory Data:

Radiologic/Diagnostic Testing Data:

Impression/Plan:

Several areas for improvement can be identified from the brief note presented in question 2. First, even a brief note must include a review of systems that documents positives and relevant negatives. To enhance brevity, it may be helpful to use the statement "review of remaining systems is negative" to indicate that a comprehensive review of systems was performed during the examination. In addition, even a brief note should include some assessment of the psychosocial dimension, whether that is mood, coping, or current concerns. It is not necessary to wait to document the plan until all data have been obtained; however, it is important to include a summary assessment or impression along with the plan. In the preceding example, that summary impression and plan could be stated as follows: Patient tolerating consolidation therapy well. No new problems on interval history, review of systems, and physical examination. Will review complete blood count if within normal limits, will proceed with cycle 2 of consolidation chemotherapy. *Answer 2:* **c.** *Answer 3:* **b.** *Answer 4:* **a: 4; b: 2; c: 6; d: 7; e: 8; f: 9.**

QUESTIONS

5. All of the following statements regarding procedure notes is true *except:*

   a. APNs do not need to prepare procedure notes unless they are performing surgical procedures such as chest tube insertion, first assist in the operating room, and so on.

   b. For billing purposes, a note summarizing the procedure performed should be prepared when the provider performs any invasive or diagnostic procedure.

   c. Procedure notes are necessary both to ensure quality care and to meet the requirements for reimbursement.

   d. In the event of an adverse occurrence, procedure notes are necessary to document care provided.

ANSWERS

5. A note summarizing the procedure performed should be prepared when the provider performs any invasive or diagnostic procedure, whether in the clinic, on the inpatient unit, or in the operating room. Procedure notes are needed both to ensure quality of care and to meet the requirements for reimbursement. In addition, in the event of an adverse occurrence, procedure notes provide evidence that a standard of care was followed in performing the procedure or in monitoring the patient after the procedure. An example of a procedure note is given in Box 27-3. *Answer 5:* **a.**

> BOX **27-3** | **Sample Procedure Note**
>
> Procedure: Bone marrow aspirate and biopsy
> Date of Procedure: March 6, 2002
> Indication for Procedure: Reevaluate disease status following 2 cycles of VAD chemotherapy
> After obtaining informed consent and administering premedication of Ativan 1 mg IV and morphine 10 mg IV, the patient was placed in the prone position. The left posterior iliac crest was prepped and draped in an aseptic fashion. Using 2% lidocaine, I administered subcutaneous anesthesia and infiltrated up to the level of the periosteum.
> The posterior iliac crest was accessed, and bone marrow aspiration was performed. The samples were sent for hematopathologic review FISH, flow, cytogenetics, and molecular diagnostics. Following aspiration, a biopsy of the left posterior iliac crest was obtained, with samples sent for routine hematopathologic review.
> A sterile pressure dressing was applied to the left posterior iliac crest, and the patient was observed in the clinic for 45 minutes after the procedure. He tolerated the procedure well, without excessive pain or bleeding. Postprocedure self-care instructions were provided to the patient.
> *Jane R. Doe, CRNP, AOCN*

QUESTIONS

6. What is the *major* format difference between a consultation note and a progress note?

   a. A consultation note and a progress note follow an identical format.

   b. A consultation note should document only suggestions or recommendations.

   c. A consultation note is focused only on the problem for which help is being sought.

   d. A consultation note should follow the same SOAP format as progress notes but should include recommendations rather than a plan.

ANSWERS

6. Consultation notes may be somewhat more limited in scope than a comprehensive progress note because consultants are usually involved in evaluating one or two focused patient problems, such as pain, nutritional issues, psychosocial concerns, or rehabilitation needs. Consultations can follow the same SOAP format as progress notes; however, because consultants usually do not take over the responsibility for care, they make suggestions or recommendations rather than a plan.

BOX **27-4**   **Consultation Note**

Mrs. Brown is seen in consultation at the request of the team regarding pain control options for her postherpetic neuralgia.

She is a 71-year-old with relapsed stage IIIB multiple myeloma currently receiving salvage therapy with thalidomide. She developed an outbreak of herpes zoster in the right T1-T4 dermatome approximately 3 months ago. Although the lesions resolved nicely with intravenous acyclovir, she has been left with residual pain in the area.

She describes the pain as shooting and stabbing in quality, radiating across the axilla and the inner aspect of her upper arm. She rates the pain as a 5 on a 0-10 scale and indicates that it interferes with sleep and mental concentration. In addition, she has extreme and painful sensitivity to light touch in the area of dermatomal involvement, and this can make it painful to wear other than extremely loose clothing. Whereas she felt better able to cope with the pain a few weeks ago, the news of her disease relapse has made this more difficult for her, and she reports feeling depressed and tearful, particularly at night. She denies suicidal thoughts. She denies changes in appetite but does note that her energy level has declined significantly over the past 3 months. She has good family support from her daughter and son-in-law, who live close to her home.

LIMITED PHYSICAL EXAMINATION

Lymph: right supraclavicular and axillary regions are without lymphadenopathy.

Skin: without rashes, bruising, or petechiae; painful hyperesthesia of the skin in the right T1-T4 dermatome

Musculoskeletal: range of motion of the right upper extremity without pain or deficit

CURRENT MEDICATIONS

Elavil 25 mg PO qhs, oxycodone 5-10 mg PO q4h prn for pain, thalidomide 300 mg PO qd

ASSESSMENT AND RECOMMENDATIONS

Postherpetic neuralgia, uncontrolled by antidepressants and opioids. The patient has painful skin hyperesthesia in the previously involved dermatome as well as residual neuralgia. All lesions are well healed. In the setting of relapsed disease, her risk of recurrence of zoster is high. Suggest consideration to restart preemptive/prophylactic coverage with famciclovir, valacyclovir, or acyclovir. Suggest EMLA cream to skin for hyperesthesia and gabapentin 300 mg PO tid for postherpetic neuralgia. If tolerated, within 5 days I would begin escalating gabapentin dose by 100 mg tid every 5 days to a maximum daily dose of 1800 mg tid. Would suggest having physical therapy see the patient regarding TENS. Referral to psychooncology team for supportive psychotherapy for depression is also recommended.

I appreciate the opportunity to participate in the care of this patient and will continue to follow her with you.

Jane Doe, CRNP, AOCN
Nurse Consultant, Pain Control Team

Nevertheless, the relevant subjective and objective data, as well as the impression, should be included, along with the recommendations of the consultant. A sample consult note for pain control is given in Box 27-4. *Answer 6:* **d.**

QUESTIONS

7. Which of the following *best* describes the purpose of the discharge summary?
   a. The discharge summary lists all of the events of the patient's hospitalization.
   b. A discharge summary is a legal requirement for all hospitalizations.
   c. The discharge summary summarizes the events of the hospitalization and contributes to continuity of care, smooth transitions from one care setting to another, and coordination of postdischarge follow-up.
   d. The discharge summary justifies the need for hospital admission to third-party payers.

ANSWERS

7. The discharge summary summarizes the events of the patient's hospitalization. Justification of the need for hospitalization to third-party payers is a separate process from the discharge summary. If the patient has been hospitalized for more than 48 hours or if the patient's hospitalization has been complicated, a dictated summary is generally required. The discharge summary should be written in narrative format, but it does not need to list all of the events of a patient's hospitalization. The discharge summary is important not only because it is a legal requirement of all hospitalizations but also because it can contribute to continuity of patient care, facilitate a smooth transition of care from the inpatient to the outpatient setting or from the hospital to another care setting such as hospice or long-term care, and ensure coordination of postdischarge follow-up. *Answer 7:* **c.**

BOX 27-5 | **Components of the Discharge Summary**

The discharge summary should contain the following elements:
- Patient name and medical record number
- Admission and discharge dates
- Discharge diagnoses, including active and resolved problems
- Procedures/major diagnostics tests/ operations performed during admission
- Transfusion
- Consultations
- Discharge medications
- History of present illness, concluding with the reason for admission
- Review of systems of the day of discharge
- Physical examination on the day of discharge
- Laboratory tests on the day of discharge
- Summary of results of major diagnostic tests, including any positive culture results
- Summary of course of hospitalization
- Plans for follow-up
- Discharge instructions

QUESTIONS

8. All of the following are components of the discharge summary *except:*
- **a.** Medications on admission
- **b.** Discharge diagnosis or diagnoses
- **c.** Discharge medications
- **d.** Discharge instructions and plans for follow-up

ANSWERS

8. The components of the discharge summary are given in Box 27-5. A sample discharge summary is given in Figure 27-1 at the end of the chapter. *Answer 8:* **a.**

Case Study continued

The state nurse practice act, delineation of privileges, and the clinical practice agreement guide the APN when writing orders and prescriptions. All prescriptions require the date; the patient's name and address; and the provider's phone number, license number, DEA number, and signature. The prescription or medication order is traditionally written in Latin (Logan, 1999), and the name of the medication, strength, and administration instructions must all be writ-

ten. Outpatient prescriptions should also include the quantity to be dispensed and whether there are to be any refills. Legible handwriting and the avoidance of shortcuts or abbreviations that are not accepted or uncommon should be avoided.

QUESTIONS

9. Review the following orders or prescriptions, and identify the missing or problematic elements.
- **a.** Tobramycin (2.5 mg/kg) 300 mg IV
- **b.** Neupogen
  Sig: One vial SC qd
  Dispense: 14
- **c.** Insulin
  Sig: 10U SC ac meals
  Dispense: 4 vials
- **d.** Compazine 10 mg
  Sig: 10 mg q6h prn for nausea
  Dispense: 200
  Refills: Three
- **e.** Klor-Con 10 mEq
  Sig: Take 20 mEq PO qd for 1 month
  Dispense: 30
- **f.** Ativan .5 mg
  Sig: .5 mg PO qhs prn for sleep
  Refills: Three

ANSWERS

Answer 9: **a: No interval for administration is specified. b: No strength for the vial of Neupogen is specified. Therefore the expected dose is unknown. Neupogen is available in vials containing either 480 μg or 300 μg. c: The type of insulin (e.g., regular Humulin, NPH) is not specified. Also, the "10U" could be misread as "100." The word** units **should be written out. d: The route for administration is not specified (e.g., PO, PR, IV). e: The number of doses to be dispensed is less than a 1-month's supply because the patient will need to take 2 tablets per day to achieve a daily intake of 20 mEq. In addition, the qd could be mistaken for qid. It would be better to state "daily." f: A tenfold overdose could occur if the decimal point is not seen. If the dose is less than 1, a zero should precede the decimal point. In addition the number to be dispensed is not provided. Refills cannot be prescribed for controlled substances.**

QUESTIONS

10. Review the admission orders written in Box 27-6 for a patient admitted for febrile

BOX **27-6** | **Admission Order**

Admit to 6C, Oncology Unit, Attending Physician: Dr. John Smith
Diagnosis:
 Recurrent non-Hodgkin's lymphoma—large cell
 Day +9 following cycle 2 of ESHAP chemotherapy
Condition: stable
Activity as tolerated
Diet: low-microbial diet
Isolation: neutropenic precautions
Medications:
 Imipenem 500 mg IV q6h
 Vancomycin 1 g IV q12h
 Compazine 10 mg IV/PO q6h prn for nausea
 Klor-Con 20 mEq PO tid
 Neupogen 480 μg SC qd
Chest radiograph on admission
Access Mediport for vascular access; dressing change to accessed Mediport as per University Hospital policy
Notify MD/APN for temperature >38° C, pulse >120 or <60 beats/min, respirations >30 or <12 breaths/min, systolic blood pressure >160 or <90 mm Hg, diastolic blood pressure >90 or <50 mm Hg, pulse oximetry <92%

BOX **27-7** | **Admission and Transfer Orders**

Usual categories for admission or transfer orders include the following:
- Admit/transfer: floor, room, service, attending
- Diagnoses: list in order of priority
- Condition: good, fair, guarded, critical
- Allergies
- Vital signs and pulse oximetry: every shift, q4h
- Diet
- Activity level
- Isolation
- Intake and output every shift
- Daily weight
- Medications: antibiotics, antiemetics, pain medications, insulin, bedtime sedation, electrolyte supplementation
- Intravenous fluids
- Transfusion support
- Laboratory tests on admission
- Diagnostic tests and consultations on admission
- Daily/routine laboratory tests
- Dressing care
- Vascular access care instructions
- Respiratory care: suctioning, oxygen
- Notify instructions: Notify MD/APN for temperature >100.5° F or 38.2° C, pulse >120 or <60 beats/min, respirations >30 or <12 breaths/min, systolic blood pressure >160 or <90 mm Hg, diastolic blood pressure >90 or <50 mm Hg, pulse oximetry <92%

neutropenia and identify five or more elements that were not included:

a. _____
b. _____
c. _____
d. _____
e. _____

——————————————————— **ANSWERS**

10. Admission/transfer orders have a number of standardized elements to ensure that the care provided is organized and delivered to achieve the goals of the hospital admission. The following elements are missing from the above order set:
- Admission diagnosis of febrile neutropenia
- Allergies
- Hydration/IV fluids
- Frequency for monitoring vital signs
- Intake and output

- Laboratory studies to be obtained on admission and daily

The usual elements to be included in admission or transfer orders are summarized in Box 27-7. *Answer 10:* **See text.**

REFERENCES

Buppert, C. (1999). *Nurse practitioner's business practice and legal guide.* Gaithersburg, MD: Aspen.
Logan, P. (1999). Principles of practice for the acute care nurse practitioner. Stamford, CT: Appleton and Lange.

Discharge Summary

Kline, Amelia
MR #3456789
Date of Admission: May 13, 2002
Date of Discharge: May 15, 2002

Discharge Diagnoses:
1. Status post consolidation chemotherapy, cycle 2 with Taxol and cisplatin
2. Stage IIIB kappa multiple myeloma, diagnosed in January 2001
3. Status post autologous peripheral blood stem cell transplantation on 9/10/01, following conditioning chemotherapy with BCNU 300 mg/m^2 and Melphalan 140 mg/m^2
4. Steroid-induced hyperglycemia, resolving
5. Postherpetic neuralgia
6. History of herpes zoster reactivation
7. Depression
8. Anemia
9. Osteolytic bone lesions of the skull, bilateral humeri, and iliac bones
10. Hypokalemia
11. History of renal insufficiency

Procedures: Chemotherapy Administration 5/13/01-5/15/01

Consultations: None

Transfusions: None

Discharge Medications: Levaquin 500 mg PO qd, Diflucan 400 mg PO qd, Famvir 500 mg PO tid, Klor-Con 20 mEq PO bid, Neurontin 900 mg PO tid, nortriptyline 100 mg PO qhs, folic acid 1 mg PO qd, Multivites without iron 1 tab PO qd, Axid 150 mg PO bid

HISTORY OF PRESENT ILLNESS; ALLERGIES; PAST MEDICAL, FAMILY, AND SOCIAL HISTORY; AND CURRENT MEDICATIONS: Remain the same as documented by Dr. Smith in his admission note of 5/13/01.

Review of Systems: On the day of discharge, the patient denied fevers, chills, cough, shortness of breath, dyspnea, or chest pain. She has had no nausea, vomiting, or diarrhea. Her appetite remains good, and her energy level is also quite good. Her mood is upbeat. She continues with some pain in her left buttock and the thigh, which is residual to her recent outbreak of herpes zoster. She continues with fairly severe postherpetic neuralgia requiring Neurontin and Elavil for pain control. Review of remaining systems is negative.

Physical Examination: Temperature 36.6° C, pulse 98 beats/min, respirations 20 breaths/min, blood pressure 127/53 mm Hg, pulse oximetry 98% on room air, weight 69.2 kg, performance status 80%-90%. HEENT: Pupils are equal, round, and reactive to light bilaterally; extraocular movements intact; sclerae and conjunctivae are clear bilaterally. Oral cavity is smooth, moist, pink, and without open lesions. The neck is supple and without adenopathy. The dentition is in good repair. The lungs are clear to auscultation and percussion; no wheezing, rales, or rhonchi. Cardiac S_1, S_2, regular rhythm; no murmur, rub, or gallop. Mediport is in situ in the left chest; the pocket is without erythema or tenderness. Abdomen is soft, flat, nontender, with positive bowel sounds ×4 quadrants; there is no organomegaly. Neurologic: Alert and oriented ×3; there is no focal neurologic deficit. Extremities/musculoskeletal: Range of motion without pain or deficit; there is no clubbing, cyanosis, or edema. Skin has healing lesions consistent with recent herpes zoster reactivation noted over the left sciatic region; there are no new active skin lesions noted. There is no bruising and no petechiae noted. Psychologic: The patient is in good spirits.

Laboratory Data: WBC count of 2.4 with 74% granulocytes, hemoglobin 9.3, hematocrit 25.7, platelets 37,000/mm^3. Sodium 142, potassium 3.3, chloride 112, CO_2 21, glucose 207, BUN 20, creatinine 1.4, calcium 7.3, phosphorus 4.6, magnesium 2.5, total protein 4.6, albumin 2.3, alkaline phosphatase 108, AST 30, ALT 101, total bilirubin 0.7, LDH 560.

Hospital Course: The patient was admitted and began intravenous hydration at 125 ml/hr. After premedication with Benadryl 50 mg IV, dexamethasone 40 mg IV, and Zantac 50 mg IV, Taxol 135 mg/m^2 was administered over 6 hours intravenously. Cisplatin 75 mg/m^2 was then commenced as a continuous intravenous infusion over 24 hours. Dexamethasone and Kytril were used to achieve antiemesis.

The patient tolerated the chemotherapy well, without problems such as nausea, vomiting, or significant fluid or electrolyte imbalance. She did experience mild steroid-induced hyperglycemia, which was resolving at the time of her discharge. Her BUN and creatinine remained stable throughout her hospitalization.

On the day of discharge, the patient was feeling well, and she was subsequently discharged home accompanied by her husband. She will begin therapy with Neupogen 480 µg/day subcutaneously to begin on 5/16/01.

Follow-Up Plans: The patient will return to oncology clinic on 5/20/01 for labs and reevaluation. She will have interim counts and chemistries evaluated at her local laboratory on 5/17/01 with results faxed to our office. The patient is knowledgeable regarding subcutaneous injection technique and was therefore provided with appropriate prescriptions for Neupogen and subcutaneous injection supplies, but will not require home nursing services. Given her ongoing low CD4 lymphocyte count, the need for her to resume prophylaxis against *Pneumocystis carinii* pneumonia with pentamidine or Bactrim will be reviewed at her next follow-up appointment.

Discharge Instructions: The signs and symptoms for which the patient should contact the health care team were reviewed in detail and include fevers, chills, shortness of breath, dyspnea, chest pain, nausea, vomiting, diarrhea, or inability to drink fluids or take oral medications. In addition, she is aware to notify us for any worsening of her skin lesions or the development of any new skin blisters. Self-care strategies during periods of neutropenia and thrombocytopenia were also reviewed. The patient and her husband verbalized understanding of these instructions. Appropriate telephone contact numbers for daytime and after-hours assistance were provided, and the written discharge instructions were reviewed. The patient was discharged in good condition, accompanied by her husband.

If you have any questions or require any additional information, please do not hesitate to contact us.

Sandra A. Mitchell, CRNP, MScN, AOCN
Advanced Practice Nurse-Oncology

John G. Smith, MD
Attending Physician, Hematology Oncology

c.c. Dr. Referring Oncologist
Primary Care Provider, FNP
Dr. John Brain, Division of Infectious Disease
Oncology Follow-up Clinic

Figure 27-1 Sample discharge summary.

Doe, Jane
MR #1220099
Date of Service: April 8, 2002

Jane is seen in the stem cell transplant unit during a 23-hour admission following vertebroplasty to T12 and L1 vertebrae. She is day +61 status post related, T-cell depleted, peripheral blood stem cell transplantation for AML, subtype M-4. She was transplanted in second complete remission. Her posttransplant course has been complicated by CMV reactivation, for which she completed a course of ganciclovir on 1/28/01; steroid-induced diabetes requiring treatment with oral hypoglycemic agents and now insulin; osteoporosis, with fractures of T12 and L1 vertebrae, necessitating vertebroplasty; and poor graft function of unclear origin. In addition, she has experienced acute graft-versus-host disease of the skin.

Review of Systems
On review of systems, Jane denies fever, chills, cough, shortness of breath, dyspnea, or chest pain. She has had no nausea, vomiting, diarrhea, or abdominal pain. She has no skin rashes and no joint or muscle pains. She has had no bleeding problems. She denies pain around her double-lumen PICC line located in the right upper extremity. Appetite is good, and energy level is fair. She continues to experience intermittent spasmodic back pain, usually brought on by activities and for which she is now taking Flexeril, as well as intermittently using narcotic analgesics.

Physical Examination
On examination, temperature is 37.2° C, pulse 100 beats/min, respirations 20 breaths/min, blood pressure 123/86 mm Hg, pulse oximetry is 98% on room air, weight is 70 kg, performance status is an 80%. **HEENT:** Pupils are equal, round, and reactive to light bilaterally; extraocular movements are intact; sclerae conjunctivae are clear bilaterally; oral cavity is smooth, moist, and pink, without erythema or open lesions; there are severely cushingoid facial features. The neck is supple and without adenopathy.
Lymph: There is no cervical, supraclavicular, axillary, or inguinal lymphadenopathy.
Lungs: Clear to auscultation and percussion anteriorly and posteriorly; no wheezing, rales or rhonchi.
Cardiac: S_1, S_2, regular rhythm; no murmurs, rub, or gallop.
Abdomen: Soft, flat, nontender; bowel sounds are positive ×4 quadrants. There is no organomegaly.
Extremities/MSK: Range of motional without pain; there is mild proximal muscle weakness in the lower extremities bilaterally. Strength is 4+ and equal bilaterally. A double-lumen PICC line is in situ in the right upper extremity; site is without erythema, tenderness or discharge.
Neurologic: Alert and oriented ×3; there is no focal neurologic deficit. Skin is without rashes, bruising, or petechiae. Vertebroplasty site overlying T12 and L1 is without erythema, tenderness, or discharge.
Skin: Without rashes, bruising, or petechiae.
Psychologic: The patient is in good spirits.

Labs
WBC count is 2.4 with 74% granulocytes, hemoglobin 9.3, hematocrit 25.7, platelets 37,000/mm^3. Sodium 138, potassium 3.6, chloride 102, CO_2 22, glucose 170, BUN 10, creatinine 0.6, calcium 7.3, phosphorus 4.6, magnesium 1.6, total protein 4.6, albumin 2.3, alkaline phosphatase 108, AST 30, ALT 101, total bilirubin 0.7, LDH 560.

Current Medications
Prilosec 20 mg PO qd, magnesium oxide 400 mg PO tid, Klor-Con 20 mEq PO tid, pentamidine 300 mg by inhalation (next due on 5/3/01), Sporanox 200 mg PO q12h, Valtrex 500 mg PO q12h, Medrol 20 mg PO qAM and 4 mg PO qPM, Levaquin 500 mg PO qd, glyburide 5 mg PO qd, IVIG 30 g IV qmo (next due on 4/12), Aredia 90 mg IV qmo (next due on 4/23)

Assessment and Plan
1. **Acute myelogenous leukemia, subtype M-4, in second complete remission, and now day +106 status post matched, related, T-cell depleted peripheral blood stem cell transplantation.** Jane's white blood cells count is decreased today at 1.4, with an ANC of approximately 1000. She received a dose of Neupogen 480 μg SC today. In addition, her hematocrit is low, and she received a transfusion of one unit of packed red blood cells as well as Epogen 40,000 units SC. She will continue support with Epogen weekly. We have also transfused one single-donor platelet product today for her platelet count of 30,000. The indication for this platelet transfusion was that she is status post vertebroplasty, and we wish to avoid the possibility of the development of a hematoma at the operative site. We will continue to monitored her counts closely to evaluate the need for ongoing support with platelets, packed cells, and cytokines.
2. **Graft-versus-Host-Disease.** Jane continues on Medrol 20 mg PO qAM and 4 mg PO qPM for treatment of her graft-versus-host disease of the skin. She has no GI symptoms such as nausea, vomiting, or diarrhea. Her liver function tests are at her baseline. She will begin therapy with tacrolimus 1 mg PO qd so that we can begin a taper of her steroids as soon as possible. We will check a tacrolimus level at her clinic visit on 4/12/01, and adjust the dosage as indicated. Jane is experiencing a number of side effects from high-dose steroids, including osteoporosis and insulin-dependent diabetes. She began therapy with insulin today as discussed below.
3. **Infection.** Jane is afebrile, nonneutropenic, taking steroids, with no recent positive culture data. She continues on weekly CMV screening, and her most recent CMV antigen remains negative. She continues on antimicrobial prophylaxis with Valtrex, Levaquin, itraconazole, and pentamidine.
4. **Fluids, Electrolytes, and Nutrition.** Jane is taking a soft, no concentrated sugar diet in adequate quantities. She is drinking at least 2 quarts of fluid daily. Her weight, BUN, and creatinine are stable. She continues on oral electrolyte supplementation with magnesium and potassium. In addition, she was noted today to have a low ionized calcium and received an ampule of calcium gluconate IV in clinic. Given her osteoporosis, future consideration should be given to beginning calcium supplementation to at least 1200 mg of oral calcium with vitamin D supplementation. In addition, Jane's phosphorus level was also noted to be low, and she received 40 mmol of K-Pho IV today. Jane is on gastric cytoprotection with Prilosec 20 mg PO qd.
5. **Diabetes Mellitus.** Jane's hyperglycemia is poorly controlled on Diabeta. She begins therapy today with NPH insulin 12 units qAM and 8 units qPM. We will escalate this therapy as needed. She will be monitoring her capillary blood glucose levels at home so that her insulin dosages can be further adjusted. Arrangements were made for her to obtain a glucometer, and she will receive home care follow-up for diabetic teaching, including self-injection of insulin, monitoring of capillary blood glucose levels, and reinforcement of the signs and symptoms of hyperglycemia and hypoglycemia and the principles of the diabetic diet. In addition, an appointment has been made for Jane to attend the diabetic education center on 4/15/01 for additional education.
6. **Osteoporosis.** Jane has developed osteoporosis, likely secondary to her long-term treatment with steroids. She has begun therapy with Aredia 90 mg IV qmo and should also begin supplementation with calcium and vitamin D. She underwent a vertebroplasty today, in treatment of her compression fractures of T12 and L1. The postvertebroplasty self-care instructions were reviewed with Jane and her husband, and they were provided with written instructions as well. Jane continues on a slow steroid taper, and tacrolimus has recently been added to facilitate a more rapid tapering schedule.

Jane will return to clinic on 4/14/01 for labs and reevaluation. In addition, she will be seen by the home care nurses for diabetic teaching and is scheduled to be seen in the diabetic education center. In the meantime, she and her husband are aware of the signs and symptoms for which they should contact the health care team.

The patient was seen and examined with Dr. John G. Smith; labs and plan of care reviewed.

Sandra A. Mitchell, CRNP, MScN, AOCN
Advanced Practice Nurse-Oncology

John G. Smith, MD
Attending Physician, Hematology Oncology

c.c. Dr. Referring Oncologist
Primary Care Provider, FNP
Dr. John Brain, Division of Neuroradiology
Diabetic Education Center

Figure 27-2 Sample progress note.

Consultant, Researcher, and Educator Roles

CHAPTER

28 Consultation

Jennifer L. Aikin

CASE | STUDY

ESTABLISHING THE CONSULTANT ROLE

You are hired to work as an oncology clinical nurse specialist at a large urban hospital. In this new role, you will serve as a resource for three oncology units: a surgical oncology inpatient unit, a hematology/oncology inpatient unit, and an outpatient chemotherapy clinic. You are new to the city as well as the hospital.

QUESTIONS

1. As you seek to establish your role as consultant, what should be your priorities during the first few months in your new position?

    1. Meet with key administrators, physicians, and other members of the interdisciplinary team (i.e., social workers, physical and occupational therapists, dietitians) to describe your role and areas of expertise.

    2. Identify patients who may benefit from your expertise.

    3. Be visible on the oncology units.

    4. Before seeing patients on the units, wait to receive a formal consultation request so that nurses do not feel threatened by your presence.

    a. 1 & 2
    b. 1, 2, & 3
    c. 1, 3, & 4
    d. 3 & 4

ANSWERS

1. Initially, consultants must market their services (Barron & White, 1996). To do this, they must identify their own areas of expertise and what consultative services they will provide. When entering a new organization, it is important that you meet with key administrators, physicians, and other members of the interdisciplinary team to learn more about the organization, to identify key players, and to describe your role and areas of expertise. You need to be visible on the oncology units daily and attend interdisciplinary team meetings and in-services. During nursing rounds or

report, you may initially need to identify patients with complex clinical needs who will benefit from a consult. These cases will give you an opportunity to demonstrate your experience and areas of expertise, educating staff nurses about what types of cases are appropriate for future consultations. This active approach is essential: Advanced practice nurses (APNs) who wait for consultations will get off to a very slow start. *Answer 1:* **b.**

QUESTIONS

2. What key characteristics should you cultivate and demonstrate to facilitate your consultant role?

    1. Respect the expertise of consultees

    2. Communicate warmth and acceptance to nursing staff

    3. Possess clinical expertise in an area of advanced practice

    4. Demonstrate skill in the consultative process

    a. 1 & 2
    b. 1, 2, & 3
    c. 2, 3, & 4
    d. All of these

3. What important principles must you keep in mind as you work as a consultant?

    1. To be respected, you should have line authority over the staff nurses on the unit.

    2. When consulted, you will assume professional responsibility for the patient.

    3. The consultee needs to identify the problem.

    4. The staff nurse is free to accept or reject your recommendations.

    a. 1 & 2
    b. 1, 2, & 3
    c. 1, 3, & 4
    d. 3 & 4

ANSWERS

2. To be successful as a consultant, you must have experience, identify your areas of expertise, and demonstrate effective communication skills

(Beyers, 1986). According to Barron and White (1996), the APN should establish warm, accepting, and respectful relationships with consultees; avoid stereotyping and suspend judgment; communicate the belief that the problem identified by the consultee is important; and communicate confidence that the consultee can overcome any difficulties associated with the problem. Skill in the consultation process will also enhance your effectiveness. *Answer 2:* **d.**

3. Barron and White (1996) outline key principles for successful consultation (Box 28-1). According to these authors, there should *not* be a hierarchical relationship between the consultant and consultee (i.e., the consultant should not have line authority) because this could prevent the free exchange of ideas and diminish the consultee's freedom to accept or reject the consultant's recommendations. *Answer 3:* **d.**

QUESTIONS

4. During the first 6 months of your new position, what kinds of consultations should you expect?
   1. Formal client-centered consultations
   2. Informal client-centered consultations
   3. Consultee-centered case consultations
   4. Consultee-centered administrative consultations
      a. 1 & 2
      b. 1, 2, & 3
      c. 3 & 4
      d. All of these

ANSWERS

4. Caplan describes four types of consultation. *Client-centered case consultation,* the most common type of consultation, assists the consultee to develop an effective plan of care for a patient with a complex problem (Barron & White, 1996). This type of consultation may be formal or informal. In

---

| BOX **28-1** | **Consultation: Key Characteristics** |

1. The problem is always identified by the consultee.
2. The relationship between the consultant and the consultee is nonhierarchical.
3. Professional responsibility for the patient remains with the consultee.
4. The consultee is free to accept or reject the ideas and recommendations of the consultant.

Adapted from Barron, A. M., & White, P. (1996). Consultation. In Hamric, A. B., Spross, J. A., & Hanson, C. M. (Eds.). *Advanced nursing practice* (p. 170). Philadelphia: WB Saunders.

consultee-centered case consultation, the focus is on a consultee: The consultant assists the consultee to overcome specific deficits, which may include a lack of knowledge, skill, confidence, or objectivity. An example of *program-centered administrative consultation* is when an APN receives a request from the hospital's nursing administration to develop a new clinical program. Finally, *consultee-centered administrative consultation* focuses on the consultee's difficulties in meeting the organization's objectives. As an APN serving as a resource in the clinical setting, it is most likely that you will initially be involved in consultations that directly or indirectly affect patient care: client-centered consultations (formal and informal) and consultee-centered case consultations.

You will move through several phases as you develop your consultant role. Initially, the consultant focuses on proficiency in the client- and consultee-centered clinical consultations. However, as you become recognized as a credible and successful expert and gain knowledge about the organization's structure and culture, the role will evolve to include more administrative consultations. *Answer 4:* **b.**

CASE 2 STUDY

CLIENT-CENTERED CASE CONSULTATION

A new staff nurse on the medical oncology unit is passing medications. As you walk by, the nurse asks, "Mrs. Miller began taking morphine 3 days ago, and she's experiencing nausea. Is that normal?"

QUESTIONS

1. What would be the *best* response to this question?
   a. "If you would like me to assess Mrs. Miller, I can see her later this afternoon."
   b. "I can't answer that question without seeing Mrs. Miller and evaluating her for myself."

c. "Tell me a little bit more about Mrs. Miller's situation. What is her diagnosis? What other medications is she taking?"

d. "Usually, patients experience nausea for the first few days after beginning narcotics. An antiemetic should take care of the nausea."

1. Consultation may be either formal or informal. You need to determine whether casual questions asked in passing can be answered quickly and immediately or whether the answer is more involved. In this case, although answer d is technically correct, other issues need to be considered, such as the patient's diagnosis, medications, and other contributing factors. When considering this informal consultation, it is important that you do not take control of the situation or move ahead to assess the patient independently of the staff nurse, as in answers a and b. In this case, you need to determine what the nurse knows about Mrs. Miller's situation and gather more information before answering the nurse's question. *Answer 1:* **c.**

Case Study continued
The staff nurse explains that Mrs. Miller is a 52-year-old woman with metastatic breast cancer who was hospitalized with a spinal cord compression. From report, the nurse knows that Mrs. Miller's appetite has been poor but that she has not vomited; there is no standing order for an antiemetic, and Mrs. Miller has not had a bowel movement since her admission 4 days ago. The staff nurse admits that thus far in the shift she has not had time to perform a physical assessment because she has been too busy.

QUESTIONS
2. Given this additional information, what should be your response?

a. Call the physician to request that an antiemetic be ordered

b. Explain that the nausea is probably caused by her morphine and will eventually pass

c. Ask the nurse to call you after she performs a physical assessment to discuss her question then

d. Ask the nurse how you can be most helpful in this situation

2. During the assessment phase of this consultation, you need to consider the request and clarify the nature of the consultative relationship: What kind of assistance is the staff nurse requesting? Rushing ahead to identify a problem or suggest solutions is premature in this situation. You should ask the staff nurse how you can be most helpful. The staff nurse may choose to consult with you after she performs a physical assessment, or she may request that you help evaluate Mrs. Miller. Does the staff nurse want to maintain responsibility for this situation or is she asking for you to be more involved? The first option would allow the staff nurse to maintain more independence and responsibility for the situation, whereas the second would involve you to a greater degree. If you and the staff nurse determine that a more formal consultation is appropriate in this situation, then together you could complete an assessment of the problem. *Answer 2:* **d.**

Case Study continued
The staff nurse says that she is new to oncology and would like you to be involved in the evaluation of Mrs. Miller. You review Mrs. Miller's chart and note that laboratory results are within normal limits. Then, you and the staff nurse go into Mrs. Miller's room together. You conduct a physical assessment and question the patient about her symptoms. The assessment reveals that Mrs. Miller's abdomen is distended and firm, and bowel sounds are very faint. She says that she has not had a bowel movement since her admission, but she claims that is partly because she is not allowed to get up to the bathroom without assistance and she does not want to use a bedpan. Mrs. Miller rates her pain as a 6 on a 0 to 10 scale. She says that her nausea is intermittent and that she has not vomited. She says, "I don't know what is worse—the pain or the queasiness." A neurologic assessment reveals weakness and some numbness and tingling in her extremities. Mrs. Miller has a urinary catheter in place.

QUESTIONS
3. You and the nurse leave the room. What should be your response based on this new information?

1. You should assist the staff nurse to develop a plan of care for Mrs. Miller's pain, nausea, and constipation.
2. You should call the physician to report these findings.
3. You should instruct the staff nurse to call the physician to request an order for an antiemetic and stool softener.

4. You should document the assessment and consultation in the patient's record.
   a. 1 & 2
   b. 1, 2, & 3
   c. 1 & 4
   d. 2 & 4

3. After a thorough assessment, problems can be identified. The process of problem identification needs to be collaborative. Therefore you and the staff nurse should meet together to discuss the assessment and identify Mrs. Miller's problems, which include nausea, pain, and constipation. You can make recommendations for interventions, such as recommending an antidepressant for neuropathic pain, an antiemetic, and stool softener; further monitoring; patient education; and other comfort measures; but ultimately, patient care remains the responsibility of the staff nurse. You and the staff nurse should mutually decide how the interventions will be evaluated and what role you are to play in the future care of Mrs. Miller. Because APNs are accountable for their practice, it is important that you document your interaction with Mrs. Miller in the progress notes. According to Barron and White (1996), a progress note may not be required when the patient is not seen directly by the consultant; however, consultants should document all consultations in their own records. *Answer 3:* **c.**

For the following questions, identify whether the scenarios presented are examples of consultation (a), collaboration (b), or referral (c).

4. You call the psychiatric clinical nurse specialist to assess and follow a patient for depression.

5. You counsel and support the family while the staff prepare the patient for transfer to the medical intensive care unit.

6. The physician contacts you to discuss the feasibility of home total parenteral nutrition (TPN) in a frail patient who lives alone.

4-6. As mentioned earlier, in consultation the consultee maintains responsibility for patient care, and the consultee may accept or reject the recommendations of the consultant. In collaboration, responsibility for patient care is shared by the staff nurse and APN, so there is comanagement of patients. During a referral, responsibility for care is relinquished to another health care professional, either on a temporary or permanent basis. *Answer 4:* **c.** *Answer 5:* **b.** *Answer 6:* **a.**

CASE 3 STUDY

CONSULTEE-CENTERED CASE CONSULTATION

You receive a call from a nurse in the outpatient chemotherapy unit. The nurse states that a patient will be seen the next day who will be receiving an investigational agent as part of a clinical trial. The nurses on the unit are anxious about administering the drug because there is the potential for infusion-associated reactions and other unique neurologic side effects. This investigational agent has never been administered at this hospital, and the nurses are asking if you have experience with the agent. You have experience with other investigational agents but not the agent in question.

1. How should you respond to this request?
   1. Offer to consult with the investigational drug pharmacist and obtain a copy of the research protocol
   2. Offer to conduct an in-service for nurses on the outpatient unit about the study drug and nursing implications
   3. Offer to be available on the unit the next day when the patient is treated
   4. Explain that you have no experience administering the drug and suggest that they call the investigational drug pharmacist for assistance
   a. 1 & 2
   b. 1, 2, &3
   c. 1 & 3
   d. 3 & 4

1. This is an example of a consultee-centered case consultation. Although you may not have experience administering this particular investigational agent, you have administered other investigational agents and understand the outpatient nurses' anxiety. You also have expertise in assessing and managing neurologic toxicities. The investigational pharmacist and the research proto-col are good resources for learning more about administering the investigational agent. You may offer to conduct an in-service and to be avail-able the next day when the patient is treated. *Answer 1:* **b.**

Case Study continued

The outpatient nursing staff requests that you provide an in-service about the investigational drug. The in-service will be held the next morning from 8:00 to 8:30 in the conference room. Six nurses are working that day, and patients will be arriving at 8:30 AM.

QUESTIONS

2. What steps can you take to ensure a successful in-service?
   1. Invite the investigational drug pharmacist to attend
   2. Prepare a lecture to ensure that all of the important information is covered
   3. Ask the outpatient nurses what information they would like to learn during the in-service
   4. Allow time for discussion
      a. 1 & 2
      b. 1, 2, & 3
      c. 1, 3, & 4
      d. 2 & 3

3. What method will be *most* effective for evalu-ating the success of this consultation?
   a. Informal conversations about the nurses' level of comfort administering the new drug
   b. Brief written evaluation of the in-service
   c. Chart review to determine whether the drug was administered correctly
   d. Patient interviews to ensure that their side effects were managed properly

ANSWERS

2. At times, consultation and education go hand in hand. As a first step, you should conduct an informal needs assessment by asking the outpa-tient nurses about what information they would like to have addressed at the in-service. Although the amount of time allotted for the in-service is brief, a didactic presentation is not the most effective strategy to use with adult learners. A better strategy is to allow time for discussion and provide written information about the drug that can be referred to after the in-service if questions arise. It is a good idea to include the investiga-tional pharmacist in the discussion to role model collaboration and teamwork, as well as to ensure that all resources are used for educating the staff. *Answer 2:* **c.**

3. Although the in-service is an effective strat-egy for meeting the needs of the consultees, a written evaluation of the program will not be sufficient to evaluate the success of the con-sultation. The primary problem identified by the outpatient nurses was anxiety related to ad-ministering a new agent. Chart reviews and questionnaires are appropriate for determining whether learning occurred, but informal conversa-tions are more appropriate for evaluating a consul-tation. According to Barron and White (1996), evaluation discussion should ask whether the problem was solved; if not, why not and what next? If the problem was solved, you should review why and confirm the new skills and abilities resulting from the interaction. Finally, the overall process of the consultation should be reviewed. *Answer 3:* **a.**

CASE 4 STUDY

PROGRAM-CENTERED ADMINISTRATIVE CONSULTATION

You have been hired to develop a comprehensive breast care center for a large hospital located in the suburbs of a major metropolitan area. This new center will expand the hospital's current mammography services. Currently under con-struction, the new center will be staffed with mammography technicians, an on-site radiolo-gist, receptionist, office staff, and nurses. Two days every week, a medical oncologist and surgical oncologist will see patients in the center. You are responsible for making recommenda-tions about the layout, developing clinical policies and procedures, hiring and training the nursing staff, facilitating interdisciplinary team meetings, and putting systems in place to ensure continuity of care.

QUESTIONS

1. What should be your priorities during your first month in this new position?
1. Meet with key administrators and physicians to learn about their expectations for the new breast center
2. Develop a breast health questionnaire for women to fill out while they wait for their mammograms
3. Establish relationships with key personnel in other departments who will interact with the breast center staff (e.g., pathology, laboratory, operating room)
4. Conduct an assessment of the community to learn about the target population for the breast center's services
   a. 1 & 2
   b. 1, 2, & 3
   c. 1, 3, & 4
   d. 2 & 4

ANSWERS

1. When beginning a program-centered administrative consultation, a thorough organizational assessment is an important first step. This includes learning about the organization's history, culture, structure, goals, and priorities; assessing the surrounding community to determine the target population for the hospital's service; meeting with people in key leadership positions to learn about their expectations for the program; and establishing relationships with personnel in other departments that will interact with the breast center. Beyers (1986) emphasizes this point by saying, "Always obtain information from individuals and groups directly involved and those that surround the subject of the consultation, including those that interface with or that impact the consultation situation" (p. 26). Although a breast health questionnaire will be a useful clinical tool, this should not be as great a priority as the other items listed. *Answer 1:* **c.**

QUESTIONS

2. What factors will contribute to your success in this new role?
1. Support from the hospital administration
2. Your experience, expertise, and effective communication skills
3. Adequate funding to support the new breast center
4. Your flexibility and willingness to adapt to changing situations
   a. 1 & 2
   b. 1, 2, & 3
   c. 2 & 4
   d. All of these

BOX **28-2** | **Principles for Effective Consultations**

1. The consultant must have expertise, experience, and effective communication skills.
2. The purpose of the consultation must be mutually understood by the consultant and the group or person engaging the consultant.
3. Resources adequate for the consultative experience must be available at the appropriate time to achieve the purposes of the consultation.
4. The consultant must be supported by top administration, governing bodies, and others. Consistent definition of the consultant's role and purpose and open lines of communication throughout the consultation are essential to a healthy, ongoing relationship.
5. Flexibility and a willingness to adapt to changing situations that inevitably occur during a consultative experience must be shared by the client and the consultant engaged.
6. Parties in the consultative experience need to accept the ambiguity inherent in most consultation situations.

Adapted from Beyers, M. (1986). On the scene: corporate nursing and consulting. Corporate consultation: the opportunities and the challenges. *Nurs Admin Q, 10*(4), p. 26.

ANSWERS

2. Beyers (1986) describes six principles for effective consultations. These principles are outlined in Box 28-2. All of the factors listed will contribute to your success. *Answer 2:* **d.**

QUESTIONS

3. When meeting with a key medical oncologist, the physician criticizes your supervisor, saying that the whole concept for the breast center is too grandiose and not feasible given the institution's financial problems. He says, "This program is doomed to fail." What is the *best* response to this comment?
   a. "I am interested in hearing all perspectives on this new center, so I am pleased that you would share your thoughts and concerns with me."
   b. "It sounds like you've given a lot of thought to this."
   c. "I can tell you're unhappy with the way the breast center is being developed."
   d. Ignore the comment and change the subject.

ANSWERS

3. According to Norris (1977), it is important that the consultant listen to everyone because each person has a different perception that can be valuable in developing the program. Norris cautions consultants to take care not to agree or even give the impression of agreeing with those who have opinions or have identified problems with the program. Self-affirming statements such as, "It sounds like you've given a lot of thought to this" or "I can tell that you're unhappy," may be comforting, but they are likely to be misinterpreted. The best response is, "I'm interested in hearing all perspectives on this new center, so I am pleased that you would share your thoughts and concerns with me." *Answer 2:* **a.**

Case Study continued

During her assessment, you learn that the breast center will service a largely middle-class population from a variety of racial and ethnic groups (Caucasian, Hispanic, and African American). Many of the women in the neighborhood are professional women who commute to the city. Most have private health insurance.

QUESTIONS

4. How will this information affect your plans for the breast center?
1. When hiring, you should consider employees who can speak both English and Spanish.
2. The breast center should be open from 8 AM to 5 PM, Monday through Friday.
3. Marketing efforts should focus on the convenience of having all breast health services in one location.
4. Educational materials should be at or below a fifth grade level.
   a. 1 & 2
   b. 1 & 3
   c. 2 & 4
   d. 3 & 4

ANSWERS

4. The community assessment provides valuable information as you develop your plan for marketing the center, hours of operation, and educational strategies. A bilingual staff will enhance communication with women who use the breast center's services. Because most of the women commute to the city to work, evening and weekend hours will be essential to attract women to the center. When targeting professional women, television advertisements should be aired during evening and weekend hours as well.

Educational materials in English and Spanish should be at an educational level no lower than a fifth grade level so as not to offend professional women who may be at a higher educational level. *Answer 4:* **b.**

QUESTIONS

5. You plan to implement a primary nursing model in the breast center. What is necessary to make primary nursing successful?
1. Physicians must understand and support the role of the primary nurse.
2. Nurses must have experience working with this model of care.
3. Only bachelor's-prepared nurses should be hired to work as primary nurses.
4. Nurses must have an adequate knowledge base about risk factors, early detection strategies, and diagnostic procedures, as well as effective interpersonal skills.
   a. 1 & 2
   b. 1 & 4
   c. 2 & 3
   d. 3 & 4

ANSWERS

5. The two factors that will affect the success of primary nursing are (1) nursing knowledge (the nurses must be familiar with risk factors, early detection strategies, and diagnostic procedures) and skills related to developing the nurse-patient relationship, and (2) physicians understanding and support of the new model of care. The other factors (experience in primary nursing and bachelor's degree) are not as important. *Answer 5:* **b.**

QUESTIONS

6. Once the comprehensive breast care center is up and running, list three methods that could be used to evaluate the program.
   a. _____
   b. _____
   c. _____

ANSWERS

6. A number of objective parameters may be used to evaluate the success of the comprehensive breast care center. These include the number of mammograms performed, the number of physician visits, and the revenue generated by the breast center each year. A more subjective method for evaluating the quality of care would be a patient satisfaction questionnaire. Quality control measures can be instituted for mammography and patient management by selecting individual cases for peer-review at the multidisciplinary team meeting. *Answer 6:* **See text.**

CASE 5 STUDY

INDEPENDENT NURSE CONSULTANT PRACTICE

You are an oncology clinical nurse specialist who has worked in the hospital setting for 15 years. During your tenure there, you have been responsible for both oncology nursing and patient education. The hospital is currently experiencing some financial problems, and there are rumors that many jobs will be eliminated. Over the last few years, you have considered leaving your position to establish your own nursing consultation practice.

QUESTIONS

1. List two benefits of an independent nursing consultation practice.

    a. _____

    b. _____

2. What should you consider before you leave your hospital position to work independently as a consultant?
    1. Identify your skills and areas of expertise
    2. Consider your financial resources
    3. Establish a fee schedule
    4. Write a business plan
      a. 1 & 2
      b. 1, 2, & 3
      c. 3 & 4
      d. All of these

3. Challenges of working as an independent nurse consultant include:
    1. Keeping focused if working alone at home
    2. Maintaining contact with nursing colleagues
    3. Creating a market for one's services
    4. Negotiating the terms of an agreement
      a. 1 & 2
      b. 1, 2, & 3
      c. 3 & 4
      d. All of these

ANSWERS

1. In today's health care environment, many clinical nurse specialist positions are being eliminated or changed to case manager positions. Those who wish to work in the role may look beyond traditional clinical settings (hospitals and outpatient clinics) in order to practice as clinical experts, educators, consultants, and researchers. Starting a nursing consultation practice is one

way to expand the clinical nurse specialist role. *Answer 1:* **Advantages include autonomy, opportunities in many settings, and more flexible work schedules.**

2. Schulmeister (1999b) identified a number of important questions to answer before starting a nursing consultation practice (Box 28-3). An APN must identify personal strengths and areas of expertise, consider financial resources (as he or she may need to rely on personal savings or a loan to get started), contact potential sources of consultation work, and write a business plan. Sometimes, the APN will choose to remain employed during the start-up phase. After the decision is made, fees for consultation may be determined based on community standards. *Answer 2:* **d.**

3. There are a number of challenges for nurses who work as independent consultants. According to Norris (1977), two challenges include creating a market for one's services and negotiating the terms of a consultation agreement. Schulmeister (1999a) describes the challenges of working independently at home. He includes the challenges of (1) keeping focused (avoiding distractions), (2) staying connected (professional interaction with nursing colleagues or

---

BOX 28-3 | **Important Questions to Answer Before Starting a Nursing Consultation Practice**

1. Why does starting a consultation practice interest me? Is this something I really want to do, or am I reacting to something else going on in my life?
2. What are my clinical strengths and areas in which growth is needed?
3. What are my personal strengths and areas in which growth is needed?
4. How well do I cope with uncertainty?
5. How essential is a steady income?
6. Do I have the necessary reserves (financial, emotional, physical) to cope if the business is a failure?
7. Do I have the support of those closest to me?
8. Do I have the time and energy required to get the business off the ground?
9. What sacrifices am I willing to make in order to devote time and attention to starting and growing the consultation business?

Adapted from Schulmeister, L. (1999b). Starting a nursing consultation practice. *Clin Nurs Spec, 13*, pp. 94-100.

potential clients), (3) locating resources, and (4) frequently examining business costs and expenses. *Answer 3:* **d.**

REFERENCES

Barron, A. M., & White, P. (1996). Consultation. In Hamric, A. B., Spross, J. A., & Hanson, C. M. (Eds.). *Nursing advanced practice: An integrative approach* (pp. 165-183). Philadelphia, WB Saunders.

Beyers, M. (1986). On the scene: Corporate nursing and consulting. Corporate consultation: the opportunities and challenges. *Nurs Admin Q, 10,* pp. 25-29.

Norris, C. M. (1997). A few notes on consultation in nursing. *Nurs Outlook, 24,* pp. 756-761.

Schulmeister, L. (1999a). The challenges of a home-based nursing consultation business. *Clin Nurs Spec, 13,* pp. 101-103.

Schulmeister, L. Starting a nursing consultation practice. *Clin Nurs Spec, 13,* pp. 94-100.

29 Utilization and Conduct of Research

Mary E. Cooley
Dana N. Rutledge

CASE 1 STUDY

Rachel, an oncology clinical nurse specialist in a small community hospital in a large western city, was unable to attend the Oncology Nursing Society (ONS) Congress in 1998 but had reviewed the published abstracts in the April issue of the *Oncology Nursing Forum*. She was particularly interested in those on the outpatient management of febrile neutropenic patients because physicians in her institution were still admitting these patients for inpatient care. In the past few years, management, both nursing and nonnursing, had discussed trying to use outpatient services when possible for things currently done on an inpatient basis. When she went to Congress in 1999, she was able to hear presentations by two groups of nurses doing outpatient management and was very encouraged that this practice was scientifically valid.

After attending Congress, Rachel asked a faculty friend to do a Medline literature search back to 1992 on neutropenia, oncology patients, and outpatient management. There were 22 citations that seemed pertinent to the topic (Table 29-1). Of these, 4 described randomized control trials (RCTs), 4 described non-RCT studies, and 14 were reviews.

QUESTIONS

1. After studying Table 29-1, think about the following questions. How much work has been done in this area? What indications can be drawn from the fact that only two U.S. studies were published during this time?

ANSWERS

1. Rachel decided that a lot of work must have been done in the area before 1992 to enable 14 reviews to be written. The fact that only two U.S.

studies were published during this time (1992 to 1999) implied that most U.S. work had been done earlier. Based on the titles of the articles and the information Rachel had heard at Congress, she determined the following regarding outpatient therapy for febrile neutropenic patients:

1. It must benefit a specific group of patients (probably those not quite as sick and those with good home support or home care).
2. It probably would necessitate regular clinic visits and/or home care visits.
3. It might use oral and/or intravenous antibiotics.

Rachel did not know how to validate that outpatient management of febrile neutropenic patients was scientifically sound, was unsure how to go about tackling this if it led to a practice change, and wondered if her small hospital would even be interested. Rachel's role at the hospital covers all oncology care across four medical-surgical units, a small bone marrow transplant unit, pediatrics (inpatient/outpatient), and the outpatient chemotherapy clinic.

QUESTIONS

2. A process Rachel might consider in approaching the issue of outpatient management of febrile neutropenic cancer patients is:
1. Research utilization
2. Evidence-based practice
3. Quality improvement
4. Benchmarking
   a. 1 & 2
   b. 2 & 3
   c. 1 & 4
   d. 3 & 4

TABLE 29-1 Selected Articles Related to Outpatient Management for Febrile Neutropenic Cancer Patients

AUTHOR	YEAR	TITLE	JOURNAL INFORMATION	TYPE	IF STUDY, COUNTRY
Martino P, Girmenia C, Raccah R, et al.	1992	Single daily dose ceftriaxone plus amikacin treatment of febrile episodes in neutropenic patients attending day hospital for hematologic malignancies	*Oncology, 49*(1), pp. 49-52	One-group study	Italy
Buchanan GR	1993	Approach to treatment of the febrile cancer patient with low-risk neutropenia	*Hematology Oncology Clinics of North America, 7*(5), pp. 919-935	Review	
Rubenstein EB, Rolston K, Benjamin RS, et al.	1993	Outpatient treatment of febrile episodes in low-risk neutropenic patients with cancer	*Cancer, 71*(11), pp. 3640-3646	Randomized controlled trial	United States
Rubenstein EB, Rolston K	1994	Outpatient management of febrile episodes in neutropenic cancer patients	*Supportive Care in Cancer, 2*(6), pp. 269-273	Review	
Talcott JA, Whalen A, Clark J, et al.	1994	Home antibiotic therapy for low-risk cancer patients with fever and neutropenia: A pilot study of 30 patients based on a validated prediction rule	*Journal of Clinical Oncology, 12*(1), pp. 107-114	One-group study	United States
Malik IA, Khan WA, Karim M, et al.	1995	Feasibility of outpatient management of fever in cancer patients with low-risk neutropenia: Results of a prospective randomized trial	*American Journal of Medicine, 98*(3), pp. 224-231	Randomized controlled trial	Pakistan
Escalante CP, Rubenstein EB, Rolston KV	1996	Outpatient antibiotic treatment in low-risk febrile neutropenic cancer patients	*Supportive Care in Cancer, 49*(5), pp. 358-363	Review	
Freifeld AG, Pizzo PA	1996	The outpatient management of febrile neutropenia in cancer outpatients	*Oncology, 10*(4), pp. 599-612	Review	
Rolston KV, Rubenstein EB, Freifeld A	1996	Early empiric antibiotic therapy for febrile neutropenia patients at low risk	*Infectious Disease Clinics of North America, 10*(2), pp. 223-237	Review	

Continued

TABLE 29-1 Selected Articles Related to Outpatient Management for Febrile Neutropenic Cancer Patients—cont'd

AUTHOR	YEAR	TITLE	JOURNAL INFORMATION	TYPE	IF STUDY, COUNTRY
Rubenstein EB, Escalante CP, Rolston KV	1997	Outpatient antibiotic therapy for febrile episodes in low-risk neutropenic patients with cancer	*Cancer Investigation, 15*(3), pp. 237-242	Review	
DeLalla F	1997	Antibiotic treatment of febrile episodes in neutropenic cancer patients: Clinical and economic considerations	*Drugs, 53*(5), pp. 789-804	Review	
Talcott JA	1997	Outpatient management of febrile neutropenia: Should we change the standard of care?	*Oncologist, 2*(6), 365-373	Review	
Davis DD, Raebel MA	1998	Ambulatory management of chemotherapy-induced fever and neutropenia in adult cancer patients	*Annals of Pharmacotherapy, 32*(12), pp. 1317-1323	Review	
Karthaus M, Carratala J, Jurgens H, Ganser A	1998	New strategies in the treatment of infectious complications in haematology and oncology: Is there a role for out-patient antibiotic treatment of febrile neutropenia?	*Chemotherapy, 44*(6), pp. 427-435	Review	
Rolston KV	1998	Expanding the options for risk-based therapy in febrile neutropenia	*Diagnostic Microbiology in Infectious Disease, 319*(2), pp. 411-416	Review	
Tice AD	1998	Outpatient parenteral antibiotic therapy for fever and neutropenia	*Infectious Disease Clinics of North America, 12*(4), pp. 963-977	Review	
Hidalgo M, Hornedo J, Lumbreras C, et al.	1999	Outpatient therapy with oral ofloxacin for patients with low risk neutropenia and fever: A prospective, randomized clinical trial	*Cancer, 85*(1), pp. 213-219	Randomized controlled trial	Spain
Minotti V, Gentile G, Bucaneve G, et al.	1999	Domiciliary treatment of febrile episodes in cancer patients: A prospective randomized trial comparing oral versus parenteral empirical antibiotic treatment	*Supportive Care in Cancer, 7*(3), pp. 134-139	Randomized controlled trial	Italy

| TABLE **29-1** | Selected Articles Related to Outpatient Management for Febrile Neutropenic Cancer Patients—cont'd |

AUTHOR	YEAR	TITLE	JOURNAL INFORMATION	TYPE	IF STUDY, COUNTRY
Papadimitris C, Dimopoulos MA, Kostis E, et al.	1999	Outpatient treatment of neutropenic fever with oral antibiotics and granulocyte colony-stimulating factor	*Oncology, 57*(2), pp. 127-130	Clinical trial	Greece
Westermann AM, Holtkamp MM, Linthorst GA, et al.	1999	At home management of aplastic phase following high-dose chemotherapy with stem-cell rescue for hematological and non-hematological malignancies	*Annals of Oncology, 10*(5), pp. 111-117	Three-group study	The Netherlands
Rolston KV	1999	New trends in patient management: Risk-based therapy for febrile patients with neutropenia	*Clinical Infectious Disease, 298*(3), pp. 515-521	Review	
Uzun O, Anaissie AJ	1999	Outpatient therapy for febrile neutropenia: who, when, and how?	*Journal of Antimicrobial Chemotherapy, 43*(3), pp. 317-320	Review	

3. According to the Iowa Model of research utilization (Table 29-2), the impetus, or "trigger," that led Rachel to consider the possibility of a practice change is:
  a. Problem focused
  b. Knowledge focused
  c. Trend focused
  d. Patient focused

4. Given the articles listed in Table 29-1, Rachel can follow several courses of action to search for the scientific basis for outpatient management of these patients. Which of the following would be the best use of her time?
  1. Pulling together a work team for this project
  2. Ordering copies of only the most recent (1999) review articles and read them to get an overview of the science
  3. Assuming that outpatient management of febrile neutropenic patients will work and begin to work toward changing practice
  4. Beginning to plan how to describe current practice at the hospital with febrile neutropenic cancer patients

  a. 3 & 4
  b. 1, 2, & 3
  c. 2, 3, & 4
  d. 1, 2, & 4

ANSWERS

2. Research utilization, evidence-based practice, quality improvement, and benchmarking are all processes used to improve patient care. *Research utilization* involves using findings following a systematic implementation of a scientifically sound research-based practice protocol within a health care setting with an evaluation of outcomes (Rutledge, 1995). Slightly different is *evidence-based practice*, which integrates current best scientific evidence with a clinician's expertise (Madigan, 1998), pathophysiologic principles, and patient preferences (Sackett, Rosenberg, Gray, et al., 1996). Evidence-based practice began in medicine as an attempt to reduce variability among physician practice patterns and aims to improve appropriateness of services by using research-based clinical protocols and decision-making algorithms. Evidence-based practice in nursing is rooted in nursing's research utilization initiatives (Barnard, 1986; Cronenwett, 1995;

TABLE 29-2	Characteristics of Three Research Utilization Models		
	CURN PROJECT	**STETLER MODEL**	**IOWA MODEL**
Origin	Inductively developed to bridge gap between research and practice	Inductively developed to bridge gap between research and practice	Inductively developed outgrowth of the Quality Assurance Model Using Research
Goal	Change practice	Facilitate application of research findings	Change practice
Stimulus	Problem focused	Problem focused	Knowledge or problem focused
Perspective	Organizationally focused	Individually focused	Organizationally focused
Assumptions	1. Organization must be committed to the process	1. Formal organization may or may not be involved	1. Research can be applied to practice
	2. Visible, potent, and enduring mechanisms must be in place, i.e., standing committees, policies and procedures, and so forth	2. Research usually provides probabilistic information, not absolutes	2. A link between academia and practice potentiates success of use of this model
	3. Substantive resources, including personnel, equipment, time, and funds, must be provided	3. Experiential and theoretical information are more likely to be combined with research information	3. Creating an environment in which inquiry and critical thinking are valued enhances the effectiveness of this model
	4. Planned change is essential	4. Lack of knowledge regarding utilization can inhibit appropriate, effective use	4. Expectations of involvement in research must be communicated in job descriptions, clinical ladders, and merit programs
	5. Two or more studies are required to support practice change	5. User of model must have sound research knowledge of the research process, research utilization process, and substantive area under review	
Process	1. Systematic identification of patient care problems	1. Preparation	1. Identification of problem- or knowledge-focused triggers
	2. Identification and assessment of research base	2. Validation	2. Assemble relevant research literature
	3. Transformation of the knowledge into a solution or clinical problem	3. Comparative evaluation	3. Critique
	4. Clinical trial and evaluation	4. Decision making	4. Determine sufficiency of research base
	5. Decision	5. Translation/application	5. If insufficient, conduct research, consult with experts, and determine scientific principles
	6. Develop means to extend or diffuse the new practice	6. Evaluation	6. If sufficient, identify outcomes, design intervention(s), conduct pilot and evaluation, and modify as needed
	7. Develop mechanisms to maintain the innovation over time		7. Decision making
			8. Change practice
			9. Monitor outcomes
Evaluation	1. Determination as to whether predicted result was obtained	1. Informal self-monitoring of individual patient responses	1. Effect on patient and family
		2. Ongoing assessment at the individual level	2. Effect on staff
		3. Formal monitoring of effectiveness of innovation	3. Fiscal implications

From White, J. M., Leske, J. S., & Pearcy, J. M. (1995). Models and processes of research utilization. *Nurs Clin North Am, 30*(3), pp. 409-420.

Donaldson, 1992; Funk, Tornquist, & Champagne, 1989; Horsley, Crane, Crabtree, & Wood, 1983; Rutledge & Donaldson, 1995; Stetler, 1994; Titler, Kleiber, Steelman, et al., 1994). Institution-specific *quality improvement* or systemwide *benchmarking* efforts may or may not involve research utilization or evidence-based practice, depending on the clinical problem and the processes used. Quality improvement data showing a clinical problem that necessitates practice change may trigger an initiative that leads to a research utilization or evidence-based practice process. Similarly, benchmarking trends among similar clinical agencies may indicate that a particular institution or unit has outcomes different from those of similar institutions. That institution may then initiate a search for practices that may have led to differences. At this point, Rachel does not have either quality improvement data or benchmarking trends to indicate any problem with caring for febrile neutropenic patients. Having a quality improvement or benchmarking effort turn into a research utilization or evidence-based practice initiative is most likely when the problem is one that has a substantial research base (e.g., pain management, skin integrity) and when the institution has a history of such efforts. *Answer 2:* **a.**

3. Management efforts and the trend to do more care on an outpatient basis created Rachel's heightened interest in febrile neutropenia and its management. However, this case does not describe a problem-focused trigger or clinical problem that might stem from risk management data, quality improvement data, or an institution-specific quality initiative (Titler, et al., 1994). In 1998, Rachel saw three abstracts describing outpatient management and subsequently heard two presentations on a similar topic. This "trigger" is considered *knowledge focused* because it stemmed from new information gained both from the literature and from a conference. Other knowledge-focused triggers might come from national agency (e.g., ONS or Agency for Health Care Policy & Research) standards and/or guidelines, philosophies of care, and questions from institutional committees (Titler, et al., 1994). *Answer 3:* **b.**

4. In her master's program, Rachel had studied the Michigan Nurses Association Conduct and Utilization of Research in Nursing (CURN) model of research utilization (Horsley, Crane, Crabtree, & Wood, 1983). In this research utilization model (see Table 29-2), research findings are used to define new practices, whereas research methods

are used to assist in practice change implementation and evaluation. Important throughout research utilization is *planned change.*

Activities in the CURN research utilization model (see Table 29-2) include identifying and synthesizing multiple research studies in one area (research base), transforming useful knowledge from the research base into a clinical solution or protocol, translating the protocol into directed nursing actions, and evaluating the practice change in the clinical area (Horsley, Crane, Crabtree, & Wood, 1983). Research utilization is viewed as an organizational process, not a process carried out by an individual nurse.

Rachel remembers that reading the literature is only one of many steps in the research utilization process. She knows that finding out if there are others interested in this clinical area is very important because she will not be able to make this type of complex change alone—even if the literature did support it. Thus it is important to get a team together. Because the potential change involves a knowledge-focused trigger (see Table 29-2) (Titler, et al., 1994), Rachel knows there is a need to assess and describe current practice at her hospital regarding febrile neutropenia patients. At the same time, Rachel can begin reading the most recent review articles before or while getting the group together. To do the third choice would be premature because health care providers in this institution have not investigated the scientific basis nor has this practice been standardized. *Answer 4:* **d.**

QUESTIONS

5. What questions does Rachel need to answer, and what information is necessary before practice can be changed?

ANSWERS

5. Because Rachel needs to be able to describe current practice to be able to differentiate it from any proposed practice change, she must decide how detailed the answers need to be. As a start, Rachel can pull a few old charts of patients with suspected infections to outline how patients were managed. She believes she can delineate the high-risk patients based on comorbid conditions and treatment regimens. Outcomes of and resources for current care may be more difficult to obtain.

Answers to the following questions would help Rachel describe current practice.

- How are neutropenic patients treated when fever or suspected infection occurs in the hospital? When they are at home and call in or visit the clinic with an elevated temperature?

- What are the outcomes of current care that could be assessed? Patient mortality and morbidity may be looked at; that is, which patients survive these suspected infections according to what treatment protocols? Do different treatment protocols have different clinical sequelae? What factors might suspected infections and their treatment affect? Would they alter cancer treatment regimens? length of stay? number of clinic visits? and so on.

- What resources are required to accomplish current care—costs/charges, staffing requirements, family requirements, supplies, and so on.

- What is the infection rate in neutropenic and in nonneutropenic cancer patients at this community hospital/clinic? Is this something that is currently known, or will data need to be collected? What is the admission rate for infection for oncology patients? How many of these patients are neutropenic?

- Are there certain groups of patients who are more at risk for this condition (e.g., bone marrow transplant recipients, those with leukemia)? What assumptions does the APN make when he or she divides the oncology population into treatment modalities and disease states? *Answer 5:* **See text.**

QUESTIONS

6. Rachel needs to organize her thoughts and then prioritize actions necessary for this project. Which of the following activities do you believe will help her find out about current practice?
1. Noting trends in charts of appropriate patients as she goes about her daily practice
2. Discussing fever incidence with the inpatient units and clinic nurses
3. Finding out who else might be interested in the project; calling the local school of nursing to see if there might be a faculty member or student who might be interested in assisting with this project; asking staff nurses in the hospital if they want to get involved
4. Getting administrative support to do a chart review based on pharmacy records
   a. 1, 2, & 3
   b. 2, 3, & 4
   c. 1, 3, & 4
   d. All of these

7. For this change project, identify how a specifically designed data collection sheet could be used.
1. Chart review
2. Pilot testing
3. To describe current practice
4. To plan the information gathering aspect of the project
   a. 1, 2, & 3
   b. 2, 3, & 4
   c. 1, 3, & 4
   d. All of these

8. To achieve success, what must Rachel be sure she has as she begins this project?
1. Protected time each week
2. Administrative authority
3. Secretarial support
4. Physician support
   a. 1, 2, & 3
   b. 2, 3, & 4
   c. 1, 3, & 4
   d. All of these

ANSWERS

6-8. To begin a research utilization project, one must establish the current state of care. Answers to some or all of the preceding questions will do this. Although this involves collection of data, either from a prospective sample of patients (inpatient/clinic) who are expected to become neutropenic or from chart review (inpatient/clinic), the purpose of this data collection is not research (which would be generalizable to other settings); rather, the purpose is to help establish institutional practices and outcomes. This information will help staff at this institution decide whether a new way of caring for patients with suspected infection (outpatient management) should be considered. Answers to some of the questions may not involve collecting data but may require looking at the literature. For example, incidence of infection rate may be available through the literature, depending on the protocols being used for patients at Rachel's hospitals.

All activities may assist in assessing current practice. Trend identification would probably be a good use of time because Rachel already knows the patients and could assess the case for issues related to fever management. By discussing why she is interested in fever/infection incidence, Rachel would be getting the discussion out into the hospital, thus creating awareness that a potential change might be in the works. By enlisting the assistance of others in gathering this data, Rachel can spread herself further. Administrative approval of a chart review brings the project to the attention of administration and can assist "buy-on." By finding out about antibiotic regimens used with febrile neutropenia in both the inpatient (including bone marrow transplant unit) and outpatient setting, Rachel would gain information that assists in establishing current practice. Because Rachel works in a small community hospital, she probably needs to discuss the research utilization process and this clinical idea with her supervisor so that way she can gain administrative approval and assurance of resource allocation for developing a work group. Because a major barrier for oncology staff nurses and nurse specialists/managers in doing research utilization is lack of authority to change patient care (Rutledge, Ropka, Greene, et al., 1998), Rachel needs to discuss this barrier with her supervisor and others she believes can influence this barrier. *Answer 6:* **d.** *Answer 7:* **a.** *Answer 8:* **b.**

Case Study continued

Rachel begins discussing her interest with others in her hospital.

QUESTIONS

9. Because of the nature of the potential change, which group of persons does Rachel *not* need to include in the work group?
  a. Quality assurance staff
  b. Pharmacists
  c. Patients
  d. Inpatient nurses

10. What personality characteristics or skill sets would optimize the effectiveness of a successful change?
  a. Energy and persistence
  b. Long-time employee and hesitant to new ideas
  c. Problem solver and novice nurse
  d. Loner and persistent

11. Besides problem solving and critically evaluating this possible new practice, what critical roles will the team members serve in the future as the new practice is adopted?
  1. Team leaders
  2. Change agents
  3. Triage roles
  4. Opinion leaders
    a. 1 & 2
    b. 2 & 3
    c. 2 & 4
    d. None of these

12. What resources will be needed to get this project off the ground and then to proceed?
  a. Time, additional registered nurse (RN) staff, Internet access
  b. Consistent/same meeting space, secretarial support, overtime budget
  c. Graphics department, secretarial and RN staff support
  d. Time, money, secretarial support

ANSWERS

9. At minimum, key stakeholders in a practice change regarding outpatient management of febrile neutropenia would come from nursing administration, quality assurance, physicians, pharmacists, home care nurses, inpatient care nurses, and clinic nurses. If available, a medical librarian might work with the group on finding and retrieving articles to establish the scientific basis for the practice change. Also, if members of the group do not feel comfortable reviewing/synthesizing research literature, assistance of a nurse researcher would be invaluable. Oncology staff nurses and clinical nurse specialists (CNS)/managers reported lack of familiarity with statistical analyses in research reports as one of the top five barriers to using research (Rutledge, et al., 1998). *Answer 9:* **c.**

10. Helpful attributes for group members are "interest, time and energy, persistence, flexibility, interpersonal abilities, problem-solving skills, group skills, and experience within the organization and/or with change" (Horsley, Crane, Crabtree, & Wood, 1983, p. 12). *Answer 10:* **a.**

11. Persons in this group will serve as change agents, so they must be interested in promoting research-based changes. Some in the group will have formal leadership roles (e.g., nurse manager). Often, however, opinion leaders, or those who have informal leadership skills, can have major influences with staff as changes are implemented. Change agents and opinion leaders can be from any discipline. *Answer 11:* **c.**

12. Fortunately, Rachel's environment is very supportive of making systematic changes, and the hospital philosophy embraces evidence-based practice. In recent years, several changes have been implemented based on the Agency of Health Care Policy & Research guidelines (e.g., new protocols for pain management, skin integrity), and a research-based falls prevention program is currently being trialed on several units. These changes were made based on problem-focused triggers—quality improvement data (e.g., poor patient satisfaction with pain management and high fall rates). No existing research utilization committee exists.

As Rachel proceeds, she should try to discuss this project with as many persons as possible, including nurses, physicians, and those from other disciplines. She should try to get an idea of which groups may be resistant to change and perhaps gain some insights into why. Then she can help the implementation group prepare strategies to decrease this resistance.

Resources needed to implement a research utilization project vary from institution to institution and may include time for work group meetings, monies for literature search and article retrieval (and copying), time for article reading/synthesis, secretarial support for minutes/write-ups, and secretarial support (or Internet access) for communication among members. Time is especially problematic, for both reading the literature and for implementing the proposed change (Rutledge, et al., 1998). *Answer 12:* **d.**

Case Study continued

Rachel discusses her ideas with her supervisor, Mary Jean, the vice president of patient services of the hospital. Mary Jean advises Rachel to call this the Febrile Neutropenia Work Group, gives her some suggestions for members, asks her to prepare a budget and timeline, and urges her to begin.

QUESTIONS

13. In their discussion, what advantages or benefits of this project can Rachel point out to Mary Jean?
1. A well-publicized research utilization project could give the oncology services some needed visibility.
2. The topic necessitates bringing a multidisciplinary group together.
3. The topic necessitates physician dominance in the project.
4. A new protocol could decrease costs if patients do not have to be hospitalized or have shorter lengths of stay.
   a. 1, 3, & 4
   b. 1, 2, & 3
   c. 1, 2, & 4
   d. All of these

14. What specific things could Mary Jean do in her administrative position to facilitate this change effort?

1. Allocate resources as the proposal is being written
2. List on agendas all managerial meetings
3. Discuss the project at weekly tumor board
4. Provide protected time to Rachel for project work
   a. 1 & 4
   b. 2 & 3
   c. 3 & 4
   d. 2 & 4

ANSWERS

13-14. Rachel believes this project could benefit the hospital in several ways. Visibility for the oncology service could be an outcome of a successful project. This is especially important when disease management exists in an institution and staff and physicians work together by clinical specialty. When a multidisciplinary group from both inpatient and outpatient settings works together on a clinically important issue, communication among group members is enhanced, which can improve patient care outside of the project. Also, all can benefit from discussing issues from disciplinary/setting perspectives and thinking about patient and institution benefits. Physician dominance is unlikely because the project is being initiated from within nursing. If patients with suspected infection are treated successfully outside the hospital inpatient setting and clinical outcomes are good, cost savings are possible through decreased length of stay in the inpatient facility with less expensive resources used (clinic visits and home care).

Mary Jean should begin discussing the project with members of her administrative team, especially nurse managers and those in disciplines involved with oncology. She also should mention it in all committees she sits on so that she can begin enhancing awareness of the potential change in practice and listen for people's responses. When she receives a written proposal from Rachel (with timeline and budget), she can begin allocating resources for the project. *Answer 13:* **c.** *Answer 14:* **d.**

Case Study continued

Two months go by. The Febrile Neutropenia Work Group has met every 2 weeks. Based on the wishes of the group, the group divided into two teams with Rachel, an inpatient staff nurse, and the two graduate students on both. The two teams are as follows:
1. Literature team: to work on the literature synthesis and write up a suggested protocol

2. Implementation team: to carry out the proposed change

QUESTIONS

15. Based on your understanding of the research utilization process, place the following people on the appropriate team: three staff nurses (two inpatient nurses, one from the clinic), the nurse manager of the bone marrow transplant unit, a nurse from quality assurance, a pharmacist, a nurse researcher from the school of nursing, two graduate nursing students, the medical librarian, and the director of a home care agency.

Literature Team	Implementation Team

16. Given the literature in Table 29-1 and reviewing responses to question 4, which steps must be taken by the literature group?
   1. Rerun literature search
   2. Analyze integrative reviews
   3. Develop an evaluation form
   4. Identify strategies or development
      a. 1 & 2
      b. 1, 2, & 3
      c. 2, 3, & 4
      d. All of these

ANSWERS

15-16. The literature group needs people who have the time and interest to read research reports. These readers either need to have expertise doing this or need some instruction and guidance. The nurse researcher is a must for this group. Although perhaps not knowledgeable in research utilization, the nurse researcher should at least have research critiquing as a skill. Nurses with a master's degree (or graduate students) are often knowledgeable about research utilization and the review process (Stetler, Morsi, Rucki, et al., 1998). The physician probably should be on this group because his or her interpretation (representing medicine) of the scientific merit of any proposed protocol is vital to any change effort. At least one other staff member should be reading the literature, especially to represent staff. If this person were a known opinion leader, this would be a plus. Rachel chose one of the inpatient staff RNs whom she knows is well respected by her peers and interested in pursuing this type of activity. The medical librarian should be asked to meet with this group when possible.

The implementation team should be composed of those who know the system and who know how to get things done. Because the importance of planning and the amount of time required to develop an adequate plan are often underestimated (Horsley, Crane, Crabtree, & Wood, 1983), institutional leaders and those who can think strategically should be on this team. The nurse manager, quality assurance nurse, and home care agency director would be helpful for planning and developing strategies. Also, it is important to have the perspective of the two areas involved—inpatient and outpatient care—represented, so the other two staff nurses should be on this team.

1. First, the medical librarian should rerun a search of both Medline and CINAHL to be sure that the initial search done by a school of nursing faculty member captured all relevant articles.
2. If this search resulted in the same articles, then copies of all 14 review articles could be obtained for members of the literature group.
3. In a subject area where 14 current review articles have been done, selected members of the literature group should start by reading these reviews and synthesizing the findings.

Integrative reviews are systematic analyses with synthesis of the research in a specific area or on a topic (Stetler, et al., 1998). Usually, research utilization requires the reading of original research studies (Horsley, Crane, Crabtree, & Wood, 1983); however, there are times when enough evidence indicates that the research base is strong (e.g., clinical practice guidelines from the Agency of Health Care Policy and Research; 14 current reviews). In this case, the group should decide the scientific merit of the reviews and determine whether the review authors came to similar conclusions.

To evaluate the findings in each review, the group should develop/find an evaluation form—a checklist for this effort that all readers could use. Stetler et al. (1998) discuss desirable attributes of integrated reviews. These attributes include sufficient operational detail about studies reviewed, indication of study quality using specific evaluation criteria, inclusion of tables with information relative to research utilization (application of findings), and communication with recognized researchers in the area under review. Although any one review may not have all of these characteristics, the readers can discuss the strengths and weaknesses of each review using the form/checklist as a point of discussion (Stetler, et al., 1998). Stetler et al. include an evaluation tool in their article for existent integrative reviews. One of the important decision points in the tool asks the reader whether the integrative review findings/recommendations are based on sufficient scientific rationale, and if yes, how should the findings/recommendations be used?

Next, the group must integrate these findings in a meaningful and organized way (Stetler, et al., 1998). *Answer 15:* **See text.** *Answer 16* **b.**

Case Study continued

Rachel has a debate with the nurse researcher over the point of reviewing original research studies. The researcher believes the group should read all of the original studies.

QUESTIONS

17. What is a pro and a con for reading/reviewing the original research studies and a pro and a con for reading/reviewing the 14 reviews?

Pro	Con
Original:	
Review:	

18. What tools could be used for evaluating the implementation of outpatient management of febrile neutropenic patients?
   1. Temperature
   2. Blood
   3. Clean-catch urine
   4. Outpatient visits

   a. 1, 2, & 4
   b. 1, 2, & 3
   c. 2, 3, & 4
   d. All of these

ANSWERS

17. The CURN guidelines (Horsley, Crane, Crabtree, & Wood, 1983) for assessing relevant research-based knowledge presume that original studies will be read and evaluated to determine replication, scientific merit, and potential risk to patients. This first set of criteria establishes the validity and generalizability of the knowledge. By reviewing the original studies, the reviewers can truly assess the scientific merit of each one (Table 29-3). However, given the relative inexperience of the work group regarding this type of review, Rachel believes that reading the 14 reviews and evaluating them with the Stetler criteria is the best use of time. The group will be able to look for replication and potential risk issues as they read the reviews.

Another set of criteria suggested for determining the practice relevance of the research base (Horsley, Crane, Crabtree, & Wood, 1983) includes evaluation for clinical merit, clinical control, feasibility, and cost benefit. Rachel believes this set can be evaluated from the reviews as well as it could be from the original studies, especially given the composition and practical nature of her work group. A final set of criteria that may be used for evaluating a research base relates to measurement instruments that might be used in conducting an evaluation of the practice change (Horsley, Crane, Crabtree,

TABLE 29-3 Pros and Cons of Reviewing Original Research Studies When Multiple Review Articles Have Been Done

PROS	CONS
READING THE ORIGINAL STUDIES	
• True assessment of scientific merit of each study • Better feel for breadth/depth of research base • Learning by group members of how to read original research literature	• Need for huge number of manuscripts to be pulled, read, and critiqued • Instruction and guidance required for inexperienced group doing literature synthesis for research utilization • Very time-consuming
READING THE 14 REVIEWS	
• Fourteen different sets of authors reviewed literature on similar topics; if findings/conclusions are similar, strong case for scientific merit of research base • Time savings • Criteria for evaluating reviews available (e.g., Stetler, et al.)	• Possibility that authors may not have done the best job possible in reviewing/critiquing the original studies (e.g., may not have included all important studies, may not have described studies well) • Need to compare/contrast the reviews according to methods and findings

& Wood, 1983). Rachel believes that the tools for evaluating the proposed practice change are already being used in the clinical setting. *Answer 17:* **See text.**

18. Clinical outcome tools such as temperature, blood, and/or other body fluid cultures can be used for evaluating the implementation of the new research utilization protocol. In Rachel's hospital, temperatures are monitored for oncology inpatients every 4 to 8 hours and every visit for clinic and oncology home care patients. When fever (as evidenced by two consecutive elevated temperature readings) is observed in neutropenic inpatients, infection is suspected and physician-directed antibiotic and antifungal protocols begin. However, the definition of fever is less clear in the outpatient setting, and care delivery is not standard. Rachel thinks a standard protocol could be developed for monitoring fever and its outcome (decreased temperature) in outpatient care. *Answer 18:* **b.**

Case Study continued

Rachel and her colleagues successfully implemented their project, Outpatient Management of Febrile Neutropenia. The literature review group took 6 months to critically review the 14 reviews, synthesize the findings, and develop a clinical protocol. The implementation team took the protocol and tried it with five patients over 6 more months. Based on the trial, the team modified the protocol, obtained appropriate institutional approvals, and did a full-scale implementation within another 6 months. The evaluation took another 3 to 4 months and indicated that these patients could safely (no increased infection rates, no increased mortality) and effectively (decreased costs, altered care delivery patterns) be cared for in the outpatient setting.

QUESTIONS

19. Which of the following are possible roadblocks and barriers that could have occurred during this process?
1. Inadequate facilities to implement the change
2. Lack of relevance of the research
3. Conflicting research results
4. Isolation from knowledgeable colleagues with whom to discuss research
   a. 1, 2, & 4
   b. 2, 3, & 4
   c. 1, 3, & 4
   d. All of these

ANSWERS

19. Barriers can be categorized as characteristics of the innovation adopters (nurses), the organization, the communication (presentation/accessibility of the research), and the innovation (the research itself) (Funk, Tornquist, & Champagne, 1995) (Table 29-4). These are based on the work of Rogers' theory of diffusion (Rogers, 1983).

In a survey of 407 oncology nurse managers and APNs (Rutledge, et al., 1998), barriers to research utilization were identified. Nurse managers and APNs perceived characteristics of the innovation adopters (nurses), the organization, and the communication (presentation/accessibility of the research) as greater barriers than the characteristics of the innovation (the research itself). The top five barriers for these advanced practice nurses were as follows:
1. Lack of awareness of research
2. Statistical analysis not understandable
3. Lack of time to implement new ideas
4. Lack of time to read research
5. Nurse not capable of evaluating the quality of the research

While these generalizations can be stated, the particular combination of barriers and roadblocks that occur are unique to an institution and to the research utilization topic. *Answer 19:* **d.**

TABLE 29-4	Barriers to Research Utilization		
		COMMUNICATION	**RESEARCH**
Resistance to change	No authority to change practice	Difficulties with the study statistics	Conflicting results
Lack of awareness of the research	No time to read or implement new practices	Unclear research reports	Lack of replication
Not feeling capable of evaluating the research	Lack of support	Difficulty obtaining the reports	Uncertainty as to findings' validity
Being isolated from knowledgeable colleagues with whom to discuss the research	Belief that research is irrelevant	Lack of relevance of the research	Methodologic inadequacies
	Inadequate facilities to implement changes		

CASE 2 STUDY

Patricia, an oncology APN, notices that a growing number of patients with head and neck cancer are receiving combined therapy with radiation and chemotherapy. These patients are experiencing multiple side effects, such as nausea, pain, and difficulty swallowing, and must manage most of their care as outpatients. Patricia would like to gain a better understanding of how treatment affects quality of life in these patients, and she approaches the nurse researcher to discuss initiating a research study. The nurse researcher advises Patricia on various ways to identify a research problem.

QUESTIONS

1. Which of the following ways are best to identify a research problem?
1. Using direct observations from your clinical practice
2. Discussing the problem with other experienced nurses
3. Reading the literature and identifying gaps in knowledge and noting any discrepancies in the literature
4. Using a theoretical framework to guide problem identification
   a. 3 only
   b. 1, 2, & 3
   c. 3 & 4
   d. All of these

2. Once the research problem has been identified, it is essential to develop a research purpose. The research purpose is a clear, concise statement of the specific aim or intent or the study. The purpose of the study should include:
1. Variables that will be studied
2. Population of interest
3. Data analysis method
4. Data collection instrument
   a. 1 only
   b. 1, 2, & 3
   c. 1 & 2
   d. All of these

The purposes of a study may be to describe, explain, or predict a solution to the problem. Match each purpose of a study to the appropriate definition.

3. Descriptive

4. Explanatory

5. Predictive

a. Estimate the probability of a specific outcome in a given situation.
b. Identify the nature and attributes of the phenomenon.
c. Clarify relationships among variables or identify why certain events occur.

ANSWERS

1. APNs commonly identify clinical problems that need to be resolved. Various research skills or competencies are needed to address these problems. McGuire and Harwood (1996) have identified three research competencies for APNs: interpret and use research, evaluate practice, and conduct research (see Table 29-4). The first competency, interpret and use research, is also known as *research utilization* and was addressed in the first section of this chapter. The second and third competencies involve using data to evaluate nursing practice or to generate new knowledge; these are best achieved through collaboration with other researchers. APNs may progress to an advanced level, however, through additional experience, continuing education, and mentorship (Table 29-5).

TABLE 29-5	Overview of Advanced Nursing Practice Research Competencies and Levels of Activity	
COMPETENCY	**BASIC LEVEL**	**ADVANCED LEVEL**
Interpreting and using research	• Incorporate relevant research findings appropriately into own practice • Assist others to incorporate research into individual or unit practice	• Develop programmatic and/or departmental research utilization process
Evaluating practice	• Use existing data to evaluate nursing practice, individual, and/or aggregate • Collaborate in conduct of evaluation studies	• Identify and/or develop practice-specific package or outcome criteria • Lead the conduct of evaluation studies
Conducting research	• Participate in collaborative research	• Participate in independent research

From McGuire, D. B., & Harwood, K. V. (1996). Research interpretation, utilization, and conduct. In Hamric, A. B., Spross, J. A., & Hanson, C. M. (Eds.). *Advanced nursing practice: An integrative approach* (p. 191). Philadelphia: WB Saunders.

APNs are in an ideal position to identify clinical problems for research because of their knowledge and direct clinical experience. Once a problem has been identified, a review of the literature can assist in identifying gaps in knowledge and need for further study. Discussion with other experienced nurses and collaboration with a nurse researcher can assist in clearly defining the problem. Often, the use of a theoretical framework can provide direction for which variables are important in investigation of the problem (McCorkle, 1990). *Answer 1:* **d.**

2. The research purpose provides a clear, concise statement of the intent of the study (Burns & Grove, 1999). The purpose of the study should include the population to be studied, the variables, and possibly the setting.

The research purpose from Sarna and Chang's (2000) article "Colon cancer screening among older women caregivers" is given as an example:

> The purposes of this exploratory study were to describe the participation in colorectal cancer screening of older women who provide the primary caregiving for an ill spouse or parent, and to investigate the relationship of the caregiving burden and general health perceptions to participation in colorectal cancer screening (p. 110).

In this example, the purpose of the study provides information about the population to be studied—older women who provide primary caregiving for an ill spouse or parent—and the variables of interest—caregiving burden, general health perceptions, and colorectal cancer screening. In addition, Sarna and Chang (2000) state the intent of the study, which is to describe participation in colorectal cancer screening by older women who provide primary caregiving for an ill spouse or parent and to explain or clarify relationships among the variables of caregiving burden, general health perceptions, and participation in colorectal cancer screening. *Answer 2:* **c.**

3-5. Table 29-6 provides a definition of descriptive, explanatory, and predictive studies and presents an example of each type of study purpose as reported in the literature (Mast, 1998; Schwartz, 1998; Weinrich, Weinrich, Boyd, & Atkinson, 1998). *Answer 3:* **b.** *Answer 4:* **c.** *Answer 5:* **a.**

Case Study continued

Patricia conducted a literature review and found that little information was available about the health-related quality of life in adults with head and neck cancer who are receiving combined therapy. She decided to collaborate with the nurse researcher and begin to develop a research proposal. The nurse researcher discussed the nature of the research question with Patricia. They discussed the differences between quantitative and qualitative research methods and that the research question helps determine the best method to use.

TABLE 29-6	Definitions and Examples of Descriptive, Explanatory, and Predictive Studies
TYPE OF STUDY	**DEFINITION**	**EXAMPLE**
Descriptive: asks the question, What is this, or what is happening here?	Identify the nature and attributes of a phenomenon	This study will describe how cancer-related fatigue affects the exercise patterns of physically active individuals who received cancer treatment (Schwartz, 1998, p. 485).
Explanatory: asks the question, What is the relationship between...?	Clarify relationships among variables or identify why certain events occur	The purpose of this report is to examine correlates of fatigue, including the relationship of fatigue with illness uncertainty, for women 1 to 6 years after the completion of treatment for breast cancer (Mast, 1998, p. 136).
Predictive: asks the question, What will happen if...?	Estimate the probability of a specific outcome in a given situation	The present study sought to determine the level of knowledge about prostate cancer screening among a cohort of men in the southeast and to identify whether knowledge was a predictor for participation in a free prostate cancer screening opportunity (Weinrich, Weinrich, Boyd, & Atkinson, 1998, p. 527).

Data from Diers, D. (1979). *Research in nursing practice.* Philadelphia: JB Lippincott; and McCorkle, R. (1990). Development of the research question. In Grant, M. M., & Padilla, G. V. (Eds.). *Cancer nursing research: A practical approach* (pp. 27-42). Norwalk, CT: Appleton and Lange.

QUESTIONS

6. Patricia was interested in learning more about the differences in the research approaches. Provide a definition for *quantitative* and *qualitative research.*

7. There are various approaches to qualitative research. Which of the following types of qualitative research studies the meaning of lived experiences?

  a. Ethnographic research
  b. Grounded theory
  c. Phenomenologic research
  d. Historical research

ANSWERS

6. *Quantitative research* is a formal, objective, systematic process used to describe and test relationships and to examine the cause-and-effect relationships among variables. *Qualitative research* is a systematic, subjective approach used to describe life experiences (Burns & Grove, 1999). Fundamental differences exist between quantitative and qualitative research approaches, and these are listed in Table 29-7 (Lewis & Haberman, 1990; Munhall & Boyd, 1993). *Answer 6:* **See text.**

7. *Ethnographic research* studies issues related to culture. An example of an ethnographic study is provided by Beck (2000):

> The purpose of this study was to describe the cultural context of cancer pain management,

| TABLE 29-7 | Characteristics of Quantitative and Qualitative Research Approaches |

QUANTITATIVE RESEARCH	QUALITATIVE RESEARCH
Control is important	Fluidity is possible
Reductionistic	Holistic
Deductive reasoning	Inductive reasoning
Truth is absolute	Truth is dynamic
Objective approach and researcher remains detached from research	Subjective approach and researcher engaged in research
Prespecify theoretical framework	Theory development

Adapted from Burns, N., & Grove, S. K. (1995). *Student study guide for understanding nursing research.* Philadelphia: WB Saunders; Lewis, F. M., & Haberman, M. R. (1990). Selection of the research design. In Grant, M. M., & Padilla, G. V. (Eds.). *Cancer nursing research: A practical approach* (pp. 75-100). Norwalk, CT: Appleton and Lange; and Munhall, P. L., & Boyd, C. O. (1993). *Nursing research: A qualitative perspective.* New York: National League for Nursing Press.

summarize the factors (barriers and facilitators) influencing cancer pain management, and recommend actions to improve cancer pain management in South Africa (p. 92).

Grounded theory studies are based on symbolic interaction theory and focus on discovering basic social psychologic processes that occur in a particular social world. Through this mode of inquiry, a theory of social process is developed. An example of a grounded theory study is provided by Taylor (2000):

> The purpose of this study was to generate a descriptive theory about the process and outcomes of searching for positive meaning from the perspectives of women with breast cancer (p. 782).

Phenomenologic research is both a research method and a philosophy used to describe the lived experiences of individuals. An example of a phenomenologic study is provided by Cohen and Ley (2000):

> Phenomenologic philosophy guided this investigation of the experience of patients undergoing autologous bone marrow transplant to better understand the effect of this treatment on their lives and how nursing care can best meet their needs (p. 474).

Historical research studies the recent or remote past. By studying the past, researchers often gain insights into present and future issues and trends. *Answer 7:* **c.**

Case Study continued

Patricia decides to ask the question, "What is the health-related quality of life in adults receiving treatment for head and neck cancer?" She and the nurse researcher decide to use a quantitative research method. Patricia and the nurse researcher need to decide on a definition of *health-related quality of life.* They choose to use the definition proposed by Cella (1994; Cella, et al., 1993), which consists of distinct areas: physical, emotional, and social well-being. This definition helps guide selection of the most appropriate instrument. The nurse researcher explains that the way health-related quality of life is defined guides selection of the items that must be included in the assessment instrument. Therefore the Functional Assessment of Cancer Therapy (FACT) is chosen to measure health-related quality of life because this instrument matches the definition proposed in Patricia's study. The FACT is a standardized questionnaire that has been used extensively in adults with cancer. The internal consistency reliability has been established to be 0.89 for the entire scale. In addition, concurrent validity has been established.

QUESTIONS

8. What type of research study design would be best in this situation?
- **a.** Experimental
- **b.** Quasiexperimental
- **c.** Descriptive
- **d.** Correlational

9. The definition of *health-related quality of life* is known as which type of variable in the study?
- **a.** Conceptual variable
- **b.** Operational definition
- **c.** Independent variable
- **d.** Dependent variable

10. Reliability of an instrument is defined as:
- **a.** The ability to measure phenomena in a consistent manner
- **b.** An attempt to measure the underlying attribute of the instrument
- **c.** Being concerned with whether the items adequately represent the domain of interest
- **d.** Establishing the relationship between the instrument and another measure

11. What is the recommended internal consistency reliability for an established instrument used for group comparisons?
- **a.** 0.60
- **b.** 0.70
- **c.** 0.80
- **d.** 0.90

ANSWERS

8. Descriptive, correlational, quasiexperimental, and experimental study designs are among the most commonly used designs in nursing research. Descriptive and correlational study designs are nonexperimental research and involve natural observation of phenomena in field settings. These designs are used when the researchers want to gain a better understanding of what is happening and understand the relationships among the variables. In contrast, the researcher introduces a treatment in quasiexperimental and experimental research designs. The purpose of these designs is to gain an understanding of the *effect* of a treatment on an observed outcome. Three conditions are needed in experimental research: manipulation, control, and randomization (Polit &

Hungler, 1995). *Manipulation* means that the researcher introduces a treatment to at least one group of subjects. *Control* means that the researcher imposes some rules to decrease the chance of error and increase the chance that the results are attributable to the treatment. *Randomization* is when the subjects are assigned to the treatment or control group randomly. This means that the subjects have an equal chance of being assigned to either group. Experimental designs are the most powerful method to understand cause-and-effect relationships. It is not always possible, however, to use an experimental design. Sometimes, the researcher cannot tightly control the treatment or randomly assign subjects to the treatment. In this case, a quasiexperimental design may be used. Figure 29-1 provides an algorithm for determining the type of study design. *Answer 8:* **c.**

9. In the example provided, Patricia and the nurse researcher are not introducing a treatment. Although subjects are receiving combined treatment for their illness, Patricia and the nurse researcher did not introduce or manipulate this treatment. A descriptive design would be used because they want to gain an understanding of the health-related quality of life in adults receiving combined treatment for head and neck cancer, and they will not be examining relationships among variables. Table 29-8 provides definitions and examples of the various types of study variables. *Answer 9:* **a.**

10-11. It is important to select instruments that are reliable and valid. *Reliability* refers to the ability of an instrument to measure phenomena in a consistent manner. Two types of reliability are often studied: internal consistency and repeatability. *Internal consistency* refers to the degree that items within an instrument (or within distinct subscales) appear to measure the same attribute. *Repeatability,* or stability of the measurement from one time to another time, is the second type of reliability and is most commonly assessed by test-retest reliability. Selecting a time interval during which the phenomena are not expected to change is important when assessing for test-retest reliability (McCorkle, 1987). *Validity* refers to the ability of an instrument to measure the phenomena it is supposed to be measuring (Lynn, 1986). Three types of validity are commonly recognized: content, construct, and criterion (Polit & Hungler, 1995). *Content validity* is concerned with whether the items adequately represent the domain of the phenomena measured by the instrument and is usually the first step in constructing a new measure. *Construct validity* attempts to measure

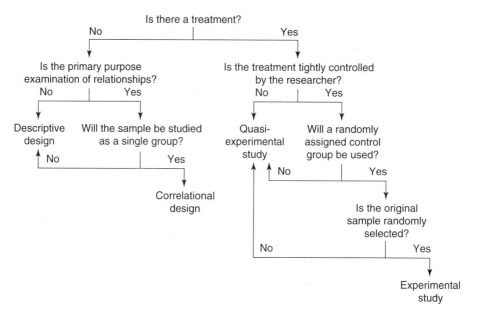

Figure 29-1 Algorithm for determining type of study design. (Modified from Burns, N., & Grove, S. K. [1999]. *Understanding nursing research* [p. 192]. Philadelphia: WB Saunders.)

TABLE 29-8	Definitions and Examples of Study Variables	
STUDY VARIABLE	**DEFINITION**	**EXAMPLE**
Conceptual	Provides the theoretical meaning of the concept or variable	*Health-related quality of life* is defined as physical, psychologic, functional, and social well-being.
Operational	Defines the procedure or way the concept or variable will be measured	Health-related quality of life will be measured by the FACT questionnaire.
Demographic	Characteristics of subjects gathered during data collection to describe the sample	Age, gender, marital status, income.
Independent	Variable thought to cause or influence the dependent variable; in experimental research, it is the treatment that is administered or manipulated by the researcher	McCorkle, Benoliel, Donaldson, et al. (1989) conducted a randomized clinical trial of home nursing care for lung cancer patients. Subjects were randomly assigned an oncology home care, home care, or office care (routine care) group. Subjects who received nursing care had less symptom distress and increased functional status for 6 wk longer than those who received office care only. Independent variable in this example is home nursing care.
Dependent	Variable thought to be influenced or caused by the independent variable; is the outcome variable of interest in a study	Dependent variable in the example provided above is symptom distress and functional status. Subjects who received home nursing care were observed to have less symptom distress and increased functional status for longer than those who did not receive this type of care.

Adapted from Burns, N., & Grove S. K. (1995). *Student study guide for understanding nursing research.* Philadelphia: WB Saunders; and Polit, D. F., & Hungler, B. F. (1995). *Nursing research: Principles and methods.* Philadelphia: JB Lippincott.

the underlying attribute (construct) of the instrument by assessing whether the measurement of one concept is logically related to another concept and behaves as expected (Frank-Stromberg & Olsen, 1997). *Criterion validity* is concerned with establishing the relationship between the instrument and another measure, usually a gold standard because it has been used successfully in the field (Polit & Hungler, 1995; Streiner & Norman, 1995). Cronbach's alpha is the most common method of measuring internal consistency. The recommended Cronbach alpha for an instrument depends on the use of the instrument. A Cronbach alpha of 0.70 is sufficient if the instrument is used to make group-level comparisons. If the data are used to make decisions about individuals, a Cronbach alpha of at least 0.90 is recommended (Nunnally & Bernstein, 1994; Polit & Hungler, 1995). A reliability of 0.80 is desirable for a well-developed instrument (Burns & Grove, 1999). *Answer 10:* **a.** *Answer 11:* **b.**

Case Study continued

Patricia and the nurse researcher discuss sampling criteria and the need to develop a sampling plan. They decide that they will approach all potential patients who are eligible to participate in the study. Patricia points out that the oncologist who is coordinating the clinical trial also admits patients to a nearby hospital. Patricia and the nurse researcher decide that it would be a good idea to discuss the potential study with the oncologist so that they can gather support for the study, coordinate efforts, and perhaps have access to a larger study population. The oncologist who is coordinating the study is enthusiastic about adding a health-related quality-of-life aspect to the ongoing study. Patricia and the nurse researcher discuss the benefits of conducting a pilot study before they piggyback the health-related quality-of-life study onto the larger clinical trial.

QUESTIONS

12. Sampling criteria would include:
1. Inclusion criteria
2. Exclusion criteria
3. Power analysis
4. Number of variables that will be used in the study
   a. 1 only
   b. 1 & 2
   c. 1, 2, & 3
   d. All of these

13. What type of sampling plan have Patricia and the nurse researcher proposed for the study?
a. Random
b. Convenience
c. Purposive
d. Network or snowball

14. The reasons for conducting a pilot study include:
1. Determining whether the proposed study is feasible
2. Refining the data collection plan
3. Clarifying relationships among variables
4. Estimating the probability of a specific outcome
   a. 1 only
   b. 1 & 2
   c. 1, 2, & 3
   d. All of these

ANSWERS

12. Sampling criteria define the characteristics that are essential for subjects' inclusion in the study (inclusion criteria) or exclusion from the study (exclusion criteria) (Burns & Grove, 1999). Once sampling criteria are established and each member or element of the accessible population is identified, a sampling plan is identified. *Answer 12:* **b.**

13. Sampling plans can be grouped into two major categories: probability and nonprobability. Probability sampling involves some form of random selection for choosing who will be included in the study, whereas nonprobability sampling involves nonrandom selection (Burns & Grove, 1999; Polit & Hungler, 1995). Random selection means that each member or element in the population has an equal chance of being selected for inclusion into the study. Simple random, stratified random, cluster, and systematic sampling are the four types of random sampling. Nonprobability sampling, however, is the most common type of sampling used in both medicine and nursing. The various types of nonprobability sampling are convenience, network (or snowball), quota, and purposive. Because nonprobability sampling techniques are used more often, each type is defined here. Convenience sampling is the use of the most readily available subjects for the study; this is the type of sampling that Patricia and the nurse researcher will use for their study. This type of sampling is inexpensive and requires less time than other methods. Snowball sampling is often used when the targeted research population has characteristics that may be difficult to identify by ordinary means. In this situation, the researcher may ask other subjects in the study to identify other people that they know who would meet the designated study criteria. This type of sampling is often used to identify populations that may be difficult to access, such as women with tattoos. Quota sampling is similar to convenience sampling except the researcher identities characteristics and proportions of elements needed from the various segments of the population. For example, the researcher may preselect how many females and/or racial minorities will be included in the study. This type of sampling helps ensure that certain types of subjects will be adequately represented. In purposive sampling, the researcher consciously selects subjects for inclusion into the study. It is important to recognize that inherent differences are involved when using a quantitative or qualitative research approach (Munhall & Boyd, 1993). Qualitative studies use the term *participant* when referring to people involved in a study. Also, nonprobability sampling methods, such as purposive or snowball sampling, are preferred, and sample sizes are usually smaller in qualitative studies (Sandelowski, 1995). *Answer 13:* **b.**

14. Pilot studies are a smaller version of the study. Pilot studies are useful because they help the researchers obtain information about whether the project is feasible and whether any revisions are needed in the data collection plan and/or the questionnaires and other instruments (Polit & Hungler, 1995). *Answer 14:* **b.**

Case Study continued

So far, Patricia and the nurse researcher have decided the research question, the design of the study, the questionnaire that will be used to measure quality of life, and the sampling plan. The next step is to determine the frequency of data collection, the organization of the data, and type of analysis. They decide to collect data at several time points: before starting treatment, before starting a second treatment (3 to 4 weeks after baseline), before starting a third treatment (6 to 8 weeks after baseline), and 3 months later. Data collection times were based on information that was available in the literature and within the time constraints for survival of the population being studied. Various demographic, clinical, and social variables, such as age, race, gender, type of cancer, stage of cancer, marital status, and income, will be collected so that Patricia and the nurse researcher can describe the characteristics of the sample group.

QUESTIONS

15. Gender is considered what type of measurement variable?
   a. Nominal
   b. Ordinal
   c. Interval
   d. Ratio

16. In the description of the data, Patricia and the nurse researcher would want to report age of the subjects in the study. A measure of central tendency would be used. Which of the following would be best to describe age of the subjects in the sample?
   a. Mean
   b. Mode
   c. Median
   d. Chi-square

17. When describing age, measures of dispersion or variability are also reported. Which of the following measures of dispersion would be best to describe age of the sample?
   a. Range
   b. Standard deviation
   c. Scatterplot
   d. Histogram

ANSWERS

15. To obtain data for quantitative research, the characteristics of people, events, and/or objects must be measured. Stevens (1946) defines *measurement* as "the assignment of numerals to objects or events according to rules." Four types or levels of measurement have been identified: nominal, ordinal, interval, and ratio. Table 29-9 defines each type of measurement and provides an example.

Knowledge of the level of measurement helps the researcher decide how to organize and display data and which statistical tests would be most appropriate to use for analysis (Munro & Page, 1993). *Answer 15:* **a.**

16. The mean, mode, and median (also known as the *average*) are measures of central tendency. These measures tell us where the values for the distribution of the variable cluster. The mean is the most commonly used measure of central tendency and is obtained by adding all of the numbers and then dividing the sum by the number of scores or subjects. The mode is the number or score that occurs most frequently, but it does not necessarily indicate the center of the data. The median is the exact center of the data set distribution; if there are an odd number of data, the median

TABLE 29-9 Levels of Measurement

LEVEL OF MEASUREMENT	DEFINITION	EXAMPLE
Nominal	Assign characteristics into numerical categories. The numbers assigned, however, do not have any meaning. It is not possible to rank, add, or subtract numbers.	Gender 1 = male 2 = female
Ordinal	Assign and order the variables along some continuum. Distance between categories is not known. It is possible to rank order the characteristics.	Income level 1 = low 2 = medium 3 = high
Interval	Attribute of variable is rank ordered on a scale that has equal distances between points on the scale. The zero point on the scale is unknown. It is possible to add and subtract across this type of scale.	Fahrenheit thermometer
Ratio	Attribute of a variable is measured, and there are equal distances between points on the scale and a true zero point. It is possible to add, subtract, multiply, and divide across this type of scale.	Weight Blood pressure

Adapted from Kerlinger, F. N. (1986). *Foundations of behavioral research*, 3rd ed. Fort Worth, TX: Harcourt Brace Jovanovich; and Munro, B. H., & Page, E. B. (1993). *Statistical methods for health care research*, 2nd ed. Philadelphia: WB Saunders.

is the exact middle, whereas in the case of an even number of data, the two middle numbers are added and then divided by 2. The mean is usually used to report age of subjects in a study. *Answer 16:* **a.**

17. Another important concept when considering measures of central tendency is the variability of the data, or how spread out the data are. Common measures of variability are the range and the standard deviation (Munro & Page, 1993). The *range* is the difference between the maximal and minimal value of the distribution. It is usually reported by providing information about the minimal and maximal values in the data set; this would be the most appropriate way to report the dispersion or variability of age in the study. *Answer 17:* **a.**

Case Study continued

Patricia and the nurse researcher are preparing the final proposal. An important step is to make sure that the rights of human subjects are safeguarded and that informed consent is obtained from all subjects before they participate in the study.

QUESTIONS

18. What committee has been established to review ethical concerns related to research studies?
- **a.** Quality assurance
- **b.** Nursing credentialing committee
- **c.** Medical review board
- **d.** Institutional review board

19. Which of the following definitions best describes informed consent?
- **a.** Agreement by prospective subject to voluntarily participate in research after he or she has assimilated essential information about the study
- **b.** Condition in which the subject's identity cannot be linked by his or her individual responses
- **c.** Freedom of the individual to determine the time, extent, and general circumstances under which private information will be shared with others or withheld
- **d.** Principles of respect for persons, beneficence, and justice that are relevant to the conduct of research

20. Which of the following are considered components of informed consent?
1. Disclosure of study information to the subject
2. Comprehension of the information by the subject
3. Competency of the individual to give consent
4. Voluntary consent by the individual to participate in research
- **a.** 4 only
- **b.** 1 & 4
- **c.** 1, 2, & 4
- **d.** All of these

TABLE 29-10 Definition of Common Concepts Used in Protecting Rights of Human Subjects

CONCEPT USED TO PROTECT HUMAN RIGHTS	DEFINITION
Anonymity	Condition by which the subject's identity cannot be linked by his or her individual responses
Benefit:risk ratio	Ratio considered by researchers and reviewers as they weigh the potential benefits and risks in a study
Confidentiality	Management of data in research in such a way that subject responses are not linked with their responses
Ethical principles	Principles of respect for persons, beneficence, and justice that are relevant to the conduct of research
Privacy	Freedom of an individual to determine the time, extent, and general circumstances under which private information will be shared with or withheld from others

Adapted from Burns, N., & Grove, S. K. (1999). *Understanding nursing research*, 2nd ed. Philadelphia: WB Saunders.

TABLE 29-11 Rights of Research Subjects

The following rights are the rights of every person who is asked to be in a research study:
• To be told what the study is trying to find out
• To be told what will happen to me and whether any of the procedures, drugs, or devices is different than would be used in standard practice
• To be told about the frequent or important risks, side effects, or discomforts of the things that will happen to me for research purposes
• To be told if I can expect any benefit from participating, and if so, what the benefit might be
• To be told of other choices I have and how they may be better or worse than being in the study
• To be allowed to ask any questions concerning the study both before agreeing to be involved and in the course of the study
• To be told what sort of medical treatment is available if any complications arise
• To refuse to participate at all or to change my mind about participation after the study is started; the decision will not affect my right to receive the care I would receive if I were not in the study
• To receive a copy of the signed and dated consent
• To be free of pressure when considering whether I wish to agree to be in the study

From Anderson, P. (1990). Strategies for project implementation. In Grant, M. M., & Padilla, G. V. (Eds.). *Cancer nursing research: A practical approach* (p. 187). Norwalk, CT: Appleton and Lange.

ANSWERS

18. It is important for APNs to be aware of the ethical arena of research. Important aspects of ethical research include making sure that subjects rights are protected, that benefits and risks of a study are balanced, that informed consent has been obtained, and if institutional review is needed within your institution, that it has been obtained (Burns & Grove, 1999). An institutional review board (IRB) is a committee of peers established to review research and determine whether rights and welfare of subjects are protected, whether methods to obtain informed consent are appropriate, and whether the potential benefits of the study are greater than the risks (Martin, 1996). Table 29-10 provides definitions of common terms that are important in protecting the rights of subjects in research. Table 29-11 provides information about the bill of rights for individuals who participate in research. *Answer 18:* **d.**

19-20. Informed consent is agreement by the potential subject to participate in the research after having had a chance to assimilate information about the study. Informed consent consists of four related but distinct components: provision of information to the potential subject about the study, comprehension of the information about the study by the subject, competency of the subject to give consent, and voluntary consent by the subject to participate in the research (Burns & Grove, 1999). *Answer 19:* **a.** *Answer 20:* **d.**

REFERENCES

Anderson, P. (1990). Strategies for project implementation. In Grant, M. M., & Padilla, G. V. (Eds.). *Cancer nursing research: A practical approach* (pp. 175-192). Norwalk, CT: Appleton and Lange.

Barnard, K. E. (1986). Research utilization: The clinician's role. *MCN Am J Matern Child Nurs, 11*(3), p. 224.

Beck, S. L. (2000). An ethnographic study of factors influencing cancer pain management in South Africa. *Cancer Nurs, 23*, pp. 91-99.

Burns, N., & Grove, S. K. (1995). *Student study guide for understanding nursing research*. Philadelphia: WB Saunders.

Burns, N., & Grove, S. K. (1999). *Understanding nursing research*, 2nd ed. Philadelphia: WB Saunders.

Cella, D. F. (1994). Quality of life: Concepts and definitions. *J Pain Sympt Manage, 9*, pp. 186-192.

Cella, D. F., Tulsky, D. S., Gray, G., et al. (1993). The functional assessment of cancer therapy scale: Development and validation of the general measure. *J Clin Oncol, 11*, pp. 570-579.

Cohen, M. Z., & Ley, C. D. (2000). Bone marrow transplantation: The battle for hope in the face of fear. *Oncol Nurs Forum, 27*, pp. 473-480.

Cronenwett, L. R. (1995). Effective methods for disseminating research findings to nurses in practice. *Nurs Clin North Am, 30*, pp. 429-438.

Diers, D. (1979). *Research in nursing practice*. Philadelphia: Lippincott.

Donaldson, N. E. (1992). If not now, then when? Nursing's research utilization imperative. State of the Art Paper. *Communicating Nurs Res, 25*, pp. 29-44.

Frank-Stromberg, M., & Olsen, S. (1997). *Instruments for clinical health care research*. Boston: Jones and Bartlett.

Funk, S., Tornquist, E. M., & Champagne, M. T. (1995). Barriers and facilitators of research utilization. An integrative review. *Nurs Clin North Am, 30*, pp. 395-407.

Funk, S. G., Tornquist, E. M., & Champagne, M. T. (1989). A model for improving the dissemination of nursing research. *West J Nurs Res, 11*(3), pp. 361-367.

Horsley, J., Crane, J., Crabtree, M., & Wood, D. (1983). *Using research to improve nursing practice: A guide*. New York: Grune & Stratton.

Kerlinger, F. N. (1986). *Foundations of behavioral research*, 3rd ed. Fort Worth: Harcourt Brace Jovanovich College Publishers.

Lewis, F. M., & Haberman, M. R. (1990). Selection of the research design. In Grant, M. M., & Padilla, G. V. (Eds.). *Cancer nursing research: A practical approach* (pp. 75-100). Norwalk, CT: Appleton and Lange.

Lynn, M. R. (1986). Determination and quantification of content validity. *Nurs Res, 35*, pp. 382-385.

Madigan, E. A. (1998). Evidence-based practice in home healthcare: A springboard for discussion. *Home Healthcare Nurse, 16*(6), pp. 411-415.

Martin, P. A. (1996). Member responsibilities on a nursing research committee. *Appl Nurs Res, 9*, pp. 153-157.

Mast, M. E. (1998). Correlates of fatigue in survivors of breast cancer. *Cancer Nurs, 21*, pp. 136-142.

McCorkle, R. (1990). Development of the research question. In Grant, M. M., & Padilla, G. V. (Eds.). *Cancer nursing research: A practical approach* (pp. 27-42). Norwalk, CT: Appleton and Lange.

McCorkle, R. (1987). The measurement of symptom distress. *Semin Oncol Nurs, 3*, pp. 248-256.

McCorkle, R., Benoliel, J. Q., Donaldson, G., et al. (1989). A randomized clinical trial of home nursing care for lung cancer patients. *Cancer, 64*, pp. 199-206.

McGuire, D. B., & Harwood, K. V. (1996). Research interpretation, utilization, and conduct. In Hamric, A. B., Spross, J. A., & Hanson, C. M. (Eds.). *Advanced nursing practice: An integrative approach* (pp. 184-212). Philadelphia: WB Saunders.

Munhall, P. L., & Boyd, C. O. (1993). *Nursing research: A qualitative perspective*. New York: National League for Nursing Press.

Munro, B. H., & Page, E. B. (1993*). Statistical methods for health care research*, 2nd ed. Philadelphia: WB Saunders.

Nunnally, J. C., & Bernstein, I. H. (1994). *Psychometric theory*, 3rd ed. New York: McGraw-Hill.

Polit, D. F., & Hungler, B. F. (1995). *Nursing research: Principles and methods*. Philadelphia: JB Lippincott.

Rogers, E. M. (1983). *Diffusion of innovations*. New York: Free Press.

Rutledge, D. N. (1995). Research utilization in oncology nursing. *Oncol Nurs, 4*(2), pp. 1-14.

Rutledge, D. N., & Donaldson, N. E. (1995). Building organizational mechanisms for research utilization. *J Nurs Admin, 25*(10), pp. 12-16.

Rutledge, D. N., Ropka, M., Greene, P. E., et al. (1998). Barriers to research utilization for oncology staff nurses and nurse managers/clinical nurse specialists. *Oncol Nurs Forum, 25*(3), pp. 497-506.

Sackett, D. L., Rosenberg, W. M. C., Gray, J. A. M., et al. (1996). Evidence based medicine: what it is and what it isn't. *Br Med J, 312*, pp. 71-72.

Sandelowski, M. (1995). Sample size in qualitative research. *Res Nurs Health, 18*, pp. 179-183.

Sarna, L., & Chang, B. L. (2000). Colon cancer screening among older women caregivers. *Cancer Nurs, 23*, pp. 109-116.

Schwartz, A. L. (1998). Patterns of exercise and fatigue in physically active cancer survivors. *Oncol Nurs Forum, 25*, pp. 485-496.

Stetler, C. B. (1994). Refinement of the Stetler/Marram model for application of research findings to practice. *Nurs Outlook, 42*(1), pp. 15-25.

Stetler, C. B., Morsi, D., Rucki, S., et al. (1998). Utilization-focused integrative reviews in a nursing service. *Appl Nurs Res, 11*(4), pp. 195-206.

Stevens, S. S. (1946). On the theory of scales of measurement. *Science, 103*, pp. 677-680.

Taylor, E. J. (2000). Transformation of tragedy among women surviving breast cancer. *Oncol Nurs Forum, 27*, pp. 781-788.

Titler, M. G., Kleiber, C., Steelman, V., et al. (1994). Infusing research into practice to promote quality care. *Nurs Res, 43*, pp. 307-313.

White, J. M., Leske, J. S., & Pearcy, J. M. (1995). Models and processes of research utilization. *Nurs Clin North Am, 30*(3), pp. 409-420.

Weinrich, S. P., Weinrich, M. C., Boyd, M. D., & Atkinson, C. (1998). The impact of prostate cancer knowledge on cancer screening. *Oncol Nurs Forum, 25*, pp. 527- 534.

30 Educator Role

Jeanne Erickson

CASE 1 STUDY

STAFF DEVELOPMENT: AN ORIENTATION PROGRAM

In your advanced practice nurse (APN) role, you are responsible for the orientation of six new staff nurses who will work on the oncology unit. Two of the new staff nurses are recent graduate nurses, and two are nurses who have worked on general medical and surgical units in the same hospital for approximately 1 year. The remaining two nurses have worked in oncology for an average of 18 months in other settings. Your unit orientation program will cover principles of oncology nursing, including intravenous (IV) therapy and venous access devices, transfusion therapy, symptom management, and chemotherapy administration.

QUESTIONS

1. Orientation for new staff nurses is divided into centralized and decentralized content. What content belongs in the centralized orientation program for all nurses who are new to your institution?
   1. Patient population served at the institution
   2. Personnel and employment policies
   3. Medication administration policies and procedures
   4. Universal precautions and infection control policies
   a. 1 & 2
   b. 1, 2, & 4
   c. 2, 3, & 4
   d. All of these

ANSWERS

1. Orientation for new nursing staff is one of the most critical activities implemented in a health care setting. If orientation is a positive learning experience for new staff members, it can enhance retention, future recruitment, staff morale, and quality of care on the unit. The APN often has a position with responsibility for the orientation

process, either at the centralized organizational level or at the decentralized, or specialty, level. *Answer 1:* **d.**

QUESTIONS

2. You decide to use a preceptor-based program for your unit-based orientation because you believe it has many benefits. Which of the following are true of preceptor programs?
   1. Preceptors have a formal and long-term relationship with the orientee.
   2. Precepting is usually a one-to-one relationship; the orientee is less likely to "feel lost" on the unit.
   3. Preceptors can provide accurate and ongoing evaluation of the orientee's progress.
   4. Preceptors are often motivated to maintain and upgrade their own clinical skills and knowledge.
   a. 1 & 2
   b. 1, 2, & 3
   c. 2, 3, & 4
   d. All of these

3. List at least three criteria that you would use to select staff nurses to be preceptors.

ANSWERS

2. The preceptor method has become a popular and effective method of orientation in the recent past (Abruzzese & Quinn-O'Neal, 1996; Giles & Moran, 1989; Mackin & Studva, 1997). Precepting is a one-to-one, short-term, contractual, and formal relationship between an experienced practitioner and a neophyte. The preceptor serves as a teacher to provide the orientee with the clinical experiences necessary to acquire the knowledge and skills to be a competent practitioner.

The APN can have many roles in a preceptor program. The APN may function as a preceptor but may also serve to coordinate preceptor selection and training, to develop orientation goals and objectives, and to participate in the appraisal process with the orientee, preceptor, and manager. *Answer 2:* **c.**

3. Many factors must be considered when choosing nurse preceptors. Nurses chosen as preceptors must have considerable experience and expertise in their specialty and show a commitment to professional development. They should demonstrate a higher level of communication, organization, and interpersonal skills. Effective preceptors are sensitive to others' feelings and cultural differences, and they create a supportive environment for learning. Last, but not least, nurses should be chosen as preceptors because of their willingness and interest to teach (O'Mara, 1997). *Answer 3:* **See text.**

Case Study continued

You review the performance and qualifications of the 25 nurses who work on the oncology unit, and you consider the Dreyfuss Model of skill acquisition, as applied by Benner (1984) to the nursing profession.

QUESTIONS

Match each level of proficiency with key aspects of performance at that level.

4. Novice

5. Advanced beginner

6. Competent

7. Proficient

8. Expert

    a. Anticipates events and modifies plans in response to each situation

    b. Has intuitive grasp of each situation

    c. Uses experience to note important aspects of each situation and is learning to prioritize

    d. Performs rule-governed behaviors that are often limited and inflexible

    e. Has mastery of skills and makes deliberate plans, including long-range goals

9. You choose and assign preceptors based on which of Benner's suggestions (1984)?
    1. Competent nurses may be appropriate as preceptors for new graduate nurses.
    2. Advanced beginners may be appropriate as preceptors for new graduate nurses.
    3. Proficient and expert nurses are preferred as preceptors for experienced new employees.

    4. Only proficient and expert nurses should be chosen as preceptors.
    a. 1 & 3
    b. 1, 2, & 3
    c. 2 & 3
    d. 4 only

ANSWERS

4-8. A nurse's expertise may be interpreted using Benner's five levels of clinical nursing practice (Table 30-1). New employees are likely to be at the novice or advanced beginner levels, whereas nurses who have been in a consistent practice situation for 2 to 3 years are likely to be at the competent level. Proficient and expert nurses have extensive experience. *Answer 4:* **d.** *Answer 5:* **c.** *Answer 6:* **e.** *Answer 7:* **a.** *Answer 8:* **b.**

9. Competent nurses are often ideal preceptors for novice and advanced beginners because they are likely to remember their own learning experience and are able to teach decision making based on objective data. Proficient and expert nurses may have already forgotten steps and cues necessary for a beginning level of practice and may not relate as well to entry-level orientees. Proficient and expert nurses are better used as preceptors for competent or experienced nurses (Avillion & Abruzzese, 1996). *Answer 9:* **a.**

Case Study continued

You choose a group of six nurses to act as preceptors. You schedule a 1-day seminar for preceptors to cover content that you believe is important to the success of the preceptor role.

TABLE 30-1	Benner's Concepts of Practice Levels
LEVEL	**CHARACTERISTICS**
Novice	Has little or no experience and knowledge; performs rule-governed behavior
Advanced beginner	Has minimal experience but able to integrate guidelines; unable to prioritize
Competent	Has mastery of skills; practices with deliberate planning
Proficient	Perceives whole situation and anticipates events
Expert	Intuitively grasps situation and identifies critical areas

From Benner, P. (1984). *From novice to expert: Excellence and power in clinical nursing practice.* Menlo Park, CA: Addison-Wesley.

10. Which of the following topics would be appropriate to include in the preceptor workshop?

1. Principles of adult learning
2. Strategies to promote critical thinking skills
3. Methods to evaluate learning
4. Group process skills

   a. 1, 2, & 3
   b. 1, 3, & 4
   c. 1 & 4
   d. All of these

ANSWERS

10. Preceptors require support to be effective in their teaching role. An initial workshop for preceptors should include an overview of the preceptor program as well as preceptor responsibilities. Other content can include principles of adult learning, individualized teaching strategies, the importance of giving feedback, and performance evaluation (O'Mara, 1997). *Answer 10:* **a.**

Case Study continued

You develop learning objectives and competencies for the clinical orientation and discuss them with the preceptor group.

QUESTIONS

11. Which of the following principles should guide you when writing these goals?

1. Clinical objectives are broad statements that will help preceptors select specific learning strategies.
2. Competencies outline specific actions needed to perform a particular task.
3. Objectives can address knowledge, attitudes, and skills.
4. The objectives should be flexible so that the new staff can have some input into what will be learned.

   a. 1 & 2
   b. 1, 2, & 3
   c. 2 & 3
   d. All of these

Educational objectives can be ordered into a hierarchy, in which higher-level objectives involve more complex behaviors and build on the lower-level objectives. The cognitive domain can be divided into six categories, ranging from simple to complex behaviors. List the six categories of cognitive domains in order of increasing complexity.

12.

13.

14.

15.

16.

17.

a. Analysis
b. Evaluation
c. Knowledge
d. Synthesis
e. Comprehension
f. Application

18. Which educational objectives are the most difficult to measure and evaluate?

   a. Cognitive
   b. Psychomotor
   c. Affective

ANSWERS

11. Clinical objectives specify what cognitive, affective, and psychomotor learning will be the focus for the educational program. *Cognitive* learning is the acquisition of knowledge and concepts. *Affective* learning is the acquisition of new values and attitudes. *Psychomotor* learning is gaining specific skills necessary to complete a task. *Clinical objectives* are broad statements that outline the content to be learned. *Competencies* are specific abilities to be demonstrated by the learner and may be broken down into even more specific performance criteria (Gaberson & Oermann, 1999a). *Answer 11:* **d.**

12-17. A hierarchy for educational objectives may be helpful when considering levels of complexity in clinical learning (Itano, 1987). Taxonomies for proposed levels of cognitive, affective, and psychomotor domains of learning are outlined in Table 30-2. *Answer 12:* **c.** *Answer 13:* **e.** *Answer 14:* **f.** *Answer 15:* **a.** *Answer 16:* **d.** *Answer 17:* **b.**

18. Objectives for clinical practice should be discussed with the preceptors to be sure they are valid and measurable. Preceptors should be clear about what behaviors the orientee needs to demonstrate to meet the objective. Affective behaviors are the most difficult to evaluate because they often express attitudes, values, and interests (Itano, 1987). *Answer 18:* **c.**

QUESTIONS

19. The new staff nurses represent a diverse group of individuals, with varied backgrounds and life experiences. Which strategy would best determine the learning needs of this diverse group?

TABLE **30-2** **Taxonomy of Educational Objectives**

DOMAIN	LEVEL	DEFINITION
Cognitive	Knowledge	Recalls previous material
	Comprehension	Grasps meaning of material
	Application	Uses new material in a new situation
	Analysis	Breaks down material into components and understands structure
	Synthesis	Puts components together to form a whole
	Evaluation	Judges the value of material based on defined criteria
Affective	Receiving	Is aware of and listens to new information
	Responding	Actively reacts to a phenomenon
	Valuing	Attaches value to a phenomenon or behavior
	Organization	Concerned about the relationships between values
	Characterization by a value	Holds value system that controls behavior
Psychomotor	Imitation	Begins crude and imperfect form of skill after observation
	Manipulation	Practices to improve performance
	Precision	Performs refined, accurate skill
	Articulation	Efficiently coordinates skill with other activities
	Naturalization	Automatically proficient on cue

From Reilly, D. E., & Oermann, M. H. (1992a). *Clinical teaching in nursing education*, 2nd ed. New York: National League for Nursing.

a. Review the clinical objectives for orientation with them and ask if they have questions
b. Ask them what knowledge, skills, and attitudes they believe they need to learn to be a competent nurse on this unit
c. Conduct a written pretest to determine their current level of knowledge
d. Ask them to introduce themselves and describe their nursing experience

ANSWERS

19. The program coordinator must also assess the learning needs of the orientees, including their current level of knowledge and experience, as well as other characteristics that will influence their learning (Gianella, 1996). It is likely that the group of orientees will represent diverse cultural backgrounds and learning styles that must be taken into consideration. In addition, this group might also have personal experiences that will influence how they view new content, such as having a family member with a new diagnosis of cancer or past involvement with end-of-life issues. Asking for input from the orientees with regard to clinical objectives, learning opportunities, skills, values, and attitudes can give important information about the learning needs of the group to verify that the proposed objectives and learning experiences are planned at the appropriate level. An important principle of adult learning is that learners learn best if they par-

ticipate fully in the learning experience (Manley, 1997). *Answer 19:* **b.**

QUESTIONS

20. You discuss with the preceptor group what teaching methods are appropriate to use to achieve the orientation objectives. Preceptors should choose teaching activities that are:
a. Based on the preceptor's interest and skills
b. Consistent throughout the orientation period
c. Based on the orientee's level of ability and experience
d. Based on the resources of the clinical setting

21. You collaborate with the nurse manager and the preceptor group to develop a comprehensive orientation skills checklist. The skills checklist is a critical tool for your unit because it:
1. Will document the orientee's progress
2. Provides evidence of staff competency to meet the Joint Commission on Accreditation of Healthcare Organizations (JCAHO) requirements
3. Will define accurate and current competency requirements on the unit
4. Can be used to plan unit continuing education activities
a. 2 & 3
b. 1 & 4
c. 1, 2, & 3
d. All of these

22. You meet with the nurse manager to decide whether to develop a lecture or a self-learning module to meet the learning objectives related to documentation. Which of the following statements are *true* about these teaching strategies?

1. A lecture efficiently provides information to the entire group.
2. In a lecture, educators can reinforce important information and correct misinformation.
3. Self-learning modules require additional time for educators to develop.
4. Self-learning modules offer more flexibility to educators and learners.
    a. 1, 2, & 3
    b. 2 & 3
    c. 1 & 4
    d. All of these

23. The preceptors decide to use computer-assisted instruction (CAI) to meet some of the objectives related to IV therapy. The advantages of this teaching method include all the following *except:*
    a. CAI provides individualized instruction.
    b. CAI can be appropriate for all levels of learning, from basic to mastery.
    c. CAI is time-efficient and cost-effective.
    d. CAI can address cognitive, affective, and psychomotor objectives.

24. The orientation program contains learning objectives related to symptom management. To develop critical thinking abilities of new orientees in this area, you suggest that preceptors may want to:
    a. Use a multiple-choice posttest
    b. Discuss typical scenarios
    c. Develop a self-learning packet
    d. Use return demonstrations

25. You observe a preceptor discussing a packed red blood cell (PRBC) transfusion procedure with a new staff nurse. Which question does not reflect a question to evaluate higher-level critical thinking skills?
    a. What are the types of transfusion reactions you will watch for?
    b. How much of a temperature increase would define a febrile transfusion reaction?
    c. How will you assess the effectiveness of the PRBC transfusion for your patient?
    d. In what sequence should we administer this blood transfusion and the IV antibiotics?

ANSWERS

20. JCAHO requires documentation of an employee's competency to practice. The essential elements of competent practice must be identified for each practice setting, and these elements form the basis for the learning needs of new employees. An orientation checklist should be developed to document the orientee's progress. The checklist can also be used as a basis for annual competency validation, as defined by the organization, as well as a tool to plan future continuing educational activities. *Answer 20:* **c.**

21. The APN should guide the preceptors to use a variety of teaching strategies. The differences in learners, teachers, clinical settings, and clinical objectives require that a variety of teaching methods be used. The choice of a teaching method is based on a variety of criteria, including the content of the objective, appropriateness for the learner's ability, compatibility with the teacher's skill, and availability of resources. A flexible learning environment that offers learners a choice of strategies for learning would be ideal. Box 30-1 lists examples of teaching strategies. *Answer 21:* **d.**

22. Clinical teaching strategies commonly used on the unit include role modeling, demonstration, and questioning. Learning activities may also be self-directed, such as a self-instructional manual or CAI. These methods have the advantages of allowing learners at any level to proceed at their own pace and providing educators flexibility with other projects while learners are learning. However, self-instructional modules require more time for development and do not allow educators to verbally reinforce material or immediately address concerns. *Answer 22:* **d.**

BOX 30-1	Teaching and Learning Strategies

Case study discussions
Computer-assisted instructions
Demonstrations
Games and simulations
Lectures
Programmed instructions
Role modeling
Questioning
Seminars and symposiums

From Gianella, A. (1996). Effective teaching and learning strategies for adults. In Abruzzese, R. S. (Ed.). *Nursing staff development: Strategies for success,* 2nd ed. (pp. 223-241). St. Louis: Mosby.

23. CAI has become a popular learning tool. It can cover a wide variety of content, including psychomotor skills, value concepts, and application of concepts to a clinical setting. Cost is one potential disadvantage of CAI and other multimedia products. Computer hardware and software programs are expensive, and using these resources for a large group of learners is often impractical or not time-efficient (David & Dowling, 1995). *Answer 23:* **c.**

24-25. As educators, preceptors should be competent to infuse critical thinking skills into all learning experiences (Avillion & Abruzzese, 1996). Experiential learning, such as case study scenarios and critical incident techniques, are useful to encourage critical thinking. Preceptors should strive to ask thought-provoking questions to elicit higher-level thinking skills, which test more than recall of factual information and focus on the learner's problem-solving, decision-making, and clinical judgment skills (Oermann, 1997). *Answer 24:* **b.** *Answer 25:* **d.**

QUESTIONS

26. Your chemotherapy competency module is based on the *ONS Cancer Chemotherapy Guidelines and Recommendations for Practice,* which includes a self-learning didactic component and a clinical practicum component. What will be an effective measure of the knowledge obtained in the didactic component?
   a. Multiple-choice pretests and posttests
   b. A skills checklist
   c. Performance appraisal
   d. Skills simulation

27. To pass the age-based competency module developed to meet JCAHO requirements in your organization, nurses must pass a multiple-choice test with an 85% minimum score. This is an example of:
   a. A norm-referenced evaluation
   b. A criterion-referenced evaluation

28. You plan weekly group evaluation sessions with the new staff during the orientation period to discuss their progress, answer their questions, and make any revisions in the orientation schedule. This is an example of:
   a. Summative evaluation
   b. Formative evaluation
   c. Structured evaluation
   d. Clinical performance evaluation

29. You ask preceptors to document clinical examples of how each new staff nurse has met

each clinical objective. Orientation will be completed when each clinical objective is met. This is an example of:
   a. Summative evaluation
   b. Formative evaluation
   c. Structured evaluation
   d. Process evaluation

ANSWERS

26. Evaluation of the teaching process tracks progress toward meeting the learning objectives of the educational program. Evaluation strategies, such as tests, performance checklists, and return demonstrations, need to be chosen to match the learning objectives and should be planned into the program. For example, administering a multiple-choice posttest is a common way to measure whether the learner has met the objectives of a didactic program, such as in a chemotherapy course. Such multiple-choice tests are usually criterion referenced rather than norm referenced. *Answer 26:* **b.**

27. On criterion-referenced tests, learners must achieve a preset score for competency. Norm-referenced tests relate the achievement of the learner as compared with a larger group of learners, as in national standardized examinations (Abruzzese, 1996). *Answer 27:* **b.**

28-29. Evaluation strategies may be viewed as formative or summative. Formative evaluation gives information about the learning process and identifies what additional teaching might be needed. Formative evaluation is not intended to be used for a grade or to determine completion of the orientation. In contrast, summative evaluation occurs at the end of a course or program and determines what has been learned (Gaberson & Oermann, 1999b). *Answer 28:* **b.** *Answer 29:* **a.**

QUESTIONS

You plan evaluation of your orientation program on four levels and will use this information in your own annual performance evaluation. Match each level of evaluation with the appropriate strategy.

30. Process   **a.** Administer a chemotherapy module posttest.

31. Outcome   **b.** Audit nursing documentation for selected pain assessment

32. Content   criteria.

           c. Measure orientee's level of

33. Impact   satisfaction with the orientation program.

           d. Measure preceptors' level of job satisfaction.

30-33. Comprehensive and expensive educational programs need a total program evaluation at several higher and progressively more complex levels (Abruzzese, 1996). The first and most basic level of evaluation is process evaluation, which measures learners' satisfaction with the learning experience. The second level is content evaluation, which measures the knowledge attained by participants of the program. The third level is outcome evaluation, which measures a behavioral change related to the learning process. The final and highest level of evaluation is impact evaluation, which is the operational result of the program on the whole organization.

For the APN with responsibility for comprehensive educational programs, total program evaluations that demonstrate positive outcome and impact evaluations are powerful data to document the value and contributions of the APN position in the organization. *Answer 30:* **c.** *Answer 31:* **b.** *Answer 32:* **a.** *Answer 33:* **d.**

CASE 2 STUDY

INDIVIDUAL PATIENT EDUCATION: TEACHING GRANULOCYTE COLONY-STIMULATING FACTOR ADMINISTRATION

Han Nguyen, a 52-year-old man with non-Hodgkin's lymphoma and osteoarthritis, has completed three cycles of chemotherapy with the CHOP regimen. His last cycle was complicated by a neutropenic fever, which required 4 days of hospitalization. He is now ready to begin his fourth cycle of chemotherapy, which will include granulocyte colony-stimulating factor (G-CSF), to reduce the chance of subsequent neutropenic complications.

You need to teach Mr. Nguyen about G-CSF during his clinic visit today. Mr. Nguyen is Vietnamese and emigrated to the United States 15 years ago. He tells you that he understands some English but that he does not speak or write it well. His wife, who also speaks limited English, accompanies him. Their 17-year-old daughter, Kim, is in school today, but they tell you they can depend on her for translation and assistance.

QUESTIONS

1. To provide culturally sensitive nursing care to Mr. Nguyen, it is important to consider information about which of the following factors when planning your interventions?
   1. Biologic variations
   2. Environmental control
   3. Time and space
   4. Social orientation
     a. 1, 2, & 4
     b. 1 & 4
     c. 1, 3, & 4
     d. All of these

2. You attempt to locate a professional interpreter from a directory at your institution. You locate an interpreter, aware that which of the following characteristics may influence the effectiveness of the communication?
   1. Gender differences between the patient and interpreter
   2. Socioeconomic differences between the patient and interpreter
   3. Age differences between the patient and interpreter
   4. Interpreter's skill and fluency
     a. 1 & 4
     b. 2 & 4
     c. 1, 3, & 4
     d. All of these

1. Immigrants from a variety of countries, especially the Asian-Pacific islands (API), Mexico, and the Caribbean, are redefining the composition of the U.S. population (Taoka & Itano, 1997). Nurses are challenged to understand the impact of ethnic minority cultures as these patients interact with U.S. health care providers.

Various cultural assessment models can provide a systematic approach to enable nurses to gain the cultural information necessary for sensitive health care planning and intervention. The Giger and Davidhizar Transcultural Assessment Model, for example, identifies six essential cultural phenomena evident in all cultural groups (Giger & Davidhizar, 1995):
   1. Communication
   2. Space
   3. Social organization
   4. Time
   5. Environmental control
   6. Biologic variations

Although recognizing that each individual is unique, knowledge of general cultural characteristics can initiate culturally competent care. Using this model, for example, the nurse can base care for an API patient on cultural characteristics, such as the importance of family and patrilineal authority (social organization), politeness and respect (communication), and privacy and modesty (space) (Taoka & Itano, 1997). *Answer 1:* **d.**

2. A language difference between the patient and nurse is an obvious obstacle to communication and patient teaching. Professional interpreters are an optimal choice to facilitate communication when language differences exist. However, the interpreter's skill and fluency as well as the patient's personal level of comfort in using the interpreter can limit their effectiveness. The nurse should take the culture's social organizational forces, such as gender, age, and socioeconomic status, into consideration when planning interactions between a patient and interpreter. *Answer 2:* **d.**

QUESTIONS

3. To determine Mr. Nguyen's emotional readiness to learn about G-CSF therapy, you speak with him to obtain information about his:
- **a.** Experience with injections
- **b.** Level of education
- **c.** Motivation and willingness to perform subcutaneous injections
- **d.** Financial status

4. Examples of intrinsic factors that may motivate Mr. Nguyen to learn this new information about G-CSF include all of the following *except:*
- **a.** A little anxiety about performing subcutaneous injections
- **b.** A personality that is open to learning new self-care measures
- **c.** A history of asking lots of questions before chemotherapy begins
- **d.** A positive and informal relationship with you and the other nurses

5. List some assessment data you would obtain to determine whether Mr. Nguyen is capable of performing subcutaneous injections.

ANSWERS

3. Once the need for patient education is identified, the nurse needs to assess two components of the patient's readiness to learn: emotional readiness and experiential readiness (Redman, 1988c). Emotional readiness, or motivation, includes both intrinsic and extrinsic factors. *Answer 3:* **c.**

4. Although intrinsic motivating factors relate to the person's own set of values and attitudes, extrinsic factors relate to the environment and can be manipulated by the nurse to promote learning. A person's experiential readiness provides a picture of the individual's background, which will enable him or her to learn the new skill. Emotional readiness and experiential readiness are closely related. *Answer 4:* **d.**

5. In addition to the patient's readiness, the nurse must assess the patient for any barriers to learning (Agre, 1993). A patient's ability to learn may be affected by a physical condition, such as pain, nausea, weakness, altered mental status, loss of fine motor coordination, or vision or hearing impairment. Psychosocial influences may relate to high levels of anxiety, lack of reading skills, low educational level, or a language barrier. Nurses need to collect and analyze comprehensive assessment data to determine and promote the patient's ability to learn. *Answer 5:* **See text.**

QUESTIONS

6. Based on the Health Belief Model, which of the following statements made by Mr. Nguyen would cause you to be concerned about his compliance with giving the G-CSF injections and following other self-care measures to prevent infections?
- **a.** "So these shots are going to keep me from getting an infection?"
- **b.** "I didn't feel that sick when I had that infection."
- **c.** "I know another guy in this clinic who takes these shots."
- **d.** "I was afraid that this chemotherapy could cause a lot of problems."

7. Which of the following examples illustrates effective cognitive teaching methods?
- **a.** Mr. Nguyen watches a short video that demonstrates drug preparation and administration and has the opportunity to ask questions.
- **b.** You describe G-CSF preparation and administration, and then Mr. Nguyen practices drawing up the medication from the vial and giving the injection to a model arm.
- **c.** Mr. Nguyen has the opportunity to practice the G-CSF skills for a few days in the clinic.
- **d.** Mr. Nguyen watches another patient prepare and administer a G-CSF injection.

8. With the help of the interpreter, you ask Mr. Nguyen to identify on himself the possible locations for subcutaneous injections. When he appears reluctant to answer your question, which of the following actions would be most appropriate?

1. Rephrase and repeat the question because he may not have understood it.
2. Review this content to be sure that he has learned it.
3. Repeat the question, but consider that the lack of privacy may be an obstacle because of the interpreter's presence.
4. Review the benefits of G-CSF because he does not seem to grasp the importance of the injections.
   a. 1 & 2
   b. 1 & 3
   c. 1, 2, & 4
   d. All of these

9. What are the two most appropriate methods you can use in the clinic today to evaluate the effectiveness of Mr. Nguyen's learning?

1. Observe him preparing a G-CSF injection and administering it into a model.
2. Ask him "what if?" questions to determine his understanding of aseptic technique and management of side effects.
3. Write a note to document the teaching process you used to teach Mr. Nguyen about G-CSF therapy and his response.
4. Arrange for a home health nurse to visit Mr. Nguyen and observe him self-administer a G-CSF injection.
   a. 1 & 2
   b. 2 & 3
   c. 3 & 4
   d. 1 & 3

ANSWERS

6-8. The Health Belief Model is often used as a predictive theory regarding readiness to perform a health action (Rosenstock, 1960). The model is based on individuals' beliefs about susceptibility, seriousness, and threat of disease, as well as their beliefs about the benefits and barriers of health care behaviors. If the person perceives that he or she is susceptible to a disease and believes that the disease is harmful, and if he or she believes that health behaviors are effective and worthwhile, that person is likely to perform the health care behavior. Based on this model, Mr. Nguyen's statement that he did not feel sick with his infection may indicate that he does not perceive the seriousness of infectious complications from chemotherapy; therefore he may be less likely to understand the importance of preventive infection measures, such as G-CSF injections.

Mr. Nguyen is an example of a significant percentage of Americans who lack necessary literacy skills. Patients with low literacy skills need especially short, concrete, vivid demonstrations of the content (Fisher, 1999). In this situation, the videotape would provide the preferred method of teaching because it is the only method that includes a demonstration of both drug preparation and administration. Teaching is also most effective when patients have the opportunity to immediately apply learning to their situation (Redman, 1988b). For the nurse, this means answering questions and giving immediate feedback to the patient. *Answer 6:* **b.** *Answer 7:* **a.** *Answer 8:* **b.**

9. Evaluation of the teaching process will determine whether the goals of patient education have been met. For motor skills, direct observation of the skill with specific steps whenever possible is an effective measurement of the correctness of what the patient learned. Questioning the patient about hypothetical situations, such as "What if you contaminated the syringe before administration?" can verify the patient's understanding of cognitive learning, although what people say they would do and what they actually do may be different (Redman, 1988a).

Evaluation of teaching in a transcultural setting presents additional challenges. When learning objectives are not met, the nurse needs to consider whether teaching and/or evaluation were affected by cultural issues. Obstacles to teaching and evaluation may relate to communication difficulties, privacy and modesty issues, or time orientation. *Answer 9:* **a.**

CASE 3 STUDY

PATIENT EDUCATION: GROUPS

You are an APN based on an inpatient medical oncology unit and an inpatient hospice unit. You observe that the staff on both units spend a significant amount of time teaching family caregivers strategies to manage physical symptoms after discharge. You decide to design a group education program on these units to provide information about at-home care for family members who will be the primary caregiver.

BOX **30-2** **Learning Needs Assessment Strategies**

Advisory groups
Anecdotal notes
Brainstorming
Checklists
Critical incident technique
Delphi technique
Focus groups
Interviews
Nominal group process
Professional standards
Questionnaires
Rating scales
Surveys

QUESTIONS

1. You see a small group of family members of several patients talking over coffee in the lounge area. You ask them for their opinions about your idea for the program. They think it is a great idea, and over the next 30 minutes, they give you some ideas about questions that they would like to have answered. They also suggest times when the sessions could be held. What type of learning needs assessment just took place?
   a. Critical incident technique
   b. Focus group
   c. Interview
   d. Nominal group process

ANSWERS

1. Patient education programs may be designed to meet a specific, individualized need. Six steps are involved in the development of patient education programs (Padberg & Padberg, 1997):
   1. Planning and strategy selection
   2. Selection of processes and materials
   3. Development of materials and pretesting
   4. Implementation
   5. Assessment of effectiveness
   6. Program refinement

The planning stage includes a needs assessment to clearly define the education goals of the program and to identify the target audience. A variety of techniques may be used to define learning needs, and the use of multiple techniques is recommended to give a more accurate picture of what needs to be taught (Wise, 1996) (Box 30-2). The situation described in this scenario most closely resembles a focus group, where a small group of consumers may formally or informally provide information about a specific topic. *Answer 1:* **b.**

Case Study continued

Based on the input you received from these family members, you design an educational program consisting of four weekly sessions to be held on the unit at 11:30 AM. The first session covered symptom management of fatigue, infection, and bleeding, and the second session covered management of gastrointestinal symptoms. You were pleased with attendance and participation at the session.

QUESTIONS

2. Which principles of adult learning explain the success of your program so far?
   1. Adults need to know why they should learn something.
   2. Adults are ready to learn when they experience the need to know.
   3. Both extrinsic and intrinsic motivators motivate adults.
   4. Adults have a need to be self-directed.
      a. 1 & 2
      b. 1, 2, & 3
      c. 2 & 3
      d. All of these

3. Identify at least five sources where you can obtain printed patient education materials for use in your classes.

ANSWERS

2. Characteristics of the target audience should be understood so that appropriate objectives and teaching materials can be chosen. When possible, education programs should be held in the places where the target audience is located. Although some programs are hospital based to meet the needs of hospital and clinic patients, others can serve target audiences in community settings.

Principles of the Adult Learning Theory emphasize the characteristics of adults as learners (Knowles, 1980). This theory gives implications for nurses to use in patient education, as outlined in Table 30-3. The adult learner is usually independent and motivated by the need to know. Adults learn out of interest and by doing, and they need to apply what they learn immediately. Teaching strategies that are based on these guidelines are likely to be successful. *Answer 2:* **d.**

3. Today, nurses and patients can find a tremendous quantity of patient education materials and information sources. Advances in computer technology and electronic communication can deliver answers to both common and challenging learning

---

TABLE 30-3 **Principles of Adult Learning and Their Implications for Nursing Practice**

Adults are independent learners.	Respect adult learners' independence and ability to control their learning. Facilitate active learning.
Adults' past experiences are resources for learning.	Value and use past experiences to enhance learning.
Adults' readiness to learn emerges from developmental stages.	Teach information in the context of life's tasks or problems.
Adults' learning is task- or problem-oriented.	Teach in response to adult learners' perceived needs.

Padberg, R. M., & Padberg, L. F. (1997). Patient education and support. In Groenwald, S. L., Frogge, M. H., Goodman, J., & Yarbro, C. H. (Eds.). *Cancer nursing: Principles and practice*, 4th ed. (pp. 1642-1665). Boston: Jones and Bartlett.

needs directly to nurses and patients in a matter of minutes. The American Cancer Society, National Cancer Institute, Oncology Nursing Society, and Leukemia and Lymphoma Society provide a wide variety of free patient education products related to cancer, both written and online. Other organizations provide disease-specific information (e.g., the Brain Tumor Society and the National Prostate Cancer Coalition), information about symptoms (e.g., CancerFatigue.org), and specific pharmacologic information (e.g., www.aredia.net). Nurses are challenged to keep informed about new sources of patient education, to incorporate them into their practice, and to guide patients who may be interested in exploring information sources on their own. *Answer 3:* **See text.**

Case Study continued

You note that at the conclusion of the first two sessions, family members remained to discuss some of the emotional challenges of the role of caregiver. When you reflect this observation to the participants, they admit that they find support when they share their stories with each other.

QUESTIONS

4. Based on your feedback from the group, you suggest that part of the fourth session could include a discussion of the psychosocial issues that families experience rather than only physical symptoms. This is an example of using:
   a. Summative evaluation
   b. Formative evaluation
   c. Process evaluation
   d. Structural evaluation

5. During their discussion of the emotional challenges of caregiving, several family members indicate difficulty with communication and conflict resolution within their family. What teaching strategy could you use that would best address this identified learning need?

   a. Explaining typical emotional responses to illness and the principles of conflict resolution
   b. Role-playing
   c. Role modeling
   d. Reading a patient education booklet that gives strategies for more effective communication

---

ANSWERS

4. Formative evaluation occurs during the learning experience and may lead to revision of learning objectives and content. In this case, your evaluation led an education group to also incorporate objectives related to coping. Grassman (1993) reports that it is common for groups to have both educational and psychosocial objectives. *Answer 4:* **b.**

5. Support groups will likely deal with content related to expression of emotions and feelings and the ability to cope with the cancer experience. Role-playing can be an effective intervention when meeting such affective objectives. *Answer 5:* **b.**

Case Study continued

Following this education series, one family member, Mr. Holly, approaches you to share how valuable he found the sessions. He was sure that similar classes would be helpful for other families in his community who were caring for a person with cancer in the home. You decide to investigate whether there is an interest for your program in the community outside of the hospital.

You recall that the local senior center presents frequent health education series. When you contact the director to ascertain possible interest, the director is interested in the program.

QUESTIONS

6. Before you can make plans to implement the program at the senior center, you need information about which of the following?

BOX 30-3 | **Strategies for Teaching the Elderly**

Address misperceptions and fears about cancer.
Customize assessment and teaching to accommodate for aging changes.
Enter into partnerships with families.
Provide frequent review and reinforcement.

Boyle, D. M., Engelking, C., Blesch, K. S., et al. (1992). ONS position paper on cancer and aging. *Oncol Nurs Forum, 19*, pp. 913-933.

1. Target audience, such as size, age, gender, and sociocultural factors
2. Setting, such as space, equipment, and other resources
3. Educational materials available
4. Success of previous health education classes
   a. 1, 2, & 3
   b. 1, 2, & 4
   c. 1 & 2
   d. All of these

7. What barriers should you consider when planning education for an elderly audience?
   1. The elderly often have misperceptions and fear of cancer.
   2. Declining neurosensory function may inhibit learning by the elderly.
   3. Printed education materials are often not suitable for the use with the elderly.
   4. The elderly often require more repetition and reinforcement of teaching.
   a. 1 & 2
   b. 1, 2, & 3
   c. 2 & 3
   d. All of these

8. If you were planning the educational sessions for an elderly rural community, what resources and settings could you explore?

ANSWERS

6. With the U.S.'s rapidly aging population, nurses will commonly be caring for elderly persons with cancer. Nurses must become skilled at meeting the unique needs of this population, including age-related factors that affect learning. *Answer 6:* **b.**

7. Boyle, Engelking, Blesch, et al. (1992) outline barriers to learning in the elderly and recommend teaching strategies in an ONS Position Paper (Box 30-3). *Answer 7:* **d.**

8. Nurses need to offer creative educational programs that fit with the lifestyle of selected elderly populations. These populations may be most likely to attend programs during the day, for example, and be less likely to travel outside their own community because of limitations with transportation. Educational projects for the elderly in rural settings may include outreach programs that network through community centers, churches, general stores, county fairs, or farm cooperatives. *Answer 8:* **See text.**

REFERENCES

Abruzzese, R. S. (1996). Evaluation in nursing staff development. In Abruzzese, R. S. (Ed.). *Nursing staff development: Strategies for success,* 2nd ed. (pp. 242-258). St. Louis: Mosby.

Abruzzese, R. S., & Quinn-O'Neal, B. (1996). Orientation for general and specialty areas. In Abruzzese, R. S. (Ed.). *Nursing staff development: Strategies for success,* 2nd ed. (pp. 259-280). St. Louis: Mosby.

Agre, P. (1993). *Guidelines for patient education.* New York: Triclinica Communications.

Avillion, A. E., & Abruzzese, R. S. (1996). Conceptual foundations of nursing staff development. In Abruzzese, R. S. (Ed.). *Nursing staff development: Strategies for success,* 2nd ed. (pp. 30-43). St. Louis: Mosby.

Benner, P. (1984). *From novice to expert: Excellence and power in clinical nursing practice.* Menlo Park, CA: Addison-Wesley.

Boyle, D. M., Engelking, C., Blesch, K. S., et al. (1992). ONS position paper on cancer and aging. *Oncol Nurs Forum, 19*, pp. 913-933.

David, C. L., & Dowling, J. S. (1995). Computer-assisted instruction. In Fuszard, B. (Ed.). *Innovative teaching strategies in nursing,* 2nd ed. (pp. 135-141). Gaithersburg, MD: Aspen.

Fisher, E. (1999), Low literacy levels in adults: Implications for patient education. *J Contin Educ Nurs, 30,* pp. 56-61.

Gaberson, K. B., & Oermann, M. H. (1999a). Preparing for clinical learning activities. In Gaberson, K. B., & Oermann, M. H. (Eds.). *Clinical teaching strategies in nursing* (pp. 22-39). New York: Springer.

Gaberson, K. B., & Oermann, M. H. (1999b). Process of clinical teaching. In Berson, K. B., & Oermann, M. H. (Eds.). *Clinical teaching strategies in nursing* (pp. 68-75). New York: Springer.

Gianella, A. (1996). Effective teaching and learning strategies for adults. In Abruzzese, R. S. (Ed.). *Nursing staff development: Strategies for success,* 2nd ed. (pp. 223-241). St. Louis: Mosby.

Giger, J. N., & Davidhizar, R. E. (1995) *Transcultural nursing: Assessment and interventions,* 2nd ed. St. Louis: Mosby.

Giles, P. F., & Moran, V. (1989). Preceptor program evaluation demonstrates improved orientation. *J Nurs Staff Dev, 5,* pp. 17-24.

Grassman, D. (1993) Development of inpatient oncology educational and support programs. *Oncol Nurs Forum, 10,* pp. 669-676.

Itano, J. (1987). Developing educational objectives. *Oncol Nurs Forum, 14*, pp. 62-65.

Knowles, M. S. (1980) *The modern practice of adult education: From pedagogy to andragogy*, 2nd ed. Upper Saddle River, NJ: Globe Fearon Cambridge.

Mackin, J., & Studva, K. (1997). An on-the-job preceptor model for newly hired nurses. In Flynn, J. P. (Ed.). *The role of the preceptor: A guide for nurse educators and clinicians* (pp. 75-118). New York: Springer.

Manley, M. J. (1997). Adult learning concepts important to precepting. In Flynn, J. P. (Ed.). *The role of the preceptor: A guide for nurse educators and clinicians* (pp. 15-46). New York: Springer.

Oermann, M. H. (1997). Evaluating critical thinking in clinical practice. *Nurse Ducator, 22*, pp. 25-28.

O'Mara, A. M. (1997). A model preceptor program for student nurses. In Flynn, J. P. (Ed.). *The role of the preceptor: A guide for nurse educators and clinicians* (pp. 47-74). New York: Springer.

Padberg, R. M., & Padberg, L. F. (1997). Patient education and support. In Groenwald, S. L., Frogge, M. H., Goodman, J., & Yarbro, C. H. (Eds.). *Cancer nursing: Principles and practice*, 4th ed. (pp. 1642-1665). Boston: Jones and Bartlett.

Redman, B. K. (1988a). Evaluation of health teaching. In Redman, B. K. (Ed.). *The process of patient teaching in nursing*, 6th ed. (pp. 220-259). St. Louis: Mosby.

Redman, B. K. (1988b). Learning. In Redman, B. K. (Ed.). *The process of patient teaching in nursing*, 6th ed. (pp. 83-124). St. Louis: Mosby

Redman, B. K. (1988c). Readiness for health education. In Redman, B. K. (Ed.). *The process of patient teaching in nursing*, 6th ed. (pp. 21-48). St. Louis: Mosby.

Reilly, D. E., & Oermann, M. H. (1992a). *Clinical teaching in nursing education*, 2nd ed. New York: National League for Nursing.

Rosenstock, I. M. (1960). What research in motivation suggests for public health. *Am J Public Health, 50*, pp. 295-302.

Taoka, K. N., & Itano, J. K. (1997). Cultural diversity among individuals with cancer. In Groenwald, S. L., Frogge, M. H., Goodman, M., & Yarbro, C. H. (Eds.). *Cancer nursing: Principles and practice*, 4th ed. pp. 1691-1735. Boston: Jones and Bartlett.

Wise, P. S. (1996). Learning needs assessment. In Abruzzese, R. S. (Ed.). *Nursing staff development: Strategies for success*, 2nd ed. (pp. 188-208). St. Louis: Mosby.

INDEX

Page numbers followed by f indicate
figures; t, tables; b, boxes.

I

Ibuprofen, 141, 236t
Idiopathic pneumonitis, 193
Ifosfamide, 161t
Imipramine, 257t
Immunosuppressive therapy, 180, 183-184. *See also specific agent.*
Impact evaluation, 449-450
Inapsine. *See* Droperidol.
Incident pain, 262
Incisional biopsy, 9t, 80t
Increased intracranial pressure, 361-368
Independent nursing consultation, 420-421
Independent variables, 438t
Infection. *See also specific infection.*
    bacteria commonly associated with, 335, 337
    chemotherapy-related, 98-99
    diagnostic assessments, 99
    hypothermia signs of, 334
    nosocomial, 86
    postoperative, 83, 85-86
    posttransplant, 164, 165t, 184-185
    risk factors, 336t
    transfusion-related, 171
    wound, 86
Inflammatory bowel disorders, 47
Informational power, 390, 390t
Informed consent
    components of, 155, 441-442
    definition of, 155
    description of, 114, 441-442
    process of, 143-144, 144b
In-service consultation, 417
Insomnia, 142-143
Institution
    conflicts in, 381-382
    environment of, 380-381
    productivity and resource assessments, 380
    staff, 382-383
Integrative reviews, 431-432
Interferon therapy
    classification of, 136-137
    contraindications, 137
    description of, 72-74
    half-life of, 139
    patient education, 139
    side effects of
        capillary leak syndrome, 142
        depression, 143
        fatigue, 139-140
        fever, 137-139, 142
        hypotension, 145
        management of, 144-145
        myalgias, 137-138
        neurologic, 143
        renal toxicity, 141

Interleukin-6, 99
Internal consistency, 437
Interpreters, 450-451
Interval level, 441t
Intestine. *See* Bowel.
Intracranial pressure, increased
    clinical manifestations of, 367t
    corticosteroids for, 365
    definition of, 364
    metastatic brain lesions associated with, 364
    patient education regarding, 366-367
    recurrent, 366
    sequelae of, 367-368
    symptoms of, 364
    treatment of, 367-368
Intrarenal renal failure, 167-168
Intravenous immunoglobulin, 165-166
Invasive ductal carcinoma, 12
Invasive lobular carcinoma, 12
Irinotecan, 116-117
Iron deficiency anemia, 286t

J

Jaundice
    causes of, 292
    differential diagnoses, 291-292
    signs and symptoms of, 289, 291, 292b

K

Kaolin/pectin, 117
Ketoconazole, 64
Ketoprofen, 237t
Ketorolac. *See* Toradol.
Kidneys
    failure of. *See* Renal failure.
    insufficiency of. *See* Renal insufficiency.
    nonsteroidal antiinflammatory drug effects, 235
    potassium depletion, 279
Klonopin. *See* Clonazepam.
Knowledge-focused triggers, 427
Kytril. *See* Granisetron.

L

Laboratory tests. *See* Diagnostic and evaluative tests.
Lactulose, 350t
Laparoscopic biopsy, 80t
Large cell carcinoma, 28
Laxatives, 239t, 245-246, 350t
Leading, 379t
Learning
    adult learning theory, 453, 454t
    assessment of, 449, 453b

Learning—cont'd
    computer-assisted instruction, 448-449
    critical thinking skills, 448-449
    formative evaluation, 454
    self-learning modules, 448
    strategies for, 448b
    types of, 446
Legitimate power, 389-390, 390t
Lentigo maligna melanoma, 68, 68t
Leucovorin, 52-53
Leukocyte depletion, 171
Levorphanol (Levo-Dromoran), 251, 252t
Licensure, 395, 397-398
Li-Fraumeni syndrome, 268t-269t
Linear accelerators, 126
Lioresal. *See* Baclofen.
Lipid profile, 101-102
Lipids, 305-306
Literature searches, 431
Liver
    anatomy of, 77
    enlargement of, 138-139, 285
    hepatitis of, 285
    hepatocellular death, 285
    length of, 77
    metastases, 49, 53, 89-90, 284
    pre-existing conditions, 78t
    venocclusive disease of, 166-167
Liver function tests, 138-139, 283-285
Loperamide, 124
Lorazepam, 97t
Low-microbial diet, 176
Lumpectomy
    complications of, 11b
    modified radical mastectomy vs., 9-10
Lung cancer
    dyspnea symptoms, 35-36
    hospice care, 42-43
    metastases, 27t, 28-29, 31t, 41, 90
    non–small cell. *See* Non–small cell lung cancer.
    primary prevention, 23
    risk factors, 26t. *See also* Smoking.
    small cell. *See* Small cell lung cancer.
    smoking and. *See* Smoking.
    superior vena cava syndrome caused by. *See* Superior vena cava syndrome.
Lupron, 62, 64
Lymph nodes
    elective dissection of, 68-69
    sentinel mapping of, 69
Lymphoma, 268t
Lynch II syndrome, 46

Surgery—cont'd
  colorectal cancer, 51-52
  colostomy, 88-89
  complications of
    infection, 83, 85-86
    paralytic ileus, 87
    postoperative, 32-34, 83, 85
    prophylaxis strategies, 81-82
  hemicolectomy, 52, 83
  hydration guidelines, 82
  informed consent for.
    See Informed consent.
  laboratory studies before, 79
  management principles, 79b
  melanoma, 70
  palliative, 90
  preoperative assessments and
    evaluations, 76, 78t
  prophylactic uses of, 81-82
  resective, 83, 84f
  spinal cord compression treated
    using, 300
Susceptibility genes
  age-related penetrance of, 267
  breast cancer, 5-6, 266-272,
    273-274
  inheritance patterns, 267
  types of, 268t-270t
Swallowing
  assessments of, 306
  difficulties in. *See* Dysphagia.
Syndrome of inappropriate
    secretion of antidiuretic
    hormone (SIADH)
  causes of, 330b
  description of, 41, 109
  diagnostic criteria, 329, 330t
  fluid management of, 163
  in hematopoietic stem cell
    transplantation patient, 162
  in lung cancer, 39, 41
  physical findings of, 330
  risk factors, 329-330
  treatment of, 331-332
Systemic inflammatory response
    syndrome, 334, 335b,
    337-338
Systems-oriented team, 385

T

Tachyphylaxis, 138
Tacrolimus
  drug interactions, 183t
  side effects of, 180, 181t-182t
Tamoxifen, 6-7, 14t, 102, 285
Taxol. *See* Paclitaxel.
T-cell depletion, 179-180
Teaching
  activities for, 447-448

Teaching—cont'd
  assessment of, 452
  cognitive methods of, 451-452
  cultural considerations,
    450-452
  elderly patients, 454-455, 455b
  strategies, 454
Team
  actions that interfere with, 388
  assessments of, 386
  barriers to, 386, 388
  building of, 385-386, 388
  collaborative care, 399-400
  dysfunctional roles in, 386,
    387t
  functional roles in, 386, 387t
  function-oriented, 385
  interdisciplinary, 130, 385
  leadership in, 387, 389
  meeting of, 385
  mentors, 393-394
  negativism in, 390
  norms, 387-388
  power in, 389-390, 390t
  research utilization implementa-
    tion, 430-432
  systems-oriented, 385
  territoriality, 99
Tegretol. *See* Carbamazepine.
Territoriality, 399
Testicular cancer, 91
Tests. *See* Diagnostic and evaluative
    tests; *specific test.*
Thalassemia, 286t
Thiethylperazine maleate, 97t
Thiotepa, 161t
Thorazine. *See* Chlorpromazine.
Thrombosis
  deep venous. *See* Deep venous
    thrombosis.
  in disseminated intravascular
    coagulation patient, 316
Tobacco use. *See also* Smoking.
  ethnic minority groups affected
    by, 24-25
  populations affected by, 24
  prevention programs, 24
Tolerance, 247-248
Tomography. *See* Computed
    tomography; Positron
    emission tomography.
Tongue, 96, 98
Toradol, 237t
Torecan. *See* Thiethylperazine
    maleate.
Total body irradiation, 161t
Tramadol, 249
Transfer order, 407b
Transverse colon, 77

Trastuzumab
  description of, 10
  toxicities associated with,
    103-104
Treatment. *See specific treatment
    modality.*
Trend identification, 428
Trials. *See* Clinical trials.
Tricyclic antidepressants, 219-220,
    255, 257t
Trigeminal nerve, 42t
Trilafon. *See* Perphenazine.
Trilisate. *See* Choline magnesium
    trisalicylate.
Trimethoprim-sulfamethoxazole,
    194-195
Trismus, 135
Trochlear nerve, 42t
Trofanil. *See* Imipramine.
Tumor lysis syndrome
  assessments of, 354-355
  clinical manifestations of, 356b
  description of, 148, 150
  diseases associated with, 353
  hyperkalemia findings, 358-359
  hypocalcemia findings, 353-354
  laboratory tests and findings,
    356t
  management of, 354-355,
    355b
  metabolic abnormalities associated
    with, 353
  organ systems commonly affected,
    355-356
  pathogenesis of, 353
  patient education regarding,
    359-360
  prevention of, 354-355
  renal failure secondary to,
    357-358
  risk factors, 354b
  signs and symptoms of, 354,
    359-360, 360b
Tumor markers, 49-50
Tylenol. *See* Acetaminophen.

U

Ultram. *See* Tramadol.
Uric acid nephropathy, 357
Urinary alkalinization, 357

V

Vaccinations, 206-208
Vagus nerve, 42t
Validity, 437, 439
Valproic acid (Valproate), 257t
Varicella-zoster virus reactiva-
    tion. *See* Herpes zoster
    reactivation.